ASSOCIATE EDITORS

PAUL S. CASAMASSIMO, D.D.S., M.S.

Professor and Chairman,
Department of Growth and Development
University of Colorado, School of Dentistry
Denver, Colorado

HENRY W. FIELDS, Jr., D.D.S., M.S., M.S.D.

Professor
Departments of Pediatric Dentistry and Orthodontics
University of North Carolina, School of Dentistry
Chapel Hill, North Carolina

DENNIS J. McTIGUE, B.S., D.D.S., M.S.

Professor and Chairman
Department of Pediatric Dentistry
Ohio State University, College of Dentistry
Columbus, Ohio

ARTHUR J. NOWAK, D.M.D.

Professor
Departments of Pediatric Dentistry and Pediatrics
University of Iowa, Colleges of Dentistry and Medicine
Iowa City, Iowa

PEDIATRIC DENTISTRY
INFANCY THROUGH ADOLESCENCE

SENIOR EDITOR

J. R. PINKHAM, B.S., D.D.S., M.S.

Professor and Department Head
Department of Pediatric Dentistry
University of Iowa, College of Dentistry
Iowa City, Iowa

1988 Som
W. B. SAUNDERS COMPANY
Harcourt Brace Jovanovich, Inc.
Philadelphia ■ London ■ Toronto
Montreal ■ Sydney ■ Tokyo

W. B. SAUNDERS COMPANY
Harcourt Brace Jovanovich, Inc.

The Curtis Center
Independence Square West
Philadelphia, PA 19106

Library of Congress Cataloging-in-Publication Data

Pediatric dentistry.

1. Pedodontics.   I. Pinkham, J. R.
[DNLM: 1. Pedodontics.   WU 480 P371]
RK55.C5P448   1988   617.6′45   87-4952
ISBN 0-7216-2106-6

Editor: Darlene Pedersen
Developmental Editor: Kathleen McCullough
Designer: Karen O'Keefe
Production Manager: Carolyn Naylor
Manuscript Editor: Tom Stringer
Illustration Coordinator: Walt Verbitski
Indexer: Nancy Weaver & Nelle Garrecht

5-15-91

Pediatric Dentistry: Infancy Through Adolescence   ISBN   0-7216-2106-6

Last digit is the print number: 9   8   7   6   5   4   3

Contributors

STEVEN M. ADAIR, BS, DDS, MS
Senior Clinical and Research Associate and Chairman, Department of Pediatric Dentistry, Eastman Dental Center, Rochester, New York; Associate Professor, Clinical Dentistry, University of Rochester School of Medicine and Dentistry, Rochester, New York; Associate Dentist, Strong Memorial Hospital, Assistant Attending Pediatric Dentist, The Genesee Hospital, Rochester, New York.
Epidemiology and Mechanisms of Dental Diseases in Children

JAY A. ANDERSON, BS, DDS, MD
Assistant Professor, Department of Anesthesiology, School of Medicine, Department of Oral and Maxillofacial Surgery, School of Dentistry, University of North Carolina at Chapel Hill, Chapel Hill, North Carolina; Attending in Anesthesiology and Oral and Maxillofacial Surgery, North Carolina Memorial Hospital, Chapel Hill, North Carolina.
Physiologic Principles in Pediatric Dentistry; Pain and Anxiety Control (Parts I and II); Antibiotics in Pediatric Dentistry; Medical Emergencies in Pediatric Dentistry

JAMES A. BARTLEY, PHD, MD
Associate Professor of Pediatrics, University of Iowa Hospitals and Clinics, Iowa City, Iowa.
Congenital Genetic Disorders and Syndromes

GARY K. BELANGER, DDS
Chairman, Pediatric Dentistry, University of Colorado School of Dentistry, Denver, Colorado.
Pulp Therapy for the Primary Dentition; Pulp Therapy for Young Permanent Teeth

SIDNEY L. BRONSTEIN, DDS, MScD
Associate Professor and Chairman, Division of Oral and Maxillofacial Surgery, University of Colorado School of Dentistry, Denver, Colorado.
Periodontal Disease and Temporomandibular Joint Disorders

PAUL S. CASAMASSIMO, DDS, MS
Associate Professor and Chairman, Department of Growth and Development, University of Colorado School of Dentistry, Department of Dentistry, University Hospital, University of Colorado Health Science Center, Denver, Colorado.
Examination, Diagnosis, and Treatment Planning; Periodontal Considerations; Periodontal Disease and Temporomandibular Joint Disorders

JOHN R. CHRISTENSEN, DDS, MS, MS
Clinical Assistant Professor of Pediatric Dentistry and Orthodontics, University of North Carolina, Chapel Hill, North Carolina.
Examination, Diagnosis, and Treatment Planning; Space Maintenance in the Primary Dentition; Oral Habits; Orthodontic Treatment in the Primary Dentition; Treatment Planning and Treatment of Orthodontic Problems; Periodontal Disease and Temporomandibular Joint Disorders

JAMES J. CRALL, DDS, MS, SM
Assistant Professor, Department of Pediatric Dentistry, University of Connecticut Health Center, Farmington, Connecticut; Staff Appointment, John Dempsey Hospital, University of Connecticut Health Center, Farmington, Connecticut.
Prevention of Dental Disease

CLIFTON O. DUMMETT, JR., DDS, MSD, MEd
Professor and Coordinator, Postgraduate Pediatric Dentistry, Louisiana State University School of Dentistry, New Orleans, Louisiana; Chief, Pediatric Dentistry Section, Charity Hospital at New Orleans; Staff, Children's Hospital of New Orleans; Staff, New Orleans Adolescent Hospital, New Orleans, Louisiana.
Anomalies of the Developing Dentition

HENRY W. FIELDS, JR., DDS, MS, MSD
Professor of Pediatric Dentistry and Orthodontics, School of Dentistry, University of North Carolina, Chapel Hill, North Carolina; North Carolina Memorial Hospital, Chapel Hill, North Carolina.
Examination, Diagnosis, and Treatment Planning; Space Maintenance in the Primary Dentition; Oral Habits; Orthodontic Treatment in the Primary Dentition; Treatment Planning and Treatment of Orthodontic Problems; Periodontal Disease and Temporomandibular Joint Disorders

CATHERINE M. FLAITZ, BA, DDS, MS
Assistant Clinical Professor, Department of Growth and Development, University of Colorado Health Sciences Center, Denver, Colorado; Dental Staff Associate, St. Joseph's Hospital, Denver, Colorado.
Oral Pathologic Conditions and Soft Tissue Anomalies in Children

CLEMENS A. FULL, BS, DDS, MS
Professor, Department of Pediatric Dentistry, University of Iowa College of Dentistry, Iowa City, Iowa; University of Iowa Hospitals and Clinics, Department of Hospital Dentistry, Iowa City, Iowa.
The Dynamics of Change

STEPHEN J. GOEPFERD, DDS, MS
Associate Professor, Department of Pediatric Dentistry, University of Iowa College of Dentistry, Iowa City, Iowa; Staff, University of Iowa Hospitals and Clinics, Iowa City, Iowa.
Examination of the Infant and Toddler

M. JOHN HICKS, BS, DDS, MS, PhD
Associate Clinical Professor, Department of Growth and Development, Oral Sciences Research Center, University of Colorado School of Dentistry, Denver, Colorado; St. Joseph's Hospital, Children's Hospital, University of Colorado Hospital, Denver, Colorado.
The Acid-Etch Technique in Caries Prevention

DENNIS J. McTIGUE, BS, DDS, MS
Professor and Chairman, Department of Pediatric Dentistry, Ohio State University College of Dentistry, Columbus, Ohio; Active Staff, Children's Hospital, Columbus, Ohio.
Introduction to Dental Trauma; Managing Traumatic Injuries in the Young Permanent Dentition

R. DENNY MONTGOMERY, DDS, BS
Assistant Professor, Oral and Maxillofacial Surgery, Ohio State University, Columbus, Ohio; Ohio State University Hospitals, Children's Hospital, Riverside Methodist Hospital, Columbus, Ohio.
Local Anesthesia and Oral Surgery in Children

ARTHUR J. NOWAK, DMD
Professor, Department of Pediatric Dentistry, University of Iowa College of Dentistry, Iowa City, Iowa; Department of Pediatrics, University of Iowa College of Medicine, Iowa City, Iowa; University of Iowa Hospitals and Clinics, Iowa City, Iowa.
Prevention of Dental Disease

WILLIAM H. OLIN, DDS, MS
Professor, Departments of Otolaryngology and Orthodontics, Colleges of Medicine and Dentistry, University of Iowa, Iowa City, Iowa; University of Iowa College of Dentistry, Iowa City, Iowa; University of Iowa Hospitals and Clinics, Iowa City, Iowa.
Sports Injuries/Mouth Protectors

J. R. PINKHAM, BS, DDS, MS
Professor and Department Head, Department of Pediatric Dentistry, University of Iowa College of Dentistry, Iowa City, Iowa; University of Iowa Hospitals and Clinics, Iowa City, Iowa.
The Practical Importance of Pediatric Dentistry; The Dynamics of Change; Patient Management

JOHN W. REINHARDT, BS, DDS, MS
Associate Professor, Department of Operative Dentistry, University of Iowa College of Dentistry, Iowa City, Iowa.
Esthetic Restorative Dentistry for the Adolescent

ANDREW L. SONIS, DMD
Assistant Clinical Professor of Dentistry, Harvard School of Dental Medicine, Boston, Massachusetts; Associate Professor of Pediatric Dentistry, Children's Hospital, Associate Professor of Surgery, Brigham and Women's Hospital, Boston, Massachusetts.
Childhood Diseases and Oral Manifestations of Systemic Disease

WILLIAM F. WAGGONER, DDS, MS
Assistant Professor, Department of Pediatric Dentistry, Ohio State University College of Dentistry, Columbus, Ohio.
Restorative Dentistry for the Primary Dentition

JERRY D. WALKER, BS, DDS, MA
Professor, Department of Pediatric Dentistry, University of Iowa College of Dentistry, Iowa City, Iowa; University of Iowa Hospitals and Clinics, Iowa City, Iowa.
The Dynamics of Change

STEPHEN WILSON, BS, DMD, MA, PhD
Assistant Professor, Pediatric Dentistry, Ohio State University College of Dentistry, Columbus, Ohio; Staff, Children's Hospital, Columbus, Ohio.
Hospital Dentistry; Local Anesthesia and Oral Surgery in Children

Preface

Why has this book been written? Why has energy been directed to the development of another textbook on dentistry for the child patient? What is the rationale behind the organization of this book?

These are relevant questions to anyone who has seriously watched the evolution of contemporary pediatric dentistry. They are particularly important to those people with a keen interest in the information that is taught in dental colleges to prepare dental students for a career of service to children. The frank and simple answer to all these questions, which were asked by the members of the editorial team before one word of this text was written, is that pediatric dentistry now approaches children of varying ages with such specificity that a book portraying the realistic differences between dentistry for various age groups was needed.

What contemporary dentistry can afford a parent and a child that favorably impacts on the dental and oral health of the child is today an aggregation of information and techniques that is extensive, effective, and diverse. Dentistry for children today embodies such abundant clinical science and technique that it presents organizational dilemmas to those who seek to logically portray this arena of dentistry. Unquestionably, to be an effective clinician for all challenges presented by any possible child patient requires a dentist to coordinate his approach and clinical cleverness to the child according to the needs of the child at his particular age. For instance, the behavior management of a 3-year-old is quite different than that of a 13-year-old. Orthodontic considerations also vary dramatically with age. A long list of age-related differences would be easy to develop.

This book exists because the editors believe that a reference textbook on dentistry for children was needed that was, by design, developmentally organized. This book has been written in the belief that age is so incredibly relevant to pediatric dentistry that by presenting information according to a developmental organization, a student's appreciation of the science and techniques needed to effectively practice dentistry for children will be enlarged.

In the Orientation to the Text, the reader will be told how to approach finding information in this book. It may become apparent, then, that this textbook on pediatric dentistry will emphasize two groups of children perhaps more earnestly than has been traditional for basic textbooks on dentistry for children. One of these groups will be adolescents. Adolescent children are sometimes overlooked in pediatric dental curricula, since they do not present typical pediatric dental problems. However, they *are* children, albeit children in rapid transition to adulthood. It is entirely appropriate that their peculiarities and needs be specified in a textbook that addresses dentistry for children.

The other group emphasized in this text, more so than in previous references in this field, is the child under age 3 years. The section of the book that handles the child from conception to age 3 mirrors a dramatic change in the dental profession over the

past 10 years in regard to the ideal age for getting children started in dentistry. No longer is it reasonable to wait until 3 or 4 years of age to design a prevention program for a child. How utterly silly it was for a child to arbitrarily be withheld to 36 or 40 months of age to study his fluoride supplementation needs. Shouldn't any concerned dentist be able to give a reasonable portrayal of what a pregnant mother should be aware of in the dental development of her fetus? Is it not intelligent for parents to learn about appropriate non-cariogenic snacks for their nursing infant before snacking becomes a potential problem?

In summary, this book is designed to approach dental information relevant to all children regardless of age. Basic information is presented, and then the art and science of dentistry for children is categorized by a four part design reflecting dentistry by developmental hallmarks. Specifically, this will be the child from conception to age 3; the child from 3 to 6 years — the primary dentition years; the child from 6 to 12 years — the transitional dentition years; and the adolescent child.

As senior editor, I wish to thank Drs. Casamassimo, Fields, McTigue, and Nowak for the tremendous contributions that they have made in the design and coordination of this book. In fact, without their enthusiasm for a book of this sort of design and their willingness to take on such a substantial role in organizing, editing, and writing this book, I doubt if this book would have ever been done. These four associate editors are friends and colleagues of mine, and I regard them as elite pediatric dentistry educators. The two years that we spent in the generation of this textbook, although they meant a lot of work, will certainly be remembered fondly by me because of the dedication we had to our effort and our unanimous belief that a textbook organized the way that we have organized this one was needed.

I am also deeply appreciative for the expertise, organization, and work that each associate editor lent the particular section they designed and directed at the beginning of this project. Outlining this textbook was quite an adventure. These sectional responsibilities were as follows: Dr. Arthur Nowak: Section I: Conception to Age Three; Dr. Dennis McTigue: Section II: The Primary Dentition Years: Three to Six Years; Dr. Henry Fields: Section III: The Transitional Years: Six to Twelve Years; Dr. Paul Casamassimo: Section IV: Adolescence.

In addition to sectional responsibilities, each of these editors lent their expertise in organizing the information of certain recurrent themes in the book. Obviously, in a book designed to address some topics up to four different times, this was a considerable responsibility. These assignments were as follows:

Dr. Paul Casamassimo — Examination, diagnosis, and treatment planning and periodontal disease

Dr. Henry Fields — Orthodontic diagnosis, treatment planning and treatment, and related themes

Dr. Dennis McTigue — Pulp therapy, including management of trauma and restorative dentistry

Dr. Arthur Nowak — Prevention of dental disease

Again, the effort it took by these editors to coordinate these topics throughout this book is appreciated.

The entire editorial team offers our profound gratitude for the efforts of the contributing authors. Every author was recruited not only because of the author's expertise but also because of our belief that each author would have the ability to portray the information that he or she would address in a way that would be educationally relevant to the student who wanted growth or refreshment in this field of dentistry. Obviously, we knew that no matter what the elegance of the design of this book was, in the final analysis its quality would be word, sentence, paragraph,

and chapter dependent. I think the authors of this textbook have done a tremendous job in designing and writing their chapters.

Also, I am appreciative of the W.B. Saunders Company for sponsoring this book. This company's reputation in the field of health science publications is most prestigious, and it has been a joy to work with true professionals. Particularly, I want to thank Ms. Darlene Pedersen for understanding the editors' enthusiasm for a pediatric textbook based on a developmental organizational philosophy.

My last acknowledgment is to the people who have worked clerically on the preparation of this text. First, I would like to thank the clerical staff of the Department of Pediatric Dentistry at Iowa, which helped me and my associate editor, Dr. Arthur Nowak, as well as our Iowa colleagues, Drs. Full, Goepferd and Walker, in preparing our manuscripts. These staff members are Ms. Julie Lemke, Ms. Anita Forbes, Ms. Cindy Becker, and Ms. Sharon Gaffney. From our word processing group in the College of Dentistry at Iowa, I thank Ms. Judy Norris and Ms. Vicki Hudachek. At Colorado, Dr. Casamassimo extends his appreciation to Ms. Denise Marie Richardson. At North Carolina, Dr. Fields recognizes Ms. Carolyn Gravely for her efforts. At Ohio State, Dr. McTigue thanks Ms. Cynthia Walland.

Finally, the editors and authors thank our supportive families, friends, and colleagues, who were patient with our efforts to produce this book.

JIMMY R. PINKHAM

Orientation to the text

Pediatric Dentistry: Infancy Through Adolescence is divided into a section of introductory chapters and four major age-related sections. The introductory chapters deal with basic information and themes pertinent to dentistry for children at virtually all ages. Ten chapters are included in this division of the book.

In inspecting the information covered in the introductory chapters of this book, a student will readily see that much of the information has been, or likely will be, covered in other aspects of his dental school's curriculum. However, because of the uniqueness of children, their physiological differences from adults, and other age-related issues, no textbook on pediatric dentistry would be complete without a discussion of the themes covered in this section of the textbook. Oral pathology in children, the use of drugs for a pediatric population, and the oral effects of systemic disease are themes very relevant to understanding the dental needs of children. In addition, the student needs to appreciate the epidemiology and mechanisms of dental diseases in children and other dental findings that require diagnostic as well as treatment considerations.

The four remaining sections of the textbook divide childhood into four age groups and address each of these age groups according to the changes the child will experience physically, cognitively, emotionally, and socially; his examination requirements; prevention needs; and possible treatment considerations. These four age groups are as follows:

- CONCEPTION TO AGE THREE
- THE PRIMARY DENTITION YEARS: THREE TO SIX YEARS
- THE TRANSITIONAL YEARS: SIX TO TWELVE
- ADOLESCENCE

The division of the textbook according to these age groups was a deliberate decision. The editors felt that a discussion of dentistry for children should be divided into logical age-related categories, since each age range has certain themes that should be emphasized. The child from conception to age 3 has historically been one who has not been involved in professional dental supervision. In fact, until recently dentistry has never actively encouraged this child to be involved in professional care. Age 3 has for many years been a customary entry age of children to the dental experience. This textbook certainly does not encourage this tradition. It is deeply believed by the editors and authors that prevention programs have to be started well before age 3 to ensure success. Therefore, Section I, Conception to Age Three, exists to focus on the needs of an age group that has been virtually overlooked previously.

Section II, The Primary Dentition Years: Three to Six Years, deals with a child with a complete primary dentition who generally is capable of going into the dental office as a cooperative patient. Indeed, most of the literature on techniques for the behavior management of children are directed to this young age group. The clinician who works with this age group will need to understand the morphology and anatomy of the primary dentition, how to preserve dental arch integrity if teeth are lost, and the interception of malocclusions in the primary dentition. The primary dentition presents its own challenges regarding restoration and pulpal therapy. The primary dentition also serves as a template for the permanent dentition and contains many clues as to the final form of the permanent dentition. Because of management concerns related to age and the importance of maintaining an intact primary dentition, the information in this section is critical to the family dentist.

Section III, The Transitional Years: Six to Twelve Years, is so labeled because between 6 and 12 years of age the majority of children will shed all of their primary teeth and will gain all of their permanent teeth except their third molars. With this "transition" to the permanent dentition comes the responsibility of the clinician of understanding the treatment needs of young permanent teeth. Orthodontic considerations and esthetic considerations become more and more important in this age group also. Although the prevention needs of the preschool child remain pertinent in the transitional years, the transitional years also see the child taking on more and more responsibility for his own oral hygiene.

The last section, Section IV, deals with adolescence. The adolescent is also a child who many involved in dentistry for children feel has been largely overlooked by the profession. The needs of the adolescent regarding prevention and treatment planning considerations, the seriousness of dental and facial esthetics at this age, as well as increasing concerns about periodontal disease certainly justify a major section in any pediatric dental textbook.

Although redundancy can have educational merit, the editors have tried to provide for the least redundant textbook possible. Obviously, there are certain examination considerations or preventive issues that are pertinent for all four age groups. In such situations, relevant information will addressed again if necessary. However, as much as possible an issue will be discussed one time and one time only at that point of a child's development at which it is first most appropriate, in the editors' judgement, to be discussed. For instance, fluoride supplementation, which certainly is pertinent for the very young child, will be discussed in Section I, Conception to Age Three. It will only be referred to in following sections, even though supplementation is certainly a fundamental feature of many children's prevention program from 3 to 6 and even in the first several years of adolescence. Using the same guideline, stainless steel crown technique will be discussed in the restorative chapter of Section II, The Primary Dentition Years: Three to Six Years. This is because it is rare for dentists to restoratively treat children younger than 3 years of age but commonplace after age three.

The following represent the locations of themes that occur in at least two of the sections:

Dynamics of change: Chapters 11, 16, 28, 35
Examination: Chapters 12, 17, 29, 36
Treatment planning: Chapters 12, 17, 29, 36
Radiographic concerns: Chapters 17, 29, 36
Prevention: Chapters 13, 18, 30, 37
Trauma: Chapters 14, 33, 39
Restorative dentistry: Chapters 19, 31, 38
Pulp therapy: Chapters 20, 32

Periodontal disease: Chapters 23, 40
Orthodontic therapy: Chapters 26, 34
Orthodontic diagnosis: Chapters 17, 29, 36

If a student is using the text as a reference and wants to find out where a certain issue or technique is covered, he or she is encouraged first to look at the table of contents, and if not successful there, to check the index. A quick perusal of the text should also help in orienting a student to where certain information may be.

Contents

section **III**

THE TRANSITIONAL YEARS: SIX TO TWELVE YEARS   325

Introduction

chapter *1*

The practical importance of pediatric dentistry

J. R. Pinkham

Pediatric dentistry is synonymous with dentistry for children. Pediatric dentistry exists because children have dental and orofacial problems. The genesis of dentistry for children unquestionably is allied to dental decay, pulpitis, and the inflammation and pain associated with infected pulpal tissue and suppuration in alveolar bone.

From its extraction-oriented beginnings, pediatric dentistry phased into an interception of decay era that also featured a heavy emphasis on diagnostic procedures and maintenance of arch integrity when, because of decay or trauma, one or more teeth in the arch were lost. Restorative techniques, pulpal therapy, space maintenance, and interceptive orthodontics were the main themes of this era. This era has not gone past us. Tooth decay still exists, although its incidence is significantly less in certain areas of the United States than several decades ago. Therefore, these restorative techniques will be covered in detail in this book.

Today, however, pediatric dentistry also emphasizes prevention. Unquestionably, the prevention of dental diseases is a primary focus of this book.

In addition, this text on pediatric dentistry seeks to explain the following:

- The history of dentistry for children in the United States.
- The pertinence of other dental curricular offerings to the child patient.
- Informing the student of the great changes happening in this area of dentistry.
- Acquainting the student to the legal and professional responsibilities of the dentist in protecting children from abuse and neglect.
- Educating the student in informed consent.

Historical Perspective

In at least one state of the United States, a major dental supplier, up until the middle 1950's, gave all new clients who were opening their offices a very handsome sign that said: *No children under age 13 treated in this office.* Fortu-

3

nately, such attitudes and such signs are gone. Over the past several decades, very specific educational guidelines for pediatric dentistry have been adopted and are imposed upon all dental schools accredited by the American Dental Association's Commission on Accreditation. Graduates of all accredited dental schools have not only a didactic education in dentistry for children but also a clinical education. Furthermore, through efforts of organized dentistry and other organizations and individuals interested in the oral health of children, the ignorant notions that the "baby teeth don't deserve care because you lose them anyway" have largely disappeared save for the most uninformed individuals.

Indeed, at the writing of this book, it would seem that dentistry is on the brink of even yet another remarkable new advance in the care of the oral health of American children. This advance is the cessation of considering the 3-year-old as the ideal-aged child to enter into a program of professional dental care. For many years now, there have been voices within the dental profession that have questioned the best age for a child to enter into professional supervision. As shall be discussed later, because of communication and other behavioral reasons, the customary age of the first dental appointment became the third birthday. However, the editors and authors of this book believe that in this age of preventive dentistry when we are hoping to raise all children free of significant dental decay, age 3 is far too late an entrance date into the professional supervision of children by the dentist. The prevention of disease can never be started too early.

Milestones in Dentistry for Children in the United States

1900   Few children are treated in dental offices.
Little or no instruction in the care of "baby teeth" is given in the 50 dental schools in the United States.
1924   First comprehensive textbook on dentistry for children is published.
1926   The Gies Report on dental education notes that only 5 of the 43 dental schools in the United States have facilities especially designed for treating children.
1927   After almost a decade of frustration in

getting a group organized to promote dentistry for children, the American Society for the Promotion of Dentistry for Children is established at the American Dental Association's (ADA) meeting in Detroit, Michigan.
1932   A report of the College Committee of the American Society for the Promotion of Dentistry for Children states that in 1928, 15 dental schools provided no clinical experience with children and 22 schools had no didactic information in this area.
1935   There exist six graduate programs and eight post-graduate programs in pedodontics.
1940   The American Society for the Promotion of Dentistry for Children changes its name to the American Society of Dentistry for Children (ASDC).
1941   Children's Dental Health Day is observed in Cleveland, Ohio, and Children's Dental Health Week is observed in Akron, Ohio.
1942   The effectiveness of topical fluoride applications at preventing caries is described.
The Council on Dental Education announces that all dental schools have pedodontics as part of their curriculum.
1945   First artificial water fluoridation plant is begun at Grand Rapids, Michigan.
1947   The American Academy of Pedodontics is formed. To a large degree, the start of the Academy was prompted by a need for a more scientifically focused organization concerned with the dental health of children.
1948   The American Board of Pedodontics, a group formulated to certify candidates in the practice of dentistry for children, is formally recognized by the Council on Dental Education of the American Dental Association.
1949   The first full week of February is designated as National Children's Dental Health Week.
1955   The acid-etch technique is described.
1960   There exist 18 graduate programs and 17 post-graduate programs in pedodontics.
1964   Crest becomes the first ADA-approved fluoridated toothpaste.
1974   The International Workshop on Fluorides and Dental Caries Reductions recommends that appropriate fluoride supplementation begin as soon after birth as

possible. (This was later modified by authorities to start at 6 months of age.)

1981   February is designated as National Children's Dental Health Month.

1983   A Consensus Development Conference held at the National Institutes of Dental Health endorses the effectiveness and usefulness of sealants.

1984   The American Academy of Pedodontics changes its name to the American Academy of Pediatric Dentistry.

Application of Other Disciplines

Unquestionably, pediatric dentistry as a body of knowledge and as a clinical discipline has borrowed heavily from many other aspects of dental schools' curricula and from breakthroughs in other specialty areas of dentistry. To be a complete clinician capable of handling the majority of needs of the children of any community, a dentist will need to know thoroughly preventive dentistry techniques, pulpal therapy, instrumentation and restoration of teeth, dental materials, oral surgery, preventive and interceptive orthodontics, and the principles of prosthetics. In addition, to really be knowledgeable about the best needs of child patients, the dentist needs to know certain basics in pediatric medicine, general and oral pathology, and growth and development. Nutrition and understanding of both systemic and topical fluorides are essential in the development of appropriate prevention strategies for the child patient. Lastly, it is inconceivable that a person would be happy dedicating a significant amount of practice time to children without understanding their emotional and psychological needs and processes of emotional change and social maturation. The child has to be managed differently than the adult, and, in fact, the modes of management are extremely age related.

In short, pediatric dentistry does in fact borrow a lot from other disciplines, but beyond this borrowing it is a discipline unto itself. The student who wishes to master intellectually and clinically the challenges that this age group presents must understand and accept when simple transfers from one discipline can be made to the child patient and when transfers must be modified because of the age requirements or limitations that the child patient presents. The student must also understand that these requirements and limitations may vary from one age group to another.

Some Recent Trends in Dentistry for Children

1. Over the last 20 years, a number of themes have become more and more dominant in the field of pediatric dentistry. Certainly, prevention has become an important theme, and prevention-oriented practitioners have become more and more the desired product of dental schools' curricula. This emphasis on prevention, when paired with better understanding about home care, motivating parents to take care of their children, understanding the caries process as it relates to nutrition, the use of sealants, the fluoridation of water by communities, the utilization of topical fluorides by the dentist, and the use of fluoride in home care products such as toothpastes, has brought about the cavity free child. Such a child was a rarity 20 years ago. Today, such a child is commonplace in preventively oriented practices.

Closely allied to the prevention movement in dentistry has been interest in the development of vaccines to protect the teeth from bacterial destruction. Research on animals has led to optimism by some scientists that humans one day may be protected from dental decay by vaccination.

2. As attested to by the overall organization of this book, there has recently been a growing emphasis on the development of prevention strategies for children younger than age 3. Dentistry is now often a subject covered in prenatal classes for expectant mothers. Increasing emphasis for infant oral health by dental educators and concerned private practitioners is emerging.

3. The techniques of acid-etching and the use of sealants and composite resins on etched enamel and dentin have certainly been major and dramatic changes in dentistry's approach to the restoration of teeth. The uses of gold, dental amalgam, and porcelain are all being challenged by the new resin-sealant materials and techniques. Unquestionably, today resins are being used in clinical situations that were not taught, condoned, or understood 20 years ago. The cosmetic dentistry movement has been a part of this new generation of techniques and materials. The prevention of pit and fissure caries by sealants is another extremely important aspect of these relatively new techniques.

4. Dentistry for the disabled and for other patients with special needs has been an area of development in contemporary dental education during the past 20 years. Twenty years ago there were no curricular guidelines or recommendations regarding this subject. Today these guidelines exist. Indeed, the disabled child and young adult are patients that a community's dentist must not overlook or be unprepared to examine and treat when appropriate.

5. Increasingly, dental practitioners who treat children are more aware of the problems of malocclusions and are seeking information on how to intercept and correct orthodontic problems. The term "orthopedic therapy," a seldom heard or discussed philosophy-technique 20 years ago for the treatment of malocclusion, is certainly not a rarity in its use and discussion today. Unquestionably, the dental profession will continue to be interested in methods to manage dental and facial esthetics and to achieve harmonious occlusion in children because these problems are of concern to parents and because these problems are not preventable under the conditions that pathologies such as caries and periodontal disease are.

6. Pain and anxiety control has had considerable emphasis in dentistry in general and in dentistry for children as well in the past two decades. Although this area of patient management has always been important, more specific curricular guidelines, more modalities of pharmacologic control and patient monitoring, and more educational time are spent on these issues today than at any other time in the past. Allied to this emphasis has been an increasing scrutiny of the legal liability of the dentist to any mismanagement of the patient by the use of drugs. This phenomenon has been, in instances, paralleled by increases in malpractice insurance for practitioners who use drugs in managing patients.

7. Diagnostic information obtained by radiography has also been a major area of progress and debate over the last decade. As compared with dental x-ray machinery and film two decades ago, today's machinery and film are certainly safer for the patient in terms of radiation exposure per film. Also, useful and protective guidelines exist today for the taking of films in children that were not available 20 years ago.

8. Although there is no way to really substantiate this conclusion, dentistry, the dentist, and the dental experience are probably dreaded less today by children than they were 20 years ago. As will be discussed in Chapter 21, children who are genuinely and dreadfully afraid of dentists are rare today. There are, no doubt, a lot of reasons for this finding. However, unquestionably, the greater emphasis on prevention rather than on restoration and extraction of teeth is at least a part of the reason for this change.

9. Lastly, the dentist's responsibility to the abused and neglected child has been legally defined in the past 20 years.

Child Abuse

Child abuse and neglect are sick and very ugly emotional aspects of the more general problem of family dysfunction in our society and are themes that have in the past 20 years received increased legal and health science professional attention. By 1966, each of the 50 states had drafted legislation describing the responsibilities of professionals to report suspected abuse of children. These same laws that mandate that a dentist is required to report suspected abuse often also protect the dentist from legal litigation from angry and revengeful innocent parents.

These laws also spell out the legal implications to the dentist who knowingly and willfully does not report suspected child abuse. Although the law varies from state to state, generally the dentist who fails to report such cases is guilty of a simple misdemeanor and is subject to a fine and/or jail sentence, generally 30 days in length. The law usually also makes the dentist civilly liable for any damages to the child caused by a failure to report. In other words, litigation for damages can be conducted against the dentist for any further abuse received by the child.

If while performing an examination on a child something questionable like a bruise becomes apparent, the child should be interviewed for his or her analysis and explanation of the injury. Obviously, this is more effective for the older child. Next, after this examination is completed, the parents should be interviewed separately from the child to see if the two stories correlate. If there is no correlation of the two accounts of the injury, the appropriate authorities should be informed.

Abuse can be documented because of the trauma that burning, slapping, hitting, choking, twisting, pulling, and pinching cause. Broken teeth, burns, lacerations, bruises, and broken bones alert the dentist that something may be wrong. Neglect, however, is more subtle. The dentist should look for overall hygiene as well

as for dental hygiene and adequate clothing. Suspicion of poor nutrition, apparent lack of medical care, and an absence of previous dental care are situations that should alert the dentist to think about neglect. The dentist is responsible to take the same approach for neglect as for abuse. Reporting of such cases is mandatory. The American Academy of Pediatric Dentistry defines dental neglect as failure by a parent to seek treatment for untreated caries, oral infections, and/or oral pain, or failure of the parent or guardian to follow through with treatment once he or she is informed that the above conditions exist.

Milestones in the American Recognition and Approach to Family Dysfunction and Other Cruelties to Children

19th Century	House of refuge movement: This movement occurred in many major cities and enabled the state to place abandoned or neglected children somewhere safe.
1870's	Formation of the New York Society for the Prevention of Cruelty to Children: This was the first of many groups that worked in cooperation with the houses of refuge for the rescue of endangered children.
1899–1920	Establishment of juvenile courts: The first juvenile court was begun in Illinois in 1899. By 1920, all but three states had such courts.
1946	Medical discovery of child abuse: A paper by Caffey (Caffey J: Multiple fractures in the long bones of infants suffering from chronic subdural hematoma. Am J Roentgenol 56:163, 1946) concludes that many long bone fractures in children could not be specifically documented as to their origin.
1957	Caffey asserts that such injuries as fractures in long bones of infants have been deliberately inflicted.

1961	First conference is held on the battered child syndrome.
1962	Article on battered children is published in the Journal of the American Medical Association. (Kempe CH, Silverman EN, Steele BF, Dragmueller W, and Silver HK: The battered child syndrome. JAMA 181:17, 1962.) The concept of parental cruelty is now made public. By this time, there is a movement toward doing something about this problem.
1966	All 50 states have passed laws describing the responsibilities of health science professionals to report suspected abuse.
1971	Fontana proposes a more global definition of the mistreatment of children. Neglect is now considered a potential parental shortcoming. (Fontana V: The Maltreated Child: The Maltreatment Syndrome in Children. Springfield, IL, Charles C Thomas, 1971.)
1974	A National Center on Child Abuse and Neglect is established by Congress to give further leadership toward improving the potential protection of children.
1976–1979	The number of cases of child abuse reported nationally rose 71% from 1976 to 1979, when 711,142 cases were reported. (American Humane Association: National analysis of official child neglect and abuse reporting [1979]. DHHS Publication No. [OHDS] 81-30232, revised 1981.)

Informed Consent

Informed consent is the legal issue that protects a patient's right not to be touched or in any way treated without the patient's authorization. The issue assumes that it is a right of a mentally competent adult human being to determine what, if anything, a practitioner of health sciences can do to his or her body.

There are two kinds of consent, expressed and implied. Implied consent is determined by the behavior of the patient. For instance, the patient got in the chair, opened his mouth, but said nothing. Expressed consent is written or

oral. A signed written consent to treatment is the most substantial consent for protecting a dentist from litigation.

Informed consent also implies that the patient is aware of the nature of the treatment, alternatives to treatment, probably sequelae to treatment, and the potential benefits and possible risks of any treatment. In other words, an "uninformed" patient is incapable of giving informed consent. His signature, if the patient is uninformed, is legally useless also.

The law assumes that minors cannot take the responsibility for informed consent. To avoid liability, the dentist must secure consent from the parent or the person acting *in loco parentis.* An exception to this would be the rendering of emergency care that preserves life or avoids severe compromise to the child's health when the parents could not be located in the time available.

Obtaining informed consent can be a difficult problem for the dentist who treats children. It is not unusual for older children and adolescents to come to the dental office unaccompanied by a parent. In such cases, it is advised that only very safe, limited-risk procedures be performed.

Epidemiology and mechanisms of dental diseases in children

Steven M. Adair

Much progress has been made in the last two decades in understanding the complex interactions of the dental caries process. However, because of its multifactorial nature, there is still much to be learned regarding the initiation, progression, and prevention of tooth decay. The relationships to caries between diet, microflora, saliva, host response, demineralization-remineralization phenomena, fluoride and other trace elements, and other factors all require further study.

Current knowledge has led to a wealth of preventive regimens that can be applied on an individual or a public health basis. This has led to a dramatic reduction in the prevalence of dental caries in children in the United States (Brunelle and Carlos, 1982). A caries free teenager is no longer a rarity. Such a finding is not an unrealistic goal for the dental practitioner to hold for most child patients in the practice, par-

ticularly for children whose prevention programs were initiated early in life.

This chapter reviews the caries process and the current epidemiology of dental disease in children. It also touches on water fluoridation and dietary factors related to dental decay.

Current Concepts of the Caries Process

Dental caries is a complex, multifactorial disease that has been studied by epidemiologists, pathologists, microbiologists, immunologists, biochemists, physical chemists, and biophysicists. A detailed discussion of the current knowledge is not possible in the context of this chapter, but the following brief review should orient the reader as to the major areas of study engaged in by cariologists.

Dental caries is a disease of the dental hard tissues, characterized by the decalcification of the inorganic portions of the tooth. Loss of the mineral content is then followed by breakdown of the organic portions of the tooth. This destructive process results from the actions of microorganisms on carbohydrates. In its most simplified terms, the process can be visualized by a Venn diagram illustrating the following requirements: (1) a susceptible tooth; (2) presence of bacteria; (3) access to refined, fermentable carbohydrate; and (4) time. These requirements were first proposed in 1890 by Miller (Fig. 2–1). This diagram is the basis of the acidogenic, or chemicoparasitic, theory of dental caries. It is currently the most widely accepted model. In this model, bacteria utilize dietary carbohydrates, principally sucrose, as a substrate for acid production. It is this acid that begins the process of demineralization.

MICROBIOLOGY OF DENTAL CARIES

To participate in the caries process, bacteria must be aciduric with or without being acidogenic. This means that the given microorganism must be able to withstand a low pH environment and that it may contribute to that environment by producing acid. Of the many organisms present in the oral cavity, the genus most frequently implicated as a cause of caries is *Streptococcus*.

Several species of streptococci are known to be cariogenic in laboratory animals. These include *Streptococcus mutans, sanguis, salivarius,* and *milleri* (Fitzgerald, 1968; Drucker and Green, 1978). *Lactobacillus acidophilus* and *casei* have also been associated with the decay process. Some strains of *Actinomyces* are also capable, to a lesser extent, of producing coronal caries in some animal models as well as root surfaces caries in humans (Syed et al., 1975).

In humans, *S. mutans* has been correlated with caries in numerous cross-sectional epidemiologic studies and is currently presumed to play the major role in the initiation of the lesion (Loesche et al., 1975). Lactobacilli have been known for years to be correlated with dental caries. Currently, those species are thought to be minimally involved in the initiation of caries, but they are believed to play a role in the progression of the lesions. Increasing attention is being given to the relative cariogenic potential of various combinations of plaque bacteria in recent cariologic research.

FORMATION OF PLAQUE

The initial colonization of teeth probably begins with organisms other than *S. mutans* (van Houte et al., 1971), which does not have great ability to adhere to teeth by itself. The mechanisms of initial colonization include (1) adherence of bacteria to pellicle or the enamel surface, (2) adhesion between bacteria of the same or different species, and (3) subsequent growth of bacteria from small enamel defects and from cells initially attached to tooth structure (Gibbons and van Houte, 1973). Plaque formation continues with the formation of extracellular polymer chains via the breakdown of sucrose into its two main components, glu-

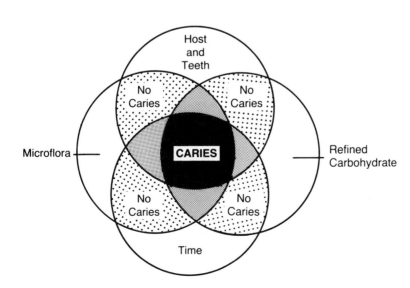

Figure 2–1 ■ Venn diagram, illustrating the relationship of the major factors involved in the caries process.

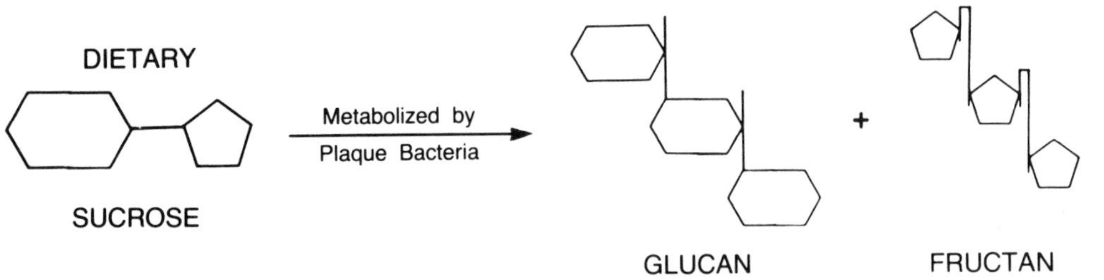

DIETARY

SUCROSE

→ Metabolized by Plaque Bacteria →

GLUCAN   +   FRUCTAN

Figure 2-2 ■ The breakdown of dietary sucrose into glucan and fructan.

cose and fructose (Fig. 2–2). The polymers are synthesized from each of these components. Chains of glucose are termed glucans (formerly called dextrans), whereas those of fructose are termed fructans (formerly called levans). These polysaccharides, especially glucans, are sticky, gelatinous substances that further enhance the bacteria's ability to adhere to the tooth and to each other. These polysaccharides also affect the rate at which saliva can enter the plaque to buffer the acid and reverse the demineralization process.

Intracellular metabolism of carbohydrates leads to the production of acids, chiefly lactic acid. This can depress the plaque pH from its resting level of around 6 to a value of 4 within minutes of coming in contact with a fermentable carbohydrate. Fructans are more soluble than glucans. They may also serve as a reservoir

of easily catabolized polysaccharide for the bacteria to utilize when other substrates are not available.

HISTOPATHOLOGY OF SMOOTH SURFACE LESIONS

The earliest clinical sign of the caries process on smooth enamel surfaces is the white spot lesion (Fig. 2–3). This is an area of white, chalky, opaque enamel, typically seen under a layer of plaque at the gingival margin of facial or lingual tooth surfaces. It can also be seen on proximal surfaces that become exposed after exfoliation of an adjacent primary tooth. The white spot lesion is an indication that the underlying enamel has become decalcified. In cross-section the lesion is conical, with its apex pointing toward the dentin. Depending on its depth, the lesion may or may not be visible on a bitewing radiograph.

Histologically, the enamel lesion has been divided by Silverstone and coworkers (1981) into zones that correspond to the changes produced in the enamel (Fig. 2–4).

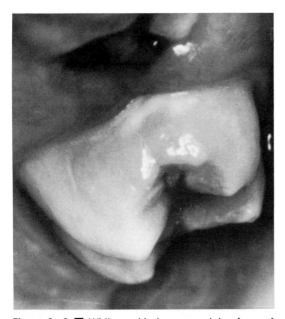

Figure 2-3 ■ White spot lesion on mesial surface of permanent first molar, below the contact area. Created by long-standing plaque, it is now visible after exfoliation of primary second molar.

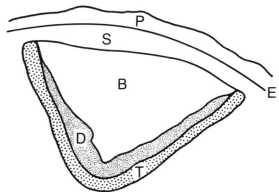

Figure 2-4 ■ Diagrammatic representation of an early enamel (white spot) lesion, illustrating: plaque (P), enamel surface and pellicle (E), intact surface layer (S), body of the lesion (B), dark zone (D), and translucent zone (T).

The surface zone is the relatively unaffected superficial enamel, which acts as a diffusion gradient, allowing minerals (fluoride, calcium, phosphate, and other ions) to pass in and out of the enamel. Only 5–10% of the mineral content is lost from the surface layer. Below this zone is the body of the lesion. This is the principal area of demineralization, representing about 60% mineral loss. The third zone, called the dark zone because of its appearance under polarized light microscopy, represents an area of mineral loss intermediate to the two preceding zones. The advancing front of the lesion, the translucent zone, has sustained a mineral loss similar to the surface zone (5–10%). Unless steps are taken to arrest and reverse this process, the lesion will continue to advance toward the dentin. As it approaches the dentino-enamel junction it spreads laterally, and the previously intact surface layer breaks down, creating clinically detectable cavitation.

The histopathology of pit and fissure caries is somewhat different from that of smooth surface lesions, and indeed approaches to the prevention of the two types of caries are different. The use of fluoride in its various forms, oral hygiene, and dietary control is primarily effective in combating smooth surface lesions, whereas sealants and the preventive resin restoration techniques are used to control pit and fissure lesions. The histopathology and prevention of pit and fissure lesions is discussed in Chapter 31.

DEMINERALIZATION-REMINERALIZATION

One of the most important concepts that has evolved in cariology in recent years involves a new view of the role played by enamel in the caries process. No longer can enamel be thought of as a solid, amorphous material that undergoes irreversible dissolution. Instead, it is being viewed as a diffusion matrix made up of crystals surrounded by a water-protein-lipid matrix that makes up 10–15% of the volume of enamel (Guggenheim, 1984). This matrix provides relatively large channels through which acids, minerals, fluoride, and other substances may pass in both directions.

Acids produced by plaque bacteria diffuse into the enamel via these channels to begin the process of demineralization below the surface layer. Once demineralization has begun, remineralization takes place. The two processes occur simultaneously in a dynamic fashion. The more soluble minerals in the enamel dissolve first, and they are replaced by the more insoluble minerals. Thus, crystals are created that are larger and now more resistant to dissolution (Feagin et al., 1971). This process occurs on almost all proximal surfaces continuously, as long as calcium and phosphate ions are available from the saliva. The presence of even very low levels of fluoride ions in this system will accelerate the remineralization process and reduce the rate of further demineralization.

Thus, dental caries must be viewed as a dynamic process taking place on all plaque-covered surfaces. The initial demineralization is followed by remineralization, a process that is enhanced by fluoride ions in the saliva, plaque, and enamel. The resultant "repaired" crystals are less soluble than the original crystals. As long as the surface layer remains intact, remineralization of the lesions is always possible. The clinician must recognize the importance of the surface layer of the white spot lesion and avoid the temptation to penetrate it with the explorer. Doing so will create an irreversible lesion that must be restored. The lesion in its early stages may not be detectable on a radiograph. However, many small lesions radiographically limited to enamel can be treated non-invasively with fluoride. This is predominantly true in permanent teeth, which have a much thicker enamel layer than primary teeth.

Epidemiology

The most recent, comprehensive data on the caries experience of United States school children were compiled by the National Caries Program of the National Institute of Dental Research (NIDR) in a nationwide study conducted in 1979–1980. Approximately 38,000 children, aged 5 to 17, were examined. Only visual-tactile criteria were used for caries determinations. No radiographs were taken. Thus, the findings are probably conservative compared with what would have been determined had the criteria applied in routine office examinations been used. The 48 contiguous states were divided into seven geographic regions. Each region was further subdivided into urban and rural areas.

Figure 2–5 shows the mean number of decayed, missing, and filled permanent tooth surfaces (DMFS) for children by age and sex. The DMFS for 5-year-olds, who as a group have few erupted permanent teeth, was 0.1. For 12-year-olds, this figure had risen to slightly more than 4, and at age 17 the mean DMFS was slightly in

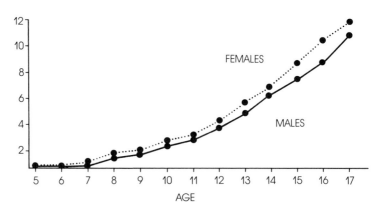

Figure 2–5 ■ Mean DMFS for children in the United States by age and sex. (Redrawn from The National Dental Caries Prevalence Survey, National Center for Health Statistics, 1981.)

excess of 11. The mean DMFS for all ages was 4.8. Females had slightly higher DMFS scores than males.

The mean number of decayed and filled primary tooth surfaces (dfs) for the 5- to 9-year-olds was 5.3. Caries free children constituted 36.6% of the sample. Another 39.8% had between 1 and 4 decayed, missing, or filled teeth (DMFT). Table 2–1 illustrates the percentage of caries free children at each age in the sample.

On a geographic basis, the highest mean DMFS, 6.1, was found in the Northeast, whereas the Southwest was lowest at 3.4. One possible explanation for this is that Boston, the largest urban center in the Northeast section, has only recently had its water fluoridated, whereas the Southwest has extensive areas high in naturally occurring water-borne fluo-

ride. Urban areas tended to have a lower prevalence of caries than rural areas, 4.7 vs. 5.0 DMFS. Exceptions to this were again the Northeast and Southwest, for the same reasons as cited above. Figure 2–6 illustrates the mean DMFS by region.

In general, the 1979–1980 survey found that the prevalence of decay in whites was slightly higher than in non-whites, although this estimate cannot be made with great precision because the study sample was not stratified by race. The mean DMFS for whites was 4.89, and for non-whites it was 4.15.

An indication of the level of care and need for care can be determined by examining the proportion of the total DMFS contributed by each component. The national survey revealed the contributions to be 16.8% decay, 7.1% missing, and 76.1% filled teeth. Similar data for the primary teeth were 37.3% decayed and 62.7% filled. This indicates a rather high level of care among United States school children.

Table 2–1 ■ **Percentage of caries free children aged 5–17**

Age	Per Cent Caries Free*
5	95
6	90
7	77
8	56
9	51
10	38
11	34
12	27
13	21
14	20
15	15
16	12
17	11

* Permanent teeth only.
From National Caries Study, 1979–1980.

COMPARISONS

The real significance of these data can be best appreciated if they are compared with earlier similar surveys. Table 2–2 compares the findings of four such studies, those conducted by the National Center for Health Statistics (NCHS) in 1963–1965, 1966–1970, 1971–1974, and the NIDR 1979–1980 study. Data for the 1963–1965 and 1966–1970 studies have been combined to cover ages 6 through 17. Although the earlier two studies reported findings in terms of DMFT only, the diagnostic criteria used were practically identical in all four studies. As Table 2–2 illustrates, the 1979–1980 survey has documented a substantial reduction in caries prevalence over the preceding two decades. This difference would be more striking if comparisons of DMFS could be made. This can

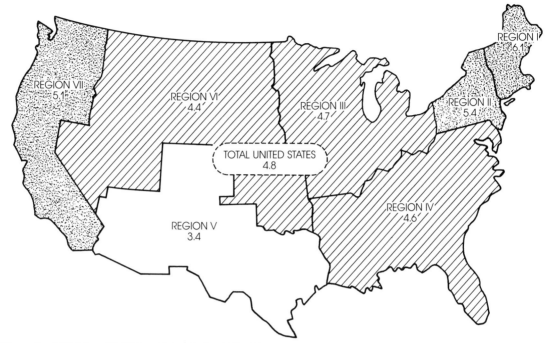

Figure 2 – 6 ■ Mean DMFS for children in the United States by geographic region, 1979 – 1980. (Redrawn from The National Dental Caries Prevalence Survey, National Center for Health Statistics, 1981.)

only be done for the 1971 – 1974 NCHS and 1979 – 1980 NIDR studies. The mean DMFS for ages 5 through 17 in the 1971 – 1974 study was 7.06. The mean DMFS in 1979 – 1980 was 4.8. This represents a 32% reduction in the mean DMFS. In a similar comparison (Table 2 – 3), the 1979 – 1980 survey has documented a significant increase in the proportion of caries free children, particularly in the 12- to 17-year-old age group.

Table 2 – 4 demonstrates the mean DMFS and percentage of caries by surface, comparing the 1971 – 1974 and 1979 – 1980 studies. The greatest proportionate reduction in DMFS prevalence was for proximal surfaces, a decrease of over 50%. Reductions of about 25% were seen for occlusal and facial-lingual surfaces. This

differential in DMFS reduction has meant that the percentage of caries by surface has shifted slightly, with the occlusal surface showing an increase in involvement from 49% to 54%.

BASIS FOR CARIES REDUCTIONS

We have seen that caries results from the interaction of specific microflora with fermentable carbohydrate on a susceptible tooth surface. There is no evidence to suggest that *Streptococcus mutans* has become less pathogenic or less prevalent in the population, although it has been proposed that the increased use of antibiotics may have some effect on the oral microflora. Similarly, there seems to be no evidence that per capita consumption of sugar

Table 2 – 2 ■ Mean DMFT in four national caries surveys

Age	NCHS 1963*– 1970†	NCHS 1971 – 1974	NIDR 1979 – 1980
6 – 11	1.4	1.7	1.1
12 – 17	6.2	6.2	4.6

* 1963 – 1965 children aged 6 – 11 years.
† 1966 – 1970 youths aged 12 – 17 years.
From Brunelle JA, Carlos JP: J Dent Res *61*(Sp Issue): 1346 – 1351, 1982.

Table 2 – 3 ■ Percentage of caries free children in four national studies

Age	NCHS 1963*– 1970†	NCHS 1971 – 1974	NIDR 1979 – 1980
6 – 11	51.1	43.6	56.7
12 – 17	10.4	9.7	17.2

* 1963 – 1965 children aged 6 – 11 years.
† 1966 – 1970 youths aged 12 – 17 years.
From Brunelle JA, Carlos JP: J Dent Res *61*(Sp Issue): 1346 – 1351, 1982.

Table 2–4 ■ Mean DMFS and percentage of total DMFS by surface type

Surface	NCHS 1971–1974	NIDR 1979–1980
Occlusal	3.5 (49%)	2.6 (54%)
Proximal	1.7 (24%)	0.8 (16%)
Facial-lingual	1.9 (27%)	1.4 (30%)

From Brunelle JA, Carlos JP: J Dent Res 61(Sp Issue) 1346–1351, 1982.

has decreased during the past 10 years (U.S. Dept. of Agriculture, 1981). However, it is possible, though unlikely, that the frequency of sugar ingestion has decreased. Therefore, it is unlikely that there has been any discernible change in the disease process itself.

The best explanation for the reduction in caries prevalence is the increased use of fluoride in its various forms, such as community water fluoridation, fluoride-containing dentifrices, and self-administered fluoride supplements. Evidence for this view is supported by the fact that the major caries reductions have occurred on proximal surfaces. These smooth surfaces benefit the most from fluoride's protective effects.

In the United States, the population exposed to optimally fluoridated water supplies doubled from 40 million to 80 million during the 1960's. Many of the children examined in 1979–1980 had the benefit of lifetime exposure to fluoridated water. Further evidence for this is found in comparing the caries scores of the Northeast, which is relatively unfluoridated, with those of the Southwest, which contains areas high in naturally occurring water-borne fluoride. In fact, the pattern of rural areas displaying higher caries rates than urban areas was reversed in these two geographic locations.

Increases in the numbers of school children who participate in school fluoride mouthrinse programs and other caries prevention programs have occurred to the point at which the effect can be seen on the national prevalence figures.

Other miscellaneous factors have been speculated to contribute to the reduction in caries prevalence. These include a presumed increase in the distribution of fluoride through foods and beverages prepared with fluoridated water. A general improvement in education and socioeconomic status may also lead to a more health conscious population with concomitant changes in dietary patterns. It is also possible that other as yet unclear factors contributing to increased human life span may have some in-

fluence on oral health, just as it is possible that improved oral health can contribute to increased longevity.

Dental caries continues to be a major health problem among children. The progress made in the past two decades is significant and encouraging, but further substantial reductions in caries prevalence will require redoubled effort. There is a limit to the number of community water systems that can be fluoridated. However, reductions in caries prevalence have been observed in communities that have maintained their current fluoridation status for many years. This makes it difficult to estimate the true contribution of fluoridated water supplies to the current DMFT scores. Increasing the use of self-applied fluoride supplements, especially through organized programs in schools, should be beneficial, even in fluoridated communities. It is obvious, too, that pit and fissure sealants are underutilized. Maximizing their use could greatly reduce that 54% of the caries that is minimally affected by fluoride.

It is interesting to note that although the prevalence of dental caries has been decreasing in the United States, it is increasing rapidly in developing nations. This has been attributed to an increase in refined carbohydrate in the diet as well as to a lower level of knowledge of oral health care in the general population of these nations.

Water Fluoridation

No single preventive dentistry measure has had the impact and success in reducing disease that has been afforded by the adjustment of the fluoride concentration in community drinking water supplies. In addition to providing caries reductions in the range of 50–70%, water fluoridation is the most cost effective means of caries prevention. It has been estimated that the annual per capita cost of water fluoridation in the United States is probably between $.15 and $.25.

HISTORY

According to Sognnaes (1979), the first observation of dental mottling was probably that reported by Kuhns in 1888. He described a dark enamel discoloration in a family that had resided in Durango, Mexico. Better known, however, is the 1901 publication by Eager describing the various enamel imperfections in the teeth of Italian emigrants bound for the United

States from Naples. He described a wide range of clinical features, from minor imperfections, to "browning" of the teeth, to a lack of enamel accompanied by extreme darkening. Eager speculated that the cause might be volcanic fumes or subterranean fires that contaminated the air or entered the drinking water. The condition was termed "denti di Chiaie" after a Professor Stefano Chiaie, who was credited with first describing it. Other terms applied to the various forms of the mottling were "denti neri" (black teeth) and "denti scritti" (teeth written upon). Most importantly, Eager realized that the condition seemed to occur in certain locations and that the incidence among children greatly diminished when the water supply was changed.

That same year, Dr. Frederick S. McKay began practicing in Colorado Springs and noticed staining in the enamel of many of his patients. Further investigation led him to the conclusion that this "Colorado brown stain," as it became to be known, followed a distinct geographic pattern. McKay invited G. V. Black to join in the investigation. The result was a full report of their clinical and histologic findings, published in 1916. The term "mottled enamel" was used to describe an endemic condition affecting 87.5% of the population in specific regions. McKay and Black advanced the idea that the causative factor, still undetermined at that time, was present during the development of the enamel, and further, that in children who resided in these locations for specific periods of time, only certain groups of teeth were affected.

Black and McKay described the appearance of affected teeth as ranging from paper-white, to brown, to black, with every conceivable intermediate degree represented. They noted that the general morphology of the teeth was nor-mal. Perhaps their most important observation was that these teeth seemed remarkably resistant to decay.

The histologic analysis of the teeth showed that the abnormal enamel was generally confined to the outer one third, with less involvement of the inner layers and dentin. Both the enamel interprismatic substance and the enamel rods were found to be affected. Some dentin involvement was noted.

Although both Eager and McKay had speculated on the possible causative factors, it was not until 1926 that McKay openly implicated drinking water supplies, although he was unsure as to what substances (or the absence of them) might contribute to mottling. It is interesting to note that in 1925, a study was published by McCollum and colleagues in which it was found that rats on high fluoride diets developed staining in their incisors. This fact was not related to human enamel mottling for years.

In 1930, Kempf and McKay demonstrated that enamel mottling in people living in Bauxite, Arkansas, disappeared only after the town changed its community water supply. There followed several studies in the 1930's conclusively linking water-borne fluoride with both enamel mottling and resistance to decay. The character of the studies of mottling, which now was termed "dental fluorosis," began to change, emphasizing whether a fluoride concentration could be found that would balance the benefits of caries protection with the risk of enamel discoloration.

By employing a system of fluorosis classification, Dean and others were able to determine that in communities with about 1.0 part per million (ppm) fluoride in the drinking water, fluorosis was not an esthetic problem. Moreover, these communities had a lower caries

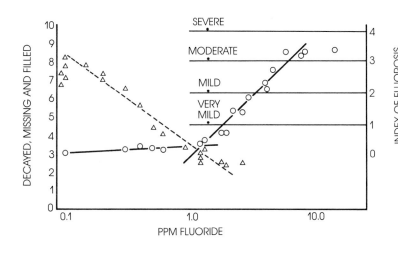

Figure 2–7 ■ Relationship between the fluoride content of the drinking water, caries prevalence, and the index of dental fluorosis. (Redrawn from Hodge HC, Smith FA: Some public health aspects of water fluoridation. *In* Shaw JH (ed): Fluoridation As a Public Health Measure. Washington, DC, © AAAS, Pub. No. 38, 1954, p. 88. Used by permission of SCIENCE.)

Table 2–5 ■ Comparison of caries scores and per cent reductions in 12- to 14-year-old children in communities with and without water fluoridation

City	Fluoride Status	Year	DMFT per Child	Per Cent Caries Reduction
Kingston	No F	1960	12.46	
Newburgh	F	1960	3.73	−70.1
Sarina	No F	1959	7.46	
Brantford	F	1959	3.23	−56.7
Grand Rapids	No F	1945	9.50	
	F	1959	4.26	−55.2
Evanston	No F	1946	9.03	
	F	1959	4.66	−48.4

From Newbrun E (ed): Fluorides and Dental Caries, 3rd edition, 1986, Courtesy of Charles C Thomas, Publisher, Springfield, Illinois.

prevalence than similar communities without fluoride. The relationship between fluoride content of the drinking water, caries prevalence (DMFT), and dental fluorosis is demonstrated in Figure 2–7.

At this point, fluoride research took a logical but dramatic turn. The emphasis now was placed on whether fluoride could be added to community water supplies to effect caries reductions. Between 1945 and 1947, large independent clinical studies were undertaken in four pairs of North American cities to test the results of fluoridation. These studies constitute some of the best designed and controlled public health trials ever undertaken. In most cases, each city was paired with a neighboring city, similar in almost all respects except for the lack of fluoride in the water supply. Table 2–5 illustrates the results of follow-up examinations of children 12 to 14 years of age conducted about 15 years after fluoridation was begun. Children residing in the trial cities had DMFT scores 50–70% lower than their counterparts in the control cities.

Further studies of water consumption led to the recognition that fluid intake is directly proportional to the average maximum daily air temperature of the community. Thus, a range of water fluoride concentrations from 0.7 to 1.2 ppm was developed by the Public Health Service to reflect the climate of various communities. The water fluoride concentration should vary inversely with the population water consumption.

CURRENT STATUS

According to the 1980 Fluoridation Census, over 106 million United States citizens in over 8000 communities receive caries protection from optimally adjusted fluoridated water. Another 9.8 million people in 3000 communities are drinking naturally fluoridated water at a concentration of 0.7 ppm or higher. Thus, over 50% of the United States population benefits from drinking water with sufficient fluoride to provide significant caries protection.

COST EFFECTIVENESS

Although the cost of labor, equipment, and chemicals involved in fluoridation may rise, it is still the most cost effective caries preventive measure available. As stated before, the annual per capita cost of fluoridation is about $.15 to $.25. Using a very simple formula for determining the cost-benefit ratio (cost of preventive program divided by savings in cost of treatment) and assuming an expected caries reduction of 55–65%, water fluoridation has been estimated to have a 1 : 60 cost-benefit ratio. This does not even take into consideration such intangibles as less pain and discomfort from disease or treatment, less time lost from work or school, improved function and appearance, and potential reductions in the prevalence of periodontal disease or certain types of malocclusion. This 1 : 60 cost-benefit ratio can be contrasted with ratios of 1 : 18 for fluoride mouthrinsing, 1 : 3.4 for daily use of supplemental fluoride tablets, and 1 : 1 for professionally applied topical fluoride (Davies, 1973; Silverstein et al., 1975).

FUTURE OF FLUORIDATION

A generation ago it was optimistically predicted that fluoridation of almost all communal

water supplies could be accomplished in as little as 5 years. Obviously, this was not the case. Such predictions were based on unrealistic expectations of the public's and the profession's understanding of the scientific, political, and social issues involved. In the United States, this public referendum has been the most common means of introducing water fluoridation. This has undoubtedly contributed to delays in its implementation, since the referendum opens the way for public debate and gives a forum to those opposed to fluoridation on emotional or political grounds. Opponents of fluoridation have used a variety of quasi-scientific and factually deficient arguments with some measure of success when the issue has been open to public debate. Until local boards of health are empowered to make decisions regarding fluoridation, it is likely to continue to be a political issue.

Further fluoridation of public water supplies will require more effort to achieve than in the past. Most of the major metropolitan areas in the United States have been fluoridated, so there are few large populations remaining that could benefit from fluoridation of large cities. Certainly, these efforts are worth pursuing. There will always remain, however, large segments of the population using private well water supplies, and these supplies cannot be economically fluoridated. One possible solution to this is school water fluoridation, which has been shown to be effective in reducing the caries experience of children in predominantly rural areas not served by a fluoridated community water system.

EFFECT OF DISCONTINUING FLUORIDATION

A disturbing trend toward discontinuing water fluoridation has become evident in recent years. Perhaps the most widely publicized case was that of Antigo, Wisconsin, which discontinued fluoridation in 1960 after 11 years of protection. Subsequently, fluoridation was resumed in 1965. The caries experience of kindergarten children rose 92% from 1960 to 1964, and by 1966 the mean number of primary teeth decayed or treated for decay (def) increased by 112%. The caries experience of the older children, who had consumed fluoridated water during a period of tooth formation, also began to rise. This is not surprising, since it is known today that fluoride exerts a major effect through a frequent, low dose contact with teeth.

Dietary Factors and Dental Caries

As mentioned previously, sugar is one of the major etiologic factors in dental caries. Sucrose has been labeled the "arch criminal of dental caries" (Newbrun, 1969), but in fact animal studies have shown other sugars, notably glucose and fructose, to be as cariogenic as sucrose (Stephan, 1966). This poses problems in making dietary recommendations, since many fruits and vegetables contain substantial amounts of naturally occurring sugars.

SUCROSE

The role of sucrose in caries formation has been speculated upon ever since the disease began to afflict humans, but one of the first controlled studies to document sucrose as an etiologic factor was the Vipeholm study (Gustafsson et al., 1954). In this study, 436 inmates in a mental institution at the Vipeholm Hospital near Lund, Sweden, were given carbohydrates in various forms to supplement the relatively sugar free institutional diets. The carbohydrate was offered as sucrose in solution, sweetened bread, milk chocolate, caramel, and toffee. The sucrose in solution and the bread were introduced with meals, whereas the other forms were given between meals. The study showed that an increase in sucrose intake was associated with an increase in caries activity and that this caries activity decreased when the sucrose-rich foods were discontinued. The cariogenic potential of the sucrose was enhanced when it was given between meals and in a more retentive form (caramels and toffees). The time required for the sugar to clear the oral cavity was closely related to the caries activity. The study also pointed out that caries formation varied among individuals, and that caries continued to form in some individuals even after a return to low sucrose diets.

Another interesting study was a survey of the dental health of children aged 3 to 14 who resided at Hopewood House in Bowral, New South Wales, Australia (Sullivan and Goldsworthy, 1958; Sullivan and Harris, 1958). Almost all of these institutionalized children had lived there since infancy and were fed an almost pure vegetarian diet supplemented with milk and an occasional egg yolk. The vegetables were generally served raw, and refined carbohydrate was rigidly restricted. In spite of poor

oral hygiene, the caries prevalence of the children was very low. Primary dentition involvement was almost non-existent, while the caries prevalence of the permanent teeth was about one tenth that of the mean score for other Australian children. Almost one third of the children remained caries free throughout the 5 year study. Children who left Hopewood House at an older age experienced a significant increase in dental caries.

RELATIVE CARIOGENICITY OF FOODS

Further studies into the relationship between diet and dental caries have refined the knowledge given by the Vipeholm and Hopewood House data, but in general the findings of those earlier studies have been confirmed. Much effort in recent years has gone into assessing the relative cariogenicity of a variety of foodstuffs (Bibby and Mundorff, 1975; Bibby et al., 1986). Wei (1982) has listed ten methods that have been used to make these assessments.

1. Caries production in experimental animals
2. Acid formed or fermentation by oral microflora
3. Enamel demineralization by foods fermented by salivary bacteria
4. Oral clearance time and retention of foods
5. Artificial caries production using an *in vitro* apparatus simulating human oral conditions
6. Microhardness tests of enamel exposed *in vivo* to dental plaque demineralization
7. Extraoral human plaque pH measurements
8. Intraoral plaque pH measurements via antimony electrode
9. Intraoral plaque pH measurements via wire telemetry and a miniature glass pH electrode built into a prosthesis
10. Clinical trials of foods in human populations

In each method it is difficult to sort out the various food and host factors involved in the caries process. Nonetheless, such research has led to the ranking of various foods according to their cariogenic potential in the test system, such as the one illustrated by Table 2–6. This has led to some interesting challenges of preconceived notions, such as the finding that potato chips produced deeper carious lesions in an artificial mouth than did cookies, sugared

Table 2–6 ■ Comparative depths of carious lesions produced by foods in artificial mouth (OroFax).*

Food	Proportionate Depth
Caramel	46.8
Fudge	45.0
Chocolate coconut bar	31.7
Potato chips	30.3
Graham cracker	28.6
White bread	26.7
Chocolate almond bar	26.2
Whole wheat bread	18.3
Plain breakfast cereal	18.3
Sugared breakfast cereal	18.2
Chocolate chip cookie	15.8
Dark chocolate	15.0
Sweet cookie	13.7
Ginger snaps	12.3
Fruit tart	11.2
Milk chocolate	7.5

* Proportionate values calculated from common control used in separate tests.
From Bibby BG: *In* Sweeney EA (ed): The Food That Stays: An Update on Nutrition, Diet, Sugar and Caries. New York, Medcom Inc, 1977, p 53.

breakfast cereal, or one form of chocolate candy. Similarly, apples were found to dissolve more enamel than soft drinks, caramel, or sugared breakfast cereal (Bibby, 1977).

OTHER FOOD FACTORS

Obviously, there are a multiplicity of food factors that require that relative cariogenicity tests be interpreted with caution. These factors include carbohydrate-sucrose concentration, stickiness, oral clearance rate, detergent quality, texture, and pH of the food itself. For example, most fruits will depress plaque pH by virtue of their own low pH. This occurs even though the low pH of the food inhibits fermentation of its sugar content. Likewise, high concentrations of sugar can also inhibit bacterial fermentation *in vitro*. The presence of starch, however, increases the acid production from sucrose (Buehrer and Miller, 1984) and may allow fermentation to take place under otherwise inhibiting concentrations of sugar. On the other hand, high levels of sugar appear to increase the

solubility of starchy foods and hasten the clearance from the oral cavity. Clearly, no one cariogenicity test can account for all these factors, except possibly trials in humans. Even in human trials, individual variations exist in plaque composition and amount, salivary buffering capacity, and enamel resistance to dissolution with or without the ability to remineralize.

Certain food components and factors may have cariostatic or caries-inhibiting effects. Phosphates, principally sodium metaphosphate, have been shown to reduce caries in animal studies (Nizel and Harris, 1964). The effect is probably local, related to buffering capacity, a reduction of enamel solubility, and other bacterial and biochemical properties. Unfortunately, clinical trials with phosphate supplements in human diets have not proved as effective (Baron, 1977; Lilienthal, 1976). Other animal studies (Featherstone and Mundorff, 1984) have shown that foods high in fat, protein, fluoride, or calcium may protect against caries. Such foods include cheese, yogurt, bologna, and peanuts. Fats, for example, may offer protection by coating the teeth and reducing the retention of sugar and even plaque by changing the enamel surface activity. Fats also may have toxic effects on oral bacteria and may decrease sugar solubility. Protein elevates the urea level in saliva and increases the buffering capacity of the saliva. Protein may also have an enamel-coating effect. Protein and fat in combination may raise plaque pH after exposure to carbohydrate. The addition of fluoride to dietary sucrose in concentrations as low as 2 ppm has also been found to significantly reduce decay in rats (Mundorff et al., 1986). Similar studies in humans have yet to be undertaken.

It has been proposed that the fibrous quality of some foods, such as celery or apples, may have a detersive effect on the teeth (Caldwell, 1970). Such foods may remove gross debris during mastication, but they are ineffective at plaque removal. By requiring vigorous chewing, these foods may stimulate salivary flow, which, in turn, buffers acid and promotes remineralization of enamel.

DIETARY COUNSELING

Many of these findings have challenged long-accepted notions that have formed the basis of dietary recommendations to reduce the caries activity in children. Is sugared cereal really worse than plain breakfast cereal if it is cleared from the oral cavity more rapidly? Are potato chips really a viable alternative to candy as a snack food?

Stookey (1979) has enumerated the attributes of the ideal snack as follows: (1) It should stimulate salivary flow via its physical form; (2) it should be minimally retentive; (3) it should be relatively high in protein and low in fat, have minimal fermentable carbohydrate, and have a moderate mineral content (especially calcium, phosphate, and fluoride); and (4) it should have a pH above 5.5 so as not to decrease oral pH, with a large acid buffering capacity and a low sodium content. Certain foods, such as raw vegetables, meet most or all of these requirements. Present day food technology should make it possible to create snacks that are nutritious and non-cariogenic, but this will not happen until the food industry finds a reliable cariogenicity test and the incentives to invest in such production.

In the meantime, we are left with the difficult task of attempting to alter the dietary habits of our caries-susceptible patients. Although such attempts are often met with failure, we as professionals have the obligation to make dietary information available to them. Although it is neither feasible nor desirable to eliminate sugar completely from the diet, we can recommend that between meal snacks be supervised by parents and that, where possible, sugar intake be limited to mealtimes when salivary flow is higher. The point should be made that lowering the frequency of carbohydrate ingestion may be more important than reducing the total carbohydrate intake.

Reduction of dental caries in children presents a continuing challenge to the profession. Much ground has been gained, but caries remains a significant chronic disease of childhood. By reducing its prevalence we not only contribute to healthier dentitions, but we are also able to focus on the many other facets of oral health care in children that deserve our attention.

REFERENCES

Baron HJ: Modifying the cariogenicity of foods with dicalcium phosphate. *In* Proceedings of workshop on cariogenicity of food, beverages, confections, and chewing gum. Chicago, American Dental Association, 1977.

Bibby BG: Cariogenicity of foodstuffs. *In* Sweeney EA (ed): The Food That Stays: An Update on Nutrition, Diet, Sugar and Caries. New York, Medcom, 1977.

Bibby BG, Mundorff SA: Enamel demineralization by snack foods. J Dent Res 54:461–470, 1975.

Bibby BG, Mundorff SA, Zero DT, Almekinder KJ: Oral

food clearance and the pH of plaque and saliva. JADA 112:333–337, 1986.

Black GV, McKay FS: Mottled teeth: An endemic developmental imperfection of the enamel of teeth heretofore unknown in the literature of dentistry. Dent Cosmos 58:(part I) 477–484, (part II) 627–644, (part III) 781–792, (part IV) 894–904, 1916.

Brunelle JA, Carlos JP: Changes in the prevalence of dental caries in U.S. schoolchildren, 1961–1980. J Dent Res 61(Sp Issue):1346–1351, 1982.

Buehrer EA, Miller CH: Sucrose and starch synergism in Streptococcus sanguis acid production. J Dent Res 63(Sp Issue):186 (abstract No. 137), 1984.

Caldwell RC: Physical properties of foods and their caries-producing potential. J Dent Res 49:1293–1298, 1970.

Davies GN: Fluoride in the prevention of dental caries. Br Dent J 135:79–83, 131–134, 233–235, 293–297, 333–335, 1973.

Dean HT: Classification of mottled enamel diagnosis. JADA 21:1421–1426, 1934.

Drucker DB, Green RM: The relative cariogenicities of Streptococcus milleri and other viridans group streptococci in gnotobiotic hooded rats. Arch Oral Biol 23:183–187, 1978.

Eager JM: Denti di chiaie teeth (chaie teeth). US Pub Health Rep 16:2576, 1901.

Feagin F, Patel PR, Koulourides T, Pigman W: Study of the effect of calcium, phosphate, fluoride and hydrogen ion concentrations on the remineralization of partially demineralized human and bovine enamel surfaces. Arch Oral Biol 16:535–548, 1971.

Featherstone JDB, Mundorff SA: Identification of the cariogenic elements of foods. Final report for period September 1981–May 1984 prepared for National Institute of Dental Research, 1984.

Fitzgerald RJ: Dental caries research in gnotobiotic animals. Caries Res 2:139–146, 1968.

Gibbons RJ, van Houte J: On the formation of dental plaques. J Periodontol 44:347–360, 1973.

Guggenheim B: Cariology Today. Basel, S Karger, 1984.

Gustafsson B, Quensel CE, Lanke L, et al: The Vipeholm dental caries study: The effect of different carbohydrate intake on 436 individuals observed for five years. Acta Odontol Scand 11:232–364, 1954.

Hodge HC, Smith FA: Some public health aspects of water fluoridation. In Shaw JH (ed): Fluoridation As a Public Health Measure. Washington, DC, AAAS, 1954.

Kempf GA, McKay FS: Mottled enamel in a segregated population. Pub Health Rep 45:2923–2940, 1930.

Lilienthal B: Phosphates and dental caries. In Myers H (ed): Monographs in Oral Science. Basel, S Karger, 1976.

Loesche WJ, Rowan J, Straffon LH, Loos PJ: Association of Streptococcus mutans with human dental decay. Infect Immun 11:1252–1260, 1975.

McCollum EV, Simmonds N, Becker JE, Bunting RW: The effect of additions of fluoride to the diet of the rat on the quality of the teeth. J Biol Chem 63:553–562, 1925.

McKay FS: Water supplies charged with disfiguring teeth. Water Works J 79:71–72, 79–80, 1926.

Miller WD: The microorganisms of the mouth. Philadelphia, SS White Dental Manufacturing Co, 1890. Republished, K Kong (ed). Basel, S Karger, 1973.

Mundorff SA, Glowinsky D, Griffin C: Fluoridated sucrose effect on rat caries. J Dent Res 65(Sp Issue):282 (abstract No. 1017), 1986.

National Caries Program, NIDR: The prevalence of dental caries in United States schoolchildren, 1979–1980. NIH publication No. 82-2245, 1981.

National Center for Health Statistics. Decayed, missing and filled teeth among children: United States. Vital and Health Statistics, Series 11, No. 106, DHEW Pub No. (HSM) 72-1003. Washington, DC, US Government Printing Office, 1971.

National Center for Health Statistics. Decayed, missing and filled teeth among youths 12–17 years: United States. Vital and Health Statistics, Series 11, No. 144, DHHS Pub No. (HRA) 75-1626. Washington, DC, US Government Printing Office, 1974.

National Center for Health Statistics. Decayed, missing and filled teeth among persons 1–74 years: United States. Vital and Health Statistics, Series 11, No. 223, DHHS Pub No. (PHS) 81-1673. Washington, DC, US Government Printing Office, 1981.

Newbrun E: Sucrose, the arch criminal of dental caries. J Dent Child 36:239–248, 1969.

Nizel AE, Harris RS. The effects of phosphate on experimental dental caries: A literature review. J Dent Res 43:1123–1136, 1964.

Silverstein SJ, Wycoff SJ, Newbrun E: Sociological, economical and legal aspects of fluoridation. In Newbrun E (ed): Fluorides and Dental Caries, 2nd ed. Springfield, IL, Charles C Thomas, 1975.

Silverstone LM, Johnson NW, Hardie JM, Williams RAD: Dental caries: Aetiology, pathology and prevention. London, The MacMillan Press Ltd, 1981, p 137–147.

Sognnaes RF: Historical perspectives. In Johansen E, Taves D, Olsen TO (eds): Continuing Evaluation of the Use of Fluorides. Boulder, CO, Westview Press, 1979.

Stephan RM: Effect of different types of human foods in dental health of experimental animals. J Dent Res 45:1551–1561, 1966.

Stookey GK: Developing the perfect snack food. In Alfano MC (ed): Changing Perspectives in Nutrition and Caries Research. New York, Medcom, 1979.

Sullivan HR, Goldsworthy NE: Review and correlation of the data presented in papers 1–6 (Hopewood House study). Aust Dent J 3:395–398, 1958.

Sullivan HR, Harris R: Hopewood House study 2. Observations on oral conditions. Aust Dent J 3:311–317, 1958.

Syed SA, Loesche WJ, Pape HL Jr, Grenier E: Predominant cultivable flora isolated from human root surface caries plaque. Infect Immun 11:727–731, 1975.

United States Department of Agriculture: Food consumption, prices, and expenditures, 1960–80. Economic Research Service Statistical Bulletin No. 672, Washington, DC, 1981.

United States Department of Health and Human Services: Fluoridation Census 1980. Washington, DC, US Government Printing Office, 1984.

van Houte J, Gibbons RJ, Pulkinen AJ: Adherence as an ecological determinant for streptococci in the human mouth. Arch Oral Biol 16:1131–1141, 1971.

Wei SHY: Diet and dental caries. In Stewart RE et al (eds): Pediatric Dentistry — Scientific Foundations and Clinical Practice. St. Louis, CV Mosby, 1982.

chapter 3

Oral pathologic conditions and soft tissue anomalies in children

Catherine M. Flaitz

The purpose of this chapter is to review the more common oral pathoses and soft tissue anomalies that occur in children. The material has been outlined in tabular form in order to make this comprehensive subject both practical and meaningful. The brief description for each of the lesions is an attempt to make this information specific to pediatrics. The categories in-

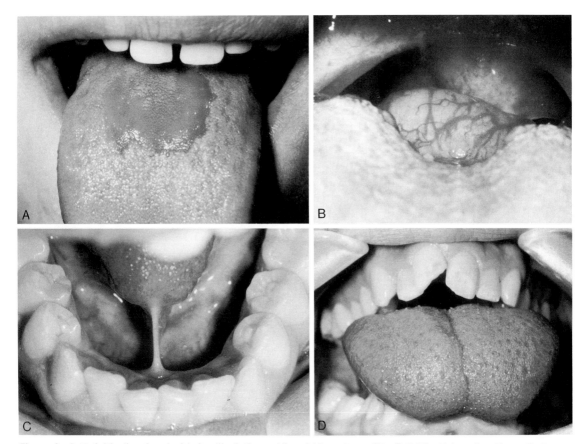

Figure 3 – 1 ■ *A,* Median rhomboid glossitis. *B,* Lingual thyroid (courtesy of Dr. G. E. Lilly, University of Iowa College of Dentistry). *C,* Partial ankyloglossia with lingual frenum attached near the tip of the tongue. *D,* Partial ankyloglossia demonstrating restricted movement of the tongue.

Table 3–1 ■ Developmental anomalies and variations of the soft tissues (Fig. 3–1)

Condition	Pediatric Age and Sex	Clinical Findings	Location	Pediatric Significance	Treatment and Prognosis	Differential Diagnosis
Fordyce granules	First and second decades No sexual predilection	Small, yellow, multifocal spots that are discrete or plaque-like; slightly elevated; asymptomatic	Bilateral buccal mucosa, labial mucosa, and retromolar pad	60% occur under 10 years of age; there is an increase in size during puberty	No treatment necessary; occasional development of pseudocysts from the ducts of these sebaceous glands	Focal keratosis
Retrocuspid papilla	First decade No sexual predilection	Soft, sessile, mucosal nodule; asymptomatic	Lingual-attached gingiva of mandibular canines; usually bilateral	Occurs in 72% of children under 10 years of age; regresses with age	No treatment necessary; normal anatomic structure	Inflammatory fibrous hyperplasia
Fissured tongue	First and second decades No sexual predilection	Small furrows or grooves of varying depths on tongue; painful if inflamed	Dorsum of tongue	Frequent oral manifestation of Down's syndrome and of mouth-breathers; occurs in 1% of children under 18 years of age	Brush tongue daily to remove debris in the grooves; may be source of halitosis	Benign migratory glossitis
Median rhomboid glossitis	First and second decades Male predilection	Varies from smooth, flat, or depressed area to an elevated nodular enlargement; ovoid or diamond shape; reddish patch devoid of papillae	Anterior to circumvallate papillae in the midline dorsum of tongue	Congenital lesion is very rare; most lesions are acquired and frequently associated with a chronic, localized candidal infection	No treatment if a developmental lesion; antifungal medication if lesion is acquired	Candidiasis Neurofibroma Granular cell tumor Lingual thyroid
Lingual thyroid	Second decade Female predilection	Nodular enlargement, with either a vascular or normal, smooth-surface appearance; may cause dysphagia, dysphonia, or dyspnea	Midline, base of tongue	Most cases arise in females during puberty or pregnancy. Majority of people with lingual thyroid lack normal thyroid tissue	If symptomatic, replacement thyroid hormone therapy and/or excision; long-term follow-up is required; adenoma or adenocarcinoma may arise from tissue	Median rhomboid glossitis Thyroglossal duct cyst Hemangioma
Partial ankyloglossia	Present at birth No sexual predilection	Short lingual frenum or anterior attachment of frenum to the tip of the tongue	Ventral surface of tongue	Rarely a problem with movement of tongue for speaking or swallowing; occasionally results in gingival recession of the mandibular incisors	Infrequently, a frenectomy is indicated	Complete ankyloglossia

cluded in the descriptions are: (1) the usual age and sex of the children that the lesion occurs in, (2) the common clinical findings of the lesion, (3) the usual location of the lesion, (4) the pediatric significance of the lesion, (5) the treatment and prognosis of the lesion, and (6) a differential diagnosis that is relevant to this age group.

The tables are arranged according to related groups of lesions for the purpose of differential diagnosis. The sequential headings for each of the tables include the following:

Developmental anomalies and variations of the soft tissues (Table 3 – 1; Fig. 3 – 1)

Benign mucosal surface lesions (Table 3 – 2; Figs. 3 – 2 to 3 – 5)

White lesions
Pigmented lesions
Ulcerated lesions
Papillary lesions

Benign mesenchymal lesions of the soft tissues (Table 3 – 3; Fig. 3 – 6)

Cysts and pseudocysts of the soft tissues (Table 3 – 4; Fig. 3 – 7)

Odontogenic cysts and neoplasms of the jaws (Table 3 – 5; Fig. 3 – 8)

Benign non-odontogenic neoplasms of the jaws (Table 3 – 6; Fig. 3 – 9)

Inflammatory lesions of the jaws (Table 3 – 7; Fig. 3 – 10)

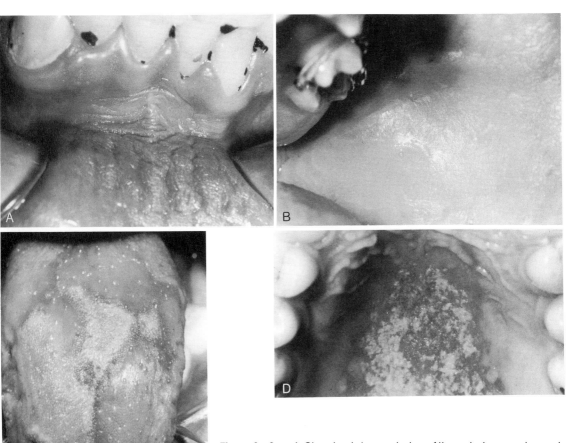

Figure 3 – 2 ■ *A,* Chewing tobacco lesion of the anterior mucobuccal fold. *B,* Leukoedema of the buccal mucosa. *C,* Benign migratory glossitis. *D,* Candidiasis of the hard palate.

Table 3–2 ■ Benign mucosal surface lesions

Lesion	Pediatric Age and Sex	Clinical Findings	Location	Pediatric Significance	Treatment and Prognosis	Differential Diagnosis
White Lesions (Fig. 3–2)						
Chewing tobacco lesions	Second decade Male predilection	White, wrinkled, corrugated, localized area with intervening pink to red furrows; translucent to opaque, rough surface	Mandibular, anterior mucobuccal fold	Mucosal lesions occur in approximately 50% of users; other health problems include periodontal disease, elevation in blood pressure, and dependence	Discontinuation of habit results in lesion reversal in 2 weeks; biopsy necessary for persistent lesions; may undergo malignant transformation	Leukoplakia Epithelial dysplasia Chemical burn
White sponge nevus	First decade No sexual predilection	White, folded, diffuse lesions; spongy texture; mucosa appears thickened; asymptomatic	Widespread involvement—buccal and labial mucosa, palate, gingiva, floor of mouth, and ventral tongue	Autosomal dominant inheritance pattern; may be present at birth but reaches full expression during adolescence	No treatment necessary; benign condition	Leukoedema Hereditary benign intraepithelial dyskeratosis
Leukoedema	First and second decade No sexual predilection	Diffuse, filmy, milky white opalescence of the mucosa; wrinkled to folded appearance; bilateral involvement; asymptomatic	Buccal mucosa, soft palate, labial mucosa	More prominent in blacks; incidence increases with age	No treatment necessary; common variant of normal mucosa	Leukoplakia White sponge nevus Hereditary benign intraepithelial dyskeratosis
Benign migratory glossitis (geographic tongue)	First and second decades No sexual predilection	Multiple areas of irregular, circular red patches surrounded by a whitish, thickened band; loss of filiform papillae; pattern changes; occasional glossodynia	Dorsum and bilateral borders of tongue	Occasionally lesions are found on buccal mucosa, lips, and ventral tongue and are called erythema migrans	No treatment necessary; bland diet if symptomatic; periods of remission	Candidiasis Fissured tongue
Candidiasis	First and second decades No sexual predilection	Soft, creamy white, slightly elevated plaque-like areas; patches wipe off, leaving erythematous mucosa; may be tender or burning sensation	Buccal mucosa, lips, tongue, palate	Contributing factors in opportunistic infection include antibiotics, diabetes, orthodontic appliance, and immunosuppressive therapy	Antifungal medications and proper oral hygiene; good prognosis if reason for infection can be eliminated or properly monitored	Plaque Superficial bacterial infection Chemical burn
Pigmented Lesions (Fig. 3–3)						
Amalgam tattoo	First and second decades No sexual predilection	Bluish-gray diffuse pigmentation; smooth surface; may	Gingiva, buccal mucosa, alveolar mucosa	Graphite tattoo has a similar appearance but is usually found on	No treatment necessary; permanent stain	Oral melanotic macule Hematoma

Lesion	Age/Sex	Clinical Features	Location	Comments	Treatment	Differential Diagnosis
		increase in size; history of amalgam restoration placement; asymptomatic; radiographs may show radiopaque particles		palate as a result of a self-inflicted pencil wound		Melanocytic nevus
Oral melanotic macule (ephelis)	First and second decades. Female predilection	Well-circumscribed, single or multiple, flat macule; brown, black, gray, or bluish in color; asymptomatic	Lip, gingiva, buccal mucosa, palate	Most common physiologic pigmentation to occur in the oral cavity of light-skinned individuals	No treatment necessary; excision if nevus cannot be excluded; no evidence of malignant transformation	Amalgam/graphite tattoo. Melanocytic nevus. Hematoma
Melanocytic nevus	Second decade. Female predilection	Well-circumscribed, raised, dome-shaped nodule; brown, blue, or black pigmentation; asymptomatic	Hard palate, buccal mucosa, lip, and gingiva	Congenital lesion; average 20 nevi on body; excision of intraoral lesions because of constant, chronic irritation of mucosa	Excision because of potential for malignant transformation; recurrence is uncommon unless incompletely excised	Oral melanotic macule. Amalgam/graphite tattoo. Hematoma
Hematoma	First and second decades. No sexual predilection	Well-circumscribed to diffuse, raised, dome-shaped enlargement; fluctuant to firm; blue, black in color; may be tender to palpation; history of trauma	Buccal mucosa, lips, soft palate, floor of mouth	Multiple and frequent hematomas may be the result of child abuse or bleeding disorders	No treatment necessary; resolution of lesion within 7–14 days	Amalgam/graphite tattoo. Oral melanotic macule. Melanocytic nevus
Ulcerated Lesions (Fig. 3–4)						
Aphthous ulcer	Usually second decade. Female predilection	Single or multiple superficial erosions; well-circumscribed and surrounded by erythematous halo; covered by white pseudomembrane; painful; heal in 7–10 days	Buccal and labial mucosa, ventral tongue, floor of the mouth, soft palate (mucosa not bound to periosteum)	Familial tendency; 20% of population affected; cause is unknown, but contributing factors include trauma, stress, allergies, and endocrine conditions	Symptomatic relief; if severe, tetracycline oral suspension rinse; variable frequency of recurrence	Traumatic ulcer. Recurrent herpetic ulcer
Traumatic ulcer	First and second decade. No sexual predilection	Usually solitary lesion; diffuse or localized; shallow or deep; covered by white pseudomembrane; painful; usually heals within 7–10 days	Lateral borders of tongue, buccal mucosa, lips, palate	Most common oral ulcer; need to rule out self-inflicted injuries or child abuse	Symptomatic relief and removal of cause; good prognosis if not inflicted intentionally	Aphthous ulcer. Recurrent herpetic ulcer

Table continued on following page

27

Table 3–2 ■ Benign mucosal surface lesions *Continued*

Lesion	Pediatric Age and Sex	Clinical Findings	Location	Pediatric Significance	Treatment and Prognosis	Differential Diagnosis
Recurrent herpes simplex infection	First and second decades No sexual predilection	Multiple small vesicles in clusters that coalesce to form ulcer; covered by white pseudomembrane intraorally; painful prodromal burning or itching sensation; heal within 7–10 days	Lips, hard palate, attached gingiva, dorsum of tongue (mucosa bound to periosteum)	Usually reactivation of herpes simplex virus type 1; contributory factors include fever, sunburn, trauma, fatigue, and menstruation; most contagious in vesicular form	Symptomatic relief; variable frequency of recurrence	Aphthous ulcer Traumatic ulcer
Angular cheilitis	First and second decades No sexual predilection	Deep fissures that bleed and ulcerate; develop superficial exudative crust; dryness and burning sensation	Corners of the mouth	Occurs most frequently in children who are mouthbreathers and in those who repeatedly moisten lips with saliva; responsible microorganisms include *Candida albicans*, staphylococci, streptococci	Lubrication of lips; antifungal or antibiotic ointment if persistent; tendency to recur	Recurrent herpetic ulcer Impetigo
Papillary Lesions (Fig. 3–5) Papilloma	First and second decades No sexual predilection	Broad-based or pedunculated, rough, corrugated, exophytic enlargement; finger-like projections; white or pink in color; usually a solitary lesion; asymptomatic	Palate, lips, dorsum of tongue, uvula	If multiple, widespread lesions are observed, then need to exclude oral florid papillomatosis or focal dermal hypoplasia syndromes	Excision; recurrence is rare if properly excised	Verruca vulgaris Giant cell fibroma
Verruca vulgaris	First and second decades No sexual predilection	Same as papilloma but may be multiple; caused by the papovavirus	Lips	Autoinoculation from sucking on fingers or thumb and nail biting	Excision; occasionally undergoes spontaneous involution; recurrence is rare	Papilloma Condyloma acuminatum
Condyloma acuminatum	Second decade No sexual predilection	Same as papilloma, but lesions are multiple; tend to enlarge and coalesce rapidly; found in diffuse clusters; caused by papovavirus	Dorsum of tongue, buccal mucosa, palate, gingiva	Sexually transmitted disease; lesions most commonly found in the anogenital region	Excision; recurrence is common	Verruca vulgaris Oral florid papillomatosis

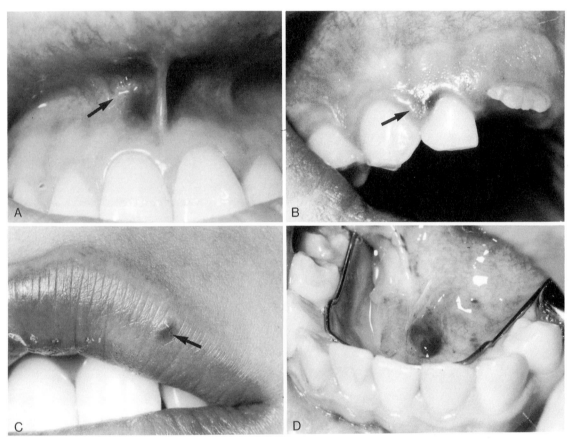

Figure 3 – 3 ■ *A,* Amalgam tattoo of the anterior mucobuccal fold *(arrow). B,* Oral melanotic macule of the gingiva *(arrow). C,* Melanocytic nevus, compound type of the maxillary lip *(arrow). D,* Hematoma of the floor of the mouth.

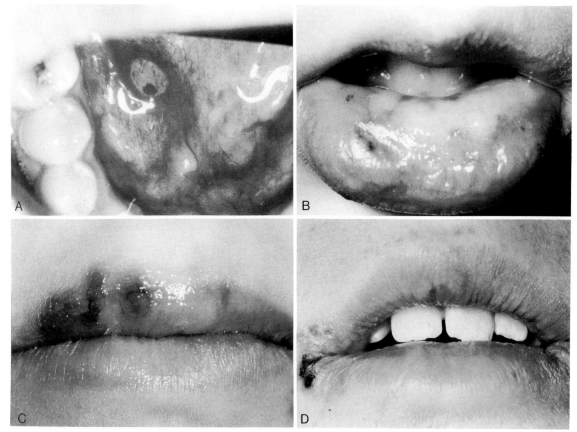

Figure 3–4 ■ *A,* Aphthous ulcer of the floor of the mouth. *B,* Traumatic ulcer of the mandibular lip as a result of macerating the tissues following a local anesthetic injection. *C,* Recurrent herpes simplex labialis. *D,* Angular cheilitis with ulcerated fissures.

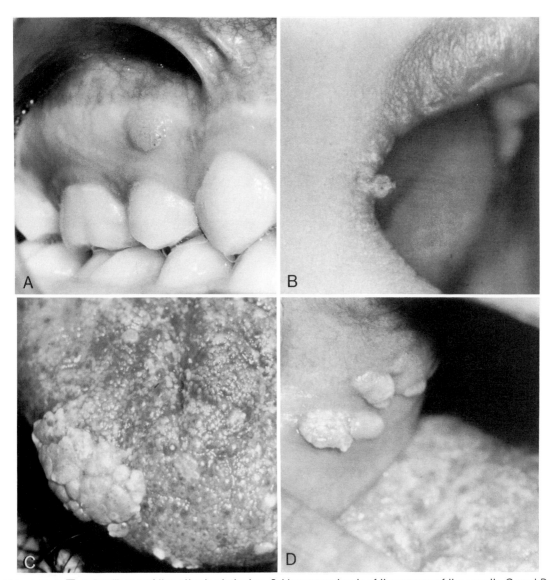

Figure 3-5 ■ *A,* Papilloma of the attached gingiva. *B,* Verruca vulgaris of the corner of the mouth. *C* and *D,* Condylomata acuminata of the lateral border of the tongue *(C)* and buccal mucosa *(D)* in the same patient (courtesy of G. E. Lilly, University of Iowa, College of Dentistry).

Table 3–3 ■ Benign mesenchymal lesions of the soft tissues (Fig. 3–6)

Lesion	Pediatric Age and Sex	Clinical Findings	Location	Pediatric Significance	Treatment and Prognosis	Differential Diagnosis
Pyogenic granuloma	Second decade Female predilection	Well-circumscribed, pedunculated or sessile, nodular enlargement; smooth or lobulated, ulcerated surface; hemorrhagic, soft consistency; red to purple in color; response to trauma or chronic irritation	Gingiva, lips, tongue, buccal mucosa	Hormonal changes during puberty and pregnancy may be responsible for an exaggerated response of gingiva to local irritation	Excision and removal of irritant; recurs if cause is not eliminated	Parulis Inflammatory fibrous hyperplasia Peripheral giant cell granuloma Capillary hemangioma
Inflammatory fibrous hyperplasia (irritation fibroma)	First and second decades Female predilection	Well-circumscribed, pedunculated or sessile enlargement; smooth to granular surface; firm, usually same color as surrounding mucosa; slow growing; asymptomatic	Lips, buccal mucosa, tongue, palate	Most common reactive lesion of the oral cavity in children	Excision and removal of irritant; recurs if cause is not eliminated	Pyogenic granuloma Peripheral giant cell granuloma Peripheral ossifying fibroma
Peripheral ossifying fibroma	Second decade; peak incidence, 13 years Female predilection	Well-circumscribed, sessile or pedunculated enlargement; smooth or ulcerated surface; firm; usually same color as surrounding mucosa; slow growing; asymptomatic	Gingiva, anterior to molar region; usually interdental papilla	Frequently causes migration of teeth	Deep excision, including periosteum and periodontal ligament; repeated recurrences are common	Pyogenic granuloma Peripheral giant cell granuloma
Peripheral giant cell granuloma	First and second decades No sexual predilection	Well-circumscribed nodular enlargement; smooth or ulcerated surface; spongy to firm; deep red to reddish-blue color; asymptomatic	Anterior mandibular and maxillary gingiva	Rarely delays eruption of teeth or causes migration of teeth	Deep excision, including periosteum and removal of local irritant; recurs if not adequately excised	Pyogenic granuloma Peripheral ossifying fibroma

Hemangioma	First decade; majority detected within the first year; Female predilection	Well-circumscribed to diffuse, lobular or dome-shaped enlargement; pedunculated or sessile; deep red to reddish blue in color; soft and compressible; blanches upon palpation; asymptomatic; 16% are multiple	Lip, tongue, buccal mucosa, and palate	May result in macroglossia or macrocheilia; hemorrhage from trauma is a common complication	Excision, sclerosing agents, cryotherapy; may undergo spontaneous regression; does not recur with adequate removal or destruction	Lymphangioma / Pyogenic granuloma / Peripheral giant cell granuloma / Hematoma / Mucous retention phenomenon
Lymphangioma	First decade; majority detected within the second year; No sexual predilection	Similar to hemangioma; color is bluish to normal mucosal pink; translucent; may have a pebbly appearance; rubbery consistency; may be multiple	Tongue, buccal mucosa, and floor of mouth	May result in macroglossia or macrocheilia; may undergo rapid enlargement during upper respiratory tract infections or menstruation	Excision, spontaneous regression is rare; high rate of recurrence	Hemangioma / Mucous retention phenomenon
Neurofibroma	Second decade; No sexual predilection	Well-circumscribed to diffuse, solitary or multiple enlargement; nodular to pendulous shape; smooth surface; same color as surrounding mucosa; soft to firm consistency; asymptomatic	Tongue, gingiva, buccal mucosa, palate	Neurofibromatosis is autosomal dominant trait characterized by neurofibromas, café au lait spots, axillary freckling, and congenital malformations. Intraoral involvement ranges from 7 to 20%.	No treatment necessary; excision if cosmetic problem or symptomatic; long-term follow-up is required; 10% undergo malignant transformation	Schwannoma / Granular cell tumor / Salivary gland neoplasms
Congenital epulis	Present at birth; Female predilection	Well-circumscribed nodular enlargement; pedunculated; firm, rubbery consistency; color the same as surrounding mucosa; smooth surface; may be hemorrhagic and ulcerated	Maxillary, anterior alveolar ridge	May cause feeding or respiratory problems	Excision with care not to disturb developing teeth; does not recur	Pyogenic granuloma / Peripheral giant cell granuloma / Hemangioma

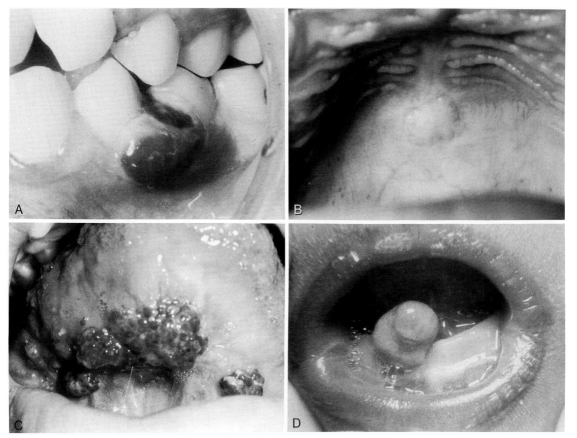

Figure 3–6 ■ *A,* Pyogenic granuloma of the gingiva (courtesy of P. S. Casamassimo, University of Colorado Health Science Center, School of Dentistry). *B,* Inflammatory fibrous hyperplasia of the hard palate. *C,* Lymphangioma of the ventral tongue. *D,* Congenital epulis of the mandibular alveolar ridge.

Table 3–4 ■ Cysts and pseudocysts of soft tissues (Fig. 3–7)

Lesion	Pediatric Age and Sex	Clinical Findings	Location	Pediatric Significance	Treatment and Prognosis	Differential Diagnosis
Palatal and dental lamina cysts of newborn	Present at birth or neonatal period. No sexual predilection	Solitary or multiple, white or grayish-white, discrete nodules; firm; small; asymptomatic	*Dental lamina cysts:* crest of alveolar ridge. *Epstein's pearls:* midpalatine raphe. *Bohn's nodules:* hard and soft palate	Found in 75% of neonates	No treatment necessary; usually slough within a few weeks	Natal/neonatal teeth
Mucous retention phenomenon	First and second decades. No sexual predilection	Compressible, dome-shaped enlargement; freely movable; fluctuates in size; translucent to bluish color; may be tender	Lower lip, buccal mucosa, ventral tongue, floor of mouth	Most common lip swelling in children; frequently associated with history of trauma	Excision; marsupialization if lesion is large; high recurrence rate if gland responsible is not removed	Hemangioma. Lymphoepithelial cyst. Mucoepidermoid carcinoma, low grade
Lymphoepithelial cyst	Second decade. No sexual predilection	Solitary, doughy, well-circumscribed nodule; smooth surface; freely movable; yellow to yellowish-white color; asymptomatic	Floor of mouth, ventral tongue, postero-lateral surface of tongue	Painful if traumatized	Excision; does not recur	Mucous retention phenomenon. Lipoma. Epidermoid cyst
Eruption cyst	First and second decades. No sexual predilection	Well-circumscribed, dome-shaped, fluctuant enlargement; bluish color; overlying an erupting tooth; usually asymptomatic	Alveolar mucosa	May occur in either dentition; tender if superimposed bacterial infection present	No treatment necessary; excision of overlying gingiva if symptomatic	Neonatal alveolar lymphangioma. Hematoma

35

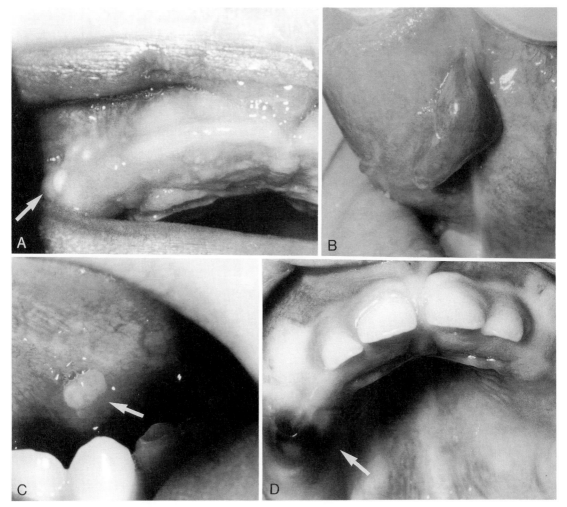

Figure 3 – 7 ■ *A,* Dental lamina cyst of the maxillary alveolar ridge *(arrow). B,* Mucous retention phenomenon of the ventral tongue. *C,* Inflamed lymphoepithelial cyst of the ventral tongue *(arrow). D,* Eruption cyst of the maxillary alveolar ridge *(arrow).*

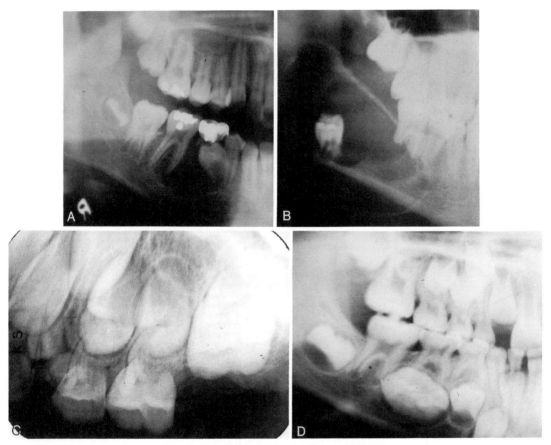

Figure 3–8 ■ *A*, Dentigerous cyst of the posterior mandible. *B*, Ameloblastoma of the posterior mandible. *C*, Compound odontoma of the anterior maxilla. *D*, Complex odontoma of the posterior mandible.

Table 3–5 ■ Odontogenic cysts and neoplasms of jaws (Fig. 3–8)

Lesion	Pediatric Age and Sex	Clinical Findings	Radiographic Findings	Location	Pediatric Significance	Treatment and Prognosis	Differential Diagnosis
Dentigerous cyst	Second decade No sexual predilection	Usually slow-growing, localized lesion associated with delayed eruption of teeth; may result in expansion of jaws; asymptomatic unless infected	Usually unilocular radiolucency around coronal aspect of unerupted tooth; well-circumscribed with sclerotic border; may displace teeth	Mandibular and maxillary third molar region; maxillary canine	Most common cyst of jaws in childhood; growth may be very rapid in this age group	Excision and curettage; recurrence is uncommon	Hyperplastic dental follicle Odontogenic keratocyst Unicystic ameloblastoma
Odontogenic keratocyst	Second decade Slight male predilection	Expansion of bone; occasional perforation of cortical plate; may be painful; large lesions may result in paresthesia of lip or teeth	Large, unilocular or multilocular radiolucency; thin, smooth border or scalloped sclerotic border; 40% associated with unerupted teeth; may cause resorption of roots or displacement of teeth	Posterior mandible	If multiple, need to rule out basal cell nevus syndrome	Excision and curettage; high rate of recurrence	Dentigerous cyst Primordial cyst Ameloblastoma
Adenomatoid odontogenic tumor	Second decade Female predilection	Slow-growing, localized, expansile lesion; associated with delayed eruption of teeth; painless	Unilocular, well-circumscribed radiolucency with variable amounts of radiopaque foci; pericoronal aspect of unerupted tooth; displacement of adjacent teeth; root resorption is rare	Anterior maxilla	80% of lesions occur between 10 and 20 years of age; behavior of lesion is very benign; occasionally found as an extraosseous lesion	Excision or curettage; does not recur	Calcifying and keratinizing odontogenic cyst Early stage of complex odontoma Cementifying and ossifying fibroma

	Age/Sex	Clinical features	Radiographic features	Comments	Treatment	Differential diagnosis
Odontoma, compound/complex	Second decade; No sexual predilection	Slow-growing; slight expansion of alveolar ridge; associated with delayed eruption of teeth; occasionally lesion erupts and results in gingival inflammation	*Compound:* radiopaque, tooth-like structures surrounded by well-circumscribed radiolucency; pericoronal position. *Complex:* radiopaque, globular mass surrounded by a well-circumscribed radiolucency; occasional sunburst pattern; pericoronal position	Most common odontogenic neoplasm; compound variety more common than complex variety	Excision and curettage; recurrence is rare	Adenomatoid odontogenic tumor; Calcifying and keratinizing odontogenic cyst; Ameloblastic fibro-odontoma
Ameloblastic fibroma	First and second decade; average age, 15 years; No sexual predilection	Slow-growing, painless expansion; cortical expansion; associated with delayed eruption of teeth	Unilocular or multilocular, well-circumscribed radiolucency with a smooth, sclerotic border; pericoronal position; may displace adjacent teeth	Posterior mandible	70% of these neoplasms occur under the age of 20	Excision; recurrence is common	Dentigerous cyst; Odontogenic keratocyst; Ameloblastoma
Ameloblastoma	Majority in first decade; No sexual predilection	Slow-growing, painless expansion; associated with displacement and loosening of teeth, paresthesia of lip; may perforate cortical bone and involve soft tissues	Unilocular to multilocular radiolucency; occasional soap-bubble appearance; pericoronal position; displacement and resorption of root; may be very extensive in size	Posterior mandible	Unicystic ameloblastoma is the most common variant of jaws in children and is the least aggressive; treatment is usually enucleation for this variant.	Excision with adequate borders of normal tissue to block resection; long-term follow-up is required; recurrence rate is high	Dentigerous cyst; Odontogenic keratocyst; Odontogenic myxoma; Central giant cell granuloma

Table 3–6 ■ Benign non-odontogenic neoplasms of jaws (Fig. 3–9)

Lesion	Pediatric Age and Sex	Clinical Findings	Radiographic Findings	Location	Pediatric Significance	Treatment and Prognosis	Differential Diagnosis
Melanotic neuroectodermal tumor of infancy	Under 1 year of age No sexual predilection	Localized, non-ulcerated, expansile, bony enlargement; blue or black areas of pigmentation; variable growth rate; displacement of maxillary lip	Diffuse radiolucency; displacement of tooth buds; floating appearance of teeth	Anterior maxilla	Dental abnormalities may be observed secondary to surgical procedure	Excision with vigorous bony curettage and long-term follow-up; local recurrence rate of 15%	Congenital epulis Large eruption cyst Pyogenic granuloma
Central giant cell granuloma	Second decade Female predilection	Slight to moderate expansion of bone; may be associated with pain; few result in perforation of cortical bone; capable of rapid growth; overlying teeth are vital	Unilocular or multilocular radiolucency; smooth or irregular borders; soap-bubble appearance; presence of faint trabeculation; displacement of teeth; may cross the midline	Anterior to first molar, mandible	Most common anteriorly located multilocular expansile radiolucency; 60% occur under the age of 20 years; need to rule out hyperparathyroidism	Excision or curettage; recurrence rate of 13%	Central hemangioma Traumatic bone cyst Ameloblastoma
Cherubism	First decade Slight male predilection	Chubby face appearance; bilateral, symmetrical, painless enlargement; malpositioned teeth;	Extensive, bilateral, multilocular radiolucencies associated with displaced teeth; teeth appear to	Bilateral involvement of angle of mandible	Autosomal dominant trait; lesions increase in size rapidly between 7 and 10 years of age and	No treatment because lesions regress with age; cosmetic treatment includes bony recontouring	Ameloblastoma

	Age/Sex	Clinical Features	Radiographic Features	Location	Comments	Treatment	Differential Diagnosis
		premature loss of primary teeth; failure of permanent teeth to erupt; hypertelorism; regional lymphadenopathy	be floating; condyle usually not involved		improve with onset of puberty	and curettage	
Traumatic bone cyst	Second decade Slight male predilection	Usually non-expansile lesion; pulps of teeth are vital; asymptomatic	Well-defined radiolucency with smooth, thin, sclerotic border; scalloped or lobulated appearance; extends between the roots of teeth; lamina dura intact; seldom displaces teeth	Premolar-molar mandible; inferior region of ramus; mandibular incisor region	May be associated with history of trauma; 75% occur within the second decade	Perform curettage and initiate bleeding; does not recur	Central hemangioma Central giant cell granuloma Odontogenic keratocyst
Fibrous dysplasia	Second decade No sexual predilection	Gradual increase in jaw size; smooth surface with normal-appearing mucosa; non-tender facial asymmetry; displaced teeth or failure of teeth to erupt	Usually a mixed radiolucent and radiopaque lesion with mottled or ground glass appearance; diffuse lesion that blends into adjacent normal bone; root of teeth may be separated or displaced	Maxilla more affected than mandible	Active growth period in adolescence; problem with facial asymmetry; need to rule out polyostotic fibrous dysplasia	No treatment except for cosmetic surgical reduction; tends to stabilize after completion of skeletal development	Cementifying and ossifying fibroma Chronic sclerosing osteomyelitis

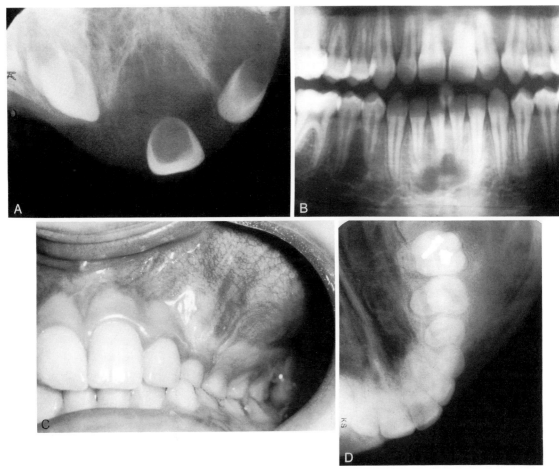

Figure 3 – 9 ■ *A,* Neuroectodermal tumor of infancy of the maxilla. *B,* Traumatic cysts of the anterior and posterior mandible. *C* and *D,* Monostotic fibrous dysplasia of the posterior maxilla, intraoral view *(C)* and radiographic view *(D).*

Table 3–7 ■ Inflammatory lesions of bone (Fig. 3–10)

Lesion	Pediatric Age and Sex	Clinical Findings	Radiographic Findings	Location	Pediatric Significance	Treatment and Prognosis	Differential Diagnosis
Focal sclerosing osteo-myelitis (con-densing osteitis)	Second decade No sexual predilec-tion	Tooth with a large carious lesion; mild pain associated with an infected pulp; tender to percussion	Well-circumscribed to diffuse radio-pacity surrounding root apex; periodontal liga-ment space and root outline intact	Mandibular first molar	Most common periapical radiopacity ob-served; most occur under age of 20; may be associated with chronic hyperplastic pul-pitis	Endodontic treatment or ex-traction of infected tooth; bone lesion does not resolve	Cementoblastoma Periapical idio-pathic osteoscler-osis
Periapical abscess	First and second decades No sexual predilec-tion	Non-vital tooth with carious lesion or intact tooth with history of trauma; mild to severe pain; tender to percussion; mobility of tooth; soft tissue swelling; lymphadenopathy	Varies from a widening of the periodontal ligament space to diffuse radiolu-cency; internal and/or external root resorption may be present	Primary dentition is most often affected in children	Children may rapidly develop cellulitis, osteo-myelitis, and bacteremia Cavernous sinus thrombosis is most serious complica-tion	Endodontic treatment or ex-traction of infected tooth; antibiotic cover-age if extensive soft tissue involve-ment	Incomplete root development of erupted tooth Periodontal abscess Periapical granu-loma
Chronic osteo-myelitis with prolifera-tive periostitis (Garré's osteo-myelitis)	First and second decades No sexual predilec-tion	Usually associated with an odonto-genic infection or trauma; localized enlargement of the outer surface of the jaw; may be tender to palpa-tion; occasional leukocytosis	Mixed radiopaque and radiolucent area with mottling; poor to well-de-fined borders; duplication of cor-tical bone with laminated or onion skin appearance	Posterior mandible	85% of these lesions occur in children under 14 years of age; may be associated with a soft tissue infection such as tonsillitis, parotid-itis, or cellulitis	Endodontic treatment or ex-traction of infected tooth; appropriate antibiotic cover-age; cosmetic recontouring may be necessary	Fracture callus Fibrous dysplasia Ewing's sarcoma Infantile cortical hyperostosis

43

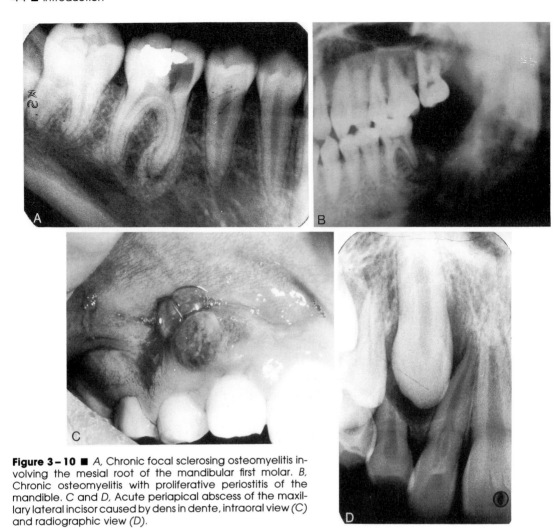

Figure 3 – 10 ■ *A,* Chronic focal sclerosing osteomyelitis involving the mesial root of the mandibular first molar. *B,* Chronic osteomyelitis with proliferative periostitis of the mandible. *C* and *D,* Acute periapical abscess of the maxillary lateral incisor caused by dens in dente, intraoral view *(C)* and radiographic view *(D).*

BIBLIOGRAPHY

Advisory Committee to the Surgeon General: The health consequences of using smokeless tobacco. U.S. Department of Health and Human Services, NIH Publication No. 86-2874, April 1986.

Batsakis JG: Tumors of the Head and Neck, 2nd ed. Baltimore, Williams and Wilkins, 1979.

Berman FR, Fay JT: The retrocuspid papilla. Oral Surg 42:80, 1976.

Bhaskar SN: Synopsis of Oral Pathology, 6th ed. St. Louis, CV Mosby, 1981.

Bouquot JE: Common oral lesions found during a mass screening examination. JADA 112:50, 1986.

Chuong R, Kaban LB: Diagnosis and treatment of jaw tumors in children. J Oral Maxillofac Surg 43:323, 1985.

Dilley DH, Blozis GC: Common oral lesions and oral manifestations of systemic illnesses and therapies. Pediatr Clin North Am 29:585, 1982.

Eversole LR: Clinical Outline of Oral Pathology, 2nd ed. Philadelphia, Lea and Febiger, 1984.

Eversole LR, Leider AS, Corwin JO, Karian BK: Proliferative periostitis of Garré: Its differentiation from other neoperiostoses. J Oral Surg 37:725, 1979.

Fromm A: Epstein's pearls, Bohn's nodules and inclusioncysts of the oral cavity. J Dent Child 34:275, 1967.

Gardner DG, Corio RL: Plexiform unicystic ameloblastoma. A variant of ameloblastoma with a low-recurrence rate after enucleation. Cancer 53:1730, 1984.

Greer RO, Mierau GW, Favara BE: Tumors of the Head and Neck in Children. New York, Praeger Scientific, 1983.

Hogan D, Wilkinson RD, Williams A: Congenital anomalies of the head and neck. Int J Dermatol 19:479, 1980.

Lack EE, Worsham GF, Callihan MD, Crawford BE, Vawter, GF: Gingival granular cell tumors of the newborn (congenital "epulis"). A clinicopathologic study of 21 patients. Am J Surg Pathol 5:37, 1981.

Page LR, Crawford BE, Giansanti JS, Weathers DR: The oral melanotic macule. Oral Surg 44:219, 1977.

Redman RS: Prevalence of geographic tongue, fissured tongue, median rhomboid glossitis and hairy tongue among 3,611 Minnesota school children. Oral Surg 30:390, 1970.

Saunders B: Pediatric Oral and Maxillofacial Surgery. St. Louis, CV Mosby, 1979.

Shafer WG, Hine MK, Levy BM: A Textbook of Oral Pathology, 4th ed. Philadelphia, WB Saunders Co, 1983.

Skinner RL, Davenport WD: Biopsied oral lesions in pediatric patients. J Dent Res 64:248, 1985.

Toretti EF, Miller AS, Peezik B: Odontomas: An analysis of 167 cases. J Pedod 8:282, 1984.

Wood NK, Goaz PW: Differential Diagnosis of Oral Lesions, 2nd ed. St. Louis, CV Mosby, 1980.

Zachariades N, Papanicolaou S, Triantafyllou D: Odontogenic keratocysts: Review of the literature and report of sixteen cases. J Oral Maxillofac Surg 43:177, 1985.

Zallen RD, Preskar MH, McClary SA: Ameloblastic fibroma. J Oral Maxillofac Surg 40:513, 1982.

Anomalies of the developing dentition

C. O. Dummett, Jr.

A variety of dental anomalies are associated with defects in tooth development precipitated by hereditary, systemic, traumatic, or local factors. Numerous systems have been used to classify dental anomalies, and each classification certainly has merit. The one that will be used in this text categorizes dental anomalies in terms of abnormalities in tooth number, size, shape, structure, and color (Stewart and Prescott, 1976). The advantage of this system is that the categories can be related to the stages of tooth development during which the respective anomalies are thought to originate. These stages of development are discussed in Chapters 1–10. The reader is also encouraged to review textbooks on dental histology, dental embryology, and orofacial genetics for more in-depth information.

Anomalies of Number

Alterations in tooth number result from problems during the initiation, or dental lamina stage, of dental development. In addition to hereditary patterns producing extra or missing teeth, physical disruption of the dental lamina, overactive dental lamina, and failure of dental lamina induction by ectomesenchyme are several examples of etiologic factors that affect tooth number (Stewart and Prescott, 1976).

HYPERDONTIA

Hyperdontia, or supernumerary teeth, describes an excess in tooth number, which can occur in both the primary and permanent den-

titions. Reports on the incidence of hyperdontia include values as high as 3%, with males being affected twice as frequently as females (Primosch, 1981). Ninety to 98 per cent of supernumerary teeth occur in the maxilla, with the permanent dentition being more frequently affected than the primary dentition. The most common supernumerary tooth is the mesiodens, which occurs in the palatal midline and can assume a number of shapes and positions relative to the adjacent teeth.

As reported by Primosch in 1981, supernumerary teeth are morphologically classified as either supplemental or rudimentary. Supplemental supernumerary teeth duplicate the typical anatomy of posterior and anterior teeth. Rudimentary supernumerary teeth are dysmorphic and can assume conical forms, tuberculate forms (Fig. 4–1), or shapes that duplicate molar anatomy. From a clinical standpoint, the tuberculate or barrel-shaped supernumeraries generate the most severe complications with respect to difficulty of removal and adverse effects on adjacent teeth such as impaction or ectopic eruption.

Cleft lip and palate commonly demonstrate alterations in the normal complement of teeth and provide clear examples of physical disruption of the dental lamina as an etiologic factor. Classic syndromes demonstrating supernumerary teeth include cleidocranial dysplasia, Gardner's syndrome, and orofacial digital syndrome.

HYPODONTIA

Hypodontia, or congenital tooth absence, represents a deficiency in tooth number. Heredity plays the largest role in precipitating patterns of hypodontia. Incidence reports identify a range of 1.5–10%, excluding third molars, in American populations (Maklin et al., 1979). The majority of studies indicate that the most frequently occurring congenitally absent permanent tooth, excluding third molars, is the mandibular second bicuspid, followed by the maxillary lateral incisor. According to Grahanen and Granath in 1961, there is a 30% correlation between primary tooth absence and permanent tooth absence. Ectodermal dysplasia is a classic syndrome that demonstrates multiple congenitally missing teeth (Fig. 4–2). Other conditions demonstrating hypodontia include Down's syndrome, Hurler's syndrome, chondroectodermal dysplasia, and cleft palate.

Anomalies of Size

MICRODONTIA AND MACRODONTIA

Abnormalities in tooth size are epitomized in microdontia and macrodontia. Hemifacial microsomia resulting from a hematoma of the stapedial artery during embryologic development can cause a deficient nutrient supply to the affected side of the face. A reduced amount of growth occurs in this less vascularized area, with smaller teeth occurring as a result. Peg-shaped lateral incisors represent examples of microdontia and are commonly seen in Down's syndrome. These abnormalities originate during the morphodifferentiation stage of tooth development.

Hemifacial hypertrophy demonstrates comparatively larger teeth on the affected side (Fig. 4–3). Of the many factors thought to cause this condition, vascular and neurogenic abnormalities are considered the most likely. In addition to an increase in crown and root size, affected teeth develop more rapidly and erupt earlier than on the uninvolved side. Isolated teeth displaying macrodontia can also result from twinning abnormalities that originate during the proliferation stage of tooth development. Fusion and gemination are the most common twinning abnormalities, and both anomalies demonstrate enlarged crowns.

FUSION

Fusion has an incidence of 0.5% and is more common in the primary dentition (Grahanen and Granath, 1961). The classic definition of fusion is the dentinal union of two embryologi-

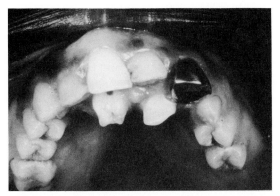

Figure 4–1 ■ Supernumerary teeth—tuberculate morphology.

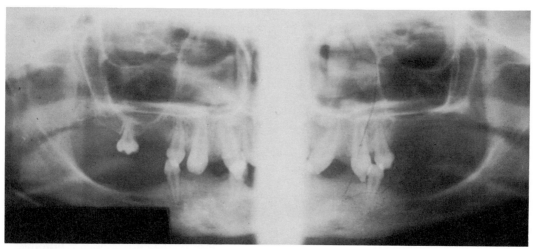

Figure 4–2 ■ Hypodontia in a child with ectodermal dysplasia. Note atrophy of alveolar ridge.

cally developing teeth. Although fused teeth can contain two separate pulp chambers, many appear as large bifid crowns with one chamber. This makes them difficult to distinguish from geminated teeth.

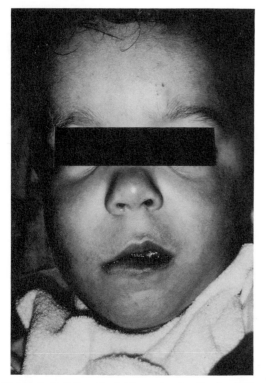

Figure 4–3 ■ Hemifacial hypertrophy. Teeth on the patient's affected side (right) are larger in all dimensions than those on the unaffected side.

GEMINATION

Gemination has a frequency similar to fusion and is also more common in the primary dentition. Conceptually, a geminated tooth represents an incomplete division of a single tooth bud resulting in a bifid crown with a single pulp chamber. Gemination tends to occur in a familial pattern, and its significance is similar to that of fusion in that both conditions may result in retarded eruption of the permanent successor. Clinically, the distinction between fusion and gemination is usually made by counting the number of teeth in the arch. If there is a deficiency in the normal complement, including the bifid crown, the condition is fusion. Fusion with a supernumerary tooth must also be considered and ruled out, since this would not affect the normal number of teeth.

Concrescence is a twinning anomaly involving the union of two teeth by cementum only. Its cause is thought to be trauma or adjacent tooth malposition. Because it can occur after root development, concrescence is technically not a developmental anomaly.

Anomalies of Shape

Abnormalities in shape originate during the morphodifferentiation stage of tooth development and are manifested as alterations in crown and root form. Modes of inheritance include both autosomal dominant and polygenic patterns.

Dens evaginatus ■ Dens evaginatus is an extra cusp, usually in the central groove or ridge

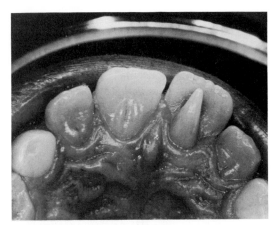

Figure 4-4 ■ Dens evaginatus—talon cusp. All three elements of dental tissues are represented in the extra cusp.

of a posterior tooth and in the cingulum area of the central and lateral incisors. In incisors, these cusps appear talon-shaped and can approach the level of the incisal edge (Fig. 4-4). This extra portion contains not only enamel but also dentin and pulp tissue as well, and therefore a pulp exposure can result from radical equilibration. It occurs with a frequency of 1-4% and results from the evagination of inner enamel epithelium cells, which are the precursors of ameloblasts (Stewart and Prescott, 1976).

Dens in dente ■ Dens in dente is a condition resulting from the invagination of the inner enamel epithelium producing the appearance of a tooth within a tooth. Thomas in 1971 reported a 7.7% prevalence of dens in dente, with the maxillary lateral incisors being the teeth most frequently affected. The clinical significance of this anomaly results from potential carious involvement through the communica-

tion of the invaginated portion of the lingual surface of the tooth with the outside environment. The enamel and dentin in the invaginated portion can be both defective and absent, allowing direct exposure of the pulp.

Taurodont teeth ■ Taurodont teeth are characterized by having a significantly elongated pulp chamber with short stunted roots, resulting from the failure of Hertwig's epithelial root sheath to achieve the proper level of horizontal invagination (Fig. 4-5). The condition can range from a 0.5-5% incidence in the population and can be classified according to the extent of the pulp chamber elongation (Mena, 1971). The syndromes that classically demonstrate taurodontism include Klinefelter's syndrome and trichodento-osseous syndrome.

Dilaceration ■ Dilaceration refers to an abnormal bend of the root during its development and is thought to result from a traumatic episode, usually to the primary dentition (Fig. 4-6). Andreason in 1971 reported a dilaceration incidence of 25% in those permanent teeth with developmental disturbances secondary to primary tooth injury.

Anomalies of Structure: Enamel

Tooth structure abnormalities are produced by disruption during the histodifferentiation, apposition, and mineralization stages of tooth development. Enamel defects are manifested as hypoplasia or hypocalcification. According to Jorgenson and Yost in 1982, they may be broadly classified as heritable defects or environmentally induced defects.

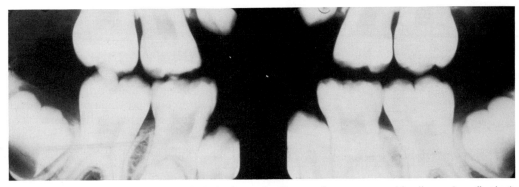

Figure 4-5 ■ Taurodont teeth. Note that primary teeth as well as permanent teeth can be affected.

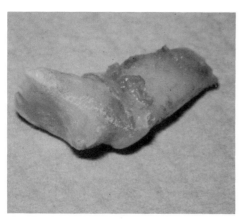

Figure 4–6 ■ Dilacerated lateral incisor.

AMELOGENESIS IMPERFECTA

Amelogenesis imperfecta represents a classic example of heritable enamel defects. Whitkop reports the incidence of this condition as 1 in 14,000 (Stewart and Prescott, 1976). There are 11 subgroup classifications of amelogenesis imperfecta, with multiple inheritance patterns represented. The three major categories will be described according to the stages of tooth development during which they are thought to occur. Further information on the subgroups can be obtained from more comprehensive resources.

Hypoplastic type ■ Heritable enamel defects occurring in the histodifferentiation stage of tooth development are exemplified by the hypoplastic type of amelogenesis imperfecta, wherein an insufficient quantity of enamel is formed (Fig. 4–7). This is due to areas devoid of inner enamel epithelium, causing a lack of cell differentiation into ameloblasts. Both primary and permanent dentitions are affected, and the condition is inherited predominantly as an autosomal dominant trait, depending on the subgroup pattern. Affected teeth appear small, with open contacts, and areas of the clinical crowns contain very thin or non-existent enamel, resulting in high sensitivity to thermal stimuli. Anterior open bite has been observed in 60% of reported cases.

Hypomaturation type ■ The hypomaturation type of amelogenesis imperfecta is an example of a heritable defect in apposition and is characterized by teeth having normal enamel thickness but a low value of radiodensity and mineral content (Fig. 4–8). The problem is related to the persistence of organic content in the rod sheath, resulting in poor calcification, low mineral content, and a porous surface that becomes stained.

Hypocalcification type ■ The hypocalcification type of amelogenesis imperfecta is an example of a heritable defect in the calcification stage of enamel formation (Fig. 4–9). Quantitatively, the enamel is normal, but qualitatively, the matrix is poorly calcified, with a resultant fracturing of the enamel surface. The hypocalcified enamel is soft and fragile, especially in the incisal regions, and is easily fragmented, exposing the underlying dentin, which produces an unesthetic appearance. Increased calculus formation and a concomitant marked delay in tooth eruption are consistent findings. Anterior open bite is seen in 60% of the cases demonstrating this defect.

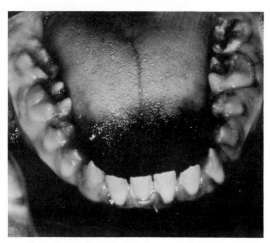

Figure 4–7 ■ Amelogenesis imperfecta—hypoplastic type.

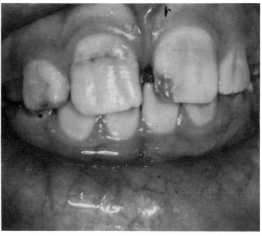

Figure 4–8 ■ Amelogenesis imperfecta—hypomaturation type.

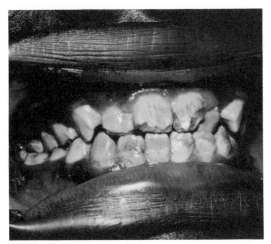

Figure 4–9 ■ Amelogenesis imperfecta—hypocalcified type.

ENVIRONMENTAL ENAMEL HYPOPLASIA

Examples of environmentally induced enamel hypoplasia can result from systemic or local causes. Examples of systemic causes producing generalized enamel hypoplasia include nutrition deficiencies, particularly in vitamins A, C, and D, as well as deficiencies in calcium and phosphorous (Jorgenson and Yost, 1982). Severe infection such as exanthamous diseases and fever-producing disorders, particularly during the first year of life, can directly affect ameloblastic activity, resulting in enamel hypoplasia. Rubella embryopathy has a high correlation with prenatal enamel hypoplasia in the primary dentition. Syphilis caused by the spirochete *Treponema pallidum* produces classic patterns of hypoplastic dysmorphic permanent teeth. The tapered and notched incisal edges of anterior teeth with screwdriver shapes are termed Hutchinson incisors, and these and the crenated occlusal patterns of posterior teeth known as mulberry molars are classic clinical findings for prenatal syphilis infection. Neurologic defects, as exemplified in children with cerebral palsy, have an increased likelihood of demonstrating generalized enamel hypoplasia. Children with asthma also demonstrate a higher frequency of enamel hypoplasia than non-afflicted children. Fluorosis, prematurity, and radiation are additional causes of systemic enamel hypoplasia that can disrupt ameloblastic matrix formation or subsequent mineralization. Syndromes demonstrating enamel hypoplasia as a consistent dental characteristic include Down's syndrome, epidermolysis bullosa, Hurler's syndrome, and hypoparathyroidism and pseudo-hypoparathyroidism.

LOCALIZED ENAMEL HYPOPLASIA

Causes of enamel hypoplasia affecting individual teeth include local infection, local trauma, iatrogenic surgery as seen in cleft palate closure, and primary tooth overretention. Turner's hypoplasia is a classic example of hypoplastic defects in permanent teeth resulting from local infection or trauma to primary precursors (Fig. 4–10).

Enamel hypocalcification can be related directly to faults in the mineralization process of the organic matrix in amelogenesis and dentinogenesis. With respect to enamel, the same factors that cause enamel hypoplasia also cause hypocalcification. The majority of localized hypocalcific defects are related to Turner's hypoplasia subsequent to localized infection and trauma.

Excess ingestion of systemic fluoride can produce enamel defects. Dental fluorosis can be manifested as a defect in the calcification of the teeth in milder forms, with significant pigmentation and enamel hypoplasia in the more severe forms. Fluorosis occurs when the concentration of ingested fluoride is above 1.8 part per million (ppm) per day (Jorgenson and Yost, 1982). There is a 90% chance of some degree of dental fluorosis when the daily amount of in-

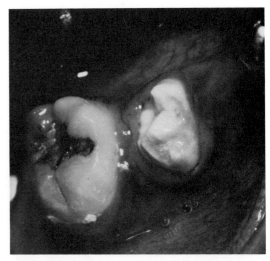

Figure 4–10 ■ Turner's hypoplasia. Note that cementum is formed on the crown areas that are denuded of enamel.

gested fluoride is greater than 6 ppm, although the severity of morphologic defects cannot be predicted from specific quantities of ingested fluoride.

Anomalies of Structure: Dentin

DENTINOGENESIS IMPERFECTA

Dentinogenesis imperfecta is an example of a heritable dentinal defect originating during the histodifferentiation stage of tooth development (Fig. 4–11). This anomaly involves a defect of predentin matrix that results in amorphic, disorganized, and atubular circumpulpal dentin. The mantle dentin is normal, in contrast to the previously described circumpulpal dentin, which is high in organic content and contains interglobular calcification. The frequency of occurrence is about 1 in 8000, and dentinogenesis imperfecta can be subdivided into three basic types (Shields et al., 1973).

Shields Type I ■ This type of dentinogenesis imperfecta occurs with osteogenesis imperfecta. Primary teeth tend to be more severely affected than permanent teeth. Periapical radiolucencies, bulbous crowns, obliteration of pulp chambers, and root fractures are evident. An amber translucent tooth color is frequently seen.

Shields Type II ■ This type, also known as hereditary opalescent dentin, tends to occur as a separate entity apart from osteogenesis imperfecta. In this case, both primary and permanent dentitions are equally affected and the characteristics previously described for Type I are the same. This condition is inherited as an autosomal dominant trait.

Shields Type III ■ This type of dentinogenesis imperfecta is quite rare and represents many of the features described previously, with a predominance of bell-shaped crowns, especially in the permanent dentition. Unlike Types I and II, Type III demonstrates teeth with a shell-like appearance with multiple pulp exposures. It has been seen exclusively in a triracial isolated group in Maryland known as the Brandywine population (Shields et al., 1973).

DENTIN DYSPLASIA

Dentin dysplasia represents another group of heritable dentin disorders resulting in characteristic features involving the circumpulpal dentin and root morphology. Shields and colleagues have proposed a classification based on characteristic patterns of dentin dysplasia.

Shields Type I ■ This type of dentin dysplasia demonstrates normal primary and permanent crown morphology with an amber translucency (Fig. 4–12). The roots tend to be short and sharply constricted. Primary teeth have obliterated pulps. Both primary and permanent dentitions demonstrate multiple periapical radiolucencies and absent pulp chambers. Cascading tubule patterns occur as a result of blockage of normal dentin tubules by calcified masses.

Shields Type II ■ This type demonstrates amber-colored primary teeth closely resembling teeth seen in dentogenesis imperfecta Types I and II (Fig. 4–13). Permanent teeth are

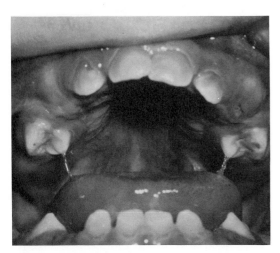

Figure 4–11 ■ Dentinogenesis imperfecta—hereditary opalescent dentin.

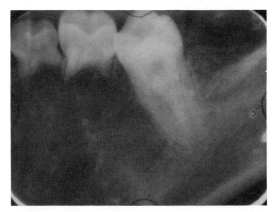

Figure 4–12 ■ Dentinal dysplasia Type I. Note rootless primary teeth.

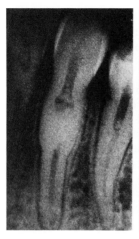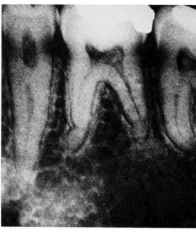

Figure 4–13 ■ Dentinal dysplasia Type II. Note thistle-tube shape to permanent pulp chambers.

normal in appearance but radiographically demonstrate thistle-tube–shaped pulp chambers with multiple pulp stones. No periapical radiolucencies are seen.

ODONTODYSPLASIA

Odontodysplasia is a condition representing a localized arrest in tooth development (Fig. 4–14). Affected teeth demonstrate thin layers of enamel and dentin with large, diffusely calcified pulp chambers and shortened poorly defined roots (Pruhs et al., 1975). The teeth have a ghost-like appearance radiographically and are susceptible to caries, fracture, and infection. No specific etiology or inheritance pattern has been identified that can explain the reported cases.

Additional conditions involving dentin abnormalities relate to systemic abnormalities that impair normal absorption and circulating serum levels of calcium and phosphorous. Vitamin D–resistant rickets, hypoparathyroidism, and pseudo-hyperparathyroidism are all conditions demonstrating characteristic dentinal abnormalities, which are summarized in Table 4–1 (Stewart and Prescott, 1976).

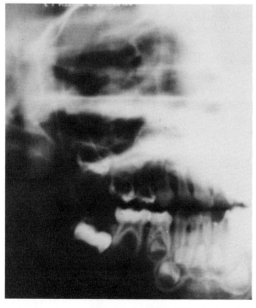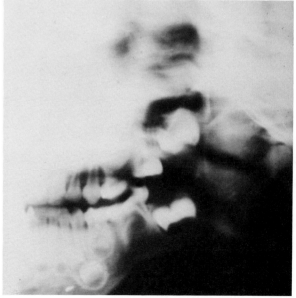

Figure 4–14 ■ Odontodysplasia in a patient's upper right maxillary area.

Table 4 – 1 ■ Conditions demonstrating characteristic dentin abnormalities

Vitamin D – Resistant Rickets
Hypomineralized dentin
Increased width to predentin
Odontoblastic disorganization
Decreased alkaline phosphatase activity in tooth
  germ

Hypoparathyroidism
Tooth defects more severe in males
Permanent teeth predominantly affected
Short, wedge-shaped roots with delayed apical
  closure
Interglobular calcification in dentin, especially at
  apices
Enamel hypoplasia

Pseudo-hypoparathyroidism
Enlarged pulp chambers
Irregular dentinal tubules
Small crowns and short, blunted roots
Pitted enamel surfaces

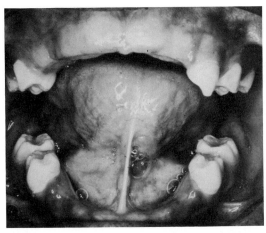

Figure 4 – 15 ■ Hypophosphatasia. Note premature exfoliation of primary anterior teeth in the upper and lower areas.

Anomalies of Structure: Cementum

Developmental defects involving cementum as an exclusive entity apart from other dental structures are rare. It is especially difficult to identify problems in cementogenesis from diseases involving the periodontal ligament. An interesting finding in Turner's hypoplasia is that in addition to coronal enamel defects of the affected permanent teeth, cementum is formed in the areas denuded of enamel (Stewart and Prescott, 1976). This finding underscores the protective role that the reduced enamel epithelium plays upon the unerupted tooth crown. Furthermore, it represents the reciprocal inductive effect of dentin when in direct contact with the mesenchymal cells of the dental follicle, which differentiate into cementoblasts. Areas denuded of enamel allow this phenomenon to occur.

Histologically, defective cementum is seen in epidermolysis bullosa dystrophica, a heritable vesicular and bullous disease of the skin and mucous membranes. Acellular cementum is fibrous in character, and an overproduction of cellular cementum occurs. The cementum that forms is poorly calcified. Cleidocranial dysplasia also displays histologic alterations in cementum formation. Extracted supernumerary teeth demonstrate layers devoid of cellular cementum.

Hypophosphatasia ■ Hypophosphatasia is a complex condition involving the failure of

bone to mineralize properly, which is associated with low serum alkaline phosphatase levels (Fig. 4 – 15). Osteoporosis, bone fragility, and premature loss of primary incisors are classic clinical features. The last-named finding is ascribed to the failure of cementum to form on the prematurely exfoliated incisors and to a decrease in cementum formation in the retained primary teeth. The condition exerts its greatest effect prenatally and during the first year of life. Bone and dentin are affected as well as cementum, so the entity is not exclusively a cementum defect.

Anomalies of Color

Both the primary and permanent dentitions can manifest significant color changes from extrinsic or intrinsic stains. Because of their developmental significance, only the intrinsic stains will be addressed. Eisenberg and Bernick in 1975 provided a detailed classification of the causes of tooth discolorations. Causes of intrinsic stains can be due to blood-borne pigments, drug administration, and hypoplastic-hypocalcified disease states. Congenital porphyria, bile duct defects, anemias, and transfusion reaction hemolysis are examples of blood-borne pigments.

A classic example of drug-induced intrinsic staining occurs from tetracycline antibiotics. Both dentitions can have severe discoloration from this antibiotic when it is given in concentrations of 21 – 26 mg/kg or higher over a period as little as 3 days (Moffitt et al., 1974) (Fig. 4 – 16). Tetracycline hydrochloride has the

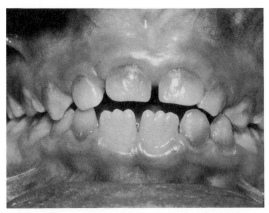

Figure 4–16 ■ Tetracycline staining of primary and permanent dentitions. Note darker hues to the primary teeth, with more diffuse yellow stain to permanent incisors.

greatest potential for staining among the tetracyclines. The agent forms an orthocalcium phosphate complex with dentin and enamel that is then oxidized by ultraviolet light. The oxidation process results in pigments that stain the hard tissues. The critical period for initiation of primary and permanent tooth staining is during the period of intrauterine development through 8 years post-partum. Tetracycline administration must be especially avoided during this time.

Systemic and localized enamel hypoplasia can result in tooth discoloration. Many of the dentin dysplasias also result in tooth color changes. Excess fluoride overlaps both the drug-induced and hypoplastic categories of agents responsible for tooth discoloration. The more severe form of dental fluorosis can produce a range of discoloration from opaque white spots with diffuse striations to a brown mottling.

REFERENCES

Andreason JO: The effect of traumatic injuries to primary teeth on their permanent successor. Scand J Dent Res 145:229, 1971.

Eisenberg E, Bernick SM: Anomalies of the teeth with stains and discolorations. J Prev Dent 2:7–20, 1975.

Grahanen H, Granath L: Numerical variations and their correlations with the permanent dentition. Odont Rev 4:348–357, 1961.

Jorgenson RT, Yost C: Etiology of enamel dysplasias. J Pedo Summer, 6(4):315–329, 1982.

Maklin M, Dummett CO Jr, Weinberg R: A study of oligodontia in a sample of New Orleans children. J Dent Child 46:478, 1979.

Mena CA: Taurodontism. Oral Surg, Oral Path, Oral Med 32:812–823, 1971.

Moffitt JM, et al: Prediction of tetracycline-induced tooth coloration. JADA 88:547, 1974.

Primosch RE: Anterior supernumerary teeth—assessment and surgical intervention in children. J Ped Dent 3:204, 1981.

Pruhs RJ, Simonsen CR, Sharma PS, Fodor B: Odontodysplasia. JADA 91:1057, 1975.

Shields ED, Bixler D, El-Kafrawy AM: A proposed classification for heritable human dentine defects with a description of a new entity. Arch Oral Biol 18:543–553, 1973.

Stewart RE, Prescott GH: Oral Facial Genetics. St. Louis, CV Mosby Co, 1976.

Thomas JG: A study of dens in dente. Oral Surg, Oral Path, Oral Med 32:812–823, 1971.

Childhood diseases and oral manifestations of systemic disease

Andrew Sonis

Herpetic Gingivostomatitis

Causative agent: herpes simplex virus type I ■ Manifestations of the infection represent the patient's primary exposure to the virus. Herpetic gingivostomatitis is most commonly observed in young children, but it may also be seen in adolescents and young adults.

Evaluation ■ Recent exposure to an infected individual should be ascertained. A lack of previous history of a similar infection is important, since infection with the virus imparts lifetime immunity. Viral cultures, serum antibody titers, and cytologic examination may aid in making the diagnosis.

Diagnosis ■ Subjective findings include a viral prodrome of malaise, arthralgia, and anorexia accompanied by fever and chills.

Objective findings ■ Initially, vesicles develop on the mucosa of the lips, tongue, and gingiva, which shortly thereafter rupture into large, painful, ulcerated areas. The gingiva is edematous, erythematous, and bleeds readily upon mild provocation. The tongue may have a white coating (Fig. 5–1).

Tzanck preparation of vesicles may reveal multinucleated giant cells with inclusion bodies. Serum antibody titers obtained during the acute and convalescent period (6 weeks later) will reveal a rise in the anti-virus antibody levels.

Therapy

1. The disease is self-limiting, and the acute phase generally lasts 7–10 days. Treatment consists of bed rest, antipyretics, and analgesics to control fever and relieve pain. Palliative mouthrinses may be helpful in offering some relief.

2. Encourage oral fluid intake, as dehydration may be a problem, particularly in the younger patient. Occasionally, intravenous fluid intake is necessary.

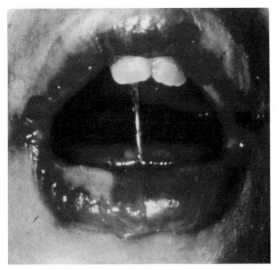

Figure 5 – 1 ▪ Herpetic gingivostomatitis: painful ulcerations involving the gingiva, tongue, and lips.

3. Isolate the patient from peers and siblings in an attempt to prevent spread of the disease.

4. Ulcers heal without scarring.

5. Antibiotics are contraindicated unless specific signs of secondary infection are present.

6. Steroids are contraindicated.

Recurrent Herpes Simplex (Herpes Labialis)

Causative agent: herpes simplex type I virus ▪ Lesions are believed to result from reactivation of the virus lying dormant in the trigeminal ganglia in a previously infected host. Approximately 25% of affected patients have one or more episodes per month. Activation of the virus may be related to cold, sunlight, or stress.

Evaluation ▪ Patients generally give a previous history of similar lesions. Look for small vesicular or ulcerative lesions involving the lips at the mucocutaneous junction, the corners of the mouth, or beneath the nose.

Diagnosis ▪ Subjective findings often include a prodrome of itchiness or a tingly sensation preceding the development of lesions. Patients may experience mild flu-like symptoms.

Objective findings include vesicles of 2 – 4 mm in diameter located at the mucocutaneous junction of the lips, corners of the mouth, and beneath the nose. Vesicles subsequently rupture and crust over in 36 – 48 hours. Healing occurs in 7 – 10 days. Viral titers peak during the first 48 hours of infection, then taper off. Tzanck preparation of vesicles may reveal multinucleated giant cells with inclusion bodies.

Therapy ▪ Numerous treatment modalities have been proposed for herpes labialis, but none are well substantiated. It is generally best to keep the lesions well lubricated with an emollient to promote healing. Isolate the patient from individuals who are at risk of developing primary herpes infection.

Ulcers heal without scarring.

Herpes Zoster (Chicken Pox)

Causative agent: variella-zoster virus ▪ Reactivation of the virus months or years after chicken pox can occur in a dorsal spinal or cranial nerve ganglion, with spread to the appropriate cutaneous dermatome and occasionally to distant sites.

Evaluation ▪ Recent exposure to an infected individual should be ascertained. Lack of previous infection is important, as infection imparts life-time immunity to the virus. Chicken pox occurs most commonly during winter and spring months.

Diagnosis

Subjective findings ▪ Patients may have a mild viral prodrome of malaise, arthralgia, and anorexia accompanied by fever and chills.

Objective findings ▪ Lesions appear as crops of vesicles on an erythematous base; the vesicles usually begin on the trunk and spread to the extremities and face. Several stages of lesions are usually present at one time. Lesions eventually crust over and heal.

Lesions involving the oral mucosa may appear as small vesicles that subsequently rupture, leaving small ulcerations with an erythematous margin. Generally, these lesions are not very painful.

Therapy ▪ The disease is self-limiting, and the acute phase generally lasts 7 – 10 days. Treatment consists of bed rest, antipyretics, and analgesics to control fever and relieve pain. Occasionally, antibiotics are necessary for secondary infection of the vesicles. The disease is contagious; therefore, isolation of an infected patient is recommended to prevent spread of disease to susceptible individuals.

Herpangina

Causative agent: coxsackie A virus ■ Herpangia is common in young children under the age of 4 years and is caused by Coxsackie A virus types 2, 3, 4, 5, 6, 8, and 10.

Evaluation ■ Recent exposure to an infected individual should be determined, as disease may occur in epidemics.

Diagnosis ■ Subjective findings include a viral prodrome of rapid onset of fever, malaise, myalgia, runny nose, throat pain, and dysphagia. Twenty-five percent of infected individuals experience vomiting and abdominal pain. The disease shows a seasonal predilection, with the highest incidence in the summer and fall.

Objective findings include multiple, small, ovoid, vesicular lesions that develop on the soft palate and tonsillar pillars. The vesicles rapidly ulcerate, leaving a gray or white central area surrounded by an erythematous base (Fig. 5–2). These painful lesions usually do not involve the anterior two thirds of the mouth. Lymphadenopathy may be present. Bacterial throat cultures may be useful to rule out bacterial pharyngitis (i.e., "strep" throat).

Therapy

1. The disease is self-limiting, and acute symptoms generally persist for about 3 days.

2. Oral lesions heal in 7–10 days without scarring.

3. Treatment is palliative and includes bed rest, antipyretics, and analgesics. A palliative mouthrinse may be helpful.

4. Oral fluids should be encouraged to prevent dehydration. A soft diet is suggested for patient comfort.

5. Isolation of the infected individual is warranted to prevent spread of the disease.

Hand, Foot, and Mouth Disease

Causative agent: coxsackie A virus ■ The disease is usually caused by Coxsackie A-16 virus and tends to occur in epidemics. Although it usually affects children between 1 and 10 years of age, it may occur in adults.

Evaluation ■ Recent exposure to an infected individual should be determined.

Diagnosis

Subjective findings ■ There is an incubation period of 2–6 days, followed by a viral prodrome of low grade fever and malaise.

Objective findings ■ Painful, multiple, small vesicles develop that subsequently ulcerate, generally involving the hard palate, tongue, and buccal mucosa (Fig. 5–3). Multiple small, painful vesicles on the palms and soles and on the ventral surfaces of fingers and toes may be seen (Figs. 5–4 and 5–5). Lymphadenopathy may be present.

Therapy ■ The disease is self-limiting and resolves spontaneously in 7–14 days. Treat-

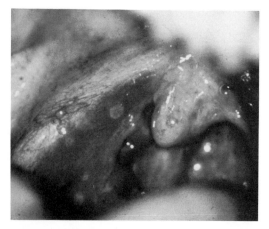

Figure 5–2 ■ Herpangia: ovoid ulcerations with whitish-gray central area surrounded by an erythematous halo involving the tonsillar pillars.

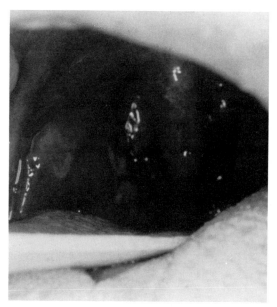

Figure 5–3 ■ Hand, foot, and mouth disease: multiple ulcerations involving the soft palate and tonsillar pillars.

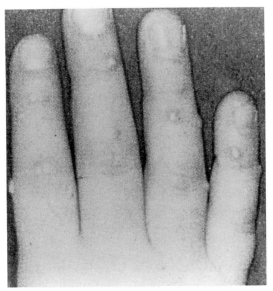

Figure 5–4 ■ Hand, foot, and mouth disease: multiple vesicles involving the fingers.

ment is palliative and may include antipyretics, analgesics, and mouthrinses. Lesions heal without scarring.

Impetigo

Causative agents: streptococci or staphylococci ■ Impetigo is classified into two distinct types: bullous and non-bullous. The non-bullous type is characterized by crusted lesions that are caused primarily by streptococci and that may be subsequently secondarily infected by staphylococci. Bullous impetigo is characterized by bullae or by relatively clean eroded lesions caused by staphylococci. Glomerulonephritis may occur as a result of the non-bullous type.

Evaluation ■ A Gram stain is helpful in bullous impetigo but not in non-bullous impetigo, since secondary infection of the latter is common. Throat and skin cultures may be indicated for family members and close contacts, as nephritogenic strains are propagated by direct contact.

Diagnosis

Subjective findings ■ There is often a history of mild trauma, insect bites, or exposure to other infected individuals. The lesions are usually asymptomatic, but occasionally pruritus may be a prominent feature.

Objective findings ■ In the non-bullous type, multiple lesions develop, which often involve the face and extremities. They are characterized by a thick, adherent, yellowish-brown crust. These lesions may spread and coalesce into large, irregularly shaped lesions. Lymphadenopathy may be present.

In the bullous type of impetigo, flaccid, large bullae may occur anywhere on the body. After 2–3 days these bullae rupture, leaving discrete, round lesions. These lesions subsequently coalesce into polycyclic areas that tend to clear centrally. Gram staining of bulla contents reveals gram-positive cocci.

Therapy

Non-bullous type ■ For minimal disease, cool water soaks are used to remove crusts, and the infected area is washed with an antiseptic cleaner. This is followed by application of a topical antibiotic two to three times a day. If lesions

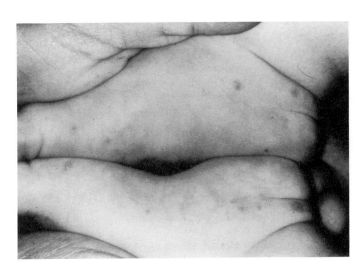

Figure 5–5 ■ Hand, foot, and mouth disease: multiple vesicles involving the feet.

do not heal quickly with this therapy, systemic antibiotics are indicated.

For moderate or excessive disease, penicillin G or erythromycin is usually effective. Even if penicillin-resistant staphylococci are present, this therapy is usually effective.

Bullous type ■ Because the causative organism is generally a penicillin-resistant strain of staphylococci, a semisynthetic penicillinase-resistant penicillin is indicated (i.e., dicloxacillin).

Scarlet Fever

Causative agents: beta hemolytic streptococci ■ Manifestations of the disease are due to a lack of immunity to erythrogenic toxins elaborated by the streptococci. However, immunity to these toxins does not protect against streptococcal infection.

Evaluation ■ Recent exposure of the patient to an individual with streptococcal infection should be determined.

Diagnosis

Subjective findings ■ Prodromal features of sore throat, fever, and vomiting are regular subjective findings.

Objective findings ■ A bright red papular skin rash beginning in skin folds and spreading to the remainder of the body is present. The rash appears 2–3 days after the initial symptoms are seen. The tongue is covered with a white coating, with the papillae being erythematous and prominent (strawberry tongue). This coating of the tongue is soon lost, leaving an erythematous, smooth, glistening surface. A grayish-white exudate may cover the tonsils and faucial pillars. Lymphadenopathy is usually present. The skin rash slowly fades and is followed by desquamation of the skin. Throat cultures will reveal streptococcal infection.

Therapy
1. Penicillin is the drug of choice.
2. Palliative mouthrinses may be helpful.
3. Early diagnosis and treatment is important to prevent complications, which include local abscess formation, rheumatic fever, arthritis, and glomerulonephritis.

Candidiasis

Causative agent: *Candida albicans* ■ Approximately 50% of the population has this organism as part of their normal oral flora. Usually, the presence of this organism is of no clinical significance. However, in newborns, debilitated patients, or individuals on long-term antibiotics whose normal oral flora has been altered, infection may occur.

Evaluation ■ It is important to identify the underlying etiology, which may include systemic diseases such as diabetes mellitus, leukemia, uremia, aplastic anemia, immune deficiency syndromes, and immunosuppression.

Diagnosis

Subjective findings ■ In cases with esophageal involvement, the patient may complain of sore throat. Otherwise, the patient may be asymptomatic or may complain of a burning or coating sensation in the mouth.

Objective findings
1. Raised, white, curdy plaques, which may appear to lump together in heaps (Fig. 5–6).
2. Scraping of the lesions leaves a raw, bleeding surface.
3. Lesions may occur on any mucosal surface.
4. Potassium hydroxide (KOH) preparation of a smear will reveal hyphae when observed microscopically.

Therapy
1. Mild disease: topical antifungal agent (i.e., nystatin).
2. Moderate disease: A systemic antifungal agent may be indicated (i.e., ketoconazole).
3. Severe disease: systemic antifungal agent (i.e., amphotericin B). This medication requires intravenous administration and is highly nephrotoxic.

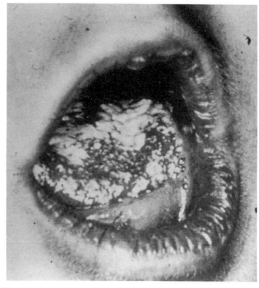

Figure 5–6 ■ Candidiasis: white, curdy plaques coating the tongue.

Diabetes Mellitus

Type I, or insulin dependent diabetes mellitus, is the most common form in children. Approximately 2 in 1000 children between the ages of 5 and 18 years have the disease.

The development of type I diabetes is the result of viral or toxic insults to the pancreatic islets in the child genetically predisposed to developing the disorder. The presence of islet cell antibodies in the newly diagnosed individual suggests an autoimmune mechanism in the destruction of the insulin-producing beta cells. Although symptoms of diabetes may develop suddenly, the initial insult may take months to years to manifest clinically.

Evaluation ■ The suspicion of diabetes usually arises by one or more of the following:

1. Family history: Relatives of patients with diabetes are two and a half times more likely to develop the disease than the population at large.

2. Symptoms: Polydipsia, polyuria, weight loss with polyphagia, enuresis, recurrent infections, and candidiasis are common findings.

3. Glycosuria may be present.

4. Ketoacidosis and coma are possible.

Diagnosis ■ Subjective findings include a history of polydipsia, polyuria, polyphagia, and weight loss.

Objective findings include a fasting blood glucose level above 120 mg/dl. There is an abnormal oral glucose tolerance test result, and elevated glycosylated hemoglobin test values are found.

Periodontal disease is the most consistent oral finding in patients with poorly controlled diabetes mellitus. These patients exhibit increased alveolar bone resorption and inflammatory gingival changes, which may mimic the clinical manifestations of juvenile periodontosis. Xerostomia and recurrent intraoral abscesses may be present. Enamel hypocalcification and hypoplasia along with reduced salivary flow can predispose these patients to an increased frequency of caries. An altered oral flora with an increase in *Candida albicans,* hemolytic streptococci, and staphylococci is also encountered. Both advanced eruption and delayed eruption of permanent dentition have been reported.

Therapy ■ The goal of treatment is to control blood glucose to as normal a level as can be obtained, and thereby reduce the potential complications of hyperglycemia and ketoacidosis. This generally involves the administration of an intermediate-acting insulin (NPH and Lente). An exciting new treatment modality currently under investigation is pancreatic transplantation.

Dental management of the well-controlled diabetic consists of the following:

1. Advise the patient to eat a normal meal before the appointment to avoid development of hypoglycemia.

2. If the dental procedure is anticipated to be stressful, consult the patient's physician regarding adjustment of the insulin dosage.

3. Consider utilization of prophylactic antibiotics for surgery, endodontics, and periodontal therapy to minimize the risk of infection.

4. Have a glucose source available to treat the onset of hypoglycemia.

Acute Lymphoblastic Leukemia (ALL)

Causative agent ■ The cause of ALL is unknown, although several theories have been postulated involving viruses and immune surveillance. This disease represents the most common childhood malignancy, occurring in approximately 4 in 100,000 children.

Evaluation ■ The manifestations of ALL are related to the functionally myelosuppressed state of the patient, which results from the overwhelming presence of malignant cells in the bone marrow. These patients demonstrate the pallor of anemia, purpura or bleeding secondary to thrombocytopenia, and prolonged or unusual infections owing to neutropenia.

Diagnosis ■ Subjective findings include fever, malaise, and occasionally bone pain.

Oral objective findings include the following:

1. Gingival oozing, petechiae, hematoma, or ecchymosis formation is commonly found.

2. Cervical and submandibular lymphadenopathy are possible findings.

3. Oral ulceration, pharyngitis, and gingival infection unresponsive to conventional therapy are also important diagnostic determinations.

Systemic objective followings include the following:

1. A peripheral blood smear may show leukoerythroblastic changes.

2. Bone marrow aspiration and biopsy will establish a definitive diagnosis.

Therapy ■ The goal of therapy is to destroy the leukemic cells and allow normal cells to repopulate the marrow. This is generally accomplished with chemotherapy, which may be supplemented with radiotherapy.

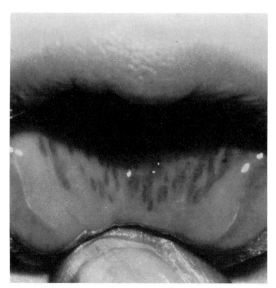

Figure 5 – 7 ■ Acute lymphoblastic leukemia: large, painful ulceration secondary to chemotherapy.

Oral complications of therapy include pain, ulceration, hemorrhage, and secondary infections. The prognosis for ALL is constantly improving, with 5 year survival rates of 60 – 80% (Fig. 5 – 7).

Sickle Cell Anemia

Sickle cell anemia is a hereditary disorder whose clinical manifestations result from an abnormality of the beta chains of the hemoglobin S molecule. Hemoglobin S forms a linear polymer upon deoxygenation, which results in sickling of the red blood cells. Approximately 10% of black Americans carry the trait, while 0.2% have the homozygous form of the disease.

Evaluation ■ There is usually no clinical manifestation of the disease until a high proportion of the red blood cells contain hemoglobin S. This generally occurs around 6 months of age. An exception to this is the increased risk of infection in infants with the disorder.

Diagnosis

Subjective findings ■ Often the earliest clinical presentation is painful swelling of the dorsum of the hand or foot owing to ischemic necrosis of the metacarpal or metatarsal bones. Other manifestations include hepatosplenomegaly, pallor, cardiomegaly, and icterus. Progressive episodes of infarction and scarring in the spleen cause it to decrease in size over time, eventually rendering the patient functionally asplenic.

Objective findings ■ Laboratory findings include severe anemia (hemoglobin 5 – 9 gm/100 ml) associated with sickled red blood cells, reticulocytosis, and variable hyperbilirubinemia.

Dental findings invariably relate to the extramedullary erythropoiesis, which is demonstrated by the following radiographic changes:

1. Decreased radiodensity with increased prominence of the lamina dura and a coarse trabecular pattern (stepladder appearance)

2. "Hair on end" effect of skull

3. Enamel hypomineralization

4. Increased prevalence of periodontal disease

Therapy ■ Infections, dehydration, acidosis, and hypoxia can all result in initiation of a painful crisis in patients afflicted with this disorder. Dental management should therefore ensure adequate hydration and the prevention of infection. Utilization of an aggressive prevention program; stress reducing protocols, including shorter appointments; and nitrous oxide sedation should be considered.

Prophylactic antibiotics are indicated for any oral surgical procedure to diminish the potential development of osteomyelitis or postoperative wound infections. (It should be noted that many children with this disorder are placed on daily prophylactic penicillin because of their splenic condition; thus some modification in antibiotic coverage may be indicated for dental procedures.)

Histiocytosis X

Histiocytosis X represents a variety of disorders of mononuclear phagocytes and related cells that resemble histiocytes. The disorder probably results from immune dysregulation rather than from a neoplastic condition. The disease is frequently indolent and relapsing, and spontaneous remissions occur.

Evaluation ■ Patients with histiocytosis X historically have been grouped into three general categories.

1. Eosinophilic granuloma: occurs in older children and adults and is characterized by localized lesion(s) confined to bone. This category is currently referred to as benign localized or polyostotic histiocytosis X.

2. Hand-Schüller-Christian disease: occurs in younger children (age 2 – 5 years) with a classic triad of manifestations of skull lesions, diabetes insipidus, and exophthalmos. Bone lesions are common, as is involvement of the

gingivae and mandible, which may result in premature loss of teeth. This disease is currently referred to as chronic progressive histiocytosis X.

3. Letterer-Siwe disease: occurs in infants and is characterized by prominent skin and visceral lesions rather than bone lesions. The spleen, lymph nodes, liver, lungs, and bone marrow are commonly involved, and organ dysfunctions are frequent. This disease is currently referred to as acute or subacute disseminated histiocytosis X.

Diagnosis
Benign localized or polyostotic histiocytosis X

SUBJECTIVE FINDINGS ■ The syndrome is found predominantly in older children as well as in adults. There is often an inability to bear weight and tender swelling owing to tissue infiltrates overlying bone lesions.

OBJECTIVE FINDINGS ■ The syndrome is characterized by solitary or multiple bone lesions. Radiographically, these lesions appear as a destructive radiolucency, usually with well-defined margins (punched-out lesions) (Fig. 5–8). Dental findings may include an intraoral mass or swelling, pain, gingivitis, and loose teeth. Oral lesions most often involve the posterior mandible. Histologic examination reveals proliferation of essentially normal, well-differentiated histiocytes. Multinucleated histiocytes are often present. Other inflammatory cells such as granulocytes, eosinophils, lymphocytes, and plasma cells are present in varying quantities. The Langerhans cell is prominent in the histologic examination of these lesions.

Chronic progressive histiocytosis X

SUBJECTIVE FINDINGS ■ The disease is found predominantly in younger children aged 2–5 years. There are multiple sites of involvement with a chronic relapsing course. Exophthalmos as a result of orbital bone involvement and loss of teeth from gingival infiltration and mandibular involvement are not uncommon.

OBJECTIVE FINDINGS ■ Diabetes insipidus with polydipsia and polyuria may occur as a result of infiltration of the posterior pituitary. Chronic otitis media owing to involvement of the mastoid and petrous portion of the temporal bone and otitis externa are not uncommon.

Dental findings include histiocytic involvement of the teeth and gingivae, often beginning in the periapical region of the teeth. Destruction of the lamina dura results in the radiographic appearance of "floating teeth." Gingival involvement may also result in premature loss of

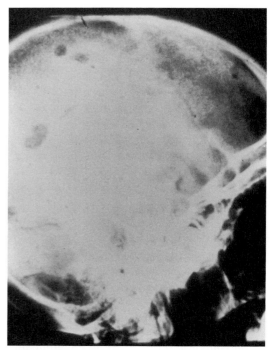

Figure 5–8 ■ Histiocytosis X: punched-out lesions involving the cranium.

teeth. The entire mandible may be involved, with bone loss leading to diminished mandibular rami height. Histologic findings are identical to those of benign localized histiocytosis X.

Acute disseminated histiocytosis X

SUBJECTIVE FINDINGS ■ Typically, an infant less than 2 years of age is presented with a scaly, seborrheic, eczematoid, sometimes purpuric rash involving the scalp, ear canals, abdomen, intertriginous areas, and face. The rash may be maculopapular or nodulopapular, with ulceration.

OBJECTIVE FINDINGS ■ Frequently, there are draining ears, lymphadenopathy, hepatosplenomegaly, and in severe cases hepatic dysfunction with hypoproteinemia and abnormal clotting factors. Pulmonary symptoms may include cough, tachypnea, and pneumothorax. Anemia and thrombocytopenia occur secondary to involvement of the hematopoietic system. Dental findings include intraosseous jaw lesions, most commonly found in the posterior mandibular region. In addition, necrotic and ulcerative soft tissue lesions involving the gingivae are common. Histologic findings are identical to those of benign localized histiocytosis X.

Therapy ■ The following therapies are used for the treatment of histiocytosis X:

1. Surgery: has a limited role, involving curettage of accessible lesions.

2. Radiotherapy: localized therapy, with care to avoid irradiating potentially sensitive normal structures.

3. Chemotherapy: Various chemotherapeutic agents have been used to treat these disorders. Careful monitoring of blood counts and clinical status is vital prior to any dental procedures, as chemotherapeutic toxicity can cause severe complications in these already compromised patients.

Prognosis ■ The prognosis for patients with histiocytosis X is dependent on three factors:

1. Age at onset: An age of 2 years portends a good prognosis, whereas patients less than 2 years of age tend to do poorly.

2. Number of organs involved: Localized disease, with less than four organ systems involved, is a good prognostic sign.

3. Degree of organ dysfunction: The specific involvement of three organ systems (hepatic, pulmonary, and hematopoietic), as manifested by organ dysfunction, has been found to be the most important prognostic indicator.

Hemophilia (Hemophilia A; Factor VIII Deficiency)

Hemophilia is an X-linked recessive deficiency of factor VIII.

Evaluation ■ A positive family history is common in most mild to moderate cases. Oftentimes, the personal history in these cases is negative unless the patient has experienced some traumatic or surgical incident, that is, a persistent oral bleeding episode. In many cases, a positive family history is often lacking, but the personal history is significant for multiple bleeding episodes dating from about age 1 year or earlier.

Diagnosis

Subjective findings ■ Mild to moderate cases may include a history of persistent bleeding, often involving the oral cavity. The sites most commonly involved are the maxillary lip, lingual frenum, and tongue. The onset of these bleeding episodes generally does not occur until the toddler stage. Subjective findings in the severe cases may include chronic joint deformities and contractures secondary to bleeding into joints and muscles.

Objective findings ■ Results of laboratory studies include normal bleeding time, normal platelet count and platelet aggregation, normal prothrombin time, and prolonged partial thromboplastin time. An assay is used to determine the severity of factor VIII deficiency. A concentration of factor VIII that is 5–30% of normal constitutes a mild deficiency, a level that is 2–5% of normal reflects a moderate deficiency, and a concentration that is less than 2% of normal constitutes a severe factor VIII deficiency.

Therapy ■ Factor VIII–containing materials raise plasma levels of factor by 2% for each unit of factor administered. Such materials include the following:

1. Fresh frozen plasma: The amount used is limited by volume considerations.

2. Cryoprecipitate: factor concentration is approximately 20 times that of fresh frozen plasma.

3. Lyophilized factor VIII preparations have concentrations of factor that vary from 20 to 100 times that of fresh frozen plasma. Preparations of pooled plasma involve a greater risk of hepatitis and acquired immune deficiency syndrome (AIDS) when compared with cryoprecipitate, which is prepared from single units of plasma.

Non-factor products ■ Epsilon-aminocaproic acid (EACA) (Amicar) inhibits fibrinolysis by blocking the activation of plasminogen to plasmin. Consequently, a formed clot will remain intact longer in the presence of EACA.

Recent reports and studies suggest that 1-desamino-8-D-arginine vasopressin (DDAVP) may be a useful adjunct in the management of hemophilia. It has been shown that the administration of DDAVP results in a transient increase in plasma factor VIII levels and is particularly effective in mild and moderate hemophilia.

Complications of therapy ■ Patients with hemophilia should avoid drugs that interfere with platelet function (i.e., aspirin, antihistamines).

Antibodies to factor VIII develop in approximately 8–16% of patients receiving factor VIII preparations. The presence of inhibitors is suggested when apparently adequate replacement therapy is ineffective. The presence of inhibitors can be documented via inhibitor assays.

Management of patients who develop inhibitors may involve the following:

1. Administration of products such as Proplex or Konyne, which have activated factors

that bypass factor VIII and allow coagulation to occur

2. Massive doses of factor VIII in an attempt to overwhelm the inhibitors

3. Plasmapheresis to remove the inhibitor, in combination with high doses of factor VIII

Dental considerations ■ The dentist must consider the severity of the hemophilia (mild, moderate, or severe) and the dental procedure to be performed. A consultation with a hematologist is mandatory prior to any treatment in these patients.

Low risk procedures generally requiring no replacement therapy in all levels of hemophilia include the following:

1. Dental prophylaxis without deep scaling

2. Infiltration, pericemental, and intrapulpal administration of local anesthesia

3. Operative dentistry during which careful consideration is given to preventing soft tissue trauma

4. Pulpotomy and pulpectomy procedures

5. Placement of orthodontic appliances

6. Normal exfoliation of primary teeth

7. Preventive program (flossing and toothbrushing)

8. Oral radiographs

Moderate risk dental procedures that may require replacement therapy include

1. Dental prophylaxis with deep scaling

2. Removal of mobile, exfoliating primary teeth

3. Operative dentistry during which soft tissue trauma is anticipated (i.e., placement of stainless steel crowns, utilization of 8A, 14A rubber dam clamps)

High risk procedures requiring replacement therapy include the following:

1. Block administration of local anesthesia

2. Simple extractions, curettage, and gingivoplasty

3. Multiple extractions, flap surgery or gingivectomy, extraction of bone-impacted teeth, and apicoectomy

4. Orthognathic surgery

5. Endotracheal or nasotracheal intubation

Precautions for hepatitis and AIDs are indicated for all hemophiliacs who have received blood products. Recent studies report that over 90% of hemophiliacs are positive for human T-cell lympotropic virus type III (HTLV-III).

BIBLIOGRAPHY

Bernick SM, Cohen W, Baker L, Laster B: Dental disease in children with diabetes mellitus. J Periodontol 46:241, 1975.

Burns JC: Diagnostic methods for herpes simplex infection: A review. Oral Surg 50:346, 1980.

Epstein JB, Pearsall NN, Truelove EL: Oral candidiasis: Effects of antifungal therapy upon clinical signs and symptoms, salivary antibody and mucosal adherence of Candida albicans. Oral Surg 51:32, 1981.

Evans BE: Dental Care in Hemophilia. New York, National Hemophilia Foundation, 1977.

Gershon AA: Management of infections due to herpes simplex virus. Pediatr Infect Dis 3(3 Suppl):S24, 1984.

Hartman KS: Histiocytosis X: A review of 114 cases with oral involvement. Oral Surg 49:38, 1980.

Huebner RJ, et al: Herpangina, etiologic studies of a specific infectious disease. JAMA 145:628, 1951.

Keys DS: Hand, foot, and mouth disease. Aust Dent J 19:1, 1974.

Kolmich JR: Oral candidiasis. Oral Surg 50:411, 1980.

Mannucci PM, Ruggeri ZM, Pareti FI, Capitanio A: 1-Deamino-8-D-arginine vasopressin: A new pharmacological approach to the management of hemophilia and von Willebrand's disease. Lancet 1:869, 1977.

Mintz GA, Rose SL: Diagnosis of oral herpes simplex virus infections. Oral Surg 58:486, 1984.

Nichols C, Laster LL, Bodak-Gyovai LZ: Diabetes mellitus and periodontal disease. J Periodontol 49:85, 1978.

Peters RB, Bahn AN, Barens G: Candida albicans in the oral cavities of diabetics. J Dent Res 45:771, 1976.

Petersen DE, Sonis ST: Oral Complications of Cancer Chemotherapy. Boston, Martinus Nijhoff Publishing, 1983.

Powell D: General dental management. In Boone DC (ed): Comprehensive Management of Hemophilia. Philadelphia, FA Davis Co, 1976.

Sanger RG, Bystrom EB: Radiographic bone changes in sickle cell anemia. J Oral Med 32:32, 1977.

Sanger RG, McTigue DJ: Sickle cell anemia—pathology and management. J Dent Handicap 3:9, 1978.

Schwentker FF, et al: The epidemiology of scarlet fever. Am J Hyg 38:27, 1943.

Ship I, Miller MF, Ram C: A retrospective study of recurrent herpes labialis in a professional population, 1958–1971. Oral Surg 44:723, 1977.

Shklar G: Oral reflections of infectious diseases. Postgrad Med 49:87, 1971.

Sonis A, Musselman RJ: Oral bleeding in classic hemophilia. Oral Surg 53:363, 1982.

Stafford R, Sonis ST, Lockhart PB, et al: Oral pathoses as diagnostic indicators in leukemia. Oral Surg 50:134, 1980.

Vierrou AM, de la Fuente B, Poole AE, Hoyer LW: DDAVP (desmopressin) in the dental management of patients with mild or moderate hemophilia and von Willebrand's disease. Pediatr Dent 7:297, 1985.

Wegner H: Increment of caries in young diabetics. Caries Res 9:91, 1975.

Physiologic principles in pediatric dentistry

Jay A. Anderson

Health care professionals are becoming increasingly aware that children require special treatment. Children are not merely smaller versions of adults, as was once assumed. Dynamic physiologic changes during growth and development require that special attention be paid to drug therapy in children. The dental practitioner needs a working knowledge of normal developmental physiology and morphology and an understanding of the relationship of disease states to these processes. Appropriate methods for prescribing and administering drugs as well as vigilant monitoring of drug effects must be understood by the practitioner who deals with children.

There are three general areas in which pediatric patients are unique that appear to increase the incidence of adverse reactions to drugs in relation to the adult population. These are pharmacokinetic differences, physiologic and anatomic differences, and psychological differences. This chapter explores the areas of pharmacokinetic, physiologic, and anatomic changes that may be expected to occur during

normal growth and development, as well as how these changes might affect drug therapy.

Pharmacokinetics

Pharmacokinetics is the dynamic process of drug turnover in the body, that is, the absorption, distribution to the tissues, biotransformation, and elimination of drugs. The pharmacokinetics of a particular drug determines its plasma concentration, duration of action, and, therefore, its effectiveness and toxicity. Pharmacokinetics is fairly well understood in adults, but the extent of the differences among infants, children, and adults was not recognized until recently. Several factors affect the kinetics of a drug, including the dose and form of the drug, plasma protein binding, ionization, lipid solubility, rate of metabolism, and volume of distribution. Many of these factors are now known to change dramatically as a result of growth and development. Some of the principal differences in pharmacokinetics when dealing with chil-

dren occur in the areas of uptake and absorption, distribution, receptor site sensitivity, metabolism, and excretion (Howry et al., 1981 (Fig. 6–1).

UPTAKE AND ABSORPTION

Drugs may be taken up by the lungs, skin, gastrointestinal tract, or via parenteral absorption (intramuscular, intravenous, or subcutaneous). Uptake of many drugs has been shown to differ in children owing to physiologic and anatomic differences.

Pulmonary uptake ■ The pulmonary uptake of inhalational agents such as nitrous oxide is more rapid in infants and children, probably as a result of higher cardiac output and alveolar ventilation as well as a higher percentage of richly perfused visceral tissues (Salanitre and Rockow, 1969).

Skin uptake ■ Topical medications may be absorbed more rapidly and completely through the skin of children as a result of its greater permeability (thin stratum corneum) and relatively inactive sebaceous glands.

Oral uptake ■ The changing characteristics of the gastrointestinal tract have a major influence on the speed and efficiency of drug absorption. Gastric emptying time in the newborn takes 6–8 hours as compared with 2 hours in the older child and adult (Morselli, 1976). Young children also have a lower gastric pH, which promotes greater absorption of weakly acidic drugs such as penicillin while delaying absorption of weakly basic drugs such as diazepam and theophylline. In young infants the transit time in the bowel is also significantly slower owing to irregular peristalsis. This produces a net effect of slower drug absorption. Some active transport mechanisms in the bowel mucosa that aid in drug absorption are known to be deficient in infants. This is thought to be the primary cause of delayed oral riboflavin uptake in infants. It also must be kept in mind that the presence of food in the gastrointestinal tract generally slows and reduces absorption of orally administered medications.

DRUG DISTRIBUTION

Protein binding ■ Once a drug has been absorbed into the blood stream, its bioavailability may be affected by plasma protein binding. Bound drug is unavailable pharmacologically, whereas unbound (free) drug is available to cross cell membranes and produce its pharmacologic effect. Neonates and infants have decreased plasma protein concentrations, especially of albumin, and therefore fewer available binding sites. Therefore, drugs that are highly protein bound have a greater effect owing to an increased free fraction and also displace other protein bound drugs and compounds such as bilirubin. Sulfonamides, vitamin K, and other drugs are known to displace protein bound bilirubin, which may lead to hyperbilirubinemia and resultant kernicterus (brain damage) in neonates (Morselli, 1977).

Blood-brain barrier ■ The central nervous system is usually protected from the influence of many drugs and metabolic products by the blood-brain barrier. Drugs are able to penetrate the blood-brain barrier in infants much more easily than in adults, probably as a result of lack of myelination of the nervous tissue and greater membrane permeability. It is not known at precisely which age blood-brain barrier permeability decreases to adult levels (Eger et al., 1971). This property can be advantageous when an attempt is made to get antibiotics into the central nervous system, or a disadvantage with the greater sensitivity that is produced to CNS depressants. Narcotics, for example, are far more toxic in infants and young children because of this effect.

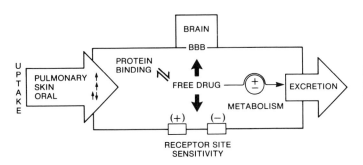

Figure 6–1 ■ Pharmacokinetic variables in children. BBB = blood-brain barrier.

RECEPTOR SITE SENSITIVITY

Many drugs interact with specific receptor sites in the body. It appears that certain receptors change in their sensitivities to drugs during a child's development. Decreased receptor site sensitivity is felt to play a role in explaining why pediatric patients require higher concentrations of the inhalational anesthetics (e.g., halothane) to achieve adequate anesthesia. MAC (minimum alveolar concentration) requirement, a measurement of the amount of anesthetic required to produce surgical anesthesia, has been found to decrease with increasing age for the inhalational anesthetics, so that neonates require the highest concentrations and the elderly the lowest (Gregory et al., 1969). Other than the notable exception of inhalational anesthetics, infants and young children are generally more sensitive and therefore more prone to drug toxicity, possibly as a result of increased receptor sensitivity. For example, non-depolarizing muscle relaxants (e.g., curare) are known to have a more profound effect in infants and small children owing to increased neuromuscular end-plate receptor sensitivity.

METABOLISM

Once drugs enter the cells in which they produce their effect, they undergo metabolism and biotransformation by enzymes produced mainly in the liver. Liver enzyme production responsible for biotransformation (detoxification) of drugs may be almost absent, reduced, or even overproduced at various stages of development. Poor oxidative rates in infants result in prolonged effects of diazepam, phenytoin, and other drugs. Poor conjugation results in prolonged effects of amphetamines and phenacetin. Low levels of glucuronyl transferase in newborn infants cause an inability to detoxify the antibiotic chloramphenicol (Done, 1964). Glucuronyl transferase deficiency also increases sensitivity to sulfisoxazole, morphine, and steroids. Glucuronyl transferase usually reaches normal levels by 1 month of age. Pseudocholinesterase levels are only 60% of normal for several months after birth, and a prolonged apneic response may be produced by succinyl choline administration. Doses of succinyl choline on an adjusted body weight scale do not reach adult levels until after 2 years of age. In summary, the dentist must be aware of the fact that various enzyme systems mature at different rates and that this may require dosing adjustments for some drugs when prescribing them for children.

EXCRETION

Drugs may be excreted by various routes, including the kidneys, biliary system, respiratory system, sweat, and feces. By far, the majority of drugs are excreted by the kidneys. At birth, the kidneys' ability to clear drugs and concentrate urine are greatly reduced, as is discussed later, especially in the preterm or sick infant. This results in prolongation of the effects of drugs that are primarily excreted by the kidneys such as pancuronium, D-tubocurarine, and ampicillin in young children.

All of these factors, as well as others, combine to produce a complicated and ever-changing system of pharmacokinetics in children, especially the very young. Although the most profound pharmacokinetic changes are usually limited to the first few months of life, significant differences in sensitivity to many drugs, including many used in pediatric dentistry, are noted throughout childhood owing to changing pharmacokinetics. The practitioner must certainly be aware of the pharmacokinetics of any drug he or she may use in treating children.

Physiologic and Anatomic Differences

In addition to these differences in pharmacokinetics, there are other anatomic and physiologic differences that impact on the management of pediatric patients. These include differences in body size and body fluids as well as physiologic and anatomic differences in various body systems (Campbell et al., 1982).

BODY SIZE

Perhaps the most obvious and significant difference between children and adults is in body size. It should be easily appreciated that for most drugs, the smaller the patient, the smaller the dose of medication should be. Less drug is needed to reach an effective plasma level and less is also needed to produce toxicity. Yet, overdoses of local anesthetics in dentistry are invariably reported with much higher frequency in children. This can occur when the dentist memorizes the maximum safe dose of

the local anesthetic (e.g., lidocaine) as "500 mg" or "14 carpules" rather than the proper weight-based dosage of 7.0 mg per kg of body weight. Five hundred milligrams may be a proper limit for lidocaine with epinephrine for a 75 kg adult, but it is far in excess of toxic levels in a 10 kg (22 pound) child. Weight-based formulas have become standard for local anesthetics used in dentistry and are appropriate for all but the very young neonate.

Not only are the height and weight of children less than those of adults, but their proportions also differ from adults. For example, a child's weight increases by about 20 times from birth to adulthood, whereas height increases only about 3½ times. This has led many professionals to advocate the use of body surface area (in square meters) for drug dosing in children. Body surface area (BSA) is estimated from the relationship between height and weight, using a nomogram. The ratio of BSA to body weight is about seven times greater for neonates than for adults, and the ratio approaches adult levels gradually during growth and development. Many physiologic functions have been shown to be proportional to BSA, including fluid volumes, metabolic requirements, metabolic rate, minute ventilation, cardiac output, and glomerular filtration rate. Because these functions affect pharmacokinetics, dosing some drugs may be done most accurately on the basis of BSA (Crawford et al., 1950). However, BSA is seldom used clinically to compute most drug doses because it is rather cumbersome and for most drugs it is not necessary. It should be kept in mind, however, that the smaller the patient, the higher the basal metabolic rate, oxygen consumption, fluid requirements per hour, and other factors, all of which relate most accurately to BSA.

BODY FLUIDS

A further basic physio-anatomic difference between adults and children relates to the volume of distribution of body fluids. The small child has a larger volume of total body water (TBW), especially in the extracellular component. For instance, for the infant TBW equals about 80% of body weight, whereas for the adult TBW equals about 50–60% body weight (male < female) (Table 6–1). This has direct bearing on pharmacokinetics, especially of water soluble (aqueous) medications. Because these drugs are distributed to a relatively larger volume once absorbed, a larger mg dose per kg

Table 6–1 ■ Differences in distribution of body fluids between infants and adults

	Infants	Adults
Total body water	80%	50%(M), 60%(F)
Extracellular fluid	35–40%	20%
Intracellular fluid	40–45%	40%

of body weight is necessary to achieve a therapeutic level in the small child.

The opposite situation exists when considering body fat. The percentage of body weight consisting of fat varies greatly in adults. However, as a general rule in children, a premature infant may have as little as 1% of body weight made up of fat. The normal newborn has about 16% fat. This increases to about 22% for the 1-year-old, again falls to about 12% for the 4-year-old, and gradually rises to levels of 18–20% by age 10 or 11. Lipid soluble drugs such as barbiturates and diazepam are distributed to fat tissues, therefore decreasing their effective plasma levels. The child with the smaller percentage of body fat thus requires a smaller dose of a lipid soluble drug.

RESPIRATORY SYSTEM

There are several anatomic and physiologic considerations of importance in the pediatric respiratory system. The head of a child is relatively large in comparison with the rest of the body, and it outgrows all other areas during infancy. This produces a situation in which the head is easily flexed at rest and predisposes the child to compromise of the airway. Children also have narrow nasal passages, a smaller diameter glottis and trachea, and further narrowing of the trachea at the rigid cricoid ring. The proportionately larger tongue, larger mass of lymphoid tissues, more copious secretions, and loose glottic areolar tissue (which is more susceptible to edema formation) combine with the other anatomic findings to produce an airway in the pediatric patient that is far more prone to obstruction and more difficult to manage during sedation, general anesthesia, or respiratory emergency.

The bony thorax of the child also presents structural difficulties. It is obviously smaller. The sternum is soft and therefore provides a less stable base for the ribs and intercostal muscles (which are also inherently weaker). The ribs are more horizontal than in the adult and

Table 6–2 ■ Physiologic variables during development

Age	Resp. Rate (brth/min)	Heart Rate (beat/min)	Systolic Blood Pressure (torr)	Blood Volume (ml/kg)	Hemoglobin (gm%)
Newborn	30–60	115–170	60–75	85	19.4
6 mo.	25–40	100–150	80–90	80	11.8
1 yr.	20–35	90–135	96	80	11.2
3 yr.	20–30	80–125	100	75	11.8
5 yr.	20–25	80–120	100	75	12.7
10 yr.	17–22	75–110	110	75	13.0
15 yr.	15–20	70–100	120	70	13.4
Adult	12–20	70	125	70	13.7(F) 15.5(M)

do not allow as much chest expansion with respiration as do the more vertically curved adult ribs. Therefore, in the event of respiratory compromise a child cannot compensate as readily as an adult by increasing ventilatory volumes by increasing chest expansion. Because of these factors, the child depends far more on the diaphragm as the primary muscle of respiration, and care should be taken not to impede diaphragmatic movement. This might occur if a small child is positioned supine (flat) with the head down, as a result of the abdominal contents placing gravitational forces on the diaphragm. This may be a particular problem when tight restraints are used.

The respiratory rate of the infant and small child is higher than that of the adult owing to an immature alveolar system and a higher basal metabolic rate. The basal metabolic rate at birth is more than double that of the adult, thus producing greater oxygen consumption and carbon dioxide production. These factors all combine to produce a respiratory system in children with far less reserve than in the adult (Smith, 1980).

CARDIOVASCULAR SYSTEM

Some basic differences exist in the cardiovascular system of infants and children when compared with that of adults (Johnson, 1978).

Blood volume ■ The relative blood volume in children is greatest at birth and decreases with increasing age. In the newborn, blood volume is about 85 ml per kg, whereas in adults it averages 70 ml per kg.

Heart rate ■ Heart rate is highest in the infant and decreases steadily throughout childhood (Table 6–2). In infants and small children, the cardiac output is dependent upon the heart rate to a much greater extent than in the adult because changes in myocardial contractility (stroke volume) cannot compensate effectively in the child's heart. Parasympathetic (vagal) tone is more pronounced in infants, probably as a result of immaturity of the sympathetic nervous system. Any vagal stimulation can cause a decrease in heart rate, resulting in decreased cardiac output and hypotension. This type of stimulation can occur especially with manipulation of the airway (endotracheal intubation), bladder distention, and pressure on the eyes. For this reason, it is often recommended that children who are to experience any of these stresses, such as with general anesthesia, be premedicated with a parasympathetic blocking drug such as atropine.

Blood pressure ■ Blood pressure is lower in children than in adults, with the lowest values being present at birth and increasing throughout childhood to reach adult levels by 13–15 years of age (Table 6–2).

Perfusion ■ Blood flow to the peripheral tissues can affect the absorption of intramuscular or subcutaneously administered medications to a great extent. In the newborn, peripheral circulation is poorly developed, causing uptake of intramuscular injections to be less effective than in the older child or adult. This is usually true only for the young infant, however. Peripheral vasoconstriction in children as a result of a cold environment or extreme anxiety can decrease the absorption of intramuscularly administered drugs, producing delayed onset of action and lower plasma levels of the drug.

When considering uptake of central nervous system–active drugs, it should also be kept in mind that in the child as much as 40% of the cardiac output contributes to the cerebral blood flow as compared with only about 20% in the adult. Because delivery of drug to the brain is the crucial factor in achieving effect, many medications, especially those given by intravenous bolus infusion or inhalation, should be expected to produce a more rapid and profound effect on the child's brain than would be true in the adult.

THE KIDNEY

The neonatal kidney is unable to concentrate urine to the same extent as the adult kidney and therefore cannot conserve water as well when deprived. The infant, therefore, requires more free water per day than the adult in order to excrete the daily solute load. The infant and young child may become rapidly dehydrated if not provided enough fluids to maintain this situation. The majority of drugs are excreted from the body primarily in the urine. The main mechanism of renal elimination of drugs is via glomerular filtration. Most drugs are readily filtered. The glomerular filtration rate of the infant, however, is only 30–50% of the adult, probably owing to less mature glomeruli and lower blood pressure. Therefore, drugs that are excreted primarily by glomerular filtration have longer half-lives (up to 50% longer) in a child. These include aminoglycoside antibiotics, digoxin, and curare. Glomerular filtration rate usually reaches adult levels by 3–6 months of age.

Other renal mechanisms such as tubular reabsorption and tubular secretion also vary in children from those of adults and may effect the half-lives of certain drugs. These mechanisms usually mature to adult levels during the first few months of life.

Further important dynamic anatomic and physiologic changes occur throughout childhood in other body systems, including the central nervous system, the gastrointestinal tract, the liver, the immune system, the eye, and the microsomal enzyme systems. Detailed discussion of these changes is beyond the scope of this text.

Summary

The basic concept that all of these physio-anatomic changes and differences should empha-size is that when administering medications of any kind to pediatric patients, extreme caution and vigilance must be practiced. The wise dental practitioner never administers a drug to a child without first investigating what is known regarding the pharmacokinetics of that drug in children. The action, route of administration, kinetics, and metabolism of each drug must be given individual consideration and related to the stage of development of the individual patient. It must be realized that for young children, especially neonates, the dose of many drugs cannot be calculated from the adult dose by the use of any single factor such as age, weight, or body surface area. Simple standardized formulas to extrapolate a pediatric dose from an established adult dose such as Clark's rule (based on weight) or Young's rule (based on age) cannot be safely applied across the board for all medications.

Proper drug doses for children of various ages should be sought on an individual basis from a reliable, current source. References such as the *Harriet Lane Handbook* (Cole, 1985) are quite useful for most drugs used in pediatrics.

REFERENCES

Campbell RL, Weiner M, Stewart LM: General anesthesia for the pediatric patient. J Oral Maxillofacial Surg 40:497–506, 1982.

Cole CH (ed): The Harriet Lane Handbook, A Manual for Pediatric House Officers, 10th ed. Chicago, Year Book Medical Publishers, Inc., 1985.

Crawford JD, et al: Simplification of drug dosage calculation by applications of the surface area principle. Pediatrics 5:783–789, 1950.

Done AK: Developmental pharmacology. Clin Pharmacol Ther 5:433, 1964.

Eger EI, Bahlman SH, Munson ES: The effect of age in the rate of increase of alveolar anesthetic concentration. Anesthesiology 35:365, 1971.

Gregory GA, Eger EI, Munson ES: The relationship between age and halothane requirements in man. Anesthesiology 30:488, 1969.

Howry LB, Bindler RM, Tso Y: Physiologic Considerations in Pediatric Medications. Philadelphia, JB Lippincott Co. 1981, pp 3–17.

Johnson TR, Moore WM, Jeffries JE: Children Are Different: Developmental Physiology. Columbus, Ohio, Ross Laboratories, 1978.

Morselli P: Clinical pharmacokinetics in neonates. Clin Pharmacokinet 1:81–98, 1976.

Morselli P: Drug Disposition During Development. New York, Spectrum Publishers, 1977.

Salanitre E, Rockow H: The pulmonary exchange of nitrous oxide and halothane in infants and children. Anesthesiology 30:388, 1969.

Smith RM: Anesthesia for Infants and Children. St. Louis, CV Mosby Co, 1980.

Pain and anxiety control (Part I: Pain perception control)

Jay A. Anderson

The overwhelming majority of pharmacologic agents used in dentistry are utilized to control pain or the fear of pain. The phenomenon of pain itself has two distinct components: pain perception and pain reaction (Bennett, 1978). Pain perception is a physio-anatomic process in which a noxious stimulus is perceived by nerve ending receptors and transmitted along neuro-anatomic pathways to the central nervous system. A threshold for pain perception exists. It is the minimum intensity stimulus that is required over a minimum time period in order to initiate a nerve impulse (action potential). This pain perception threshold can be measured and has been found to be relatively uniform for individuals who have a normal nervous system.

The second component of pain is pain reaction. Pain reaction is the response of the patient once the neural impulse has reached the brain and has been interpreted as pain. This aspect of pain is quite complex. The pain reaction threshold, or point at which a person reacts demonstrably to perceived pain, is quite variable from person to person as well as within the same person at different times. It is this component of pain that is usually referred to when discussing a person's pain threshold. Many factors affect the pain reaction threshold, including anxiety, stress, fatigue, and, of great importance in pediatric patients, past experiences and pre-conditioning by parents. The concept of pain and anxiety control acknowledges this dual nature of pain.

The complete control of pain perception in the setting of the dental operatory generally requires blocking pain perception by blocking the anatomic pain pathway. This may be accomplished peripherally using local anesthesia or centrally using general anesthesia. The pain reaction threshold is controlled using various forms of conscious sedation. With conscious sedation, the multiple factors influencing the reaction to pain may be manipulated either pharmacologically or psychologically to render the patient cooperative and comfortable. Pain control and anxiety control in actual clinical practice overlap to a significant degree. However, for the purpose of discussion, pain perception control (consisting of general anesthesia and

local anesthesia) and pain reaction control (consisting of conscious sedation) will be dealt with as separate entities.

There is no single best technique for control of pain and anxiety. No matter which technique may be a practitioner's favorite, no one technique is useful for all dental patients in all situations. The wise dentist has at least a working knowledge of several techniques and determines on an individual basis what is most appropriate for a particular patient. In some cases, this may necessitate referral.

General Anesthesia

There is a group of patients in whom the only reasonable anesthetic alternative for safe treatment is general anesthesia. Examples of such patients may include the very young precooperative child or the severely mentally retarded patient who is unable to cooperate for complicated or extensive dental procedures. General anesthesia renders the patient unconscious through depression of the central nervous system, thus eliminating patient cooperation as a factor. Pain perception as well as pain reaction are eliminated at the central level.

General anesthesia should be administered only by an individual who has completed a minimum of 1 year of residency training in anesthesiology. Rigorous patient monitoring is essential (American Dental Association, 1985).

Local Anesthesia

MECHANISM OF ACTION

Pain perception may also be altered at the peripheral level by blocking propagation of nerve impulses using local anesthesia. The process of pain perception involves production of a nerve impulse, or action potential, by a noxious stimulus that is sensed by receptors (nociceptors) at the nerve endings. This nerve impulse travels along the nerve fibers via a physiochemical conduction process involving ion transport. The primary effect of local anesthetic agents is to penetrate the nerve cell membrane and block the influx of sodium ions associated with membrane depolarization. It is currently felt that the sequence of events involved in local anesthetic block is (1) binding of the local anesthetic to a receptor site that exists on the inside of the cell membrane for the clinically useful local anesthetics, (2) blockade of sodium chan-

nels through which the sodium ions would normally enter during depolarization, (3) decrease in sodium conductance, (4) depression of the rate of electrical depolarization, (5) failure to achieve threshold potential, and (6) lack of development of a propagated action potential and thus blockade of conduction of the nerve impulse (Covino, 1976).

Local anesthetic agents are weak bases chemically, which are generally supplied as salts, such as lidocaine hydrochloride. The salts may exist in two forms, either as the uncharged free base or as the charged cation. The free base form, which is lipid soluble, is the form that must penetrate the nerve cell membrane. Penetration of the tissue and cell membrane is necessary for the local anesthetic to have an effect, since the receptor sites are located on the inside of the cell membrane. This is part of the reason why local anesthetic agents are not as effective in the area of an acute infection that renders the tissues acidic in pH. Once the free base has penetrated the cell, it re-equilibrates, and the cation is felt to be the form that then interacts with the receptors to prevent sodium conductance.

LOCAL ANESTHETIC AGENTS

Esters

The first local anesthetic discovered was cocaine in 1860. Owing to a number of adverse side effects associated with cocaine, attempts were made to develop alternatives that retained the local anesthetic properties of cocaine while eliminating the side effects. Several other benzoic acid ester derivatives were developed, including benzocaine, procaine (Novocaine), tetracaine (Pontocaine), and chloroprocaine (Nesacaine). The major problem with this chemical class of local anesthetics, the esters, is their propensity for producing allergic reactions.

Amides

In 1943, a new class of local anesthetics, the amides, was introduced with the synthesis of lidocaine. These compounds are amide derivations of diethylaminoacetic acid. They are relatively free from sensitizing reactions. Since the synthesis of lidocaine, several other local anesthetics have been introduced, all of which are amides. These include mepivacaine (Carbocaine), prilocaine (Citanest), bupivacaine (Marcaine), and etidocaine (Duranest).

LOCAL ANESTHETIC PROPERTIES

The individual local anesthetic agents differ from each other in their pharmacologic profiles (Table 7–1). They vary primarily in their potency, toxicity, onset time, and duration, all of which may be clinically important. These characteristics, in turn, vary as a function of the intrinsic properties of the anesthetic agent itself and the regional anesthetic procedure employed, and they may be modified by the addition of vasoconstrictors.

Potency

The intrinsic potency of a local anesthetic is the concentration required to achieve the desired effect of nerve blockade. Procaine has the lowest intrinsic potency; lidocaine, chloroprocaine, prilocaine, and mepivacaine have intermediate potency; and tetracaine, bupivacaine, and etidocaine are of high potency.

Onset Time

Onset time involves the time required for the local anesthetic solution to penetrate the nerve fiber and cause complete conduction blockade. It must be appreciated clinically that conduction blockade requires this time for onset, or needless pain may be produced by beginning a procedure too soon.

Duration

Duration of anesthesia is one of the most important clinical properties taken into account when choosing an appropriate local anesthetic agent for a given procedure. Generally, procaine and chloroprocaine are considered of short duration; lidocaine, mepivacaine, and prilocaine are of intermediate duration; and bupivacaine, tetracaine, and etidocaine are of long duration.

Regional Technique

The other major factor that determines drug characteristics is the type of regional (local) anesthetic procedure employed. Depending on whether topical, infiltration, or major or minor nerve block is employed, onset and duration of the various agents will vary. Potency is not affected.

Onset ■ Local anesthesia of the soft tissues by infiltration anesthesia occurs immediately with all of the local anesthetics. As more tissue penetration is necessary, the intrinsic onset latency previously discussed plays a greater role. Generally, in dentistry, for any given drug the onset time required is shortest with an infiltration block, longer with a peripheral (minor) nerve block, and longest for topical anesthesia.

Duration ■ Duration of anesthesia attained varies greatly with the regional technique performed. This profile may differ for different agents, depending on their intrinsic pharmaco-

Table 7–1 ■ Local anesthetic properties in dentistry

Generic Name	Brand Name	Type	Conc. (%)	Vasoconstrictor	Max. Rec. Dose (mg/kg)	Av. Duration of Anesthesia (min) Max. Infiltration		Mand. Bl.	
						Sft. Tsse	Pulpal	Sft. Tsse	Pulpal
Procaine	Novocain	Ester	4	1:2500 phenylephrine	15.0	90–120	30	135	30
Propoxycaine	Ravocaine	Ester	0.4 comb. with 2 procaine	1:20,000 levonordefrin (Neo-Cobefrin)	6.6	145	30	175	60
Tetracaine	Pontocaine	Ester	0.15	—	1.4	190	—	220	—
Lidocaine	Xylocaine	Amide	2	1:100,000 epinephrine	7.0	170	40–60	200	60–90
Lidocaine	Xylocaine	Amide	2	—	4.4	40–60	10	60–120	10–30
Mepivacaine	Carbocaine	Amide	2	1:20,000 levonordefrin (Neo-Cobefrin)	6.6	140	60	210	90–120
Mepivacaine	Carbocaine	Amide	3	—	6.6	85–100	20	180	40–60
Prilocaine	Citanest	Amide	4	1:200,000 epinephrine	7.9	130	60	190	90
Prilocaine	Citanest	Amide	4	—	7.9	60–85	10	175	60
Bupivacaine	Marcaine	Amide	0.5	1:200,000 epinephrine	2.0	4–9 hr	90	4–12 hr	180
Etidocaine	Duranest	Amide	0.5–1	—	4.4	4–9 hr	90–180	—	—

logic properties. Lidocaine (1%) with epinephrine (1 : 200,000), for instance, has a duration of 416 minutes for infiltration, 178 minutes for ulnar nerve block, 156 minutes for epidural anesthesia, and 94 minutes for spinal block (Covino, 1976).

Other Factors

Dose ■ The quality, onset time, and duration of a local anesthetic block may be improved by increasing the dose of local anesthetic agent by increasing either the concentration or the volume administered. Increases in dose are limited, of course, by anesthetic toxicity. However, for consistently effective local anesthetic block, an adequate concentration and volume must be administered as close to the target nerve(s) as possible.

Vasoconstrictors ■ Onset time, duration, and quality of block are also affected by the addition of vasoconstrictor agents to the local anesthetic solution. Vasoconstrictor agents, such as epinephrine, decrease the rate of drug absorption by decreasing blood flow to the tissues and thus prolong the duration of anesthesia produced and the frequency with which adequate anesthesia is attained and maintained. Toxic effects of the local anesthetics are reduced as well as a result of the delay in absorption into the circulation. Onset time of anesthesia is sometimes shortened as well. In pediatric dental patients, a vasoconstrictor is usually necessary because the higher cardiac output, tissue perfusion, and basal metabolic rate tend to remove the local anesthetic solution from the tissues and into the systemic circulation faster, producing a shorter duration of action and a more rapid accumulation of toxic levels in the blood.

It must be remembered that the vasoconstrictors are all sympathomimetic agents that carry their own intrinsic toxic effects, including tachycardia, hypertension, headache, anxiety, tremor, and arrhythmias. It has been shown that 2% lidocaine containing a concentration of 1 : 250,000 epinephrine is as effective in increasing the depth and duration of local anesthesia block as higher concentrations of epinephrine such as 1 : 100,000 or 1 : 50,000 (Keesling and Hinds, 1963). To avoid toxicity, especially in children, a concentration of 1 : 100,000 epinephrine should not be exceeded.

The pharmacologic properties of the local anesthetics commonly used in dentistry are summarized in Table 7–1.

TOXICITY

The use of local anesthetics is so common in dentistry that the potential for toxicity with these agents can be easily forgotten. Local anesthetic toxicity must especially be kept in mind by the dentist when treating pediatric patients. Toxic reactions to local anesthetics may be due to overdose, accidental intravascular injection, idiosyncratic response, or an allergic reaction. Only overdose is discussed in this section. The dental practitioner should be familiar with the maximum recommended dose for all local anesthetic agents that are used on a dose per body weight basis (i.e., mg per kg). Simply knowing a total mg (or number of carpules) "maximum safe dose" for the average adult is not adequate and may lead to overdosage in children. Maximum safe doses for local anesthetics are listed in Table 7–1.

Central Nervous System Reactions

Local anesthetic agents cause a biphasic reaction in the central nervous system as blood levels increase. Although local anesthetics have depressant effects in general, they are thought to selectively depress inhibitory neurons initially, thus producing a net effect of central nervous system excitation. Subjective signs and symptoms of early anesthetic toxicity include circumoral numbness or tingling, dizziness, tinnitus (often described as a buzzing or humming sound), cycloplegia (difficulty in focusing), and disorientation. Depressant effects may be immediately evident as well, such as drowsiness or even transient loss of consciousness. Objective signs may include muscle twitching, tremors, slurred speech, and shivering. Overt seizure activity may then ensue. Generalized central nervous system depression characterizes the second phase of local anesthetic toxicity, which may be accompanied by respiratory depression at high levels.

Cardiovascular System Reactions

The cardiovascular response to local anesthetic toxicity is also biphasic. During the period of CNS stimulation, the heart rate and blood pressure may increase. When plasma levels of anesthetic increase, vasodilatation and then myocardial depression occur, with a subsequent fall in blood pressure. Bradycardia, cardiovascular collapse, and cardiac arrest may occur at higher levels. Most of the local anes-

thetics used commonly in dentistry cause little cardiovascular alteration even at levels associated with seizure activity. The depressant effect on the myocardium is essentially proportional to the local anesthetic's inherent potency—procaine and chloroprocaine being least toxic, followed by lidocaine and mepivacaine, with tetracaine, bupivicaine, and etidocaine being the most cardiotoxic.

The use of local anesthesia in pediatric dentistry has changed the quality and quantity of procedures possible as much as any other advance in the field. In children who are properly prepared psychologically, quality local anesthesia is usually all that is necessary to eliminate pain completely. The pharmacokinetics of the agents used with children must be kept in mind. With the higher cardiac output, higher basal metabolic rate, and higher degree of tissue perfusion in children, the agents tend to be absorbed more rapidly from the tissues. Less mature liver enzyme systems, in turn, may detoxify these chemicals in young children at a slower rate than in adults, and the immature central nervous and cardiovascular systems are thought to be more susceptible to toxicity at lower levels than those of adults. For all of these reasons, a precise local anesthetic technique should be used, aspiration techniques should be practiced, a vasoconstrictor is usually necessary, and a thorough knowledge of the intrinsic properties of the local anesthetic agents to be used is essential. Above all, the recommended maximum safe dose of local anesthetic should be calculated precisely for each patient and must never be exceeded.

Analgesics

Pharmacologic relief of pain may occasionally be necessary before treatment is possible for dental conditions and may sometimes extend into the postoperative period. The agents used for these purposes are termed analgesics. Analgesic drugs should relieve pain without significantly altering consciousness. The analgesics act either in the periphery at the site of pain perception or centrally in the brain and spinal cord. The narcotic analgesics are thought to act in the central nervous system itself, and the non-narcotic analgesics, such as aspirin, are thought to act in the periphery, at the nerve endings. The great majority of dental pain in pediatrics can be managed using non-narcotic agents of relatively low potency.

NON-NARCOTIC ANALGESICS

The non-narcotic analgesics are generally useful for mild to moderate pain, which includes 90% of pain of dental origin. The non-narcotic analgesics differ from the narcotics in their site of action, lesser degree of toxicity and side effects, and in not producing drug dependence. These drugs exert their effects primarily at the peripheral nerve endings. The standard prototype drugs in this class are aspirin and acetaminophen.

Aspirin

Aspirin, a salicylate (acetylsalicylic acid), has enjoyed widespread use for its analgesic, antipyretic, and anti-inflammatory properties since its introduction in 1899. Despite the synthesis of many newer drugs, aspirin remains a standard drug of choice.

The most significant side effects of aspirin include alterations of coagulation by inhibition of platelet aggregation; gastric distress and dyspepsia; occult blood loss; and, very rarely, sensitivity reactions such as urticaria, angioneurotic edema, asthma, or anaphylaxis. The anticoagulant properties of aspirin are rarely a problem in children. However, because a single dose of aspirin can increase bleeding time, use prior to any surgical procedure is probably unwise. Aspirin should be avoided in patients with bleeding or platelet disorders and in those who are taking warfarin (Coumadin) type drugs. The gastrointestinal problems are the most commonly encountered and may be reduced by administering the drug with food or by using a buffered or enteric-coated preparation, although absorption may be affected. The more severe allergic type reactions have been shown to occur more often in patients with pre-existing asthma, atopy, or nasal polyps, and aspirin should probably be avoided in patients with such a history. The possible association of certain viral illnesses and the use of aspirin with the development of Reye's syndrome has resulted in many practitioners opting for acetaminophen as a substitute. This association, however, has not been clearly substantiated.

Dosage ■ The recommended dosage for analgesia and antipyretic purposes in children is 10–15 mg/kg/dose given at 4 hour intervals up to a total of 60–80 mg/kg/day, with a maximum limit of 3.6 gm/day.

Acetaminophen

Acetaminophen (e.g., Tylenol, Tempra, and Datril) is an effective analgesic and antipyretic that is equally as potent as aspirin. Unlike aspirin, acetaminophen does not inhibit platelet function, causes less gastric upset, and has not been implicated in Reye's syndrome. Because of these advantages, the use of acetaminophen as an aspirin substitute has risen steadily in recent years. The primary disadvantage of acetaminophen is that it has no clinically significant anti-inflammatory properties.

Toxicity as a result of overdosage may result in acute liver failure with hepatic necrosis and may be fatal. It is estimated that 15 gm of acetaminophen is required in an adult to produce liver damage, or more than 3 gm for a child under 2 years of age. Allergic reactions are very rare. Acetaminophen is a good alternative analgesic in patients who do not require an anti-inflammatory effect.

Dosage ■ The recommended dosage for acetaminophen is

Adult: 300–650 mg every 4 hours
Children: 5–10 mg/kg/dose every 4–6 hours
Maximum dose: 1000 mg every 6 hours

Non-steroidal Anti-inflammatory Agents (NSAIA)

More recently, a series of drugs called the non-steroidal anti-inflammatory agents (NSAIA), which are principally derivatives of phenylalkanoic acid, have been developed. These agents possess analgesic and anti-inflammatory properties that are superior to aspirin (especially for arthritis) and are not associated with increased side effects (Dionne, 1980). Thousands of these compounds have been tested, and several are now available clinically. Only a few have been studied for dental pain.

Ibuprofen

Ibuprofen causes somewhat less gastric upset and bleeding problems than aspirin (McIntyre et al., 1978). It has been shown to be approximately 3½ times as potent as aspirin for pain relief following oral surgery. Like aspirin, ibuprofen affects platelet aggregation, but bleeding times are not significantly altered. Side effects that have been reported include gastrointestinal upset, rash, headache, dizziness, eye problems, hepatic dysfunction, and renal dysfunction. Cross-sensitivity with aspirin may exist. Although ibuprofen was originally marketed as Motrin, which was available only by prescription, it is now available over the counter as Motrin and other brand names. It is not FDA-approved for use in children at this time.

NARCOTIC ANALGESICS

The narcotics, or opioids, have been shown to interact with opioid receptors in the central nervous system. These interactions result in the pharmacologic effects of the narcotics, including analgesia, sedation, and cough suppression. Narcotics are significantly more effective against severe and acute pain than the non-narcotic analgesics. They carry the serious drawbacks, however, of a much greater incidence of adverse effects such as sedation, respiratory depression, and dependence and abuse liability. There are many narcotic analgesics available, including morphine, meperidine (Demerol), fentanyl (Sublimaze), alphaprodine (Nisentil), codeine, and oxycodone (Percodan). Most of these drugs must be administered parenterally. Meperidine, oxycodone, and codeine are available to be given orally. Only codeine will be discussed in this section.

Codeine

Codeine is the standard of comparison for oral narcotics. It is absorbed well when given orally and may be used for more severe pain that is not responsive to aspirin or acetaminophen. Codeine is much less potent than its relative morphine and has far less addictive potential since it does not alter mood significantly. Side effects may commonly include nausea, sedation, dizziness, constipation, and cramps. If given in high doses or over prolonged periods of time, codeine is capable of producing the more serious side effects of respiratory depression and dependence seen with the other more potent narcotics. Codeine may be given alone or in combination with another analgesic. Because the narcotics act at a central site and the non-narcotic analgesics act at a separate peripheral site, it makes pharmacologic sense to combine the two types of analgesics for enhanced activity. Such drug combinations abound. An example is acetaminophen with codeine (Tylenol No. 3).

Dosage ■ It is recommended that codeine be given in combination with acetaminophen when it is given orally for pediatric analgesia.

The recommended dosage is

Children: 0.5–1.0 mg/kg/dose given at 4–6 hour intervals as needed

Adults: 30–60 mg/dose given at 4–6 hour intervals as needed.

It is rare that analgesics are necessary in pediatric dentistry. When an analgesic is required, it is rare that aspirin or acetaminophen in the recommended doses will not control dental pain. Should this situation occur, codeine in combination with acetaminophen will usually provide the needed relief. In the very rare situation in which dental pain is refractory to these modalities, a more potent agent such as meperidine may be used. This situation should always be of very brief duration and be embarked upon very carefully. Definitive dental therapy must be provided expediently.

REFERENCES

American Dental Association Council on Dental Education: Guidelines for teaching the comprehensive control of pain and anxiety in dentistry. Chicago, 1985.

Bennett CR: Conscious Sedation in Dental Practice, 2nd ed. St. Louis, CV Mosby, 1978.

Covino BG: Local Anesthetics: Mechanism of Action and Clinical Use. New York, Grune and Stratton, 1976.

Dionne RA: The pharmacologic basis of pain control in dental practice: Analgesics. The Compendium of Continuing Education, Vol 1 No 3, 191–195, 1980.

Jastak JT, Yagiela JA: Regional Anesthesia of the Oral Cavity. St. Louis, CV Mosby, 1981.

Keesling GR, Hinds EC: Optimal concentration of epinephrine in lidocaine solutions. JADA 66:337, 1963.

Malamed SF: Handbook of Local Anesthesia. St. Louis, CV Mosby, 1980.

McIntyre BA, Phelp RB, Inwood MJ: Effect of ibuprofen on platelet function in normal subjects and hemophiliac patients. Clin Pharmacol Ther 24:616–621, 1978.

chapter 8

Pain and anxiety control (Part II: Pain reaction control — conscious sedation)

Jay A. Anderson

For many patients, pain control goes beyond physio-chemical blockade of the anatomic pain pathways. Owing to any of a number of factors, a given patient may be unable to tolerate dental procedures despite adequate local anesthesia. For these patients, further steps must be taken to control anxiety. Anxiety control involves the alteration of the pain reaction threshold utilizing an array of techniques under the general heading of conscious sedation. As implied in the term conscious sedation, all of these techniques require that the patient remain conscious at all times. The spectrum of techniques available to the dental practitioner varies from psychosedation to intravenous techniques.

In 1985, the American Academy of Pediatric Dentistry and the American Academy of Pediatrics jointly endorsed a document entitled *Guidelines for the Elective Use of Conscious Sedation, Deep Sedation, and General Anesthesia in Pediatric Patients*. This document serves as a guide to those who utilize these techniques in practice, or anticipate using them. According to the guidelines, the goals of conscious sedation are (1) patient welfare, (2) control of patient behavior, (3) production of a positive psychological response to treatment, and (4) return to the pretreatment level of consciousness by the time of discharge. In the majority of instances, these goals may be achieved simply by establishing good rapport with the patient, using sound patient management techniques, and employing adequate local anesthesia. Iatrosedation, or psychosedation, involves the establishment of a trusting relationship with the patient such that he or she can cooperate and remain comfortable for a given dental procedure. The psychology of patient management is discussed elsewhere in this text (Chapter 21).

Before conscious sedation is discussed, some definitions are of utmost importance. The differences between conscious sedation, deep sedation, and general anesthesia must be clearly understood. These terms are clearly defined in

the *Guidelines for the Elective Use of Conscious Sedation, Deep Sedation, and General Anesthesia in Pediatric Patients,* adopted in 1985 as follows:

Conscious sedation

Conscious sedation is a minimally depressed level of consciousness that retains the patient's ability to maintain a patent airway independently and continuously, and respond appropriately to physical stimulation and/or verbal command, e.g., open your eyes. For the very young or handicapped individual, incapable of the usually expected verbal responses, a minimally depressed level of consciousness for that individual should be maintained.

The caveat that loss of consciousness should be unlikely is a *particularly important* part of the definition of conscious sedation and the *drugs and techniques used should carry a margin of safety wide enough to render unintended loss of consciousness unlikely.*

Deep sedation

Deep sedation is a controlled state of depressed consciousness or unconsciousness from which the patient is not easily aroused, which may be accompanied by a partial or complete loss of protective reflexes, including the ability to maintain a patent airway independently and respond purposefully to physical stimulation or verbal command.

General anesthesia

General anesthesia is a controlled state of unconsciousness accompanied by a loss of protective reflexes, including the ability to maintain an airway independently and respond purposefully to physical stimulation or verbal command.

As can be readily discerned, the patient under conscious sedation can respond *appropriately* to a verbal command and is able at all times to maintain a patent airway. If sedation techniques are practiced such that this is always the case, the patient's cardiovascular and respiratory function should always be well maintained. If, however, techniques and drug doses are used that depress consciousness further, to a point at which the patient cannot continuously respond appropriately to verbal command, a much higher risk of cardiorespiratory depression results. Such deep sedation or general anesthesia should only be administered by an appropriately trained individual who has proper resuscitation and monitoring equipment available.

Routes of Administration

The primary routes of administration for conscious sedation are (1) inhalational, (2) oral, (3) intramuscular, (4) subcutaneous, and (5) intravenous. In reviewing these techniques, only the primary advantages and disadvantages will be discussed briefly.

INHALATIONAL (NITROUS OXIDE)

For the production of conscious sedation, the inhalational route is limited to one agent, nitrous oxide. No other inhalational agent meets the guidelines for conscious sedation; all are general anesthetics. The primary advantages of nitrous oxide for conscious sedation in pediatric dentistry are as follows.

Advantages

Rapid onset and recovery time: Because nitrous oxide has a very low plasma solubility, it reaches a therapeutic level in the blood rapidly, and, conversely, blood levels decrease rapidly when it is discontinued.

Ease of dose control (titration)

Lack of serious adverse effects: Nitrous oxide is essentially considered to be inert and non-toxic when it is administered with adequate oxygen. The most commonly encountered side effect is nausea, which should be very rare unless high concentrations of nitrous oxide are used. Poor technique with high concentrations may also result in an excitement phase, in which the patient may become uncomfortable, uncooperative, and delirious.

The use of nitrous oxide in pediatric dentistry also has several disadvantages.

Disadvantages

Equipment: Must be purchased, installed, and maintained.

Weak agent: Attempts to push the concentration of nitrous oxide up in order to control moderately or severely anxious patients will be fraught with failure and will not be pleasant for the operator or the patient.

Lack of patient acceptance: There are some patients (adults and children) who do not find the effects of nitrous oxide to be pleasant. These patients may become overtly non-compliant, removing the nasal mask or becoming otherwise uncooperative.

Inconvenience: In some areas, such as the maxillary anterior teeth, the use of the nitrous oxide nasal mask may hinder exposure of the area. This may especially be problematic in small children.

Potential chronic toxicity: Retrospective survey studies of dental office personnel who were exposed to trace levels of nitrous oxide suggest a possible association with an increased incidence of spontaneous abortions, congenital malformations, certain cancers, liver disease, kidney disease, and neurologic disease. These results do point dental professionals toward the need to scavenge (remove) waste gases adequately from the dental operatory. However, it can be very difficult to scavenge nitrous oxide adequately in the uncooperative child since gases that are exhaled through the mouth cannot be effectively scavenged.

Potentiation: Although nitrous oxide is a weak and very safe agent when it is used alone (with oxygen), when it is added to the effects of other sedative drugs given by another route, deep sedation or general anesthesia may be easily produced. The combination of nitrous oxide with any other conscious sedation technique must be done with extreme care by an individual with proper training and experience.

ORAL ROUTE

A commonly used route of administration for conscious sedation in pediatric dentistry is oral premedication.

Advantages

Convenience: Oral drug administration is usually easy and convenient. The drug may be given at home or in the office. Giving it in the office has the advantages of being supervised (to be certain that the proper dose is given at the appropriate time) as well as being medico-legally safer. It usually works best to administer oral premedications in a separate, quiet, dimly lit room with a soft chair or rocking chair, where induction of sedation can be facilitated by the parent in a conducive environment.

Economical: To use oral premedications, no special office equipment needs to be purchased or maintained.

Lack of toxicity: If doses are calculated for each individual patient (keeping the previous discussion on pharmacokinetics in mind) and single drugs are used in single doses, the oral route of sedation is extremely safe. However, if drug combinations are used or two routes are combined (e.g., oral premedication followed by intravenous or inhalational medications), the chances of adverse side effects increase dramatically.

Disadvantages

Variability of effect: The biggest disadvantage of oral premedication is the fact that a standard dose must be used for all patients on a weight or body surface area (BSA) basis. Individuals of the same weight (or BSA), however, may respond quite differently to the same dose of drug, depending on many variables. Absorption of the drug from the gastrointestinal tract can be altered by several factors, such as the presence of food, autonomic tone, fear, emotional make-up, fatigue, medications, and gastric emptying time. The patient may not cooperate in ingesting the medication or may vomit, making estimation of the dose actually received impossible. If an inadequate dose has been given, a paradoxical response may be seen, which may be due to a direct effect or loss of emotional inhibitions. The patient may become agitated and more uncooperative, rather than sedated and cooperative. These factors make the oral route of administration the least dependable as far as certainty of effect is concerned. *A second dose of oral medication to "top off" a presumably inadequate dose should never be given.* Titration is not possible or safe with oral medication. If absorption of the initial dose has been delayed for any reason and a second dose is subsequently given on the assumption that the first dose was ineffective, both doses will eventually be absorbed, possibly resulting in a high serum level of the CNS-depressant drug, resulting in serious consequences such as respiratory arrest, cardiovascular collapse, and death.

Onset time: The oral route of drug administration has the longest onset time of any route of conscious sedation. A lag time of at least 45–90 minutes should be allowed from the time of administration until treatment is attempted.

Oral premedication is very useful in pediatric dentistry, but the limitations must be clearly understood. An adequate dose must be given and enough time must be allowed to elapse for absorption before the desired effect can be expected.

INTRAMUSCULAR ROUTE

The intramuscular route of administration involves the injection of the sedative agent into a skeletal muscle mass. It also involves certain advantages and disadvantages for use in pediatric dentistry.

Advantages

Absorption: Absorption from an injection deep into a large muscle mass is much faster and more dependable than absorption from the oral route.

Technical advantages: Technically, the intramuscular route of administration might be considered the easiest of all routes. It requires no special equipment except a syringe and needle. Patient cooperation is required for the oral route of administration, sometimes making it very difficult to give a full dose of a bitter-tasting medication to an uncooperative child. When intramuscular medications are administered, little or no patient cooperation is required and the full calculated dose is given with a high degree of certainty. Intramuscular injections are certainly technically easier to accomplish than the placement of an intravenous cannula, especially in children.

Disadvantages

Onset: Absorption of the injected drug can be decreased or delayed by several factors. A patient who is cold or very anxious may experience peripheral vasoconstriction in the area of the injection, significantly decreasing the rate of absorption. Perhaps the biggest variable in onset is *where* the drug actually is deposited. If the drug is deposited deep into a large muscle mass, the high degree of vascularity will allow uptake to be quite rapid. If, however, some or all of the drug is deposited between muscle layers, in the surface of the muscle, or not in the muscle at all (all distinct possibilities in small, struggling children), absorption may be quite unpredictable.

Effect: As with the oral route, a standardized dose is used, calculated on the patient's weight or BSA. Drug effect cannot be safely titrated by administering additional doses for much the same reason as with the oral route, that is, the possibility of cumulative overdose. A standard dose may have little or no effect in some children, whereas it may heavily sedate others.

Trauma: Injection sites that are devoid of large nerves and vessels are used for intramuscular injections, such as the mid-deltoid region, the vastus lateralis muscle of the thigh, and the gluteus medius muscle. Proper selection of the injection site and proper technique should minimize the possibility of tissue trauma.

Intravenous access: The potential for side effects and toxicity is higher with the intramuscular route than with the inhalational or oral routes. Compared with the intravenous route, a major disadvantage of this route is the lack of a patent intravascular access (an IV catheter) in the event of a medical emergency.

SUBCUTANEOUS ROUTE

Occasionally, the subcutaneous route of administration is utilized in pediatric dentistry for conscious sedation. In this situation, the drug is injected into the subcutaneous or submucosal space, not into muscle. Generally, similar advantages and disadvantages apply for this route as for the intramuscular route, with the following exceptions.

Advantages

Site: For dental procedures, some drugs may be injected submucosally within the oral cavity, usually into the buccal vestibule. This may be less objectionable to some patients and parents than multiple injection sites and may be more comfortable and convenient for the dentist to perform.

Disadvantages

Technical disadvantages: The rate of absorption is slower for the subcutaneous route than for the other parenteral routes. Blood supply to the subcutaneous tissue is often sparse compared with muscle. Within the oral cavity, however, vascularity is abundant and absorption is seldom a problem.

Tissue slough: Because the drug is deposited close to the surface of the skin or mucosa, the possibility of tissue sloughing is present. For this reason, only non-irritating substances should be given subcutaneously and large volumes of solution should not be injected.

INTRAVENOUS CONSCIOUS SEDATION

The intravenous route is the optimal and ideal route for administration of conscious sedation.

Advantages

Titration: Among the parenteral routes, only the intravenous route allows for exact titration to a desired drug effect. Because the drug is injected directly into the blood stream, absorption is not a factor. Within a few circulation

times, the intravenous drug will exert its maximal effect. Small, incremental doses may be given over a relatively short period of time until the desired level of sedation is achieved, thus avoiding under- or overdosing by a standardized bolus single dose, as must be given with oral, intramuscular, or subcutaneous injections.

Test dose: With the intravenous route, a very small initial test dose can be administered and a short period of time allowed to elapse to observe for an allergic reaction or extreme patient sensitivity to the agent.

Intravenous patient access: In the event that a medical emergency should occur, administration of emergency drugs is almost always best accomplished via the intravenous route. Establishing intravenous access after an emergency has occurred can be very difficult and can consume precious time.

Disadvantages

The intravenous route would be used for all conscious sedation if it did not involve some important disadvantages.

Technical disadvantages: The establishment of intravenous access (venipuncture) is technically the most difficult skill to master in the field of conscious sedation. Placing and maintaining intravenous catheters in children can be difficult even for a seasoned pediatrician. The procedure requires training and much practice.

Potential complications: Because potent drugs are injected directly into the blood stream, the intravenous route carries an increased potential for some complications. Extravasation of drug into the tissues, hematoma formation, and inadvertent intra-arterial injections are some possible complications of a misplaced intravenous catheter. If the medications are injected too rapidly, exaggerated effects may be produced. An immediate anaphylactic allergic reaction will become more rapidly life-threatening if it is due to an intravenous bolus of a drug as compared with an oral or intramuscular dose. These complications should all be avoidable by using test doses and proper, careful technique. Throm-

bophlebitis is a rare complication that is directly attributable to the intravenous cannula.

Patient monitoring: Because of the previously discussed increased potential to develop complications rapidly, the patient receiving intravenous sedation requires the highest level of monitoring.

Pharmacologic Agents for Conscious Sedation

There are a large number of drugs available for use in sedation and anesthesia. Individual drugs or techniques will not be discussed in detail here, only put into perspective. There are three primary groups of drugs used for conscious sedation in pediatric dentistry (Table 8–1). They are the sedative-hypnotics, the antianxiety agents, and the narcotic analgesics. Each of these groups acts primarily at a different area of the brain and should be expected to produce a distinctive primary effect. The wise practitioner of conscious sedation will understand which effect to expect from a given drug and will use the drug principally to achieve *that* effect.

SEDATIVE-HYPNOTICS

The sedative-hypnotics are drugs whose principal effect is sedation or sleepiness. As the dose of a sedative-hypnotic drug is increased, the patient will become increasingly drowsy until sleep (hypnosis) is produced. Further increasing the dose can produce general anesthesia, coma, and even death. It is important to note that the primary effect of these drugs is not to decrease anxiety or to raise the pain threshold (analgesia). In fact, a sedative-hypnotic used alone may lower the pain reaction threshold in some cases by removing inhibitions and in inadequate dosages may simply produce an "anxious drunk." The principal action of the sedative-hypnotics is due to the initial primary

Table 8 – 1 ■ Conscious sedation: pharmacologic agents

Group	Site of Primary Effect	Effect
Sedative-hypnotics	RAS	Sedation-sleep
Antianxiety agents	Limbic system	Decrease in anxiety
Narcotics	Opioid receptors	Analgesia

effect of these drugs on the reticular activating system, which is the area of the brain involved in maintaining consciousness. Further increases in dose will effect other brain areas, especially the cortex.

The sedative-hypnotic drugs fall into two categories: the barbiturates, such as pentobarbital, secobarbital, and methohexital; and the non-barbiturate hypnotics, which include drugs such as chloral hydrate and paraldehyde.

ANTIANXIETY AGENTS

The antianxiety agents were previously called the minor tranquilizers (the major tranquilizers being the antipsychotic drugs). These drugs have the primary effect of removing or decreasing anxiety. The primary site of action of these agents is in the limbic system, which is the "seat of the emotions." Theoretically, a dose exists for each antianxiety agent at which anxiety will be decreased without significant sedation being produced. As doses are increased, however, the reticular activating system and then the cortex are affected, producing sedation and sleep as well. Because anxiety is often the primary problem when dental phobias are dealt with, a primary effect against anxiety would appear to be desirable, especially in reasonably cooperative adults. Antianxiety drugs pharmacologically possess a flatter dose-response curve than many of the sedative hypnotics (especially barbiturates), allowing for a safer therapeutic index. This means that for most antianxiety drugs (e.g., diazepam), a larger difference exists between the dose that will produce the desired effect and the dose that will produce loss of consciousness than is the case with a rapid acting sedative-hypnotic (e.g., methohexital), which has a steep dose-response curve, the difference between a mildly sedating dose and general anesthesia being quite small. Drugs such as methohexital should not be used for conscious sedation for this reason. The antianxiety agents produce no analgesia.

The antianxiety agents consist primarily of the benzodiazepines, such as diazepam (Valium) and midazolam. This group of agents is the principal one used for conscious sedation in adults. Unfortunately, there is a lack of extensive clinical experience and research on these agents in children, but increasing clinical evidence is building for the use of these drugs in pediatric patients.

Some of the antihistamines, such as hydroxyzine (Atarax, Vistaril) and diphenhydramine (Benadryl) possess both antianxiety and sedative-hypnotic properties. They are often classified with the antianxiety agents. These drugs are not very useful alone for conscious sedation but are useful in combination with other drugs such as the sedative-hypnotics as potentiating agents.

NARCOTICS

The narcotics were previously discussed in the section on analgesics. These drugs are also used as part of conscious sedation techniques for their primary action of analgesia. The site of action of the narcotics is at the opioid receptors of the central nervous system. These drugs modify the interpretation of the pain stimulus in the CNS and therefore raise the pain threshold. As the dose of the narcotics is raised, other effects such as sedation will occur. However, it should always be realized that sedation, per se, is *not* the principal end-point being sought from a narcotic. If narcotic dosage is pushed to achieve sedation, serious side effects will be encountered, the most frequent of which is respiratory depression and apnea, which can lead to hypoxia. If sedation is desired, it should be accomplished with a drug that produces sedation as its primary effect.

Narcotics may also produce nausea and vomiting (especially when used alone), and in high doses they may produce cardiovascular depression. Narcotics are potent potentiators of other CNS depressant drugs. The principal use of narcotics in conscious sedation should, therefore, be to augment the effects of the sedative-hypnotic or antianxiety agents, as well as to contribute some degree of analgesia, which the other agents do not provide. The analgesia obtained with narcotics cannot be used as a substitute for adequate local anesthesia, which must also be attained.

Some of the narcotics utilized in conscious sedation techniques include morphine, meperidine (Demerol), fentanyl (Sublimaze), and alphaprodine (Nisentil). When considering the use of narcotics in pediatric dentistry, one is wise to remember the definition of conscious sedation from the American Academy of Pediatric Dentistry previously quoted. It states: "The caveat that loss of consciousness should be unlikely is a particularly important part of

the definition of conscious sedation and the drugs and techniques used should carry a margin of safety wide enough to render unintentional loss of consciousness unlikely." The ultra-potent narcotics such as fentanyl and alphaprodine have steep dose-response curves and, therefore, must be used with extreme caution for conscious sedation since they carry a high risk of producing respiratory depression and loss of consciousness, especially if they are combined with other agents, such as nitrous oxide.

KETAMINE

The dissociative agent ketamine has undergone periods of popularity in pediatric dental practice. It produces a cataleptic state with profound analgesia and amnesia. Ketamine acts primarily on the thalamus and cortex, not on the reticular activating system, so that the patient does not appear to be asleep, but rather dissociated from the environment. Respirations are not usually depressed with proper dosages. However, profound stimulatory cardiovascular changes are usually produced, tachycardia and increases in blood pressure being the usual case.

Ketamine is mentioned here primarily to point out that it is classified as a general anesthetic, since the patient under its influence is not capable of appropriate responses to verbal command or stimulation. It may cause respiratory depression and arrest in some patients as well as delirium and hallucinations. Ketamine should only be used by a practitioner qualified to administer general anesthesia.

Training

The level of training required for a dentist to administer sedation or anesthesia safely is currently under great debate and change throughout the United States. In some states, permits are not required in order to practice certain anesthetic techniques. The suggested minimum educational requirements for training necessary to administer conscious sedation is 60 hours of instruction and clinical experience in an accredited program (AAPD, 1985).

Deep sedation and general anesthesia are grouped together for training requirements, medico-legally, and for malpractice insurance purposes. Anyone who practices a technique from which a patient is not easily aroused and may not respond purposefully to verbal commands at all times is, by definition, practicing "deep sedation." The suggested educational requirements for the administration of deep sedation or general anesthesia is a minimum of 1 or 2 years of formal anesthesia residency training (AAPD, 1985:NIH, 1985).

REFERENCES

American Academy of Pediatric Dentistry (AAPD): Guidelines for the elective use of conscious sedation, deep sedation, and general anesthesia in pediatric patients. Chicago, 1985.

Moore PA: Monitoring and management: Adult vs. pediatric patients (scientific abstract). Anesthesia Progress 32:168–169, 1985.

NIH: National Institutes of Health Consensus Development Conference Statement: Anesthesia and sedation in the dental office. Anesthesia Progress 32:172–177, 1985.

chapter *9*

Antibiotics in pediatric dentistry

Jay A. Anderson

CHAPTER OUTLINE

■ **ANTIBIOTIC CLASSIFICATION**
    Spectrum of Coverage
    Mode of Action
    Bactericidal vs. Bacteriostatic
      Antibiotics
    Resistance

■ **ANTIBIOTIC AGENTS**
    Penicillins
    Erythromycin
    Cephalosporins
    Summary
■ **BACTERIAL ENDOCARDITIS PROPHYLAXIS**

Probably the second most commonly pre-scribed group of drugs for use in dentistry after the local anesthetics are the antibiotics. Various infections involving the teeth and oral cavity can extend to become quite severe and even life threatening if not properly treated. In dentistry, treatment of infections usually involves a definitive dental or surgical procedure and often requires the use of antibiotics. Antibiotics are substances produced by microorganisms that have the capability to produce an antimicrobial action. Antimicrobials are substances that kill or suppress the growth or multiplication of microorganisms, either bacteria, viruses, or fungi. Antibiotics are indicated for diseases in which a specific microbial agent has been identified, for a clinical situation that points clearly to a very probable microbial cause, and for use as a life-saving measure in a gravely ill patient. Prophy-lactic use is also indicated in some specific instances, such as prophylaxis against bacterial endocarditis for patients with congenital heart diesase. Antibiotic therapy will be maximally successful if the causative pathogen has been positively identified (by culture or serology), the therapeutic agent most active against that pathogen (confirmed by sensitivity testing) is utilized, and an adequate serum level of that

agent is maintained for an adequate length of time (Holroyd and Requa-George, 1978).

Antibiotic Classification

A vast array of antibiotics are available for use in pediatric dentistry. They may be classified in several different ways.

SPECTRUM OF COVERAGE

Antibiotics are considered to be either of narrow spectrum or of wide spectrum. Narrow-spectrum antibiotics are effective primarily against either gram-positive or gram-negative organisms. Broad-spectrum drugs are effective against a wider range of organisms (Table 9–1). With the broad-spectrum drugs, considerable overlap in effectiveness can exist. Generally, efficacy against a particular microorganism is ideally determined by testing the sensitivity of the actual causative pathogen (obtained by culture) to specific antibiotics. Unfortunately, this procedure may take 24 hours to several days. This requires that a best guess must be made for a specific clinical situation as to which pathogen

Table 9–1 ■ Antibiotics: spectrum of coverage

Gram-Positive
Penicillins

Erythromycin

Vancomycin

Lincomycin

Clindamycin

Bacitracin

Gram-Negative
Aminoglycosides

Polymyxin B

Colistin

Moxalactam

Nalidixic acid

Broad-Spectrum
Cephalosporins

Ampicillin

Sulfonamides

Carbenicillin

Tetracyclines

Chloramphenicol

is most likely the causative agent and which antibiotic is usually most effective against that organism. This antibiotic, or combination of antibiotics, is used until culture and sensitivity results are available.

Convenient tables listing antimicrobial treatment recommended for various clinical syndromes and sites of infection are published and updated periodically. An example is the *Pocketbook of Pediatric Antimicrobial Therapy* by J. D. Nelson. Dental and periodontal infections are primarily caused by organisms that are sensitive to penicillin.

MODE OF ACTION

Antibiotics may also be categorized according to their mode or site of action. There are five different modes of action described (Table 9–2): (1) inhibiting synthesis of the bacterial cell wall, which is required for bacterial survival; (2) inhibiting protein synthesis at one of several possible steps; (3) acting as an anti-metabolite by interfering with the metabolism of

folic acid and thus interfering with bacterial growth; (4) interfering with cell membrane permeability; and (5) inhibiting nucleic acid synthesis. By these mechanisms of action, the antibiotics produce toxic effects that selectively interfere with the life-cycle of the microorganisms while hopefully not causing significant alterations in the human host.

BACTERICIDAL vs. BACTERIOSTATIC ANTIBIOTICS

Antibiotics may also be classified as bactericidal or bacteriostatic. Bactericidal antibiotics actually kill the microorganisms, whereas bacteriostatic antimicrobials inhibit bacterial growth or multiplication and depend upon the normal host defense mechanisms (immune system) to eliminate the microorganism. Bactericidal agents are preferable in most situations. Bacteriostatic agents should not be used in immuno-compromised patients. Table 9–3 lists the agents in these categories.

Table 9–2 ■ Antibiotics: mode of action

Inhibition of Cell Wall Synthesis
Penicillins

Cephalosporins

Bacitracin

Vancomycin

Inhibition of Protein Synthesis
Bind 50s ribosome
  Erythromycin
  Chloramphenicol
  Clindamycin
  Lincomycin

Bind 30s ribosome
  Aminoglycosides
  Tetracyclines

Anti-metabolites
Sulfonamides

Alteration of Cell Membrane Permeability
Polymyxin B

Polyene agents
  Nystatin
  Amphotericin B

Inhibition of Nucleic Acid Synthesis
Rifampin

Nalidixic acid

Griseofulvin

Table 9–3 ■ Bactericidal and bacteriostatic agents

Bactericidal
Penicillins
Aminoglycosides
Cephalosporins
Bacitracin
Vancomycin
Trimethoprim
Bacteriostatic
Erythromycin
Sulfonamides
Tetracycline
Chloramphenicol
Lincomycin
Clindamycin

RESISTANCE

Spontaneous mutations may occur to produce microbial strains that are resistant to a particular antibiotic, rendering it ineffective by any of a number of mechanisms. If small numbers of resistant strains are allowed to gain dominance, they may produce clinical infections that could be very difficult to control and that could potentially cause a widespread health hazard. Development of resistant strains may be minimized by consistently using an adequate dosage of antibiotic for an adequate time period. Inappropriate use of antibiotics when the clinical situation does not warrant it, such as a probable viral syndrome, or inappropriate prophylactic antibiotic use may contribute to the development of resistant strains. Combination antibiotic therapy is sometimes indicated to prevent development of resistance; however, inappropriately combined drugs may contribute to the development of resistance, because some agents can inhibit the activity of others.

Antibiotic Agents

The antibiotic agents that may be used or considered to be used in pediatric dentistry include the penicillins, the erythromycins, and the cephalosporins.

PENICILLINS

In 1928, Sir Alexander Fleming discovered that penicillin mold lysed gram-positive microorganisms. This observation did not gain clinical usefulness until the 1940's, when the antibiotic era began. The penicillins are a group of antibiotics that differ in their pharmacologic properties. They are primarily active against the gram-positive bacteria, but their spectrums of coverage vary somewhat. They are the most allergenic antibiotics as a group, and all exhibit cross-allergenicity.

Penicillin G ■ Penicillin G was the prototype of this group of antibiotic agents and continues to be the drug of choice for many infections. Its coverage is primarily limited to gram-positive organisms and to some gram-negative cocci. It has two primary unfortunate properties. First, it is poorly absorbed orally, owing to its destruction by gastric acid, so that it is best given by the intramuscular route. Second, it is readily destroyed by penicillinase-producing microorganisms. Semi-synthetic penicillins have been developed in order to expand coverage and to overcome some of these disadvantages.

Penicillin V ■ The primary advantage of penicillin V is that it is stable at gastric pH, allowing for much improved absorption when it is administered orally. Its spectrum of coverage is the same as for penicillin G except for slightly less efficacy against *Neisseria gonorrhoeae* and some anaerobes. It also is inactivated by penicillinase. Penicillin V is the primary oral antibiotic used to treat dental infections.

Ampicillin and amoxicillin ■ Ampicillin has a broader spectrum of coverage than penicillin G, covering more gram-negative organisms, including *Escherichia coli, Haemophilus influenzae,* and *Salmonella.* It is, however, less effective against some gram-positive organisms. Ampicillin is used very commonly in pediatrics, owing to the frequency of *Haemophilus influenzae* infections. Ampicillin is absorbed better than penicillin G when administered orally, but it may commonly produce diarrhea or gastrointestinal upset. Nine per cent of children develop a maculo-papular rash after receiving ampicillin. Amoxicillin has the same spectrum of coverage as ampicillin but is absorbed better and causes less diarrhea. Despite the usefulness of these drugs in pediatrics, they are not indicated over penicillin G or penicillin V for use against dental infection. Development of resistance to these agents, especially by *Haemophilus*

influenzae, is becoming increasingly problematic.

Penicillinase-resistant penicillins ■ Some strains of staphylococci produce an enzyme, penicillinase, which destroys penicillins, resulting in drug resistance. Several penicillins have been developed that are resistant to destruction by penicillinase, including oxacillin, methicillin, nafcillin, cloxacillin, and dicloxacillin. Methicillin is not well absorbed orally. These drugs should be reserved for infections involving penicillinase-producing staphylococci and are not indicated for dental infections.

ERYTHROMYCIN

Erythromycin is a macrolide antibiotic that was introduced in 1952. Its spectrum of coverage is similar to penicillin's, with the addition of some penicillinase-producing staphylococci, chlamydiae, *Legionella,* mycoplasma, and others. It is well absorbed orally. However, the free base form is unstable at gastric pH, so it is administered with an enteric coating or in a salt form (stearate or estolate). Gastrointestinal upset is occasionally produced. Allergy is very rare, which is a major advantage over penicillin. The major disadvantage of erythromycin is that it is bacteriostatic rather than bactericidal. Despite this disadvantage, erythromycin is an effective drug for dental infections and is considered by many dentists to be the drug of choice.

CEPHALOSPORINS

The cephalosporins are a newer group of antibiotics that are chemically related to penicillin. They are broad spectrum in coverage and are divided into three "generations" by coverage. They are basically equivalent to penicillin in their activity against gram-positive organisms (except *Streptococcus faecalis*) and are resistant to penicillinase. Additionally, first generation cephalosporins have limited activity against gram-negative enterobacteria. The second generation drugs extend their spectrum to include more of these organisms, and the third generation cephalosporins have enhanced activity against many gram-negative bacilli, including most that are aminoglycoside resistant. The cephalosporins are bactericidal, and they exhibit some cross-sensitivity in penicillin-allergic patients.

The oral cephalosporins include cefaclor, cefadroxil, cephalexin, and cephradine. They have fewer side effects than oral penicillins and taste less bitter when given orally. They are, however, much more expensive. The cephalosporins are very effective against oral pathogens, but their use is highly discouraged, except as a last line of defense against serious infections. Promiscuous use of cephalosporins would certainly lead to increased development of resistant bacterial strains to these very effective agents.

SUMMARY

Most oral-dental infections are caused by gram-positive aerobes, facultative streptococci, and staphylococci, the most common organisms being streptococci (especially *Streptococcus viridans*). Other occasional pathogens include anaerobic gram-negative organisms such as *Bacteroides, Veillonella, Fusobacterium,* anaerobic peptostreptococci, and diphtheroids. The initial drugs of choice continue to be penicillin and erythromycin. Streptococci, most staphylococci, and most anaerobic pathogens continue to remain quite sensitive to both penicillin and erythromycin. Owing to their bactericidal action, penicillin V (orally) or penicillin G (intramuscular) is usually recommended as the primary drug of choice for orofacial infection, and erythromycin is usually the alternative drug of choice in patients allergic to penicillin.

Bacterial Endocarditis Prophylaxis

Bacterial endocarditis is a microbial infection of the endocardium (inner layer of the cardiac muscle). Certain patients with congenital cardiac lesions or acquired cardiac damage are felt to be at high risk for developing the condition if a procedure or manipulation causes transient bacterial seeding of the blood stream. The blood-borne bacteria may lodge in the abnormal endocardial surface and result in the infection. The cardiac conditions for which antibiotic prophylaxis is currently recommended to prevent bacterial endocarditis are listed in Table 9–4. Antibiotic prophylaxis is recommended for *all* dental procedures likely to cause gingival bleeding, including prophylaxis, in susceptible patients. Simple orthodontic adjustments that are unlikely to cause bleeding and spontaneous shedding of deciduous teeth are felt not to present a significant risk of endocarditis; there-

Table 9 – 4 ■ Cardiac conditions related to endocarditis prophylaxis*

Endocarditis Prophylaxis Recommended
Prosthetic cardiac valves (including biosynthetic valves)

Most congenital cardiac malformations

Surgically constructed systemic-pulmonary shunts

Rheumatic and other acquired valvular dysfunction

Idiopathic hypertrophic subaortic stenosis

History of bacterial endocarditis

Mitral valve prolapse with insufficiencyt

Endocarditis Prophylaxis Not Recommended
Isolated secundum atrial septal defect

Secundum atrial septal defect repaired without a patch 6 or more months earlier

Patent ductus arteriosus ligated and divided 6 or more months earlier

Postoperative coronary artery bypass graft surgery

* This table lists common conditions but is not meant to be all inclusive.
 t Definitive data to provide guidance in management of patients with mitral valve prolapse are particularly limited. It is clear that in general such patients are at low risk of development of endocarditis, but the risk-benefit ratio of prophylaxis in mitral valve prolapse is uncertain.
 (From Shulman S, et al: Prevention of bacterial endocarditis. Am J Dis Child 139:232–235, March 1985. Copyright 1985, American Medical Association.)

fore, prophylaxis is not recommended in these situations.

Bacterial endocarditis after dental manipulations is most commonly caused by alpha-hemolytic streptococci; therefore, prophylaxis is specifically directed against these organisms. In 1985, the Committee on Rheumatic Fever and Bacterial Endocarditis of the Council on Cardiovascular Diseases in the Young, American Heart Association, published updated recommendations regarding antibiotic prophylaxis of bacterial endocarditis. Their recommendations for antibiotic prophylaxis for dental and respiratory tract procedures are given in Table 9 – 5. Changes from previous recommendations are noted, including the use of a two-dose regimen.

These additional recommendations are also given:

Table 9 – 5 ■ Recommended antibiotic regimens for dental/respiratory tract procedures*

Regimen	Condition	Dosaget
Standard	For dental procedures that cause gingival bleeding, and oral/respiratory tract surgery	Penicillin V (2.0 g orally 1 hr before, then 1.0 g 6 hr later); for patients unable to take oral medications, 2 million units of aqueous penicillin G, IV or IM 30–60 min before a procedure and 1 million units 6 hr later may be substituted
Special	Parenteral regimen for use when maximal protection desired; e.g., for patients with prosthetic valves	Ampicillin (1.0–2.0 g, IM or IV) plus gentamicin (1.5 mg/kg IM or IV), half hour before procedure, followed by 1.0 g oral penicillin V, 6 hr later; alternatively, parenteral regimen may be repeated once 8 hr later
	Oral regimen for penicillin-allergic patients	Erythromycin (1.0 g orally 1 hr before), then 500 mg 6 hr later
	Parenteral regimen for penicillin-allergic patients	Vancomycin (1.0 g IV *slowly* over 1 hr, starting 1 hour before); no repeated dose is necessary

* Pediatric doses are as follows: ampicillin (50 mg/kg per dose); erythromycin (20 mg/kg for first dose, then 10 mg/kg); gentamicin sulfate (2.0 mg/kg per dose); penicillin V (full adult dose if weight greater than 27 kg (60 lb)); aqueous penicillin G sodium (50,000 units/kg; 25,000 units/kg for follow-up); and vancomycin hydrochloride (20 mg/kg per dose). The intervals between doses are the same as for adults. Total doses should not exceed adult doses.
 t IV indicates intravenous; IM, intramuscular.
 (From Shulman S, et al: Prevention of bacterial endocarditis. Am J Dis Child 139:232–235, March 1985. Copyright 1985, American Medical Association.)

1. In the case of delayed healing or other unusual circumstances, additional doses of antibiotics may be necessary, even though bacteremia rarely persists longer than 15 minutes after the procedure is completed.

2. Penicillin V is the preferred oral penicillin, owing to its resistance to gastric acid.

3. If a patient is taking penicillin chronically for some reason (e.g., rheumatic fever prevention), erythromycin or one of the parenteral regimens should be used to prevent development of resistant strains.

4. If a high risk patient (e.g., a patient with a prosthetic valve) has maintained a "high level" of oral health, oral antibiotic prophylaxis may be used for simple dental procedures, rather than the parenteral regimen. For all other patients at very high risk (those with surgical shunts or prosthetic valves), the parenteral route is still recommended (Shulman et al., 1985).

REFERENCES

Holroyd SV, Requa-George B: Antimicrobial agents. *In* Holroyd SV (ed): Clinical Pharmacology in Dental Practice, 2nd ed. St. Louis, CV Mosby, 1978.

Nelson JD: Pocketbook of Pediatric Antimicrobial Therapy, 5th ed. Dallas, Jodone Publishing Co, 1983.

Shulman ST, et al: Prevention of Bacterial Endocarditis. Am J Dis Child *139*:232–235, 1985.

Medical emergencies in pediatric dentistry

Jay A. Anderson

Dentistry is an invasive, surgical specialty that is often associated with high levels of patient anxiety. These factors combine to produce a situation that may be conducive to medical emergencies, especially those that are induced or aggravated by stress. Also, pharmacologic agents are used routinely in the dental office. All drugs, whether local anesthetics, antibiotics, sedatives, or analgesics, carry the potential of producing toxicity or allergy.

The specter of medical emergencies is often frightening and bewildering to dental students because of the implication that they will be called upon to diagnose and treat medical conditions that they are not trained or equipped to handle. It may be comforting to realize that the dentist is not expected to accurately diagnose the underlying cause of all emergencies and immediately render curative treatment. The accu-

rate diagnosis of a medical condition often, in fact, requires hours to days to determine in the hospital setting. The primary responsibilities of the dentist in the area of medical emergencies fall into the areas of prevention, preparation, basic life support, and procurement of help and transport.

Prevention of Medical Emergencies

Perhaps the most important aspect of dealing with medical emergencies is preventing their occurrence. Prevention of medical emergencies can generally be accomplished, as much as possible, by an adequate history and physical examination, medical consultation (when indicated), and vigilant patient monitoring.

HISTORY AND PHYSICAL EXAMINATION

A thorough knowledge of all existing medical conditions, physical or psychological, that may predispose the patient to development of a problem will prevent the vast majority of emergency situations. This knowledge is gained through the medical history and physical examination. The easiest way to obtain a medical history is to have the patient complete a simple medical history questionnaire, such as the short form available through the American Dental Association (ADA). Included are questions pertaining to any present or past medical conditions, allergies, hospitalizations, medications, and so forth. The dentist reviews this form, notes positive findings, and conducts a brief interview with the patient to clarify any questions and expand upon the questionnaire.

The physical examination should include baseline vital signs (heart rate, respiratory rate and character, and blood pressure in older children), a thorough head and neck examination, and observation of general appearance (gait, mental status, skin tone and color, etc.). Further physical evaluation should be dictated by the dentist's training and expertise. If a practitioner uses sedation techniques that may depress the patient's cardiovascular or respiratory function, it is recommended that the practitioner possess skills in the physical diagnosis of the cardiovascular and pulmonary systems (e.g., chest and heart auscultation).

A thorough history and physical examination should make the dentist aware of any pre-existing conditions that may lead to a medical emergency. This knowledge should allow the development of a treatment protocol for the patient that will make such an event highly unlikely. This may involve the use of conscious sedation for stress-induced conditions such as asthmatic attacks or epileptic seizures, proper timing of appointments, bacterial endocarditis prophylaxis, or even performing the needed procedures in the hospital operating room if deemed necessary.

MEDICAL CONSULTATION

If any questions arise regarding the management of a medically compromised child, it is highly desirable to contact the patient's physician by telephone for guidance.

Patient Monitoring

The level of monitoring that is necessary to treat a pediatric dental patient safely will vary, depending on the patient's condition and the patient management technique being utilized. Patient monitoring involves the observation of physiologic parameters over time in order to detect any change and deal with it before a potentially dangerous situation develops. The dentist should always monitor (observe) the general appearance of the patient, including the level of consciousness, level of comfort, muscle tone, color of the skin and mucosa, and respiratory pattern. For the majority of healthy patients being treated with local anesthesia alone, this is all the monitoring that is necessary.

When conscious sedation is used, especially in children, in whom a much narrower margin of safety often exists because of smaller degrees of respiratory and cardiovascular reserve, additional monitoring should be employed. The primary systems to be monitored during dental treatment with conscious sedation or deep sedation are the central nervous system (CNS), respiratory system, and the cardiovascular system. Pre-sedation vital signs, including heart rate, respiratory rate, blood pressure, and temperature, must always be obtained. The heart sounds and breath sounds should be continuously monitored using a precordial stethoscope in all patients undergoing conscious sedation (Fig. 10–1). This allows continuous auscultation by the dentist of the patient's heart rate and rhythm and respiratory pattern without having to look consciously at a monitor screen for data.

In addition to these essential monitors, several other devices are available that further enhance one's ability to monitor the patient's vital functions. For cardiovascular monitoring, blood pressure and heart rate may be conveniently monitored automatically utilizing automatic blood pressure devices such as the Dinamap (Critikon, Tampa, FL), which can be adjusted to measure systolic, diastolic, and mean blood pressure and heart rate at predetermined intervals and display the data digitally. The electrocardioscope is the most accurate method for monitoring cardiac rate and rhythm. Several devices have been advocated for respiratory monitoring, including the pulse oximeter, ear oximeter, impedance plethysmograph, and the transcutaneous oxygen and carbon dioxide monitors. Of these devices, the pulse oximeter appears to be the most useful

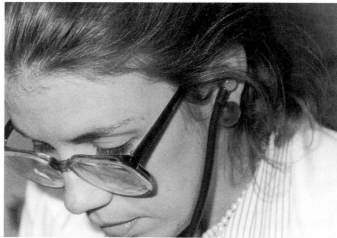

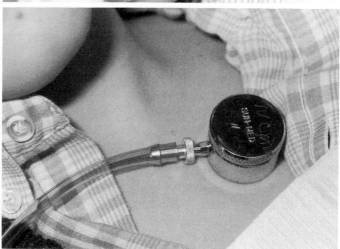

Figure 10–1 ■ Use of a precordial stethoscope.

and accurate for detecting developing hypoxia. It measures oxyhemoglobin saturation instantaneously and provides immediate feedback on the status of the patient's oxygenation.

Any time deep sedation or general anesthesia is used, more sophisticated monitoring is essential. In addition to the essential observations and precordial stethoscope, monitoring during deep sedation should include recording of vital signs at a minimum of 5 minute intervals (including blood pressure), continuous temperature monitoring, and an electrocardiogram (ECG). Placement of an intravenous catheter is also highly recommended. The use of restraining devices in small children makes monitoring especially difficult. When these devices are used, the dentist should observe at least one extremity and the face for color, check head position frequently to ensure a patent airway, and monitor heart and breath sounds with a

precordial stethoscope continuously. The use of a pulse oximeter is also highly recommended.

Preparation for Emergencies

Despite preventive measures, medical emergencies will occasionally occur. The dental practitioner must be adequately prepared for such events. Preparation involves personal, staff, and office preparation.

PERSONAL PREPARATION

As previously stated, it cannot be expected that the practicing dentist will be able to diagnose and treat every possible medical emer-

gency. It is, however, possible to anticipate with some certainty which emergency situations are most likely to arise in the dental office and be well prepared to deal with them. Examples include syncope, hyperventilation, seizures, hypoglycemia, postural hypotension, asthma, allergic reactions, and airway obstruction. Certainly, any emergency situation that might logically occur as a direct result of medications or techniques being used must be anticipated, well understood, and prepared for. Examples include local anesthetic reactions and respiratory depression secondary to sedatives. Personal preparation for the dentist should include, as a minimum, a good working knowledge of the signs, symptoms, course, and therapy for these common treatable conditions. Training in basic life support (cardiopulmonary resuscitation; CPR) should be considered essential for any practicing health professional. If conscious sedation techniques are to be used, advanced cardiac life support training is desirable.

STAFF PREPARATION

Office personnel should be trained in the recognition and treatment of common medical emergencies. It is desirable to require that all office staff members be certified in basic cardiac life support (CPR). A team approach to medical emergencies will provide for organized management of emergency situations. Each staff member should have a preassigned role in case of an emergency so that emergency equipment will be brought (and maintained) by an assigned person, emergency drugs will be prepared by another, and all tasks will be performed in an organized fashion. Because medical emergencies, fortunately, occur relatively rarely in the dental office, it is desirable to run mock medical emergency drills on a regular basis in order to keep the team protocol running smoothly and to reduce panic in an actual emergency.

OFFICE PREPARATION

Every dental office contains a great deal of equipment and supplies. There is a minimal amount of additional equipment that is essential for every office to be properly prepared for medical emergencies. These essentials can be divided into emergency equipment and emergency drugs.

Emergency Equipment

Keeping in mind the dentist's primary responsibilities of basic life support and transport in most situations, it should be apparent that very little equipment is necessary to deal with medical emergencies. First of all, oxygen must be readily available. An oxygen source capable of delivering greater than 90% oxygen at flows in excess of 5 liters per minute for a minimum of 1 hour must be available. This means that an "E" cylinder is the minimum size required. The initial primary goal of basic life support is establishment and maintenance of proper respiratory function. Hypoxemia (low oxygen content in the arterial blood) is the final common pathway leading to morbidity and mortality in the majority of severe medical emergency situations. Adequate oxygenation must be ensured by the administration of supplemental oxygen. If the patient is breathing adequately spontaneously, oxygen may be delivered by way of a face mask, nasal mask, or nasal prongs. However, the patient may cease breathing during an emergency situation, making artificial ventilation necessary. A positive pressure oxygen delivery system (bag-valve-mask) is, therefore, also considered essential equipment in order to deliver oxygen to the apneic patient.

A high volume suction device is the third piece of equipment that is considered essential to treat medical emergencies. Emergency situations, especially involving an obtunded patient, often induce vomiting. The aspiration of vomitus can be disastrous. This can usually be prevented by proper positioning and suctioning. Most dental offices, of course, contain high volume suction equipment for restorative purposes.

Other emergency equipment items that are desirable and recommended include syringes and needles, the armamentarium for establishing an intravenous line; cricothyrotomy equipment; oral and nasal airways; a laryngoscope; and endotracheal tubes.

Emergency Drugs

Most medical emergencies in the dental office do not require the use of drugs. The practitioner's thought process should be primarily directed toward basic life support measures and should turn to drug therapy only when clearly indicated. The contents of an appropriate emergency drug kit may be quite different for individual dentists, depending upon the drugs

used in the office, their individual level of training, and the level of medical support immediately available. It is expected that pharmacologic agents be available to definitely treat any medical emergency that may be expected to arise as a direct result of any drug that is utilized to treat patients. This would include the use of local anesthetics, which may produce toxic or allergic reactions.

The dentist should be well familiarized with each drug in the emergency kit. Commercially available emergency kits are not only very expensive, but also they are almost never optimal as far as which drugs are included for any individual practitioner's purposes. One of the biggest dangers of owning a commercially available emergency kit is gaining a false sense of security simply by purchasing it. If the practitioner does not know the uses, doses, and probable side effects of each drug in the kit and keep them up to date, the kit may in actuality be more dangerous than of potential benefit. A good drug kit should contain as few drugs as possible and should be simple, neat, and readily available. The dentist should be familiar with every drug, including its dose, indications, and side effects.

The following list is the author's recommendation for drugs that might be included in a basic emergency drug kit for the dentist who treats children. The list contains only superficial information and must be expanded upon as recommended previously.

DRUGS TO TREAT ALLERGY

Epinephrine

Use ■ Epinephrine is the most important drug in any emergency kit. It is the treatment of choice for life-threatening anaphylactic reactions and for severe asthmatic reactions, and it is a basic cardiac life support drug. If a dentist is administering any drugs to patients, including local anesthetics, epinephrine must be available in case of allergy.

Action ■ Epinephrine is a sympathomimetic catecholamine with both alpha and beta actions. Epinephrine increases heart rate and blood pressure, relaxes bronchial smooth muscle, and has an antihistaminic action.

How supplied ■ 1 : 1000 ampule (1 mg/ml) or 1 : 10,000 pre-loaded syringe (0.1 mg/ml).

Dose ■ 0.01 mg/kg (0.1 ml/kg of 1 : 10,000), IV or IM; may need to repeat after 5 – 10 minutes as needed.

Side effects ■ Side effects of epinephrine include hypertension, cardiac arrhythmias, anxiety, and headache.

Diphenhydramine (Benadryl)

Use ■ Diphenhydramine is used for allergic reactions of slower onset or less severity than anaphylaxis and as an adjunct to epinephrine in severe allergic reactions.

Action ■ Antihistamine.

How supplied ■ 50 mg in 1 ml ampule or 10 mg/ml vial.

Dose ■ 1 – 2 mg/kg, IV or IM.

Side effects ■ Sedation, anticholinergic.

ANTICONVULSANT

Diazepam (Valium)

Use ■ Diazepam is used for treatment of status epilepticus (recurrent seizures).

Action ■ Anticonvulsant.

How supplied ■ 5 mg/ml vials or pre-loaded syringe.

Dose ■ <5 yr: 0.3 mg/kg, slow IV (or deep IM):* maximum total dose, 5 mg.
>5 yr: 1 mg/dose, slow IV;* maximum total dose, 10 mg.
Adults: 5 – 10 mg/dose, slow IV;* maximum total dose, 30 mg.

Side effects ■ Sedation, respiratory depression.

NARCOTIC ANTAGONIST

Naloxone (Narcan)

Use ■ Naloxone is used to reverse respiratory depression or other undesirable effects of narcotic analgesics. This drug is essential if any narcotics are administered.

Action ■ Narcotic antagonist.

How supplied ■ 0.4 mg/ml ampule.

Dose ■ 0.01 mg/kg, IV or IM; may repeat dose as needed.

Side effects ■ Very rarely, cardiac arrest has been reported with the use of naloxone.

---

* May repeat dose every 15 minutes as needed, to maximum dose.

STEROID

Hydrocortisone Sodium Succinate (Solu-Cortef)

Use ■ The inclusion of a corticosteroid is recommended in order to treat acute adrenal insufficiency if it should occur in a steroid-dependent patient, or as an adjunctive treatment for a severe anaphylactic reaction or asthmatic attack.

Action ■ An adrenal corticosteroid: anti-inflammatory and membrane stabilization.

How supplied ■ 50 mg/ml in 2 ml Mix-O-Vial.

Dose ■ 3–5 mg/kg, IV.

ANTIHYPOGLYCEMICS

50 Per Cent Dextrose

Use ■ If loss of consciousness or obtundation occurs as a result of hypoglycemia, the treatment of choice is to obtain intravenous access and administer 50% dextrose to raise serum glucose levels.

Action ■ Directly raises serum glucose levels (immediately).

How supplied ■ (Dextrose 50% in sterile water—50 ml bottle (1 ml = 0.5 gm).

Dose ■ 0.5–1 gm/kg (1–2 ml/kg), IV, until patient regains consciousness.

Glucagon

Use ■ If intravenous access cannot be established, the hormone glucagon may be used. It must be kept in mind that restoration of consciousness may require a delay of 10–20 minutes.

Action ■ Raises serum glucose levels by encouraging glycogenolysis.

How supplied ■ 1 mg/ml solution.

Dose ■ 0.5–1 mg, IM (0.025–0.1 mg/kg), may repeat dose after 20 minutes if needed.

VASOPRESSORS

Especially if intravenous sedation techniques are being utilized, a drug to raise blood pressure in case of severe hypotension is advisable. If hypotension should occur, the situation must be assessed before any drug is given. If hypotension is due to a cardiac arrhythmia, the arrhythmia must first be treated with appropriate therapy. If hypotension is due to a drug effect (vasodilatation), appropriate fluid therapy with or without a vasopressor is indicated. Two possible alternative vasopressors are given.

Ephedrine

Use ■ Ephedrine is used to raise blood pressure and heart rate from shock levels.

Action ■ Indirect alpha and beta sympathomimetic actions by release of endogenous catecholamines.

How supplied ■ 25 or 50 mg/ml ampule.

Dose ■ 0.5 mg/kg, IV or IM.

Side effects ■ Hypertension, tachycardia, arrhythmias, headache.

Methoxamine (Vasoxyl)

Use ■ Methoxamine is used to raise blood pressure from shock levels.

Action ■ Methoxamine has a direct alpha sympathomimetic effect only. The drug produces an increase in blood pressure by peripheral vasoconstriction, without direct cardiac effects. Reflex bradycardia can be produced by methoxamine.

How supplied ■ 10 mg/ml vial or 20 mg/ml ampule.

Dose ■ 0.1 mg/kg, IV or IM.

Side effects ■ Bradycardia, hypertension, headache.

ANALGESIC

For acute emergencies in which the presence of pain and anxiety may significantly worsen the clinical situation, a narcotic analgesic may be indicated. This situation is primarily the case with acute myocardial infarction, which is obviously principally a problem of elderly patients. Morphine, meperidine (Demerol) or many other narcotics may be used.

ACLS DRUGS

If the dentist has training in advanced cardiac life support (ACLS), or if he or she performs deep sedation or general anesthesia, basic ACLS drugs may be included in the emergency kit. An ECG monitor and a defibrillator should be available when these drugs are used.

Atropine

Use ■ Atropine is used in the treatment of bradycardia.

Action ■ Atropine is a parasympathetic (vagal) blocking agent; therefore, it increases the patient's heart rate.

How supplied ■ 0.4 mg/ml ampules or vials.

Dose ■ 0.02 mg/kg, IV or IM.

Side effects ■ Tachycardia, arrhythmia, dry mouth.

Sodium Bicarbonate

Use ■ Acidosis, cardiac arrest.

Action ■ Raises blood pH directly.

How supplied ■ 1 mEq/ml.

Dose ■ 1 mEq/kg, IV, as needed during resuscitation.

Side effects ■ Alkalosis, hypernatremia.

Calcium Chloride

Use ■ Asystole, hypotension, electromechanical dissociation (EMD).

Action ■ Increased cardiac contractility.

How supplied ■ 10% solution (100 mg/ml).

Dose ■ 10–25 mg/kg, IV, every 10 minutes as needed.

Side effects ■ Phlebitis.

Lidocaine (Xylocaine)

Use ■ Lidocaine is used to treat ventricular arrhythmias (ventricular extrasystoles and ventricular tachycardia).

Note: Only "cardiac lidocaine" may be used for this purpose. Dental lidocaine should not be injected intravenously.

Action ■ Lidocaine depresses automaticity and suppresses ectopic ventricular pacemakers.

How supplied ■ 1% (10 mg/ml) or 2% (20 mg/ml) vials or prefilled syringe.

Dose ■ 1 mg/kg, IV.

Side effects ■ Sedation, local anesthetic toxicity in high doses (seizures).

OTHER DRUGS

Other agents that are not injectable drugs but that might be included as part of the emergency drug kit include (1) a respiratory stimulant, such as aromatic ammonia inhalants; (2) sugar (to treat hypoglycemia in an awake patient); (3) a vasodilator such as nitroglycerin; and (4) a "medihaler" of metaproterenol (Metaprel), isoproterenol (Isuprel), or isoetharine (Bronkosol) to treat an asthmatic attack.

Backup Medical Assistance

The final essential component of office preparation for medical emergencies involves securing back-up medical assistance in advance. This involves having the current telephone numbers of the nearest rescue squad and emergency room facility conveniently displayed where they will be immediately available if needed. When feasible, arrangements should be made with a physician whose office is nearby for immediate assistance should an emergency arise. Such a relationship must be prearranged, not assumed.

Management of Medical Emergencies

The management of basically all medical emergencies, especially those involving a change in the state of consciousness, should be approached in a similar fashion, keeping certain priorities in mind (Table 10–1). Not only will this approach make patient management more efficient and effective, but also it will make it less anxiety-provoking and confusing for the dentist.

POSITION

For emergencies involving obtundation of consciousness or hypotension, the best position for managing the situation is to place the patient lying flat on his or her back with the feet raised slightly above the level of the heart. This will minimize the work of the heart, increase return of pooled blood from the extremities, and increase vital blood flow to the brain. Fortunately, this position is easily accomplished in the dental chair. For medical emergencies in the conscious patient involving respiratory distress (e.g., asthmatic attack) or chest pain (angina), the semisitting position is generally preferred by the patient.

Table 10–1 ■ Management of medical emergencies

Position
Airway
Breathing
Circulation
Definitive therapy

AIRWAY ("A")

The first priority in the management of all medical emergencies is the establishment of a patent, functioning airway. If the supply of oxygen to the lungs is cut off for even a short period, especially in a child, rapid neurologic and cardiovascular deterioration will ensue, leading to cardiac arrest, brain cell damage, and death. The airway may be obstructed by progressive swelling, trauma, a foreign body, or other causes.

By far, the most common cause of airway obstruction, however, involves the tongue. When a patient becomes obtunded or unconscious, the musculature supporting the mandible and tongue becomes lax, allowing the base of the tongue to fall back against the posterior pharynx, thus blocking the airway between the oral and nasal cavities and the trachea. Extending the head on the neck and thrusting the jaw forward while opening the patient's mouth (head tilt – chin lift or jaw thrust maneuvers) is usually adequate to open the airway that is obstructed by the tongue. An oral or nasal airway device may be useful in keeping the tongue forward in the unconscious or deeply obtunded patient. These devices, however, should not be used in conscious patients, owing to their propensity to produce laryngospasm, gagging, and vomiting.

If the airway is obstructed by a foreign body, such as a cotton roll or dental restoration, management depends upon the patient's condition. In the conscious patient, the initial step should be to deliver four sharp blows with the heel of the hand to the patient's back, between the scapulae, over the spine. Sharp back blows will rapidly raise intrathoracic pressure, causing a burst of air to be expelled through the larynx, hopefully dislodging the obstruction. The four back blows should be delivered in rapid succession and should immediately be stopped if the patient begins to cough up the foreign body. If the back blows are not successful, the abdominal thrust (Heimlich maneuver) should be attempted. In the sitting or standing position, the operator positions himself behind the patient, places one fist below the xiphoid process over the mid-upper abdomen, clenches it with the other hand, and pulls up and back forcefully. This maneuver pushes the diaphragm up and produces a more sustained and forceful increase in intrathoracic pressure, expelling air through the larynx and hopefully dislodging the obstruction. Four abdominal thrusts are performed in rapid succession. The abdominal thrust may be modified for the patient who is lying down (as in the dental chair) in that the rescuer delivers the thrust with the heel of the hand from the side or front of the patient.

The abdominal thrust should not be performed with small children because of their relatively large abdominal organs (especially the liver), which could be damaged. In these cases, a chest thrust maneuver should be delivered instead, with the heel of the hand positioned over the child's mid-sternum, as would be the position for chest compressions during CPR. Chest thrusts are also used with pregnant females and the obese. The sequence of four back blows followed by four abdominal thrusts is repeated until success in dislodging the obstruction is attained or the patient loses consciousness.

In the unconscious patient with an obstructed airway, the patient is positioned supine (face up), the airway is positioned by tilting the head back and elevating the chin, and an attempt is made to ventilate the patient manually utilizing either mouth-to-mouth resuscitation or a bag-valve-mask system. Although back blows and abdominal thrusts may have been unsuccessful in dislodging an obstruction up to this point, the mechanism of positive pressure breathing is quite different because the air flow is in the opposite direction and may dislodge the obstruction. If the attempt to ventilate manually is unsuccessful, the sequence of four back blows (accomplished by rolling the patient toward the rescuer temporarily) and four abdominal or chest thrusts (from the side or front) is delivered. With an unconscious patient, these maneuvers are followed by sweeping a finger from the side of the patient's mouth deep into the oropharynx in order to remove any foreign body that may have been dislodged. An attempt at positive pressure ventilation is again made. This sequence is repeated until it is successful in establishing a patent airway or until an invasive technique is deemed necessary.

Invasive Techniques

In children, total airway obstruction will lead to cardiac arrest and brain dysfunction quite rapidly. In most small children, total airway obstruction will not be tolerated longer than 1 minute. If the above sequences are not successful in opening the airway rapidly and the patient is displaying signs and symptoms of hypoxia (cyanosis, arrhythmias), an invasive technique for opening the airway must be utilized.

The initial invasive tool in the dentist's armamentarium for dealing with airway obstruction should be direct laryngoscopy utilizing the laryngoscope. Use of the laryngoscope requires a certain amount of training and skill. With the laryngoscope, the larynx may be exposed so that any foreign body may be removed under direct vision. The trachea may then be intubated with an appropriate endotracheal tube for manual ventilation as needed.

Opening of the airway using cricothyrotomy is the last resort method of airway control. The cricothyroid membrane between the thyroid cartilage and the cricoid bone is either incised with a scalpel or punctured with a large-bore needle in order to ventilate the trachea with a flow of oxygen and/or allow respiration to be assisted. This technique, along with the critical anatomic landmarks, should be understood thoroughly by every dentist.

BREATHING ("B")

The second priority in dealing with medical emergencies, once a patent airway is established, is to ensure that adequate breathing is present. The chest should be observed for expansion and the nose and mouth observed for air flow during respiration by feeling and listening. If the patient is not breathing, rescue breathing should be initiated immediately. Initially, four rapid breaths are given in order to expand the lungs, followed by one breath every 3 seconds for children or one breath every 5 seconds for adults, until spontaneous respirations resume.

Rescue breathing may be accomplished by the mouth-to-mouth or the bag-valve-mask technique. Mouth-to-mouth ventilation is sometimes necessary in the emergency situation, but its efficacy is severely limited by the fact that exhaled air, containing a maximum of 15–18% oxygen, is delivered to the hypoxic patient's lungs.

Use of a positive pressure breathing system (bag-valve-mask), which can deliver close to 100% oxygen, is highly preferable. A mask is used, which fits tightly over the patient's mouth and nose. The mask is attached to a one-way valve, which allows oxygen to enter the patient when the reservoir bag is squeezed forceably. The empty bag then refills with oxygen only. The technique entails securing a tight mask fit on the patient's face and opening the airway with one hand and compressing the bag with the other, forcing oxygen by positive pressure

into the patient's lungs. Exhalation is passive. This technique of rescue breathing is much more efficient than mouth-to-mouth resuscitation and should be mastered by all dentists. A bag-valve-mask system, such as an Ambu bag, is considered essential emergency equipment for every dental office.

CIRCULATION ("C")

Once the airway and breathing have been established, the condition of the patient's circulatory system should be established. The most rapid, convenient, and accurate method of assessing circulation is to palpate the carotid pulse. The carotid artery should be felt just under the sternocleidomastoid muscle in the neck. One should never palpate both carotid arteries simultaneously, since pressure on the baroreceptors of the carotid sinuses may precipitate reflex bradycardia. The quality, rate, and rhythm of the pulses should be noted. If the pulse is absent, CPR should be initiated immediately. If the pulse is present, a more accurate assessment of cardiovascular status should be obtained by measuring blood pressure and heart rate.

DEFINITIVE THERAPY ("D")

Only after the "A", "B", and "C" of emergency management have been satisfied should one consider definitive drug therapy. Whether or not definitive drug therapy should be embarked upon by the dentist is dependent upon several factors, including his or her training and expertise, the availability of medical assistance, and the situation that the dentist is presented with. If the emergency is very acute and life threatening, especially if the cause is clear, or was precipitated by treatment or a drug that was administered, definitive therapy may be indicated and essential. Some common medical emergencies for which definitive therapy are indicated will be briefly discussed.

Syncope

Vasodepressor syncope, or the simple faint, is probably the most common cause of loss of consciousness in the dental office. It is, however, much less common in children than in young adults. Syncope is a maladaptive stress reaction that is usually triggered by anxiety. As the patient becomes anxious, the fight-or-flight re-

sponse of the sympathetic nervous system is triggered, and endogenous epinephrine and norepinephrine are released into the circulation. This response involves a large increase in blood flow to the muscles of the body. If the muscles are contracting, as would be the case if the individual is running, blood flow is maintained. However, in the dental chair little or no muscle contraction is occurring and the blood is, therefore, pooled in the muscles, especially in the lower extremities, effectively decreasing the relative blood volume available to the central circulation and, therefore, the brain. The heart rate will reflexively increase in an attempt to maintain the blood pressure, and the blood vessels in the periphery will constrict, producing the typical cold, pale, and sweaty skin. As blood flow to the brain decreases in the upright position, the patient feels dizzy or faint. This phase of the condition is called pre-syncope. It may begin rapidly and last a few minutes.

If it is recognized in a susceptible patient and dealt with quickly, loss of consciousness may be avoided. Management of pre-syncope consists of positioning the patient flat on the back, lowering the head, and raising the feet to augment blood flow to the brain by gravity. Encouraging the patient to contract muscles, especially in the legs, will also augment return of pooled venous blood from the musculature. Administration of oxygen is appropriate in any emergency involving a decrease in brain perfusion. The use of an ammonia inhalant to stimulate the patient may be of some benefit.

If the process of syncope continues, the sympathetic nervous system will fatigue and the parasympathetic nervous system will suddenly become dominant. This vagal response results in a sudden, severe decrease in heart rate and blood pressure, often to startlingly low levels. Blood flow to the brain is decreased, and consciousness is lost. Breathing becomes irregular, the pupils dilate, and convulsive movements are often noted. The muscles relax, and the airway may become obstructed. Loss of consciousness from syncope is usually rapidly responsive to positioning as previously mentioned. Oxygen should be administered; airway, breathing, and circulation maintained; tight and constrictive clothing loosened; and vital signs monitored.

Consciousness is usually regained fairly quickly, but heart rate and blood pressure may be quite slow in recovering. If recovery of consciousness is delayed beyond 5 minutes or is incomplete after 15–20 minutes, medical assistance should be sought. Drug therapy is usually not indicated with syncope unless the heart rate or blood pressure remain dangerously depressed after positioning. In such a case, atropine to increase heart rate or a vasopressor to increase blood pressure may be necessary.

Allergic Reaction

Allergic reactions involve hypersensitivity responses by the immune system to antigens that are recognized as foreign, with subsequent antibody formation. There are several different types of allergic responses, ranging from mild, delayed rashes to severe, sudden, life-threatening anaphylaxis. The primary agents employed in pediatric dentistry that might provoke an allergic reaction are the penicillins, intravenous sedative agents, or the ester-type local anesthetics.

The anaphylactic reaction is mediated primarily by the release of histamine from sensitized mast cells. Histamine is a potent toxic agent that produces inflammation and vascular effects. The body systems primarily involved in a clinical allergic reaction are the skin, respiratory system, and cardiovascular system. Skin involvement is the most common reaction and may range from a mild erythematous rash, to urticaria (hives), to angioedema (severe swelling).

In general, the more rapid the onset and the more intense the symptoms, the more severe the generalized reaction can be expected to become. Angioedema that involves the face and neck may be rapidly progressive, leading to airway obstruction and death. The respiratory system is usually involved after the skin reaction starts in generalized anaphylaxis. The primary problem is constriction of bronchial smooth muscle producing respiratory distress owing to airway obstruction, primarily expiratory in nature. The principal recognizable sign is wheezing, a distinctive breathing sound associated with bronchoconstriction. As the obstruction worsens, the patient has increasing difficulty in exchanging adequate volumes of air, usually becomes panicked, which worsens the situation, and may become severely hypoxic. Other smooth muscles also contract and may produce symptoms of abdominal cramps, nausea and vomiting, or incontinence. As anaphylaxis progresses, the cardiovascular system is affected. Hypotension is produced by the vasodilating effect of histamine and other mediators of the response. Reflex tachycardia, ar-

rhythmias, and eventually cardiac arrest may follow.

Management of allergic reactions depends upon the time course and severity of the symptoms. If symptoms are immediate or severe, epinephrine at 0.01 mg per kg should be administered, preferably intravenously in the 1 : 10,000 dilution or intramuscularly in the 1 : 1000 dilution. Epinephrine counteracts most of the effects of histamine. It produces bronchodilatation (countering bronchoconstriction) and raises blood pressure and heart rate by its alpha and beta effects. It also counters skin rash, urticaria, and angioedema by an unknown mechanism.

Diphenhydramine (Benadryl), a histamine receptor blocker, should also be administered. This antihistamine will not reverse to any great extent histaminic effects that have already occurred, but it may prevent further progression or recurrence of symptoms. If the reaction is delayed or mild, diphenhydramine may be all that is necessary to prevent progression of the allergic reaction. Diphenhydramine should also be administered orally at 6 hour intervals for 24 – 48 hours following any allergic reaction. Oxygen should always be administered if any respiratory symptoms are present. Use of an aerosolized sympathomimetic agent such as epinephrine, isoproterenol, or metaproterenol (Metaprel) to treat bronchospasm may also be of benefit. If the reaction is severe, the patient should be transported to the hospital, and supplemental use of a corticosteroid, such as hydrocortisone sodium succinate, should be considered. Ideally, the steroid preparation should be given early in the course of the reaction.

Seizures

Of the multiple types of seizures, the tonic-clonic (grand mal) type is the most frightening and the one that most often requires treatment. Only this type will be considered here. Grand mal seizures are manifested in four phases: the prodromal phase, the aura, the convulsive (ictal) phase, and the post-ictal phase.

The prodromal phase consists of subtle changes that may occur over minutes to hours. It is usually not clinically evident to the practitioner or the patient. The aura is a neurologic experience that the patient goes through immediately prior to the seizure. It is specifically related to the trigger areas of the brain in which the seizure activity begins. It may consist of a taste, a smell, a hallucination, motor activity, or other symptoms. A given patient's aura is often

the same for all seizures. As the CNS discharge becomes generalized, the ictal phase begins. The patient loses consciousness, falls to the floor, and tonic, rigid skeletal muscle contraction ensues. As the chest wall musculature contracts, air is expelled through the larynx, producing vocalization called the epileptic cry. Clonic movements then begin, producing rapid jerking of the extremities and trunk. Breathing may be labored during this period, and patients may injure themselves. This clonic phase usually last 1 – 3 minutes. As the clonic phase ends, the muscles relax and movement stops. A significant degree of CNS depression is usually present during this post-ictal phase, and it may result in respiratory depression. The patient has amnesia from the prodromal phase throughout the entire seizure.

Management of a seizure consists of gentle restraint and positioning of the patient in order to prevent self-injury, ensuring adequate ventilation, and supportive care, as indicated, in the post-ictal phase, especially airway management. Single seizures do not require drug therapy because they are self-limiting. Should the ictal phase last longer than 5 minutes or if seizures continue to develop with little time between them, a condition called status epilepticus has developed. This may be a life-threatening medical emergency, since the uncontrolled muscle activity can result in hyperthermia, increased oxygen consumption, tachycardia, hypertension, impaired ventilation, and cardiac arrhythmias. This condition is best treated with intravenous diazepam, and transport should be arranged to take the patient to the hospital.

Hyperventilation

Hyperventilation syndrome, like syncope, is a maladaptive anxiety reaction that primarily occurs in apprehensive young females who attempt to hide their anxiety. It is much less common in males and is rare in young children. The syndrome is often triggered by an anxiety provoking event such as the local anesthetic injection. The patient is usually unaware of the fact that she is beginning to hyperventilate. The respiratory rate may increase to 25 – 30 breaths per minute, with an increase in tidal volume as well. The patient may complain of difficulty in getting her breath. The increased ventilation causes carbon dioxide to be eliminated from the blood. The decrease in the Pa_{CO_2} in the blood (hypocarbia) will cause a physiologic vasoconstriction of the arteries supplying the brain with

a consequent decrease in blood flow to the brain. The patient will begin to feel dizzy and light-headed, which further enhances the anxiety, worsening the condition in a vicious cycle. Other symptoms that may occur include numbness and tingling of the extremities and perioral area, muscle twitching and cramping, seizures, and loss of consciousness.

Management of hyperventilation involves early recognition of the patient's anxiety and discussing it openly with the patient. Reassurance, patient rapport, and calmly coaching the patient to breathe slowly may stop the process. Oxygen should not be administered. If the cycle cannot be broken, steps should be taken to increase the arterial carbon dioxide content (Pa_{CO_2}). This can be accomplished simply by having the patient breathe into a paper bag, which causes rebreathing of exhaled CO_2-containing air, thus raising the Pa_{CO_2} and reversing the process. This should not be done for an extended period of time, of course, owing to the possibility of producing hypoxia. Occasionally, use of an antianxiety agent, such as intravenous diazepam, will be helpful.

Asthma

The primary type of asthma in children is allergic or extrinsic asthma, which is IgE antibody mediated. This type of asthma is usually outgrown by the late teens or early twenties. The asthma attack in this case is usually triggered by specific allergens, such as pollens, dust, and molds. The tracheobronchial tree is quite hyperreactive in asthma and contains increased amounts of tenacious secretions. During an acute asthmatic attack, constriction of the smooth muscle in the bronchial walls causes bronchospasm and the characteristic wheezing. Thick secretions are produced, which can plug the small airways, and bronchial wall edema may develop rapidly, further compromising the airway. This process may produce various signs and symptoms varying from mild wheezing and coughing to severe dyspnea, cyanosis, and death.

In adults, the primary type of asthma is termed extrinsic asthma. With extrinsic asthma, attacks may be precipitated by infections, irritants, exercise, and, importantly, stress. Some overlap in these asthma types certainly occurs. With any asthmatic patient, a thorough history should be taken, including how often attacks occur, how severe they have become (if hospitalization has been required, what triggers attacks, and what medications are being taken).

All attempts should be made to avoid precipitating factors. If the patient is taking medications, he or she should be instructed to continue taking them prior to the dental appointment. If patients use a Medihaler to self-administer aerosolized medications (Isuprel, Metaprel), they should bring it to their appointment.

If patients with asthma begin to wheeze and develop any respiratory distress in the dental chair, they should be given oxygen and allowed to sit up (if they are more comfortable sitting). If they have a Medihaler, they should utilize it, which will usually abort the attack. If aerosolized adrenergic agents fail to reverse the bronchospasm, 0.01 mg per kg (maximum dose, 0.5 mg) of epinephrine (1 : 1000) should be injected subcutaneously. This should reverse the attack in most cases. If no relief has been afforded after two doses of epinephrine, emergency transport to the hospital should be arranged. If the attack becomes very severe, intravenous aminophylline may be initiated in an attempt to relieve bronchospasm. A loading dose of 5.6 mg per kg is infused over 10 minutes, followed by a continuous intravenous infusion of 1 mg/kg/hour. Any patient requiring parenteral drug administration to control an asthma attack should be transported to the hospital. Early administration of a corticosteroid (hydrocortisone or dexamethasone) may also be helpful in severe attacks.

Diabetes Mellitus

Diabetes mellitus is a disorder involving poor insulin production and consequently disorders of carbohydrate, fat, and protein metabolism. It is characterized by hyperglycemia if it is untreated. Diabetes mellitus occurring in children is termed juvenile onset diabetes mellitus and usually carries the worst prognosis. These patients have little or no pancreatic beta cell function and, therefore, require parenteral insulin daily. Blood glucose levels may be very difficult to control. The principal emergencies that develop are due to either hypoglycemia or hyperglycemia. If plasma insulin levels remain low or absent for a prolonged period of time, blood glucose levels will become extremely elevated. The glucose, however, is unable to enter the cells as a result of the lack of insulin, and the cells will metabolize fat and proteins to produce more glucose as well as ketones and other metabolic acids. A condition known as diabetic ketoacidosis occurs, which may lead to coma and death if it is left untreated. The important fact to realize concerning ketoacidosis is that it re-

quires several days to develop, during which time the patient will be ill. It does not occur suddenly in a previously alert and well patient.

If a diabetic patient who is doing well has a sudden deterioration in the dental office, the condition is far more likely to be due to acute hypoglycemia, or insulin shock. The usual scenario involves a patient who has taken his or her morning insulin and has forgotten to eat a meal or has ingested inadequate carbohydrate. Exercise and stress may also increase carbohydrate utilization and lower blood glucose concentrations. Glucose and oxygen are the primary metabolites for brain cells. As the serum glucose level begins to decrease, neurologic symptoms may begin to appear. Most diabetic patients are well attuned to this phenomenon and carry a carbohydrate source to be ingested in this event. If carbohydrate is not ingested and the blood glucose concentration continues to decrease, evidence of deteriorating cerebral function will ensue. The patient may become lethargic, have a change in mood, act strangely, or become nauseated. The sympathetic nervous system becomes hyperactive in an attempt to raise the blood glucose level, producing symptoms of tachycardia, hypertension, anxiety, and sweating. The patient develops slurred speech, ataxia, mental obtundation, and eventually loss of consciousness. Seizures may occur.

Management of hypoglycemia involves the administration of glucose. The oral route is used only if the patient is fully conscious and is experiencing early symptoms. Sugar dissolved in juice or a sugar-containing soft drink may be used. If the patient has become mentally obtunded, an intravenous catheter should be established and 50% dextrose administered until consciousness is regained. Alternatively, glucagon may be administered intramuscularly if establishment of intravenous access is not possible. It must be remembered that consciousness will be regained more slowly when glucagon is utilized. The dentist should never attempt to administer glucose orally to an mentally obtunded or unconscious patient.

It is recommended that the dental practitioner further expand upon this material, becoming familiar with other medical emergency situations that may occur in the dental office, especially those drug-related emergencies that may result from pharmacologic agents being utilized in daily practice.

BIBLIOGRAPHY

Goodson JM, Moore RA: Life-threatening reactions after pediatric sedation: An assessment of narcotic, local anesthetic, and anti-anxiety drug interaction. JADA 107:239–245, 1983.

Malamed SF: Handbook of Medical Emergencies in the Dental Office, 2nd ed. St. Louis, CV Mosby, 1982.

section *I*

Conception to age three

I

Without question, the development of a child from conception to age 3 years is the most dramatic with regards to growth and development. In an approximately 3 year, 9 month period of time, a single cell, the fertilized egg, develops into a human being, complete with feelings, emotional needs, ability to communicate, gross motor skills such as walking, and fine motor skills such as piling up blocks. Dentally, the edentulous neonate will, at age 3, have a complete primary dentition consisting of 20 teeth.

From a medical standpoint, these years are very important. The obstetrician monitors the development of the fetus and the welfare of the pregnant mother and is responsible for the neonate during birthing. The pediatrician or family physician will attend to the neonate (1–4 weeks post-partum), the infant (first year of life), the toddler (1–3 years), the child (3–12 years), and the adolescent (12–19 years). To some degree, the quality of life of any culture can be measured by the health and survival rate of children under age 3. Environmental, nutritional, or disease circumstances that compromise the mother and the developing fetus and neonate can have woeful consequences. Good medical care of the pregnant mother and the neonate is essential to produce the emergence of a healthy child and adolescent.

The importance of these years dentally cannot be overemphasized. Dental conditions such as cleft palate, disturbances in calcification, unusual numbers of teeth, oral habits, caries, and the development of malocclusions start during these years. The profession of dentistry has long recognized the importance of these years. Indeed, dental students have memorized the onset of calcification dates for all the primary and permanent teeth for years. More recently, guidelines addressing fluoride supplementation for children under age 3, nursing caries, and home care techniques for the young child have been developed. However, infant oral health and care of the child patient younger than age 3 have largely been approached didactically and not clinically.

If so much could be done to enhance dental health with effective preventive strategies implemented in the first year of life, then why hasn't dentistry been doing so? The answer to this question is simple and will be addressed in another chapter of this book (see Chapter 21). First, for most of the twentieth century, dentistry was not

as prevention oriented as it was treatment oriented. The dentist who was not implementing prevention programs for patients had no reason to see patients until they had time to aggregate some disease. Because of the youth of these patients and the modest amount of time that the teeth had been in the oral cavity, it was often a poor chance that dentists could do much in children before 30 – 36 months of age. Second, if children did have teeth that needed restoration, because of their youth and inability to communicate and suppress their fears regarding a new and unknown situation, the dentist who was restoratively bound found himself with the dilemma of how to perform delicate restorative techniques on a child practicing avoidance behaviors such as crying, kicking, and wiggling.

Fortunately, contemporary dentistry is prevention oriented and most dentists today understand their disease prevention obligations to their patients and seek prevention strategies that ensure maintenance of oral health for all their patients. With this in mind, then, it is obvious that *the child in the first year of life is a most desirable preventive patient in that whatever is done preventively for this patient will have a lifetime of effect.* Also, because the dentist is seeing the child primarily to help formulate a strategy toward the prevention of dental diseases, the behavior of the child is as incidental to the dentist as it is to the physician.

Today's family-oriented dentist is active in pre-natal classes and the examination of babies. This dentist has established communications with family physicians and pediatricians within the community and stands poised and ready to dispense information that will help the physicians in the community understand what is entailed in infant oral health. In addition, children are recruited into the practice enthusiastically before the first birthday. If there are questions about oral hygiene, dietary fluoride supplementation, nutrition, and nursing, this dentist is ready to see the parents and their infant at any time. Lastly, this dentist understands the techniques of patient management and stabilization of the children in this age group so that he or she can, when needed, treat the dental disease or injuries that this age group can experience.

chapter *11*

The dynamics of change

PHYSICAL CHANGES

BODY

J. R. Pinkham

The gestation of a human being lasts approximately 9 months and begins at the moment the mother's ovum is fertilized by the father's sperm cell. At this moment of penetration of the ovum's wall, the sperm releases 23 chromosomes into the ovum, which also releases from a dissolving nucleus 23 chromosomes of its own. The human infant begins life with these 46 chromosomes. The fertilized cell begins to expand by the process of mitosis. The first division of the fertilized ovum into two cells usually takes place in 24–36 hours.

The time from conception to birth is often described in three phases. The first phase, the period of the ovum, is from fertilization until implantation. This period lasts until the dividing ovum, or blastocyst, becomes attached to the wall of the uterus. This period lasts for approximately 10–14 days. The next period lasts

2–8 weeks and is called the period of the embryo. This period is most important because of the cell differentiation that occurs during it. It is during this period that all the major organs appear. The third and last period, which starts at 8 weeks and lasts until delivery at approximately 40 weeks, is called the period of the fetus. This period is characterized by maturation of the newly formed organs.

Figure 11–1 shows the difference in the proportions of the fetus at 2 and 5 months, the newborn's body, and the changes that will be made during maturation. No year will be more dramatic in growth than will the first year of life, during which most children will undergo a 50% increase in length and almost a 200% increase in weight. Toward the end of the first year of life, the growth rate slows. After the first birthday, the growth rate will stay very stable and the height and weight increments of the child will remain relatively predictable all the way until adolescence.

There are no good predictors of the child's final height before age 3. However, at age 3,

111

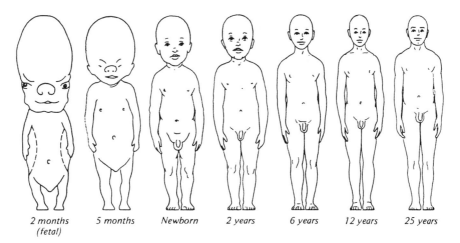

Figure 11–1 ■ The changing proportions of the human body from 2 months *in utero* to adulthood. (From Jackson CM: Some aspects of form and growth. *In* Robbins WJ, Brody S, Hogan AF, Jackson CM, and Green CW (eds): Growth. New Haven, CT, Yale University Press, 1929, p 118.)

correlations between the child's height and weight at maturity are fairly strong. The process of a newborn changing into an adult is one of elongation. The legs, at first shorter than the trunk, become longer. Also, the length of the child's trunk, when compared with his breadth, becomes considerably greater.

As the body changes and matures, the infant is afforded increasingly sophisticated postural and locomotive actions. Table 11–1 shows some of the developmental hallmarks, physically and cognitively, of a child during his first 18 months of life. (Piagetian psychology as well as object permanency and causality is discussed in this chapter's section on cognitive development.)

By age 2, a child has the gross motor skill to run, climb, walk up and down steps, and kick a ball. His fine motor skills allow him to stack blocks (up to six), make parallel crayon strokes, and turn the pages of a book one page at a time. Table 11–2 shows a variety of motor skills and the mean age they are acquired.

The nervous system of the child grows dramatically fast from birth until age 3. In fact, the child's brain by the end of his second year has attained 75% of its adult weight (Hurlock, 1950).

REFERENCE

Hurlock EB: Child Development. New York, McGraw-Hill, 1950.

HEAD AND NECK

Jerry Walker

Intrauterine Growth and Development

The miracle of growth and development is nowhere more evident than in the process and the changes that take place in the head and face (Table 11–3). The human face begins its first observable growth during the fourth week of intrauterine life with the development of the branchial apparatus. The branchial apparatus is first seen as a series of ridges on the lateral aspect of the cephalic end of the embryo at approximately the third week of intrauterine life (Moyers, 1958). A 1-month-old embryo has no real face, but the key primortia have already begun to gather. These slight swellings, depressions, and thickenings will rapidly undergo a series of mergers, rearrangements, and enlargements that will transform them from a cluster of separate masses into a face (Stewart et al, 1982) (Fig. 11–2).

The oral cavity of the embryo is bounded by the frontonasal process and by the maxillary and mandibular processes of the first branchial arch (Fig. 11–3). Each maxillary process moves towards the midline and joins with the lateral nasal fold of the frontonasal process. As this is happening, a shelf-like process (the palatal process) is developed on the medial side of each

Table 11-1 ■ Cognition, play, and language

Piagetian Stage	Age	Object Permanence	Causality	Play	Receptive Language	Expressive Language
I	Birth to 1 month	Shifting images	Generalization of reflexes		Turns to voice	Range of cries (hunger, pain)
II	1 to 4 months	Stares at spot where object disappeared (looks at hand after yarn drops)	Primary circular reactions (thumb sucking)		Searches for speaker with eyes	Cooing Vocal contagion
III	4 to 8 months	Visually follows dropped object through vertical trajectory (tracks dropped yarn to floor)	Secondary circular reactions (recreates accidentally discovered environmental effects, e.g., kicks mattress to shake mobile)	Same behavioral repertoire for all objects (bangs, shakes, puts in mouth, drops)	Responds to own name and to tones of voice	Babbling Four distinct syllables
IV	9 to 12 months	Finds an object after watching it hidden	Coordination of secondary circular reactions	Visual motor inspection of objects Peek-a-boo	Listens selectively to familiar words Responds to "no" and other verbal requests	First real word Jargoning Symbolic gestures (shakes head no)
V	12 to 18 months	Recovers hidden object after multiple visible changes of position	Tertiary circular reactions (deliberately varies behavior to create novel effects)	Awareness of social function of objects Symbolic play centered on own body (drinks from toy cup)	Can bring familiar object from another room Points to parts of body	Many single words—uses words to express needs Acquires 10 words by 18 months
VI	18 months to 2 years	Recovers hidden object after invisible changes in position	Spontaneously uses nondirect causal mechanisms (uses key to move wind-up toy)	Symbolic play directed toward doll (gives doll a drink)	Follows series of two or three commands Points to pictures when named	Telegraphic two-word sentences

(From Zuckerman BS, Frank DA: *In* Levine MD, et al: Developmental-Behavioral Pediatrics. Philadelphia, WB Saunders Co, 1983, p 91.)

Table 11-2 ■ Median age and range in acquisition of motor skills

Motor Skill	Age in Months		Motor Skill	Age in Months	
	Median	Range*		Median	Range*
Transfers objects hand to hand	5.5	4 to 8	Holds crayon adaptively	11.2	8 to 15
Sits alone 30 seconds or more	6.0	5 to 8	Walks alone	11.7	9 to 17
Rolls from back to stomach	6.4	4 to 10	Walks up stairs with help	16.1	12 to 23
Has neat pincer grasp	8.9	7 to 12	Walks up stairs both feet on each step	25.8	19 to 30
Stands alone	11.0	9 to 16			

* 5th to 95th percentile.
(Adapted from Bayley (1969). From Zuckerman BS, Frank DA: *In* Levine MD, et al: Developmental-Behavioral Pediatrics. Philadelphia, WB Saunders Co, 1983, p 89.)

maxillary process. These two palatal processes move toward the midline, where they fuse. This palatal fusion is normally completed by the eighth intrauterine week. The mandibular processes fuse at the midline somewhat before the maxillary and nasal processes (Fig. 11–4). The palate grows more rapidly in width than in length during the fetal period as a result of mid-palatal sutural growth and appositional growth of the lateral alveolar margins.

A failure in the fusion in the processes gives rise to oral or facial clefts, or both. In the mandible, the cartilaginous skeleton of the first branchial arch, known as Meckel's cartilage, provides a form for the development of the mandible (Moyers, 1958) (Fig. 11–5).

The muscles of mastication, that is, the temporalis, the masseter, and the medial and lateral pterygoids, and the trigeminal nerve also are derived from the first branchial arch. At approximately 60 days of gestation, the embryo has acquired all of its basic morphologic characteristics and enters the fetal period.

In 1978, Sperber described the presomite stage of development (21–31 days), during which the 3 mm embryo develops at its cranial end five mesenchymal elevations, or processes. The five mesenchymal elevations constitute the initial features of the face. These include the fronto-nasal process, two maxillary processes, and two mandibular arches. These processes grow differentially, and by obliterating the ectodermal grooves between them, they eventually contour the features of the face.

Rapid orofacial development is characteristic

Table 11–3 ■ Developing structures of the head and face

Developing Structures	Initiation (Weeks in Utero)
Neural plate	2
Buccopharyngeal membrane	2
Mandibular arch initiation	3
Hypoglossal muscles (tongue)	5
Medial and lateral nasal processes	5
Lens of the eye	5
Retina	5
External carotid artery	6
Eustachian tube	6
Larynx	6
Maxillary process	6
External auditory meatus	7
Nasal septum	8
Two palatal shelves fuse together	8
Palatal shelves fuse with nasal septum	10
Ossification of craniofacial skeleton	10
Eyelids completely formed and closed	10
Eyelids open	28

of the advanced development of the cranial portion of the embryo when compared with its caudal portion. The differential rates of growth result in a pear-shaped embryonic disc, with the head region forming the expanded portion of the pear. This early development of the cranial end of the embryo results in the head constituting nearly one half of the total body size during the post-somite embryonic period (fourth to eighth week).

The dominance of head growth and development in the embryonic period is not maintained in the fetal period. Accordingly, the proportions of the head are reduced from about one half of the entire body length at the end of the embryonic period to about one third at the fifth month and to about one fourth at birth.

During the fetal period, the eyeballs, following the neural pattern of growth, initially grow rapidly. This contributes to the widening of the face. Interestingly, the nasal cavity and the nasal septum have a considerable influence in determining facial form. In the fetus, the septomaxillary ligament transmits septal growth pull

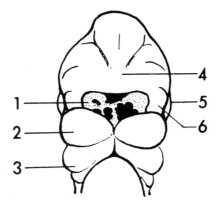

Figure 11–2 ■ Human face at about 4 weeks. 1, Stomodeal plate (buccopharyngeal membrane). 2, Mandibular arch (swelling or process). 3, Hyoid arch. 4, Frontal eminence (or prominence). 5, Optic vesicle. 6, Region where the maxillary process (or "swelling") of the first arch is just beginning to form. (From Enlow DH: Handbook of Facial Growth. Philadelphia, WB Saunders Co, 1982. Modified from Patten BM: Human Embryology, 3rd ed. New York, McGraw-Hill, 1968.)

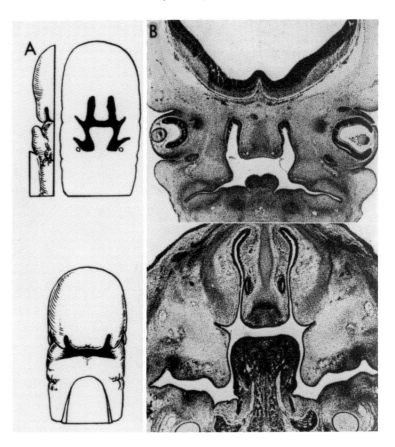

Figure 11–3 ■ *A,* Cross-section and front view of fronto-nasal process and branchial arches fusing to form the face. B, Histologic sections at approximately the same age. Note large size of tongue. The lower part of the face develops more rapidly than the upper, causing the tongue to appear to drop, so that the palatal shelves can meet at the midline. (Reproduced with permission from Moyers RE: HANDBOOK OF ORTHODONTICS, 1st edition. Copyright © 1958 by Year Book Medical Publishers, Inc., Chicago. Courtesy of Dr. James K. Avery.)

upon the maxilla. The septal cartilage directs facial growth downwards and forwards.

The thrust and pull created by the nasal septal growth separate to varying degrees the frontomaxillary, frontonasal, frontozygomatic and zygomaticomaxillary sutures. The expansion of the eyeballs, the brain, and the spheno-occipital synchondrosal cartilage also act in separating the facial sutures. The overall effect of these diverse forces of expansion is osseous buildup on the posterior and superior surface of the facial bones (Sperber, 1978).

Unlike in the embryonic period, during the fetal period the relative size of the maxilla to the mandible varies widely. Throughout the embryonic stage, the mandible is considerably larger than the maxilla. It is not until the fetal stage that the maxilla begins to overlap the mandible. Subsequent to this, the mandible grows at a greater pace and equals the size of the maxilla by 11 weeks in utero. Between the thirteenth and the twentieth week in utero, the mandibular growth again lags relative to the maxilla. At birth, the mandible tends to be retrognathic to the maxilla (Orban, 1980; Ranly, 1980).

For the remainder of its intrauterine existence, the fetus will undergo a process of growth and maturation and a reorganization of the spatial relationships between various structures (Enlow, 1982) (Fig. 11–6).

Rapid and extensive growth characterizes the ensuing 7 months of fetal life. An expansion of the cranium occurs during this fetal period as the result of a combination of growth processes, including interstitial, endochondral, and sutural or translational growth. The cartilage remnants of the chondral cranium that persist between the bones are known as synchondroses.

In addition, the cranial base undergoes selective appositional remodeling by resorption and apposition. This process is mediated by activity on the part of the bone-forming cells, the osteoblasts, as well as by bone destroying cells, the osteoclasts.

The major remodeling throughout the remainder of the early facial skeleton begins in the fetus at about 14 weeks. Before this time, the bones enlarge in all directions from their respective ossification centers. Remodeling, as a process that accompanies growth, starts when the definitive form of each of the individual bones of the face and cranium is attained (Enlow, 1982) (Fig. 11–7).

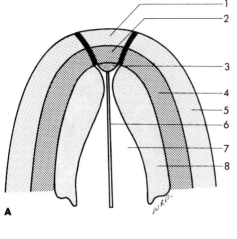

A

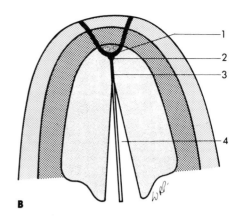

B

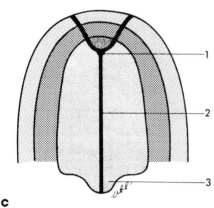

C

Figure 11–4 ■ *A,* Overview of the palatal shelves in a 7½ week embryo. 1, Philtrum of upper lip. 2, Premaxillary segment from medial nasal processes. 3, Primary palate. 4, Upper arch (part derived from maxillary swellings). 5, Cheek. 6, Nasal septum. 7, Open oral and nasal cavities. 8, Palatal shelves. In this stage, the philtrum and premaxillary segment have already merged with the maxillary swellings. *B,* Oral view of palate, showing beginning of fusion. 1, Merger of midline primary palate with bilateral secondary palatal shelves. 2, Incisive foramen. 3, Palatal raphe (midline fusion). 4, Open nasal and oral chambers. *C,* Full length palatal fusion. 1, Incisive foramen. 2, Palatal raphe. 3, Uvula. (From Enlow DH: Handbook of Facial Growth. Philadelphia, WB Saunders Co, 1982.)

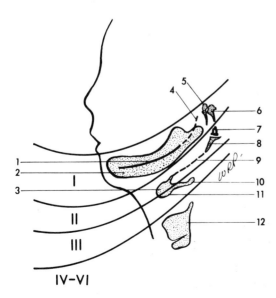

Figure 11–5 ■ Pharyngeal arch derivatives (I to VI). 1, Meckel's cartilage. 2, Intramembranous bone developing around Meckel's cartilage. 3, Superior part of body and lesser horn of hyoid. 4, Sphenomandibular ligament. 5, Malleus. 6, Incus. 7, Stapes. 8, Styloid process. 9, Stylohyoid ligament. 10, Greater horn of hyoid bone. 11, Inferior part of hyoid body. 12, Laryngeal cartilages.

The *first* pharyngeal arch gives rise to the tissues that will eventually become the mandible and its muscles. It is thus called the *mandibular arch.* A bud develops from it to become the "maxillary swelling," and this is the anlage (that is, primordium) for part of the maxillary arch that is soon to begin forming. The specific cranial nerve to the first arch is the mandibular (V), and it thus innervates the various *muscles of mastication.* The cartilage of the first arch (Meckel's cartilage) serves as the anlage for two of the ear ossicles (malleus and incus). This cartilage does not develop into the mandible itself. The bone of the lower jaw forms intramembranously *around* Meckel's cartilage, and the cartilaginous condyle develops from a separate secondary cartilage that appears later. (From Enlow DH: Handbook of Facial Growth. Philadelphia, WB Saunders Co, 1982.)

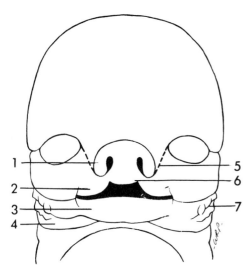

Figure 11–6 ■ The face between 7 and 8 weeks. 1, Nasolateral process. 2, Maxillary process. 3, Mandible. 4, Hyoid arch (note formation of external ear lobes). 5, Merger line of nasolacrimal groove. 6, Philtrum. 7, Hyomandibular cleft. (From Enlow DH: Handbook of Facial Growth. Philadelphia, WB Saunders Co, 1982.)

Growth and Development after Birth

At birth, the bony face and skull show little differentiation from child to child. Newborns have tiny mouths and virtually no chins. Their faces are small, although their eyes in comparison to the small face are exceedingly large. The

Table 11–4 ■ Structures of the head and face at birth

No. of Structures at Birth	Number
Bones of the skull	45
Foramina associated with floor of skull	12
Foramina associated with orbit	5
Foramina associated with face	6
Foramina associated with mouth	6
Foramina associated with exterior skull	3
Brain subdivisions	6
Facial muscles	18
Muscles of mastication	4
Cranial nerves	12
Muscles of palate	5
Muscles of tongue	5
Major facial arteries	8

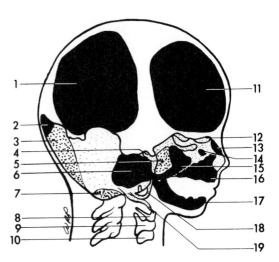

Figure 11–7 ■ Human skull at about 3 months. Intramembranous bones are shown in black. Cartilage is represented by light stippling, and bones developing by endochondral ossification are indicated by darker stippling. Approximate time of appearance for each bone is indicated in parentheses. 1, Parietal bone (10 weeks). 2, Interparietal bone (8 weeks). 3, Supraoccipital (8 weeks). 4, Dorsum sellae (still cartilaginous). 5, temporal wind of sphenoid (2 to 3 months; the basisphenoid appears at 12 to 13 weeks, orbitosphenoid at 12 weeks, and presphenoid at 5 months). 6, Squamous part of temporal bone (2 to 3 months). 7, Basioccipital (2 to 3 months). 8, Hyoid (still cartilaginous). 9, Thyroid (still cartilaginous). 10, Cricoid (still cartilaginous). 11, Frontal bone (7½ weeks). 12, Crista galli, still cartilaginous (inferiorly, the middle concha begins ossification at 16 weeks, the superior and inferior conchae at 18 weeks; the perpendicular plate of ethmoid begins ossification during the first postnatal year, the cribriform plate during the second postnatal year, the vomer at 8 fetal weeks). 13, Nasal bone (8 weeks). 14, Lacrimal bone (8½ weeks). 15, Malar (8 weeks). 16, Maxilla (end of 6th week; premaxilla, 7 weeks). 17, Mandible (6 to 8 weeks). 18, Tympanic ring (begins at 9 weeks, with complete ring at 12 weeks; petrous bone, 5 to 6 months). 19, Styloid process, still cartilaginous. (From Enlow DH: Handbook of Facial Growth. Philadelphia, WB Saunders Co, 1982. Modified from Patten BM: Human Embryology, 3rd ed. New York, McGraw-Hill, 1968.)

forehead and top of the head are big. It is difficult to imagine the diversity of individual looks that will develop over the course of childhood and adolescence from such similar little infant faces (Table 11–4; Fig. 11–8).

At birth, the maxilla frontally is very low and relatively small. By 9 months, the jaw has become considerably wider and higher. There is also a remarkable increase in the maxillary sinus. At birth, the bones that compose the cranium are not fused and are separated by six membrane-filled gaps called fontanelles (Fig. 11–9). Each of these areas is completely closed

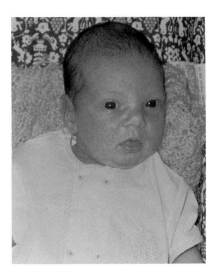

Figure 11–8 ■ The small nose, lips, jaws, ears, and chin of this 3-week-old female baby are shared with other young babies. Babies have a uniformity of appearance. With growth, of course, the subtle differences between young babies' faces will become explicit and easily recognized.

the lack of vertical growth that is yet to come. The horizontal dimensions are more nearly adult-like. The upper and total face heights are not half completed at birth. According to Ranly in 1980, they are 43% and 40%, respectively, which means that the most striking and complex growth of the head is associated with the face. After an initial spurt during the first 3 years, the rate of increase of these dimensions slows. It remains steady until the adult size is reached. The cranium as represented by cranial width and length is nearest adult size than any other part of the head. This can be explained by the development of the brain, which by the eighth month of intrauterine life has all of the nerve cells it will ever have. The symphyseal growth occurs, increasing the width of the mandible. By the second year, the synthesis is closed and growth becomes localized in the mandible as well as in the nasal-maxillary complex (Moyers, 1958). An enormous metamorphosis has taken place, but many more changes will occur before the child's adult appearance is realized.

by ossification within 2 years after birth (Moyers, 1958).

The face appears broad and flat at birth. The lower jaw seems underdeveloped and receded. The overall broadness of the face results from

REFERENCES

Caffey J: Pediatric X-Ray Diagnosis. Chicago, Year Book Medical Publishers, Inc, 1950.

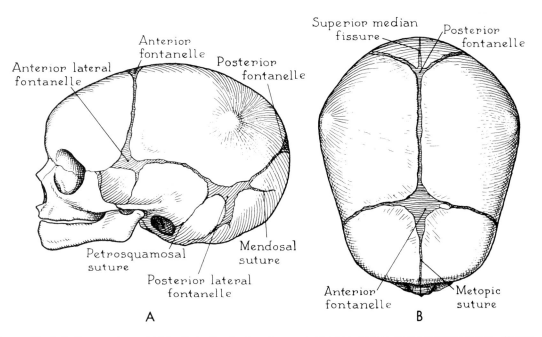

Figure 11–9 ■ The cranium at birth. Note the fontanelles, one at each corner of the parietal bones. (Reproduced with permission from Silverman FN, et al. (eds): CAFFEY'S PEDIATRIC X-RAY DIAGNOSIS, 8th edition. Copyright © 1985 by Year Book Medical Publishers, Inc, Chicago.)

Enlow DH: Handbook of Facial Growth. Philadelphia, WB
Saunders Co, 1982.

Moyers RE: Handbook of Orthodontics. Chicago, Year
Book Medical Publishers, Inc, 1958.

Orban BJ, edited by Sicher H, and Bhaskav SN: Orban's
Oral Histology and Embryology, 9th ed. St. Louis, CV
Mosby Co, 1980.

Ranly DM: A Synopsis of Craniofacial Growth. New York,
Appleton-Century-Crofts, 1980.

Sperber GH: Craniofacial Embryology. Bristol, John Wright
and Sons, Ltd, 1978.

Stewart RE, Barber TK, Troutman KC, Wei SHY: Pediatric
Dentistry: Scientific Foundations and Clinical Practice.
St. Louis, CV Mosby Co, 1982.

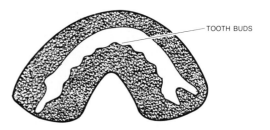

Figure 11–10 ■ Diagrammatic representation of the tooth buds — approximately 8-week-old fetus.

DENTAL CHANGES

C. A. Full

The purpose of this section is to address the growth, development, and eruption of each tooth unit from its initiation to complete eruption. By definition, *growth* signifies an increase, expansion, or extension of any given tissue. For example, a tooth grows as more enamel is deposited by ameloblasts. *Development* addresses the progressive evolution of a tissue(s). A tooth develops as the ameloblasts develop from less specific ectodermal tissue and as the dentinoblasts develop from unspecialized mesoderm.

Teeth are formed by tissues originating from both ectoderm and mesoderm. At approximately 6 weeks of age, the basal layer of the oral epithelium of the fetus shows areas of increased activity and enlargement in the areas of the future dental arches. This increase and expansion give rise to the dental lamina of the future tooth germ. As the tooth bud continues to develop, it reaches a point at which it is recognized as the cap stage. At this time, it will begin to incorporate mesoderm into its structure. Therefore, the tooth-forming organ is initially formed from ectoderm but shortly thereafter includes mesoderm.

The expansion of tissue on the epithelial borders represents the beginning of the life cycle of the tooth. The ectoderm will become responsible for the future enamel, and the mesoderm will become primarily responsible for pulp and dentin. The tooth germ is accountable for the development of the following three formative tissues:

1. Dental organ (epithelial)
2. Dental papilla
3. Dental sac

The 6-week-old fetus demonstrates ten sites of epithelial activity on the occlusal (soft tissue) border of both the developing maxilla and mandible (Brauer et al, 1959). These sites are lined next to each other and ultimately predict the position for the future ten primary teeth in both the maxilla and mandible (Fig. 11–10).

In addition to developing 20 primary teeth, each unit also develops a dental lamina that is responsible for the development of the future permanent tooth (Orban, 1957). Therefore, the primary centrals, laterals, and cuspids produce a dental lamina for the future permanent centrals, laterals, and cuspids. The first and second primary molars produce a dental lamina for the future first and second permanent premolars. The uncounted-for permanent molars develop from and on three successive locations on one dental lamina extending distally from each of the second primary molars (Fig. 11–11) (Orban, 1957).

An analysis describing the successive periods of growth of the tooth germ can be organized by the following stages of the life cycle of the tooth (Orban, 1957):

Growth
    Initiation
    Proliferation
    Histodifferentiation
    Morphodifferentiation
    Apposition
Calcification
Eruption
Attrition

Growth

INITIATION (Fig. 11–12)

The initiation stage is first noticed in the 6-week-old fetus. As the word initiation suggests, this stage is recognized by the initial formation of an expansion of the basal layer of the oral cavity immediately above the basement membrane. The basal layer is a row of organized cells

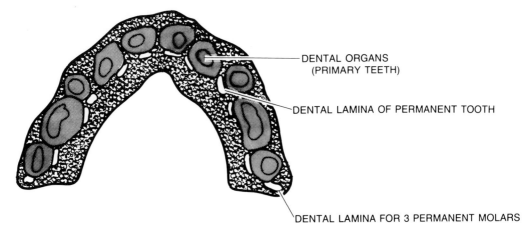

DENTAL ORGANS
(PRIMARY TEETH)

DENTAL LAMINA OF PERMANENT TOOTH

DENTAL LAMINA FOR 3 PERMANENT MOLARS

Figure 11–11 ■ Diagrammatic representation of the dental organs and dental lamina—approximately 4-month-old fetus.

lined up on the basement membrane, which is a tissue division line between the ectoderm (epithelium) and mesoderm (Fig. 11–13). The cells of the basal layer are the innermost cells of the oral epithelium (ectoderm) adjacent to the basement membrane.

At ten specific intermittent locations along the basement membrane, the cells of the basal layer multiply at a much faster rate than the surrounding cells (Schour and Massler, 1940). This development is at that point on the oral epithelium that is the tooth bud and is responsible for the initial growth of that tooth (Fig. 11–14).

It can be noted that the times of initiation of the various teeth differ (Brauer et al, 1959). This period of tooth development is also recognized as the bud stage. Such a description assists in

visually understanding the developmental process of the immature tooth.

PROLIFERATION (Fig. 11–15)

Proliferation is really only a further multiplication of the cells of the initiation stage and an expansion of the tooth bud resulting in the formation of the tooth germ. The tooth germ is a result of the prolific epithelial cells forming a cap-like appearance with the subsequent incorporation of the mesoderm. This incorporation of mesodermal tissue below and within the cap gives rise to the dental papilla.

The mesenchyme (mesoderm) surrounding the dental organ and dental papilla is the tissue that will form the dental sac. The dental sac

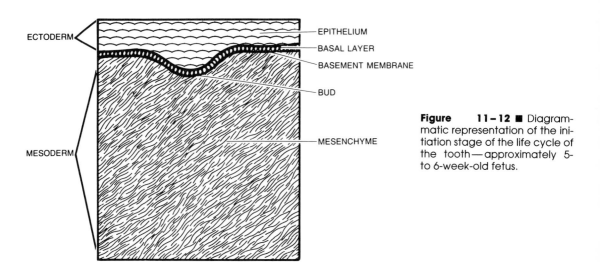

ECTODERM

MESODERM

EPITHELIUM

BASAL LAYER

BASEMENT MEMBRANE

BUD

MESENCHYME

Figure 11–12 ■ Diagrammatic representation of the initiation stage of the life cycle of the tooth—approximately 5- to 6-week-old fetus.

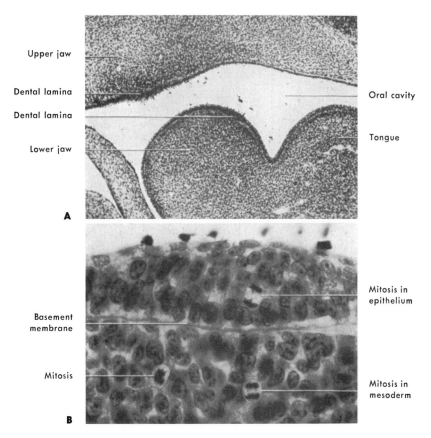

Figure 11–13 ■ Initiation of tooth development. Human embryo 13.5 mm long, fifth week. *A*, Sagittal section through upper and lower jaws. *B*, High magnification of thickened oral epithelium. (From Orban B: Dental Histology and Embryology, 2nd ed. New York, McGraw-Hill, 1929.)

ultimately gives rise to the supporting structures of the tooth. These structures are the cementum and periodontal ligament.

As the tooth germ continues to proliferate in an irregular fashion, it produces a cap-like appearance. This stage is called the cap stage because the structure takes on the form of a cap (Fig. 11–16). Like the bud stage, it is so referenced for visual identification. As the cap begins to form, the mesenchyme changes within the cap to initiate the development of the dental papilla.

The dental papilla is evolved from the mesenchyme invaginating the inner dental epithelium and specializing to form the pulp and dentin.

The dental sac also comes into being by a marginal condensation in the mesenchyme surrounding the dental organ and dental papilla.

The stellate (star-like) reticulum (network) is an organization of cells within the descending portion of the dental organ that is enamel-forming tissue and that is also called the enamel pulp.

Therefore, the tooth germ during this stage has all the necessary formative tissues to embrace the development of a tooth and its periodontal ligament (Orban, 1957).

In summary, the tooth germ consists of all the necessary elements for the development of the complete tooth. The germ is composed of the following three distinct parts: (1) dental organ, (2) dental papilla, and (3) dental sac. The dental organ produces the enamel. The dental papilla generates the dentin and pulp. The dental sac gives rise to the cementum and periodontal ligament (Orban, 1957).

HISTODIFFERENTIATION (Fig. 11–17)

The histodifferentiation stage is marked by the difference histologically in the appearance of the cells of the tooth germ because they are

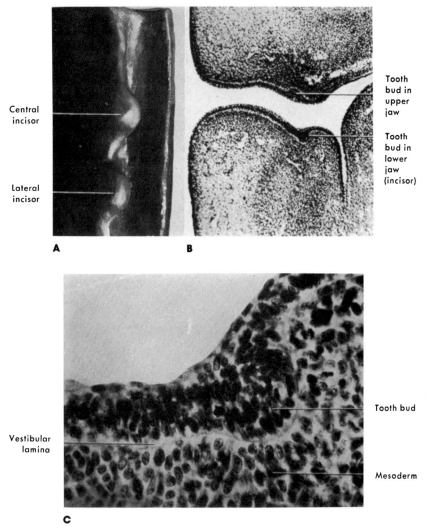

Central incisor

Lateral incisor

Tooth bud in upper jaw

Tooth bud in lower jaw (incisor)

A   B

Vestibular lamina

Tooth bud

Mesoderm

C

Figure 11-14 ■ Bud stage of tooth development (proliferation stage). Human embryo 16 mm. long, sixth week. *A*, Wax reconstruction of the germs of the central and lateral lower incisors. *B*, Sagittal section through upper and lower jaws. *C*, High magnification view of the tooth germ of the lower incisor in bud stage. (From Orban B: Dental Histology and Embryology, 2nd ed. New York, McGraw-Hill, 1929.)

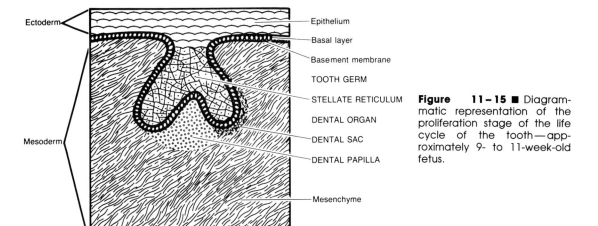

Ectoderm

Epithelium

Basal layer

Basement membrane

TOOTH GERM

STELLATE RETICULUM

DENTAL ORGAN

DENTAL SAC

DENTAL PAPILLA

Mesoderm

Mesenchyme

Figure 11-15 ■ Diagrammatic representation of the proliferation stage of the life cycle of the tooth—approximately 9- to 11-week-old fetus.

122

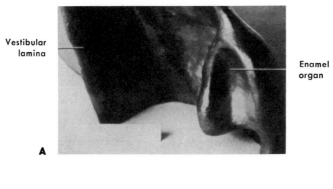

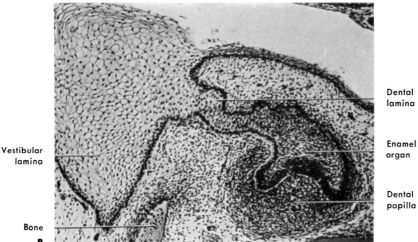

Figure 11 – 16 ■ Cap stage of tooth development. Human embryo 60 mm long, eleventh week. *A,* Wax reconstruction of the dental organ of the lower lateral incisor. *B,* Labiolingual section through the same tooth. (From Orban B: Dental Histology and Embryology, 2nd ed. New York, McGraw-Hill, 1929.)

now beginning to specialize. The cap continues to grow and takes more of the appearance of a bell. The image of a bell is registered because the extensions of the cap grow deeper into the mesoderm. This segment of development is appropriately called the bell stage. The tissue

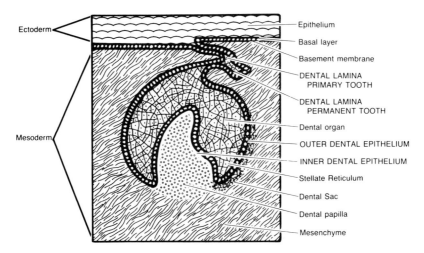

Figure 11 – 17 ■ Diagrammatic representation of the histodifferentiation stage of the life cycle of the tooth. Approximately 14-week-old fetus.

within the bell is the tissue that gives rise to the dental papilla.

The dental organ is now completely surrounded by the basement membrane and is divided into an inner and outer dental epithelium. The dental organ ultimately becomes enamel.

The condensation of the tissue (mesoderm) adjacent to the outside of the bell is responsible for the dental sac. The dental sac ultimately gives rise to the cementum, which is the covering of the tooth's root, and to the periodontal ligament, which attaches the tooth to the bone around the tooth root(s).

The dental lamina continues to shrink to look more like a cord. The dental lamina for the permanent successor becomes obvious as an extension of the primary tooth dental lamina. The basal layer continues its existence and is now divided into an inner and an outer dental epithelium. The stellate reticulum expands and or-

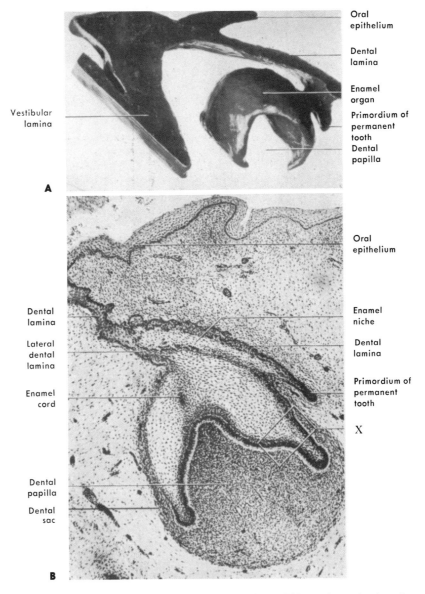

Figure 11–18 ■ Bell stage of tooth development. Human embryo 105 mm long, fourteenth week. *A,* Wax reconstruction of lower central incisor. *B,* Labiolingual section of the same tooth. "X" designates inset (see Fig. 11–19). (From Orban B: Dental Histology and Embryology, 2nd ed. New York, McGraw-Hill, 1929.)

ganizes to incorporate more intercellular fluid in preparation for the formation of enamel (Figs. 11–18, 11–19, and 11–20).

MORPHODIFFERENTIATION (Fig. 11–21)

The morphodifferentiation stage, as the name implies, is the stage at which the cells find an arrangement that ultimately dictates the final size and shape of the tooth (Brauer et al, 1959). This stage is called an advanced bell stage (Fig. 11–21). The cells of the inner dental epithelium become the ameloblasts, which produce the enamel matrix. As the ameloblasts begin their formation, the tissue of the dental papilla immediately adjacent to the basement membrane begins to differentiate into odontoblasts (Figs. 11–22 and 11–23). The odontoblasts and the ameloblasts are responsible for the formation of dentin and enamel, respectively.

Although the development of dentin is not clearly understood, structures have been identified that show progressive changes. The change in dentin formation first seen is a thickening of the basement membrane of the inner dental epithelium and the pulp developed by the dental papilla. The membrane from the mesenchyme of the pulp consists of fine reticular fibrils. A continuation of growth is noted by a formation of irregular spiraling fibers from deep in the pulp to then entangle with the reticular fibrils from the mesenchyme of the pulp. These long spiraling fibers are known as Korff's fibers and assist in the structural support of the developing dentin (Fig. 11–24) (Orban, 1957).

The specialized cells of the previous stage now arrange themselves in a manner to give each tooth its prescribed size and shape. There is a disappearance of the dental lamina except for the dental lamina proper immediately adjacent to the developing primary tooth.

The dental lamina proper continues to proliferate to the lingual of the primary tooth to begin the development of the permanent tooth. The primary tooth germ now becomes a free internal organ (Orban, 1957). The specialized cells found during the histodifferentiation stage and the organization of these specialized cells found during morphodifferentiation, respectively, prepare the tooth for the development of the various tissues of enamel, dentin, pulp, cementum, and periodontal ligament.

APPOSITION (Fig. 11–25)

Whereas the morphodifferentiation stage dictates the size and shape of the tooth, the appositional stage is when the network or tissue matrix of the tooth is formed. The cells having the potential for the deposition of the extracellular matrix fulfill the plan of the tooth germ

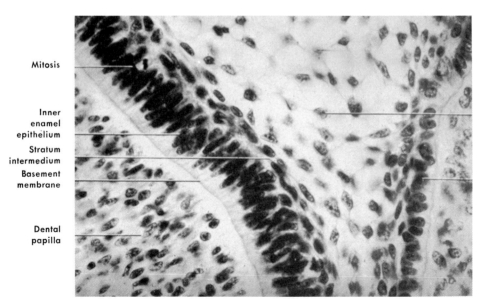

Figure 11–19 ■ The four layers of the epithelial dental organ in high magnification (area "X" of Fig. 11–18). (From Orban B: Dental Histology and Embryology, 2nd ed. New York, McGraw-Hill, 1929.)

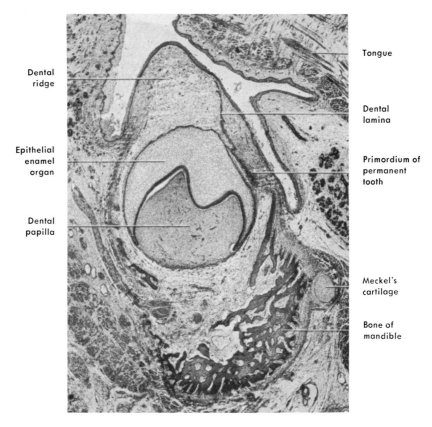

Figure 11–20 ■ Advanced bell stage of tooth development. Human embryo 200 mm long, age about 18 weeks. Labiolingual section through the first primary lower molar. (From Bhaskar, S: Synopsis of Oral Histology. St. Louis, CV Mosby, 1962, p 44.)

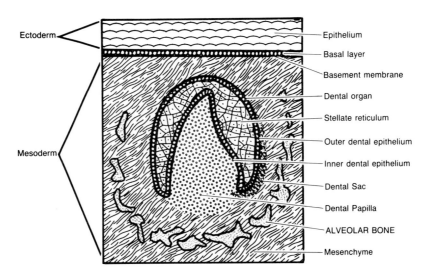

Figure 11–21 ■ Diagrammatic representation of the morphodifferentiation stage of the life cycle of the tooth. Approximately 18-week-old fetus.

established by previous stages. The growth is appositional, additive, and regular. This accounts for the layered-like appearance of enamel and dentin (Orban, 1957). The organized special tissues now deposit incremental layers of enamel and dentin matrix. The matrices layered by ameloblasts and odontoblasts begin from a growth center along the dentino-enamel and dentino-cemental junction (Figs. 11–26 and 11–27).

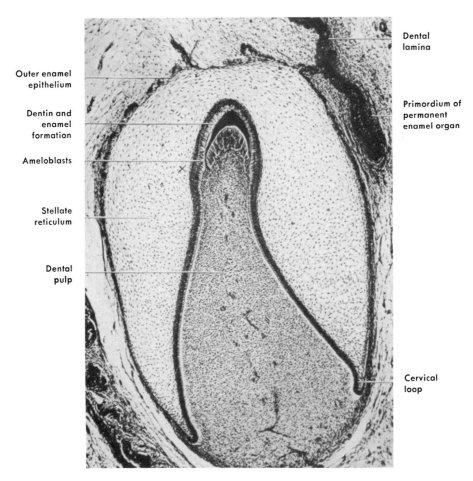

Figure 11–22 ■ Tooth germ (lower incisor) of a human fetus (fifth month). Beginning of dentin and enamel formation. The stellate reticulum at the tip of the crown reduced in thickness. "X" designates inset (see Figure 11–23). (From Diamond M and Applebaum E: J Dent Res *21*:403, 1942.)

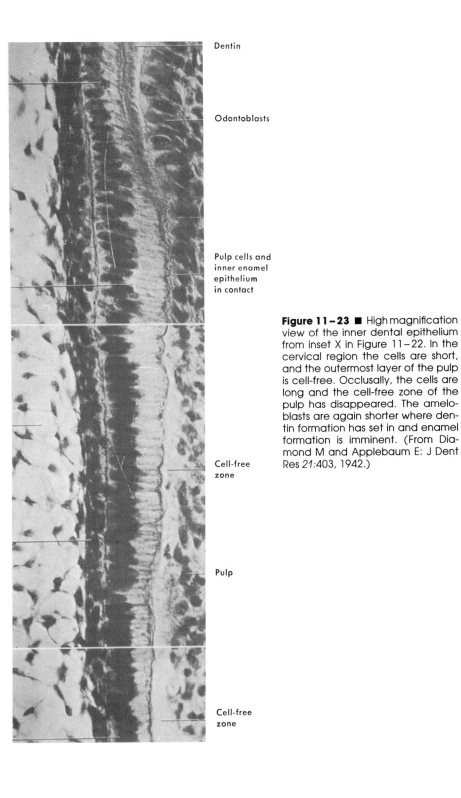

Ameloblasts

Cells of inner
enamel epithelium

Stellate reticulum

Stratum intermedium

Cells of inner
enamel epithelium

Dentin

Odontoblasts

Pulp cells and
inner enamel
epithelium
in contact

Cell-free
zone

Pulp

Cell-free
zone

Figure 11–23 ■ High magnification view of the inner dental epithelium from inset X in Figure 11–22. In the cervical region the cells are short, and the outermost layer of the pulp is cell-free. Occlusally, the cells are long and the cell-free zone of the pulp has disappeared. The ameloblasts are again shorter where dentin formation has set in and enamel formation is imminent. (From Diamond M and Applebaum E: J Dent Res *21*:403, 1942.)

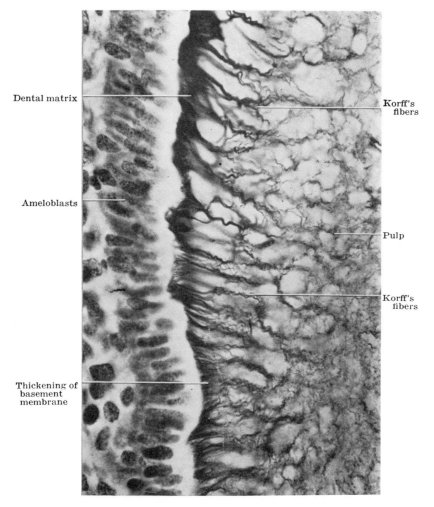

Figure 11–24 ■ Thickening of the basement membrane between pulp and inner dental epithelium— development of Korff's fibers. (Reproduced by permission from Bevelander G: *In* Sicher H and Bhaskar SN (eds): Orban's Oral Histology and Embryology, 7th ed, St. Louis, 1972, The C.V. Mosby Co.)

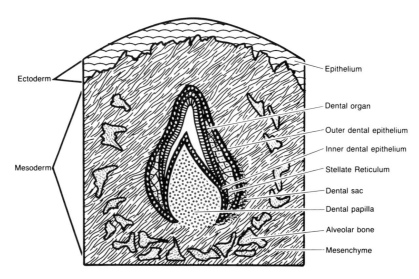

Ectoderm

Mesoderm

Epithelium

Dental organ

Outer dental epithelium

Inner dental epithelium

Stellate Reticulum

Dental sac

Dental papilla

Alveolar bone

Mesenchyme

Figure 11 – 25 ■ Diagrammatic representation of the apposition stage of the life cycle of the tooth.

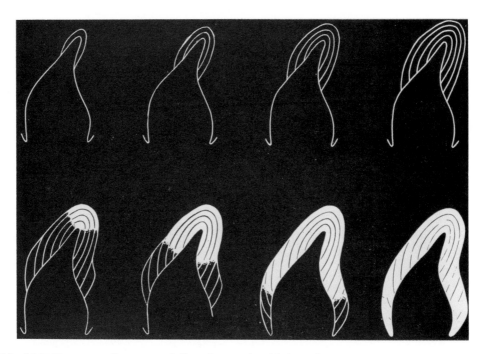

Figure 11 – 26 ■ Diagrammatic representation of enamel matrix formation and maturation. Formation follows an incremental pattern; maturation begins at the tip of the crown and proceeds cervically in cross relation to the incremental pattern. (Modified from Diamond and Weinmann. Reproduced by permission from Orban B: Oral Histology and Embryology, 4th ed, St. Louis, 1957, The C.V. Mosby Co.)

Calcification (Fig. 11 – 28)

Calcification occurs by an influx of mineral salts within the previously developed tissue matrix. The chemical structure of enamel consists of approximately 96% inorganic material and approximately 4% organic material and water. The inorganic portion is composed primarily of calcium and phosphorus, with a small portion of many other compounds and elements, such as carbon dioxide, magnesium, and sodium, to mention a few (Table 11 – 5).

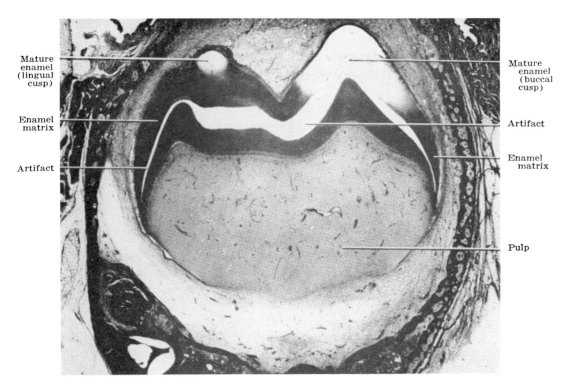

Figure 11–27 ■ Buccolingual section through a deciduous molar. Maturation of the enamel has started in the lingual cusp, while it has fairly well progressed in the buccal cusp. Note the gradual transition between the enamel matrix and the fully matured enamel. (Modified from Diamond and Weinmann. Reproduced by permission from Orban B: Oral Histology and Embryology, 4th ed, St. Louis, 1957, The C.V. Mosby Co.)

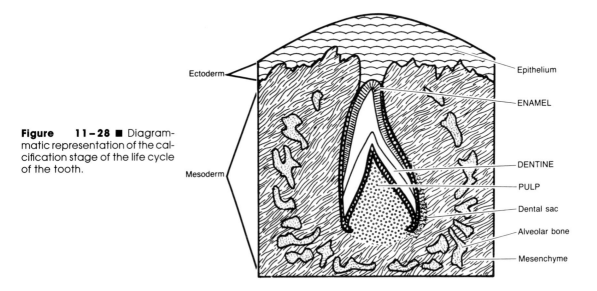

Figure 11–28 ■ Diagrammatic representation of the calcification stage of the life cycle of the tooth.

Calcification begins by the precipitation of enamel in the cusp tips and incisal edges of the teeth and continues with production of more layers on these small points of origin. Therefore, the older or more mature enamel is found at the cusp tips or incisal edges and the new enamel is at the cervical region (see Figs. 11–26 and 11–27).

The calcification of enamel and dentin is a very sensitive process that takes place over a

Table 11–5 ■ Chemical contents of enamel, dentin, cementum, and bone

	Enamel	Dentin	Cementum Compact Bone
Water	2.3%	13.2%	32%
Organic matter	1.7	17.5	22
Ash	96.0	69.3	46
In 100 Gm. of ash:			
Calcium	36.1 Gm.	35.3 Gm.	35.5 Gm.
Phosphorus	17.3	17.1	17.1
Carbon dioxide	3.0	4.0	4.4
Magnesium	0.5	1.2	0.9
Sodium	0.2	0.2	1.1
Potassium	0.3	0.07	0.1
Chloride	0.3	0.03	0.1
Fluorine	0.016	0.017	0.015
Sulfur	0.1	0.2	0.6
Copper	0.01		
Silicon	0.003		0.04
Iron	0.0025		0.09
Zinc	0.016	0.018	

	Whole Teeth	Bone
Lead	0.0071 to 0.037	0.002 to 0.02

Small amounts of: Ce, La, Pr, Ne,
Ag, Sr, Ba, Cr, Sn, Mn, Ti, Ni, V, Al, B, Cu,
Li, Se

(Reproduced by permission from Sicher, Harry: Orban's Oral histology and embryology, ed. 5, St. Louis, 1962, The C. V. Mosby Co.; compiled by Dr. Harold C. Hodge.)

long period of time. Therefore, calcification irregularities noted in any fully developed tooth can often be equated with a specific systemic disturbance (Brauer et al, 1959). In the cross section of the clinical crown of a tooth that has been prepared for histologic view, there are apparent lines or bands, which are called the incremental lines of Retzius (Fig. 11–29). Depending on how the section is prepared (either longitudinally or horizontally), the incremental lines of Retzius may appear as lines or circles (Fig. 11–30). These lines or circles represent the developmental pattern of the developing tooth.

The degree of variation of any line usually reflects a reaction to a change in the physiologic processes of growth and development of the tooth. For instance, in the primary teeth there is an incremental line of Retzius called the neonatal line or neonatal ring (Fig. 11–31). This neonatal line is due to the abrupt change in certain bodily processes of the fetus when it is born. At that time, there is enough of a change or insult to the newborn's systems to cause a growth change that is reflected dentally as a neonatal ring (Orban, 1957). This ring is actually due to disturbances in the growth and calcification of the tooth.

In summary, the aspect of enamel maturation labeled calcification involves the hardening of the already previously formed matrix by the precipitation of mineral salts (inorganic calcium salts). This calcification is a slow, gradual process beginning at the cusp tip or incisal edge of the tooth (see Fig. 11–27).

Eruption (Fig. 11–32)

It is necessary to discuss briefly root development before addressing eruption. The develop-

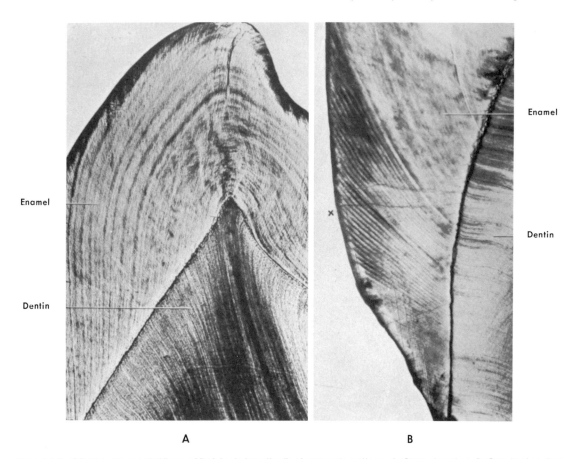

Enamel

Dentin

Enamel

Dentin

A   B

Figure 11–29 ■ Incremental lines of Retzius in longitudinal ground sections. *A*, Cuspal region. *B*, Cervical region (X). (Reproduced by permission from Bhaskar, S.N., editor: Orban's Oral histology and embryology, ed. 10, St. Louis, 1986, The C.V. Mosby Co.)

mental process of the crown of the tooth involves many overlaying processes at one time. The same is true for the root. Root development has correlations with eruption. When the clinical crown of the tooth has completed its formation, the inner and outer epithelium appear to fold over at the cemento-enamel junction and continue their growth without any tissue between them. Previously, stellate reticulum was there. The inner and outer dental epithelium without the stellate reticulum is now called Hertwig's epithelial root sheath, which is responsible for the size and shape of the root and eruption of the tooth (Fig. 11–33) (Orban, 1957).

Eruption can be categorized into three different phases: (1) pre-eruptive phase, (2) eruptive phase (prefunctional), and (3) eruptive phase (functional). The pre-eruptive phase is that period during which the tooth root begins its formation and begins to move toward the surface

of the oral cavity from its bony vault. The prefunctional eruptive phase consists of that period of development of the tooth root through gingival emergence. Most eruption tables report the time that the tooth can be first seen in the mouth (Figs. 11–34 and 11–35). The tooth root is usually approximately one half to two thirds of its final length at the time of gingival emergence.

After the tooth has erupted into the oral cavity and meets its antagonist (opposing tooth in the opposite arch), it is considered to be in the functional eruptive phase. Teeth remain a dynamic unit in that some type of movement is always taking place no matter how slight that movement might be. Teeth will continue to move and erupt as necessary as the body continues to change throughout life (Orban, 1957).

There has been considerable speculation on the causes of tooth eruption. Some examples of causes for tooth eruption often cited are (1) root

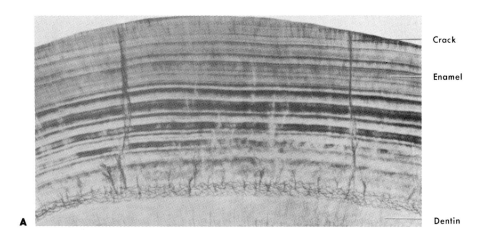

Figure 11–30 ■ *A*, Incremental lines of Retzius in transverse ground section, arranged concentrically. *B*, Decalcified paraffin section of exfoliated primary molar (×20). Heavy dark lamella runs from darkly stained dentin to surface in an irregular course independent of developmental pattern. Roughly parallel to dentin surface are seen a number of incremental lines, one of which, the neonatal line, is accentuated. (Reproduced by permission from Bhaskar, S.N., editor: Orban's Oral histology and embryology, ed. 10, St. Louis, 1986, The C.V. Mosby Co.)

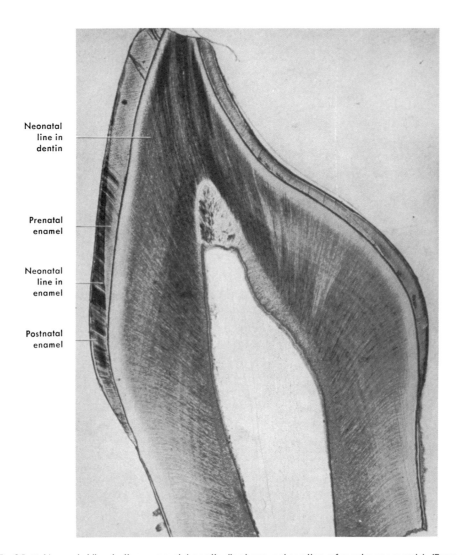

Neonatal
line in
dentin

Prenatal
enamel

Neonatal
line in
enamel

Postnatal
enamel

Figure 11–31 ■ Neonatal line in the enamel. Longitudinal ground section of a primary cuspid. (From Schour I: JADA 23:1947–1950, 1936. Copyright by the American Dental Association. Reprinted by permission.)

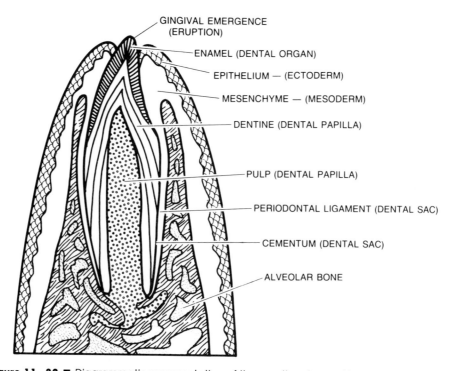

Figure 11–32 ■ Diagrammatic representation of the eruption stage of the life cycle of the tooth.

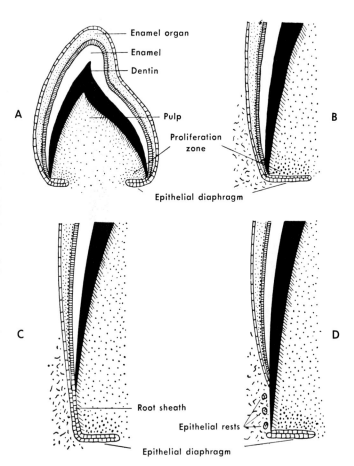

Figure 11-33 ■ Three stages in root development (diagrams). *A,* Section through a tooth germ showing the epithelial diaphragm and proliferation zone of the pulp. *B,* Higher magnification view of the cervical region of *A. C,* Imaginary stage showing the elongation of Hertwig's epithelial sheath between diaphragm and future cemento-enamel junction. Differentiation of odontoblasts in the elongated pulp. *D,* In the cervical part of the root, dentin has been formed. The root sheath is broken up into epithelial rests and is separated from the dentinal surface by connective tissue. Differentiation of cementoblasts. (Reproduced by permission from Bhaskar, S.N., editor: Orban's Oral histology and embryology, ed. 10, St. Louis, 1986, The C.V. Mosby Co.)

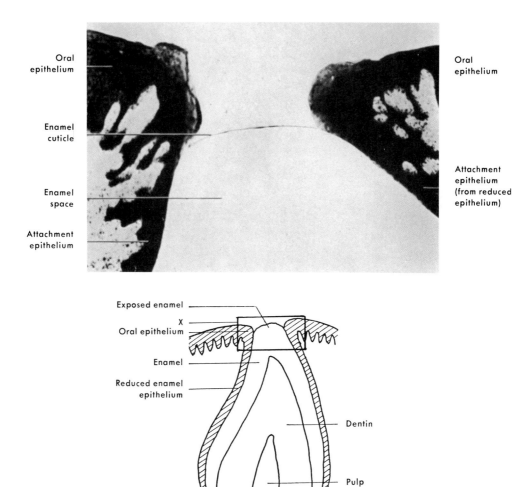

Figure 11–34 ■ Tooth emerges through a perforation in the fused epithelia. "X" in diagram indicates area from which the photomicrograph was taken. (Reproduced by permission from Bhaskar, S.N., editor: Orban's Oral histology and embryology, ed. 10, St. Louis, 1986, The C.V. Mosby Co.)

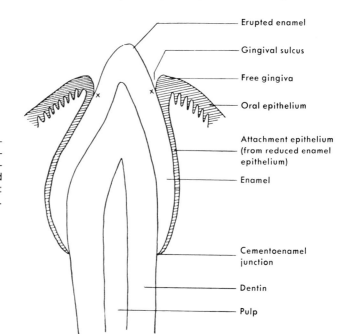

Figure 11–35 ■ Diagrammatic representation of the attached epithelial cuff and gingival sulcus at an early stage of tooth eruption. Bottom of sulcus is at "X." (Reproduced by permission from Bhaskar, S.N., editor: Orban's Oral histology and embryology, ed. 10, St. Louis, 1986, The C.V. Mosby Co.)

formation, (2) proliferation of Hertwig's epithelial root sheath, (3) proliferation of the connective tissue of the dental papilla, (4) simultaneous growth of the jaw, (5) pressures from muscular action, and (6) apposition and resorption of bone. Because of this myriad of processes happening at the time of eruption, it is difficult to single out any one process as the primary cause of tooth eruption.

The process of elimination of primary teeth is caused by the eruptive pressure of the permanent successor at the apex of the primary tooth and its surroundings. The eruptive pressure stimulates the development of osteoclasts. A progressive resorption of the tooth root, dentin, and cementum as well as adjacent bone is completed by the action of the osteoclasts.

Attrition (Fig. 11–36)

Attrition is the wearing of the teeth during function. It is the normal wearing of the teeth during contact with opposing teeth in occlusion. It is easy to understand why certain types of food and associated habits may cause more or less wear from individual to individual (Brauer et al, 1959). The effects of attrition on occlusion are adjusted for by further functional eruption.

A diagrammatic illustration summarizing the life cycle of the tooth from initiation through attrition is shown in Figure 11–37.

The Primary Dentition to Age Three

Table 11–6 demonstrates the various stages of development of the teeth from conception to adolescence (Finn, 1973). The primary teeth

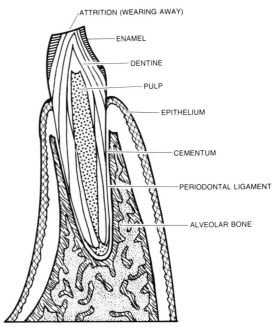

Figure 11–36 ■ Diagrammatic representation of the attrition stage of the life cycle of the tooth.

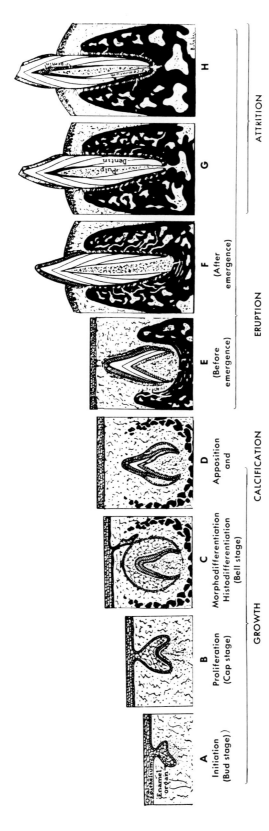

Figure 11–37 ■ Diagrammatic representation of the life cycle of the tooth. (Reproduced by permission from Sharawy, Mohamed, and Bhussry, Baldev Raj: Development and growth of teeth. In Bhaskar, S.N., editor: Orban's Oral histology and embryology, ed. 10. St. Louis, 1986, The C.V. Mosby Co.: modified from Schour, I., and Massler, M.: J. Am. Dent. Assoc., 27:1785, 1940. Copyright by the American Dental Association. Reprinted by permission.)

Table 11–6 ■ Chronology of the human dentition

Tooth	Hard Tissue Formation Begins	Amount of Enamel Formed at Birth	Enamel Completed	Eruption	Root Completed
Primary Dentition					
Maxillary					
Central incisor	4 mos. in utero	Five sixths	1½ mos.	7½ mos.	1½ yrs.
Lateral incisor	4½ mos. in utero	Two thirds	2½ mos.	9 mos.	2 yrs.
Cuspid	5 mos. in utero	One third	9 mos.	18 mos.	3¼ yrs.
First molar	5 mos. in utero	Cusps united	6 mos.	14 mos.	2½ yrs.
Second molar	6 mos. in utero	Cusp tips still isolated	11 mos.	24 mos.	3 yrs.
Mandibular					
Central incisor	4½ mos. in utero	Three fifths	2½ mos.	6 mos.	1½ yrs.
Lateral incisor	4½ mos. in utero	Three fifths	3 mos.	7 mos.	1½ yrs.
Cuspid	5 mos. in utero	One third	9 mos.	16 mos.	3¼ yrs.
First molar	5 mos. in utero	Cusps united	5½ mos.	12 mos.	2¼ yrs.
Second molar	6 mos. in utero	Cusp tips still isolated	10 mos.	20 mos.	3 yrs.
Permanent Dentition					
Maxillary					
Central incisor	3 – 4 mos.	· · · · · ·	4 –5 yrs.	7– 8 yrs.	10 yrs.
Lateral incisor	10 –12 mos.	· · · · · ·	4 –5 yrs.	8– 9 yrs.	11 yrs.
Cuspid	4 – 5 mos.	· · · · · ·	6 –7 yrs.	11–12 yrs.	13–15 yrs.
First bicuspid	1½– 1¾ yrs.	· · · · · ·	5 –6 yrs.	10–11 yrs.	12–13 yrs.
Second biscuspid	2 – 2¼ yrs.	· · · · · ·	6 –7 yrs.	10–12 yrs.	12–14 yrs.
First molar	at birth	Sometimes a trace	2½–3 yrs.	6– 7 yrs.	9–10 yrs.
Second molar	2½– 3 yrs.	· · · · · ·	7 –8 yrs.	12–13 yrs.	14–16 yrs.
Mandibular					
Central incisor	3 – 4 mos.	· · · · · ·	4 –5 yrs.	6– 7 yrs.	9 yrs.
Lateral incisor	3 – 4 mos.	· · · · · ·	4 –5 yrs.	7– 8 yrs.	10 yrs.
Cuspid	4 – 5 mos.	· · · · · ·	6 –7 yrs.	9–10 yrs.	12–14 yrs.
First bicuspid	1¾– 2 yrs.	· · · · · ·	5 –6 yrs.	10–12 yrs.	12–13 yrs.
Second biscuspid	2¼– 2½ yrs.	· · · · · ·	6 –7 yrs.	11–12 yrs.	13–14 yrs.
First molar	at birth	Sometimes a trace	2½–3 yrs.	6– 7 yrs.	9–10 yrs.
Second molar	2½– 3 yrs.	· · · · · ·	7 –8 yrs.	11–13 yrs.	14–15 yrs.

After Logan and Kronfeld: J.A.D.A., *20*, 1933 (slightly modified by McCall and Schour). Copyright by the American Dental Association. Reprinted by permission.

begin to form at 7 weeks *in utero,* and the enamel of all of the primary teeth is usually completed by the first year of age. All of the primary teeth will generally have erupted by 24–36 months of age. The root structure of these same primary teeth will be complete usually by age 3 years (Finn, 1973).

At birth, an histologic analysis of the teeth of the maxilla and mandible will in most cases show the appearance of some degree of calcification of 24 tooth units. The 24 tooth units will be all 20 primary teeth and the 4 first permanent molars (Figs. 11–38 and 11–39).

The first primary tooth to erupt is the mandibular primary incisor. This tooth usually erupts in a vertical upright position (Brauer et al, 1959). As other primary teeth erupt, they may be spaced apart from each other, particularly in the incisor area. Spaces frequently recognized in the primary dentition are the primate spaces (Fig. 11–40). Primate spaces are the spaces between the mandibular primary cuspid and first primary molar, and between the maxillary primary lateral incisor and primary cuspid. The

primary dentition remains relatively stable until it is influenced by the focus of the erupting permanent dentitions.

The Permanent Dentition to Age Three

The first permanent molar is the first tooth to show germ formation at age 3½–4 months *in utero.* It is followed by the central and lateral incisors, which demonstrate formation at 5–5½ months *in utero.* The cuspid is the only other permanent tooth that begins its formation before birth at 5½–6 months *in utero.* The first and second bicuspids and the second and third molars demonstrate germ formation after birth.

At birth, the only teeth that show a trace of hard tissue formation are the first permanent molars (Brauer et al, 1959). With the exception of the third molars, all permanent teeth demonstrate hard tissue formation by 3 years of age (Finn, 1973) (see Table 11–6).

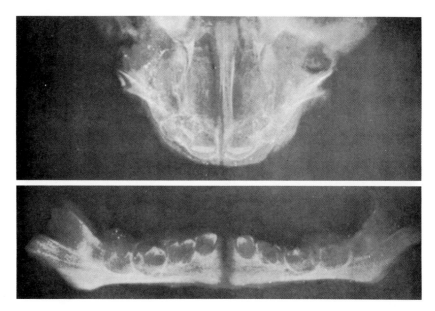

Figure 11–38 ■ Wet specimen from 8-month fetus. Note areas of dental calcification in the mandibular incisors, cuspids, and first primary molars, as well as in the maxillary central and lateral incisors and first primary molars. There is only slight calcification in the maxillary cuspids and cusp tips of the second primary molars. (From McCall JO, and Wald SS: *Clinical Dental Roentgenology,* 4th ed. Philadelphia, WB Saunders Co, 1957, p 153.)

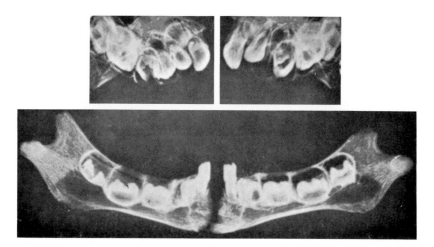

Figure 11–39 ■ Wet specimen from infant at birth. Note areas of dental calcification similar to those shown in Figure 11–38. Maxillary calcification is slightly less advanced. (From McCall JO, and Wald SS: Clinical Dental Roentgenology, 4th ed. Philadelphia, WB Saunders Co, 1957, p 154.)

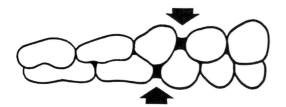

Figure 11–40 ■ Primate spaces between the maxillary primary lateral incisor and primary canine and between mandibular primary canine and mandibular first molar. (From Finn, SB: Clinical Periodontics, 4th ed. Philadelphia, WB Saunders Co, 1973; after Baume, LJ: J Dent Res *29:*442, 1950.)

GLOSSARY

Ameloblast ■ One of a group of cells originating from the ectoderm from which the dental enamel is developed; an enamel cell. The ameloblasts cover the papilla of the enamel organ.

Apposition ■ Appositional growth is that stage of the life cycle of the developing tooth during which a layer-like deposition of a non-vital extracellular secretion is laid down in the form of tissue matrix.

Attrition ■ A rubbing or friction. In dentistry, the term refers to the natural wearing away of the substance of a tooth under the stress of mastication.

Basal layer ■ Basal is an adjective meaning pertaining to or situated near a base. In the developing tooth, the basal layer is that tissue at the junction of the ectoderm and mesoderm.

Basement membrane ■ The delicate, transparent, membranous layer of cells underlying the epithelium of mucous membranes and secreting glands at the junction of the ectoderm and mesoderm.

Bud stage ■ The initial expansion of cells of the ectoderm in the developmental life cycle of the tooth.

Calcification ■ The process by which organic tissue becomes hardened by a deposit of calcium salts within its substance.

Cap stage ■ The step of tooth development after the bud stage and before the bell stage, which is caused by unequal growth of the cells of the basal layer descending into the mesoderm to form the appearance of a cap.

Cementoblast ■ One of the cells arising from the mesoderm from which the cementum of the tooth is developed.

Cementum ■ The layer of bony tissue covering the root of a tooth. It differs in structure from ordinary bone by containing a greater number of Sharpey's fibers (see *Sharpey's fibers*).

Dental lamina ■ *Dental*—pertaining to a tooth or teeth; *lamina*—a thin leaf or plate of something, such as bone; *dental lamina*—dental ridge; a band of thickening of the epithelium along the margin of the gum, in the embryo, from which the enamel organ is ultimately developed.

Dental organ (enamel organ) ■ A process of epithelium forming a cap over the dental papilla from which the enamel is developed.

Dental papilla ■ A process of condensed mesenchyme within the dental organ and cap from which the dentin and dental pulp are formed.

Dental sac ■ A process of condensed mesenchyme surrounding the dental organ and dental papilla from which the cementum and periodontal ligament are formed.

Dentinoblast ■ A cell found on the pulpal side of the dentino-enamel junction differentiated from an odontoblast to form dentin.

Ectoderm ■ The outer layer of the primitive (two-layered) embryo from which the epidermis and the neural tube are developed.

Enamel pulp ■ The soft material from which the dental enamel is developed.

Eruption ■ The act of breaking out, appearing, or becoming visible. For a tooth, it is the process of moving through alveolar bone into the oral cavity.

Hertwig's epithelial root sheath ■ An investment of epithelial cells around the unerupted tooth and inside of the dental follicle, which are derived from the enamel organ.

Histodifferentiation ■ A stage of the life cycle of the tooth identified by the cells of the embryonic tissue becoming specialized. The proliferating cells of ectoderm and mesoderm take on a definite change in this stage in order to be able to produce enamel, dentin, and cementum.

Initiation ■ A stage of the life cycle of the tooth identified as the very first point of its development.

Mesenchyme ■ The embryonic connective tissue; that part of the mesoderm whence are formed the connective tissues of the body as well as the blood vessels and lymphatic vessels.

Mesoderm ■ The middle of three layers of the primitive embryo.

Morphodifferentiation ■ A stage of the life cycle of the tooth identified as that period producing form or shape.

Odontoblast ■ One of the cylindrical connective tissue cells that form the outer surface of the dental pulp adjacent to the dentin. They are connected with each other by protoplasmic processes. Each odontoblast has a long, thread-like process, the dental fibril (or fiber of Tomes), which extends through the dentinal tubule to the dento-enamel junction.

Odontoclast ■ One of the cells that help to absorb the roots of the primary teeth. They occur between the primary teeth and the erupting permanent teeth.

Periodontal ligament ■ Periodontal—situated or occurring around a tooth; pertaining to the

periodontal membrane that attaches the tooth to alveolar bone.

Periodontal membrane ■ The connective tissue occupying the space between the root of a tooth and the alveolar bone and furnishing a firm connection between the root of the tooth and the bone.

Proliferation ■ The reproduction or multiplication of similar forms; a stage in the life cycle of the tooth bud just after the initiation stage.

Sharpey's fibers ■ Cementum is the covering of the tooth root surface. There is also a cementoid tissue covering the cementum, and it is lined with cementoblasts to maintain a dynamic state. There are connective tissue fibers passing through these cementoblasts from the periodontal ligament into the cementum. The embedded portion of the fiber in the cementum is the Sharpey fiber.

Stellate reticulum ■ *Stellate* — shaped like a star, or like stars; *reticulum* — a network, especially a protoplasmic network in cells; *stellate reticulum* — the reticular connective tissue – like epithelium forming the enamel pulp of the developing tooth.

Tooth bud ■ The very initial identification of the developing tooth by the expansion of certain cells in the basal layer of the oral epithelium (ectoderm only).

Tooth germ ■ The rudiment of a tooth, consisting of a dental sac and including the dental papilla and dental organ (enamel organ).

REFERENCES

Brauer JC, Demeritt WW, Higley LB, Lindahl RL, Massler M, Schour I: Dentistry for Children. New York, McGraw-Hill Book Co, 1959.

Finn SB: Clinical Pedodontics. Philadelphia, WB Saunders Co, 1973.

Orban BJ: Oral Histology and Embryology. St. Louis, CV Mosby Co, 1957.

Schour I, Massler M: Studies in tooth development: The growth pattern of human teeth — Part II. JADA 27:1918 – 1931, 1940.

COGNITIVE CHANGES

J. R. Pinkham

Even relatively recently, the human infant has been regarded because of his helplessness as a cognitively incompetent creature. Many psychologists now recognize that there is cognitive ability in the newborn. In fact, there now is evidence that newborns can experience sensations of pain, touch, and changes in bodily position. Also, it is now known that infants can from the first day of life smell, see, and hear. Cognitive competence explains how and why an infant explores a nursing mother's fingers and studies her face.

In 1984, Mussen and coworkers noted that there are four major areas of cognitive development during the first year of a child's life. The first is the area of perception. Even very young infants have the ability of perceiving movement, facial relationships, and color (see Table 11 – 1).

The second prominent cognitive area is recognition of information. It is now known that infants can recognize certain stimuli such as a face when viewed from various and different observational angles. In such a case, it is contended that children have developed mental schemata or representations of things encountered in their consciousness and that these schemata contain some but not all of the crucial elements of the object or event. This allows them to recognize similarity of new objects to old ones because of their ability to generalize on these crucial elements.

The third important cognitive focus is the ability to categorize. Children can group things together by way of their shape, color, and use even by age 1.

Enhancement of memory is the fourth cognitive development of the first year of life. Even very young infants can be shown to have some memory. At age 6 months and older, the ability to recall past experience appears obvious. At this age, most children have the ability to recall

a past event and to utilize the information that they gained from that event to help them pattern a reaction to things presently going on.

Two theories are of interest when studying the cognition of infants. The first is learning theory. The term conditioning is the most important concept used from that body of thought. There are two types of conditioning, classical and operant. Classical conditioning occurs when two stimuli are paired together. For instance, sucking the nipple when paired often enough with hearing a lullaby will eventually lead the infant to initiate sucking when he hears the lullaby.

Instrumental or operant conditioning occurs when a child's actions are reinforced or rewarded. This kind of learning is possible when the parents coo as a response to a child's chortles. It is also possible if the mother gives her crying daughter a cookie to quiet her down. It is contended that rewarded behavior is behavior that is likely to occur again.

The cognitive development theory of Jean Piaget is the other theory of interest when trying to understand infant cognition. According to Piaget, much of the intellectual attainments of the child between birth and age 2 happens because of actions the child has with objects in his environment.

Although piagetian theory is not without some controversy as to its exact accuracy, it is extremely useful to researchers, clinicians, parents, and other observers of infants, since Piaget based his conclusions on observations of his own children's behavior. The behaviors he saw are common to all children.

In 1954, Piaget described the first two years of life as a period of sensorimotor development, which he divided into six discrete stages. Piaget contended that during this time the child must develop knowledge in the following three areas:

1. *Object permanence:* Objects continue to exist even when they are not perceivable by the child.

2. *Causality:* Objects have uses, and events have causes. Piaget used the term circular reaction (primary, secondary, and tertiary) to describe a child's changes in this area. A primary circular reaction describes recreating an already known satisfying action, such as thumb sucking. A secondary circular reaction is the recreating of an accidentally discovered cause and effect. Tertiary circular reactions involve experimentation, and, as one might guess, such behaviors often exasperate the child's parents.

3. *Symbolic play:* One object can represent another.

The language development of the infant is, at first, very slow. The mean expressive vocabulary of an 18-month-old is ten words. At this time, the receptive vocabulary of the child is considerably higher than the expressive vocabulary.

Toward the end of the second year, the expressive vocabulary of children develops extraordinarily fast. In 1983, Levine and colleagues noted that at 3 years of age the mean vocabulary of a child is 1000 words.

Table 11–1 of the previous physical change section coordinates the six stages of the sensorimotor stage of development with cognition, play, and languages.

REFERENCES

Piaget J: The Construction of Reality in the Child. New York, Basic Books, 1954.

Levine MD, Carey WB, Crocker AC, Gross RT: Developmental Behavioral Pediatrics. Philadelphia, WB Saunders Co, 1983.

Mussen PH, Conger JJ, Kagan J, Huston AC: Child Development and Personality, 6th ed. New York, Harper and Row, 1984.

EMOTIONAL CHANGES

J. R. Pinkham

There are many human emotions, such as shame, guilt, anger, joy, fear, and sadness. Many more could be named. Emotions can be discerned by observing behavioral reactions (he cried), measuring physiologic responses (his heart rate is faster), or ascertaining an individual's thoughts and reactions ("I'm depressed").

In assessing the emotional state of young children, the latter two methods of discernment are of little or no value. As a general rule, in the first year of a child's life adults assign whatever emotion they feel that the child should feel in a particular situation. Thus, a wide range of interpretation exists. Upon the child spilling his milk, one parent of a 18-month-old may interpret the child's crying as frustration over his awkwardness, another as guilt for the mistake, and another as fear of having nothing else to drink.

It is also evident that in older children and adults, the true description of an emotion is very much influenced by how a person reacts to, analyzes, and studies his own inner feelings. Thus, for the same stimulus one person could laugh and another could cry. For very young children, ascertaining such subtleties as these are not possible. The excited babbling of a 3-month-old, which parents label as joy, may more appropriately be called simply excitement.

There appears to be an awakening of emotional states within the child between 4 months and 10 months of age. Mussen and colleagues in 1984 cited that infants were capable of displaying fearful behavior as well as anger or frustration. As a child approaches his or her first birthday, sadness upon separation from a parent, joy upon reunion, and jealousy with peers or siblings become reliable findings.

Infant and childhood fears are interesting to clinicians who must treat children and must be taken into account when formulating a strategy for dealing with the child. Uncertainty and certainty are a pair of elements that emerge early in infancy and can lead to fear or a lack of fear. For instance, if the first time the jack in a jack-in-the-box jumps up, it startles the child, the child may avoid the toy until later when he recognizes at what part of the tune the jack will jump out. Avoiding startling situations is important in helping children react with new environmental situations.

Fear of strangers is almost a universal finding after 7–12 months of age, although its intensity will vary from child to child. Another very common fear in this age group is a fear upon separation from the parents. This fear starts around 6 months of age, peaks between 13 and 18 months of life, and then declines. It is interesting to note that the onsets and peaks for separation anxiety appear to be the same for children from a variety of cultures, although the rate of diminishment of the fear varies greatly (Kagan et al, 1978). It should be noted that the problem of separation anxiety is fairly well controlled by most children by 36–40 months of age and by many children by 32–36 months of age.

REFERENCES

Mussen PH, Conger JJ, Kagan J, Huston AC: Child Development and Personality, 6th ed. New York, Harper and Row, 1984.

Kagan J, Kearsley R, Zelazo P: Infancy: Its Place in Human Development. Cambridge, MA, Harvard University Press, 1978.

SOCIAL CHANGES
J. R. Pinkham

The First Year

In the first year of life, the child is utterly and completely dependent upon the parents. Mothering is extremely important to the child at this time. In the first several months, the child will not show a clear differentiation among people. Parents as well as strangers can be cooed to or smiled at by the baby.

Non-reflexive smiling occurs at 2–3 months, and this represents the first major social behavior of the infant other than crying. With this smile, the child begins to understand what a behavior other than crying can do to expand his or her influence within the home.

The most important happenings socially during the first year of life are the development of strong and secure attachments to nurturing and caring adults. It should be noted that, according to available research, children who are started early in life in high-quality day care do not suffer developmental social consequences when compared with children raised solely by their mothers at home.

The Second Year

The 1-year-old child is capable of great social progress during his second year of development. The advent of language skills allows the child to learn and to relate to the family. Socially, children will seek to exert their will. A need to test independence will start to surface. Effective and consistent parenting strategies become very important.

Role model observation becomes important at this age and will remain so for years to come. Role models who display a consistent behavior are the most effective. Children who observe non-aggressive ways of handling frustration are likely to acquire that approach. Unfortunately, children seeing violent, aggressive behaviors consistently are just as likely to adopt those approaches.

The maintenance of affection between parent and child and increasing verbal approval and disapproval are important at this age. Discipline should be educational, not punitive.

Parents need to be reminded that 1- and 2-year-old children have not acquired internal controls and that often temper tantrums are normal and are best left unnoticed. Physical punishment, over and beyond an attention-getting technique by a parent (one painless thump on the buttocks), is usually contraindicated and actually can make a misbehaving child behave worse.

The Third Year

Depending on the individual child, late in the second year or early in the third year the child will start eating independently of the parents. The third year is when potty training generally starts. This should not be started too soon and should never become a conflict between child and parent. Parents should wait until the child is ready.

The third year is a demanding one for parents. Children between the second and third birthdays have been labeled "the terrible twos." The child in his third year may use the word "No!" anytime he cares to resist. This child is often an embarrassment to his parents, for he will not hesitate to state his observations in front of everyone ("Aunt Jane is fat!"). Genital manipulation is not an uncommon practice at this age, and this may be trying for parents also.

By the end of the third year, the child is asking how and why questions. The child's unique identity is beginning to surface, and he can integrate the standards of others into his own life. Because of this and because of increased communication skills, the child by his third birthday is capable of a variety of social interchanges with other people. Because of this ability at communication, for years the third birthday marked the entry date for many children into a program of dental care. Of course, one of the premises of this textbook is that from a prevention standpoint, age 3 is way too late for the first dental appointment.

chapter 12

Examination of the infant and toddler

Stephen Goepferd

Until recent years, tradition in dentistry for children has recommended that a child's first dental visit occur at 3 years of age. This recommendation was based upon the child's ability to cooperate in the dental setting and not upon the absence of dental disease in children under 3 years of age. Although the prevalence of dental disease in children is decreasing, infants and toddlers still experience dental disease (NIDR, 1981). One particularly destructive process in infants and toddlers is nursing caries. Additionally, dental caries seen in 3- and 4-year-old children is initiated well before age 3.

Current knowledge, modern technology such as fluorides and sealants, and advances in understanding the cariogenic potential of the diet (Newbrun, 1983), coupled with the fact that basic habits (i.e., preventive behaviors and dietary habits) are established very early in life (Anderson et al, 1977), suggest that efforts to prevent dental disease must be initiated during infancy. Furthermore, dental professionals, by virtue of early critical decision making based upon their knowledge of dental disease prevention, have been successful in producing caries-free children. It is incumbent upon the dental profession to educate parents so that they can make appropriate early decisions in an effort to prevent dental disease in their infants and toddlers.

Therefore, a child's first visit to the dentist should occur no later than 12 months of age so that the dentist can evaluate the infant's oral health, intercept potential problems such as nursing caries, and educate parents in the prevention of dental disease in their child (Goepferd, 1986). An ever-increasing demand by parents for an early dental evaluation of their infants and toddlers and for the acquisition of preventive knowledge requires the modern dental practitioner to be proficient in the examination of the infant and toddler (Goepferd, 1986).

Objectives of the Infant and Toddler Examination

The examination of the infant and toddler centers around three major objectives: preven-

149

tion, introduction to dentistry, and oral assessment.

Prevention ■ A major emphasis during the infant's initial visit should center around the counseling of parents regarding their role in preventing dental disease in the child. Preventive counseling should include diet counseling with respect to feeding practices and snacking patterns, tooth cleaning procedures (positioning and timing), and fluoride assessment resulting in the development of an appropriate fluoride program.

Introduction to dentistry ■ The modern practice of dentistry need not be unpleasant and fear producing. Rather, the initial examination of infants and toddlers should provide a foundation for the development of a positive attitude toward dentistry. The method for examining infants as well as the recommended environment should provide a pleasant, nonthreatening introduction to dentistry for the child and the parents.

Oral assessment ■ The examination of the infant begins with a thorough evaluation of the head and neck region, leading to an assessment of the child's oral development and inspection of the oral cavity to detect any pathologic process or the presence of dental disease, especially the early stages of nursing caries.

Steps of the Infant Examination

The examination of an infant should follow a logical sequence of steps that will lead to a thorough yet expedient procedure.

PREAPPOINTMENT ASSESSMENT

In order to provide the most complete and pertinent yet concise discussion during the preventive counseling portion of the visit, it is necessary to obtain and preview the following historical information. This information can be obtained from the parents through the use of a questionnaire, which is mailed to the parents and returned to the office prior to the appointment.

Biographic data and family and social history ■ This information lends insight into the family structure and provides an understanding of parent-child relationships, which is vital to the development of recommendations for di-

etary modifications and tooth cleaning procedures.

Prenatal, natal, and neonatal history ■ Information obtained in these categories is helpful in explaining dental abnormalities that occur in the primary dentition and provides a means for documenting potential causative events while they are still relatively familiar to the parents. Examples of such events would be high risk pregnancies, tetracycline ingestion during pregnancy, pre-term or low-birth-weight infants, and significant febrile episodes during early childhood.

Developmental history ■ Knowledge of the child's progress in attaining the various developmental milestones, including the eruption of the first tooth, assists the dentist in discovering significant growth alterations and provides a basis for answering the many questions that parents have regarding their child's dental development.

Medical history ■ An accurate medical history is as important for infants and toddlers as it is for older children and adults. Furthermore, a history of frequent episodes of otitis media and the accompanying frequent ingestion of antibiotic suspensions that contain high concentrations of sucrose, for example, influence the recommendations for dietary management and tooth cleaning procedures.

Dental history ■ Knowledge of episodes of previous dental trauma, teething difficulties, oral habits, and current patterns of home oral health care of the infant provides a basis for answering parents' questions and for developing recommendations for future management.

Feeding history ■ An overview of the infant's feeding history is important in assisting the practitioner in developing a relevant discussion of the dietary influences on dental caries and providing appropriate recommendations for altering potentially damaging feeding practices. Important information includes bottle versus breast feeding, frequency and duration of feedings, use of a nighttime bottle or use of the bottle as a pacifier, and the contents of the bottle.

The preappointment information aids the practitioner in tailoring the interview and counseling portion of the visit to meet the individual needs of the child and his or her parents.

INTERVIEW AND COUNSELING

Experience has shown that the interview and counseling portion of the visit is best accom-

plished prior to the examination of the infant or toddler for the following reasons.

- Specific concerns of the parents are identified so that they can be addressed during the examination, if appropriate.
- If the infant fusses during the examination (normal behavior), the parents predictably will direct their attention toward the child during the discussion following the examination and not toward the dentist.
- The child can be occupied with toys in a nonthreatening environment prior to the examination, and the parents can direct their attention toward the discussion.

Once the preappointment information has been reviewed, the dentist greets the child and the parents and confirms the preappointment information, which includes parental concerns and the reason for seeking care. At this point, an assessment is made of the family's current prevention practices. This prevention assessment includes (1) family history of dental disease; (2) fluoride inventory; (3) tooth cleaning procedures; and (4) diet history, including snacking patterns. Based upon this information, appropriate recommendations are made regarding each aspect of an overall dental disease prevention program for the child.

THE EXAMINATION PROCEDURE

The clinical examination of the infant and toddler should be accomplished with the parent's assistance in a non-threatening environment. Most often, it is neither necessary nor recommended that the dental chair be used for the infant examination. In fact, a pleasant location away from the busy dental operatory would be more appropriate. The parent and the dentist sit facing each other in a knee-to-knee position, supporting the child with the head cradled on the dentist's lap (Fig. 12–1). This position allows the parent to restrain the child gently if necessary and provides the parent as well as the dentist with good visualization of the child's oral cavity. This position is comfortable for the infant, and the parental contact provides a calming reassurance for the child. The psychological development of the child under 30–36 months of age is frequently insufficient to facilitate cooperation in a dental setting, and some of the infants and toddlers will cry or fuss during the examination, requiring minimal restraint by the parent. The dentist should reassure the parent(s) that the child's behavior is normal and should not be considered inappropriate. The parents are fully aware that their child is likely to cry in other similar situations such as during a visit to the pediatri-

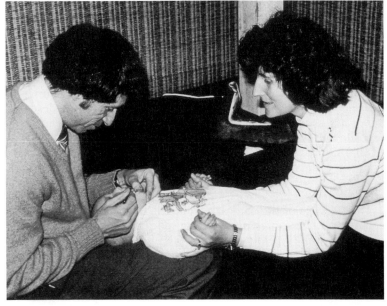

Figure 12–1 ■ Examination of an infant in the knee-to-knee position.

cian's office or the barber shop. The crying or fussing should not interfere with the examination. Initially, the practitioner will be surprised at the number of infants and toddlers who remain calm during the entire examination. This is especially true with infants 12 months of age and younger.

Once the child is positioned properly, the dentist can perform a complete head and neck and intraoral examination. The dentist should begin with a general appraisal of the child, using a warm, gentle touch in a non-threatening manner. The head and neck region should be evaluated for the presence of abnormalities in the size, shape, and symmetry of the head; lymph nodes; facial symmetry; eyes, ears, and nose; and lips and mouth. The practitioner must always be aware of the possibility of child abuse when evidence of head, neck, and facial bruising is present in the infant or toddler.

The examination of the mouth, with the aid of a penlight, should begin with palpation and inspection of the lips, gingivae, and mucosa by placing a forefinger along the cheek and positioning it on the gum pad distal to the most posterior maxillary tooth. The intraoral examination should include an evaluation of the soft tissues for the presence of any pathologic processes, such as inclusion cysts, congenital epulides, submucous clefts, traumatic ulcerations, frenum lacerations, and gingivitis. The examination of the dentition should include an evaluation of the jaw relationships, appropriate parameters of occlusion (overjet, overbite, molar relationships, midline deviations, and crossbites), presence or absence of spacing, presence of dental developmental abnormalities, hypoplastic or hypocalcified enamel, and dental caries.

Following the intraoral examination, the practitioner should demonstrate the positioning and technique for tooth cleaning in the infant. If the child exhibits proximal contacts, flossing should also be demonstrated with the aid of a floss holder. The child should then be repositioned with the head on the parent's lap so that the parent can practice tooth cleaning under the supervision and guidance of the practitioner, offering appropriate suggestions as necessary.

The findings of the clinical examination are collated with the previous information gathered, and final recommendations are offered regarding the parents' role in an optimal preventive program for their child; treatment recommendations, if any; and an appropriate recall schedule.

DETERMINING A RECALL SCHEDULE

The recall schedule's determination is based upon clinical findings, feeding practices and dietary-snacking habits, and dental development. The recall appointment may be scheduled for 3, 6, or 12 months, depending upon the child's potential risk for developing dental disease. Examples of the various criteria for each recall situation are listed in Table 12-1.

The presence of any one of the factors is sufficient to place the patient in the 3- or 6-month recall categories.

At the recall visit, in addition to the clinical examination, the practitioner should assess the parents' tooth cleaning efforts, evaluate the feeding practices and snacking patterns, and investigate the degree to which the parents are following the recommended prevention program that was previously outlined.

The Emergency Examination

Dental emergencies for infants and toddlers present a challenge for the dental practitioner. In addition to treating the particular emergency, the dentist is faced with managing the emotional upset of both the parent(s) and the child. Most of the dental emergencies occurring in children 12–30 months of age are the result of trauma. Occasionally, the emergency is related to dental caries or to some systemic condition such as primary herpetic gingivostomatitis. In the case of a traumatic injury, prior to performing the examination the dentist must obtain certain vital information, which should include (1) a thorough medical history, (2) immunization status (especially against tetanus), and (3) a complete description of the traumatic incident. If the injuries are not adequately accounted for by the description of the accident, if they are inconsistent with the reported incident, or if evidence of multiple injuries in different stages of healing is noted, there may be probable cause to suspect child abuse. The historical information will aid in the examination of the child and will provide clues to the discovery of injuries that might otherwise have gone undetected. The emergency examination of the infant and toddler is performed in the knee-to-knee position, as previously described.

The non–trauma-related dental emergencies in infants and toddlers usually concern mouth pain and are often related to dental caries, espe-

Table 12–1 ■ Criteria for recall schedule determination

	Clinical Findings	Feeding/Diet Patterns	Dental Development
3 Month	Enamel decalcification Considerable plaque build-up Amelogenesis imperfecta Dentinogenesis imperfecta	Bottle used at bedtime/nap-time Bottle used as a pacifier Bottle used past 12 months of age Frequent cariogenic snacking pattern	Stage of dental development has minimal influence on the 3 month interval recall category
6 Month	Posterior proximal contacts No previous tooth cleaning Primary dentition crowding Moderate plaque build-up	Relatively cariogenic diet/snacks	Second primary molar eruption is expected within 6 months
12 Month	Generalized spacing present Good oral hygiene exhibited Shallow occlusal anatomy	Good dietary habits exhibiting a low cariogenic potential	Second primary molar eruption is expected in 6–12 months

cially nursing caries at this age. Thorough history taking is important and often provides insight into the nature of a problem that may not be related to dental caries. It is important to remember that from the parents' perspective, most oral pain reported by their children will usually be interpreted as a toothache. Furthermore, if the history of the oral pain and symptoms suggests a primary herpetic infection, the practitioner will want to wear gloves for the examination. If the nature of the emergency (trauma, deep caries) warrants radiographs, the child is positioned on the parent's lap with the parent stabilizing the child and the film (Fig. 12–2). At all times, proper radiographic protection must be provided. If the mother brings the child to the appointment and she is pregnant, the child may have to be seen at another time as soon as possible and brought to the office by the father or other adult in the family. Alternatively, the child may be stabilized by another means, such as a papoose board.

The Management of Electrical Burns of the Mouth

Electrical burns involving children's oral and perioral tissues require both immediate and long-term management by a multidisciplinary health team, wherein the dentist plays a key role.

Most oral electrical burns are caused when a child bites on the live end of an electrical extension cord. Saliva acts as a conducting medium, producing an arc between the cord and the

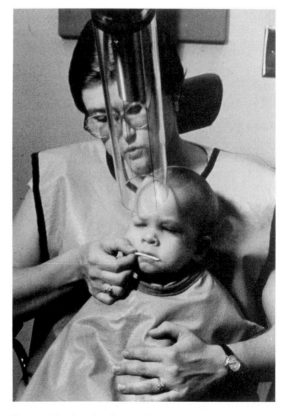

Figure 12–2 ■ Radiographic technique for infants.

child's mouth. The heat generated can reach 2500–3000° C and causes extensive tissue damage. The commissure of the lip is the most common site for oral electrical burns, which occur most often in children under 4 years of age, with a high frequency of occurrence between 18 and 24 months of age.

NATURE OF THE INJURY

Initially, the burn demonstrates charred, gray-white tissue with a centrally depressed area surrounded by elevated, erythematous margins. Swelling of the tissues begins within hours and persists up to 12–14 days. The burns are characterized by liquefaction of fat, coagulation of protein, and vaporization of fluids. Vascular damage causes further tissue damage at the borders of the wound by virtue of ischemia. Pain associated with the wound is usually minor, owing to the destruction of neural tissue. The initial wound exhibits little or no bleeding because of electrical cauterization of the surrounding blood vessels. Future bleeding from the labial artery, however, can occur with the sloughing of the necrotic tissue any time from 4 to 21 days following the injury. Sloughing of the damaged tissue is completed within 2–3 weeks, with complete re-epithelialization. Scarring of the wound results in contracture of the oral and perioral tissue and may lead to microstomia.

TREATMENT OF ELECTRICAL BURNS

An electrical burn to a child's mouth can be a severely disfiguring injury that can impede function and may result in a limited oral opening. Treatment objectives center around minimizing disfigurement and contraction. The following four main treatment approaches have been advocated: (1) immediate surgical excision of the wound; (2) delayed reconstructive surgery following 1 year of natural healing; (3) delayed primary reconstructive surgery following 2 weeks of healing; and (4) immediate postburn splinting of the oral commissure. The first three methods traditionally involve multiple surgical procedures over a period of years to achieve an esthetic result. Recent evidence indicates that immediate splinting of the commissure provides the best cosmetic result, minimizes contracture, and minimizes or eliminates the need for surgical reconstruction.

Initial Medical Management

The physician's immediate concerns are focused upon the risk of bleeding, adequate nutritional and fluid intake, risk of bacterial infection, and risk of tetanus. Although controversy exists regarding the need for systemic antibiotics, there is apparent agreement that antibiotic therapy is appropriate for the most severe burns. Daily wound débridement, followed by a topical application of an antibiotic ointment, is recommended. Diet management is aimed at minimizing trauma to the wound and depends on the severity of the injury and the child's ability to cooperate. Occasionally, the child may require hospitalization to accomplish these objectives if they cannot be attained on an outpatient basis.

Initial Dental Management

Dental management consists of fabricating a commissural splint early during the first 10 days following the injury. A number of appliance designs are available, and the selection depends upon factors such as child behavior and cooperation, dental development, stability needed, and parental compliance. The appliance may be removable, fixed, or extraoral in design, based upon the needs and demands of the given situation. (For a more in-depth discussion of the design and fabrication of the various types of appliances, the following references may be consulted: Czerepak, 1984; Holt et al, 1982; Josell et al, 1984; Silvergrade et al, 1982; Swain and Pinkham, 1983.) The functional aspect common to all of the appliances is the presence of commissural wings. Wing placement depends upon two critical measurements (Fig. 12–3). Measurement A is the distance from the midline to the unaffected commissure, and measurement B is the distance from the incisal edge to an imaginary intercommissural line, thereby producing one hori-

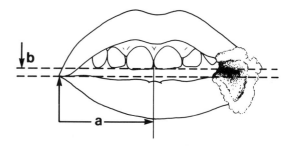

Figure 12–3 ■ Measurements for a commissural splint.

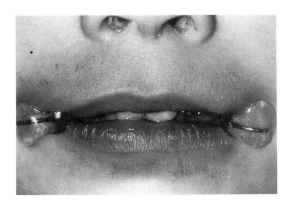

Figure 12-4 ■ Commissural splint in place.

zontal and one vertical measurement to establish the position of the commissural wings. The appliance should exert slight tension on the lips at rest (Fig. 12-4). The appliance must be worn 24 hours a day (except for cleaning and eating with a removable appliance) for a period of 6-8 months and then for 12 hours a day (nighttime) for an additional 6 months until the scar softens and loses its contractile potential.

Surgical Management

Following splint therapy, the child is evaluated by a plastic surgeon to assess whether or not any reconstructive surgery is required. Frequently, only minimal surgical intervention is required, and in many cases surgical intervention can be avoided altogether.

The management of oral electrical burns in children requires immediate and long-term management by a multidisciplinary team consisting of a physician, dentist, and plastic surgeon. The dentist plays a major long-term role in the management of oral commissural burns by preventing oral contracture and by minimizing or eliminating the need for cosmetic surgery.

Clinical Implications of Premature Birth

Premature birth (gestational age under 37 weeks) accounts for 7-10% of all live births. Prematurely born infants are subjected to a variety of metabolic stresses and exhibit a higher prevalence of oral-dental disturbances than normal full-term infants. Factors such as metabolic disorders, hypoxia, prolonged neonatal jaundice, nutritional deficiencies, and low

serum calcium levels have been implicated as causes of the enamel hypoplasia and other mineralization defects seen in the primary incisors of pre-term infants. Pre-term, low-birth-weight (LBW) infants appear to have the highest correlation (40%) with enamel hypoplasia and opacities in the primary dentition. Infants weighing less than 2500 gm are considered as having a low birth weight. Current evidence suggests that enamel hypoplasias, opacities, and other mineralization defects result from neonatal hypocalcemia during the enamel mineralization process (Melander et al, 1982).

Further evidence has demonstrated a correlation between decreased breast milk intake in LBW infants and enamel hypoplasia, opacities, and other mineralization defects. There is a remarkable association between enamel hypoplasia and mineralization defects in infants with respiratory distress, who also exhibit the least amount of breast milk intake, which is believed to contribute further to the degree of neonatal hypocalcemia.

In addition to transient neonatal hypocalcemia and enamel mineralization defects, pre-term infants are more susceptible to the development of abnormalities associated with laryngoscopy and intubation. Traumatic injury caused by laryngoscopy and endotracheal intubation at the critical period of amelogenesis appears to contribute to defects in the primary dentition of LBW infants in whom dental development is already compromised by disturbances in calcium metabolism. Intubated LBW infants exhibit a four-fold increase in primary incisor defects, occurring approximately 85% of the time. Nearly two thirds of the maxillary incisors affected are located to the left of the midline, corresponding to the greater prevalence of right-handed intubation techniques (Seow et al, 1984).

In addition to injury to the developing incisors during the intubation procedure, prolonged orotracheal intubation of infants is associated with airway damage, palatal groove formation, defective primary incisors, and acquired cleft palate (Duke et al, 1976). In 1984, Erenberg and Nowak reported a 47.6% incidence of palatal or alveolar ridge groove formation following orotracheal intubation of preterm LBW infants for a period of 1-62 days (Erenberg and Nowak, 1984b). They also noted that the incidence of palatal groove formation increased to 87.5% in infants intubated 15 days or more. To help prevent the complications associated with prolonged orotracheal intubation, Nowak and Erenberg developed an in-

traoral palatal stabilizing appliance for securing the orogastric and orotracheal tubes (Erenberg and Nowak, 1984a). Because they noticed palatal abnormalities beginning to develop as early as 12 hours following intubation, Erenberg and Nowak recommend consideration of a stabilizer for infants who will be intubated for more than 24 hours.

In addition to localized orofacial effects of the intubation process for LBW infants, systemic complications have also been identified. Approximately 30% of LBW infants experience respiratory distress syndrome (RDS), and of those infants, 16% develop bronchopulmonary dysplasia (BPD), a chronic lung disease (Koops et al, 1984). BPD places these infants at high risk for respiratory infections, increased airway resistance, and recurrent wheezing, all of which pose potential problems for the child in the dental office.

It is important for the dentist to be aware of the clinical dental implications of pre-term, LBW infants in order to offer their parents an explanation of the likely causes of any anomalies that may be present. In addition, the dentist may be in a position to act as a resource for information regarding potential dental sequelae in pre-term LBW infants or provide a service in assisting in the prevention of oral adverse sequelae to prolonged intubation of infants.

REFERENCES

Anderson TA, Fomon SJ, Wei SHY: Nutrition counseling and the development of eating habits. *In* Sweeney EA (ed): The Food That Stays: An Update on Nutrition, Diet, Sugar, and Caries. New York, Medcom, Inc, 1977, pp 22–27.

Czerepak CS: Oral splint therapy to manage electrical burns of the mouth of children. Clin Plast Surg 11(4):685, 1984.

Duke PM, Caulson JD, Santos JI, et al: Cleft palate associated with prolonged orotracheal intubation in infancy. J Pediatr 89:990, 1976.

Erenberg A, Nowak AJ: Appliance for stabilizing orogastric and orotracheal tubes in infants. Crit Care Med 12(8):669, 1984a.

Erenberg A, Nowak AJ: Palatal groove formation in neonates and infants with orotracheal tubes. Am J Dis Child 138:974, 1984b.

Goepferd SJ: Infant oral health: A rationale. J Dent Child 53(4):257, 1986.

Goepferd SJ: Infant oral health: A protocol. J Dent Child 53(4):261, 1986.

Holt GR, Parel S, Richardson DS, Kittle PE: The prosthetic management of oral commissure burns. Laryngoscope 92:407, 1982.

Josell SD, Owen D, Kreutzer LW, Goldberg NH: Extraoral management for electrical burns of the mouth. J Dent Child 51(1):47, 1984.

Koops BL, Abman SH, Accurso FJ: Outpatient management and follow-up of bronchopulmonary dysplasia. Clin Perinatol 11(1):101, 1984.

Melander M, Noren JG, Freden H, Kjellmer I: Mineralization defects in deciduous teeth of low birthweight infants. Acta Paediatr Scand 71:727, 1982.

National Institute of Dental Research (NIDR): The prevalence of dental caries in the United States children, 1979–1980. The National Dental Caries Prevalence Survey, NIH pub. no. 82-2245. Bethesda, MD, US National Institutes of Health, 1981.

Newbrun E: Cariology. Baltimore, Williams and Wilkins, 1983, pp 86–111; 308–322.

Seow WK, Brown JP, Tudehope DI, O'Callaghan M: Developmental defects in the primary dentition of low-birth-weight infants: Adverse effects of laryngoscopy and prolonged endotracheal intubation. Pediatr Dent 6(1):28, 1984.

Silvergrade D, Zacher JB, Ruberg RL: Improved splinting of oral commissure burns: Results in 21 consecutive patients. Ann Plast Surg 9(4):316, 1982.

Swain FR, Pinkham JR: Treatment of lip commissure burns with a commissural stabilizing splint. Quint Int 8:789, 1983.

chapter *13*

Prevention of dental disease

Arthur Nowak □ James Crall

Dental disease has been reported to be the most common bacterial disease affecting humans. Even though tremendous reductions in the incidence of dental caries have recently been reported, millions of children and adults are playing and working with periodontal disease, missing teeth, and malocclusions—most of which could be prevented—if only they would practice a daily preventive program and seek professional care on a scheduled basis. Dental disease is preventable! Oral pain is unnecessary! A dental disease free generation could be a reality.

The goal of this chapter is to provide the student with a plan—a plan that can provide infants, children, and young adults with a mouth that is free from disease. The plan involves many people—not only the dentist and his or her staff, but also the parents, the child, the siblings, and even the grandparents. The plan begins shortly after conception, prior to the initiation of oral disease, and it never ends. It never ends because the mouth and all of its parts were meant to last a lifetime.

The mouth plays a major role in the life of a human being. All nutrients must pass through it. Expressions of happiness, sadness, and even love and anger are developed from the actions of the lips and cheeks. Sounds and later speech are produced by the activity of the tongue, lips, and cheeks.

Therefore, a healthy mouth, with a full complement of teeth, supported by healthy gingivae and bone and in a balanced and stable occlusion, is a goal all dentists should support and promote for the patients under their care.

Pre-natal Counseling

Since the beginning of the twentieth century, the medical profession has recognized the importance of providing pre-natal counseling and care to the expectant mother. Through these efforts infant morbidity and mortality have been greatly reduced. Only recently has the dental profession become involved in this primary preventive effort.

The most common setting for pre-natal counseling is in conjunction with the programs developed in all communities in the local hospitals or the neighborhood health centers. An office-based program is yet another possibility. Wherever it may be conducted, the dentist must

157

work closely with a member of the medical profession to schedule appropriate time for the dental presentation and the questions to follow.

Although many programs have been developed in recent years, the goals of the programs are similar (Table 13–1). Depending on the setting, the time allotted, and the availability of the staff, the program should be individualized but should include information to educate parents about the dental development of the child, the dental disease process, and the preventive actions available to ensure a disease free mouth. In addition, the program should include information on the importance of the mother's diet during pregnancy, including the effects of drugs, tobacco, and alcohol; the need for professional oral supervision for the pregnant woman; and the scheduling of dental treatment during pregnancy (Table 13–2).

Most recently, there has been much discussion on the prescription of systemic fluoride during pregnancy to benefit the developing

Table 13–1 ■ A model program of pre-natal counseling

Purpose
To educate parents about dental development of the child

To educate parents about dental disease and prevention

To provide a suitable environment for the child

To strengthen and prepare the child and dentition for life

Methods
Education in development, prevention, and disease

Demonstration of oral hygiene procedures

Counseling in attitudes and motivation

Evaluation of learning, acceptance, and needs

Content
External Component (Parents)
Parents' education concerning dental disease and oral hygiene

Parents' motivation for plaque removal program

Changes in mother's oral health
    Intake of sweets
    Pregnancy gingivitis
    Myths and misconceptions about pregnancy and dentition

Parents' dental treatment

Internal Component (Parents and Child)
Parents' education—development of child

Effect of family life style on child
    Habits (smoking)
    Intake of sweets
    Exposure to disease (rubella, syphilis, etc.)

Effect of drugs on child
    Tetracyclines

Nutrition
    Calcium
    Vitamins
    Fluorides
    Essential nutrients

Child's needs after birth
    Breast feeding versus bottle
    Fluoride supplementation
    Teething
    Hygiene
    Non-nutritive sucking
    First visit

Table 13–2 ■ Dental treatment for women during pregnancy

First Trimester

Consult with woman's physician*

Emergency treatment only

Second Trimester

Elective and emergency treatment

Radiographs can be used with adequate protection

Third Trimester

Emergency treatment only

Avoid supine position

Radiographs can be used with adequate protection

Throughout Pregnancy

Plaque control program for mother and father of child

Local anesthetic is anesthetic of choice

Avoid the use of drugs if at all possible. If drugs are necessary, use only those proved safe for use during pregnancy and use in consultation with a physician.

The use of a general anesthetic for dental treatment during pregnancy is contraindicated

* The first trimester is most crucial; however, in this day of high legal "IQ," it would probably be good to consult with the woman's physician during the last two trimesters, especially if there were a major problem.

teeth. There is no doubt that fluoride passes through the placenta, but it appears that it is only a partial transfer. In 1966, the United States Food and Drug Administration (FDA) banned the manufacture of pre-natal fluoride supplements, which were claimed to prevent dental caries in the offspring. Safety was not an issue in this decision. Until recently, no additional research was available that would recommend the use of pre-natal fluoride supplementation.

In 1977, a report was published on the benefits of pre-natal exposure to dietary fluoride supplementation (Glenn, 1977). Because of the discussion and controversy that followed, it became obvious that clinical trials were necessary to decide this question. Therefore, dentists and physicians may continue to prescribe fluoride supplements for expectant mothers who reside in fluoride deficient communities, although definitive evidence regarding the cariostatic benefits of this practice is lacking at the present time.

During pre-natal counseling, some mention should be made on teething. Although the time of eruption of teeth can usually be predicted, its occurrence frequently surprises the new parents, and if the infant is demonstrating difficulty in teething, it can be a time of anxiety for them. Teething is a natural phenomenon that occurs usually without a problem. Nevertheless, some infants exhibit systemic distress, including a rise in temperature, diarrhea, dehydration, increased salivation, skin eruptions, and gastrointestinal disturbances (Honig, 1975). Treating these symptoms in the absence of upper respiratory and other infectious processes is indicated. If improvement is not seen in 24 hours, the infant should be examined by its physician. Lancing of tissues is usually not indicated. Teething rings to chew and apply pressure to the area of an erupting tooth are indicated. Increasing fluid consumption, a non-aspirin analgesic, and TLC (tender loving care) will reduce the symptoms and result in a happier infant (Carpenter, 1978).

The final comments in pre-natal counseling should provide guidelines for the parents as to the timing of the first professional dental visit. Historically, children were brought for their first dental examination between the ages of 3 and 5. Dentists now know that to prevent oral disease a comprehensive preventive program must be initiated early, at or around the time of the eruption of teeth. Dentists also know that infants can be either at low or high risk to dental disease.

CRITERIA FOR RISK OF CARIES

The criteria for a high risk caries infant include the following:

1. Child is a product of a high risk pregnancy or complicated delivery
2. Presence of a congenital or hereditary defect or developmental disability
3. No systemic fluorides given
4. A family history of severe to moderate dental disease

The criteria for a low risk caries infant are as follows:

1. Infant is a product of a normal pregnancy and delivery
2. Child receiving systemic fluoride since birth
3. A normal health history
4. No family history of severe dental disease

Therefore, the following recommendations for the first dental examination are offered:

1. For infants with an apparent dental problem that is the result of trauma, disease, or growth and developmental delays, referral should be made immediately.

2. Infants at high risk to dental disease should be referred no later than 6 months after the first tooth erupts.

3. Infants at low risk for dental disease should be referred for examination by 18 months.

Fluoride Administration

RATIONALE

Significant reductions in the prevalence of dental caries in children have been documented in the United States and in other countries during the past decade (National Caries Program, 1981). Although the exact reasons for this decline are unknown, most experts include increased availability of fluorides as one of the primary contributing factors. In spite of these advances, caries remains a relatively common yet largely preventable disease of childhood. Because of the importance of fluoride in this regard, it behooves the contemporary dental practitioner to understand the basis for using the many forms of fluoride that are available.

MECHANISMS OF ACTION

Although the precise mechanisms by which fluorides act to prevent dental caries are not fully understood, three general modes are typically considered to be involved. These include (1) increasing the resistance of the tooth structure to acid dissolution, (2) enhancement of the process of remineralization, and (3) reduction of the cariogenic potential of dental plaque.

The effects of fluoride are usually classified as either systemic or topical. Systemic effects can be obtained via the ingestion of foods that contain natural levels of fluoride, water that contains natural fluoride or to which fluoride has been added, dietary fluoride supplements, and some forms of fluoride mouthrinses that are meant to be swallowed (most fluoride rinses are intended for topical application only). Topical benefits are available from the previously mentioned sources as a result of their contact with the teeth as well as from fluoride toothpastes and other more concentrated forms that are self-administered or professionally applied.

The indications for administering the various forms of fluoride primarily depend upon the age of the child, his or her caries history and perceived susceptibility to develop caries in the future, and whether he or she drinks fluoridated water. For children in the birth to age 3 category, the principal concern is that they receive an optimal level of systemic fluoride.

SYSTEMIC FLUORIDES

Water Fluoridation

Water fluoridation remains the cornerstone of any sound caries prevention program. It is not only the most effective means of reducing caries, it is also the most cost-effective, most convenient, and most reliable method of providing the benefits of fluoride to the population, since it does not depend upon individual compliance. Numerous studies have documented caries reductions of 40–50% in the primary dentition and of 50–65% in the permanent dentition of children drinking fluoridated water from birth (U.S. Department of Health, Education, and Welfare, 1979). Over 50% of the U.S. population currently has access to drinking water containing a significant level of fluoride (greater than 0.7 parts per million). Many of these water supplies contain significant levels of natural fluoride, especially in the Midwestern and Southwestern sections of the country. Numerous fluoride deficient community water supplies have been artificially fluoridated at a cost of less than $1 per year per child (U.S. Department of Health and Human Services, 1984).

As part of their responsibility to promote oral health, dentists have the obligation to educate the public as to the effectiveness and safety of this proven preventive measure. Involvement at the local level in support of water fluoridation can be one of the major contributions a dentist can make to enhance the oral health of all children in his or her community.

Fluoride Supplementation

Fluoride supplements provide an alternative source of dietary fluoride for those children who do not have access to optimally fluoridated water. Included are those persons whose public or private water supplies are fluoride deficient, as well as individuals who reside in fluoridated communities but who do not rely on optimally fluoridated water for their primary source of fluid intake. In the latter category, particular attention should be given to infants whose primary intake consists of breast milk or formulas that are prepared with fluoride deficient water.

Because breast milk and cow's milk contain only trace amounts of fluoride, infants who derive all or most of their fluid intake from breast feeding should receive fluoride supplements, even if they reside in a fluoridated area. However, because most infants are totally breast fed for only a few months, mothers should be instructed early on to discontinue the supplements when additional foods or fluoridated water are added to the diet (Kula and Wei, 1985).

Dentists also should be aware that, even in areas where the water contains adequate amounts of fluoride, some children may derive substantially less than the average amount of their fluid intake from drinking water. Thus, even parents who reside in fluoridated areas should be questioned as to the sources of fluid in their infant's diet, realizing that fluoride supplements may be advisable for children who consume very little fluoridated water.

Supplements potentially can be as effective as fluoridated water in preventing caries (Driscoll, 1974). However, their effectiveness depends largely on the degree of parental compliance. Supplements are commercially available in liquid and tablet forms, both with and without vitamins. The fluoride-vitamin formulations are not inherently superior to supplements without vitamins in terms of reducing caries. However, the combination of fluoride and vitamins may improve parental compliance and thereby provide greater benefits (Hennon et al, 1966).

Liquid preparations are recommended for younger patients who may have difficulty chewing or swallowing tablets. Liquid supplements without vitamins are dispensed in preparations that provide dosages of 0.125 mg fluoride per drop, 0.25 mg fluoride per drop, and 0.5 mg fluoride per ml; liquid supplements with vitamins are dispensed in preparations that provide 0.25 mg fluoride per ml, 0.5 mg fluoride per 0.6 ml, and 0.5 mg fluoride per ml. Fluoride supplements in tablet form for older patients are available without vitamins in doses of 0.25, 0.5, and 1.0 mg fluoride, while fluoride-vitamin combinations are available in 0.5 and 1.0 mg doses (Kula and Wei, 1985).

In order to obtain both topical and systemic effects, fluoride supplements should be allowed to contact the teeth prior to being swallowed. For liquid preparations, this can be achieved by placing the drops directly on the child's teeth or by placing the drops in the child's food or drink, although the latter practice may reduce the bioavailability of the fluo-

ride. Older children should be encouraged to chew and swish their tablets or allow them to dissolve in the mouth prior to swallowing in order to prolong the contact of the fluoride with the outer surfaces of the teeth.

The dosage of fluoride that should be prescribed depends upon the age of the child and the fluoride concentration of his or her drinking water. The fluoride concentration of a central community water supply can be determined by contacting the local or state department of health or the local water authority. Individuals who do not obtain their water from a central supply should have samples of their water tested for fluoride content. This service is usually provided by state health departments or colleges of dentistry. Because of the potential for considerable variation in fluoride levels in the water obtained from different wells in the same area, it is important that each individual non-central source be sampled in order to determine accurately the level of fluoride for each patient. Table 13–3 gives the currently recommended daily dosage schedule for fluoride supplementation (American Dental Association Council on Dental Therapeutics, 1979).

The fluoride in most dietary supplements is incorporated as sodium fluoride (NaF). One milligram of fluoride is equivalent to approximately 2.2 mg of sodium fluoride. When prescribing fluoride supplements, the practitioner should clearly specify the dosage that is to be dispensed in terms of fluoride ion, sodium fluoride, or both. Examples of prescriptions for dietary fluoride supplements are shown in Table 13–4.

Because it is common for infants and children to experience several contacts with a physician prior to their first dental visit, dentists providing treatment for children should become aware of the prescribing practices of local physicians and be prepared to offer advice regarding appropriate fluoride supplementation. In addition, den-

Table 13 – 3 ■ Supplemental fluoride dosage schedule*

Age (yr)	Concentration of Fluoride in Water (ppm)		
	0–0.3	*0.3–0.7*	*>0.7*
0–2	0.25	0	0
2–3	0.50	0.25	0
3–13	1.00	0.50	0

* Recommended daily dosage of fluoride in mg/day; 1 mg of fluoride is equivalent to 2.2 mg sodium fluoride.

Table 13–4 ■ Sample supplemental fluoride prescriptions

1. Six-month-old whose drinking water contains <0.3 ppm fluoride

Rx:	Sodium fluoride solution 0.125 mg fluoride/drop
Disp:	30 ml
Sig:	Dispense 2 drops of liquid in mouth before bedtime

2. Three-year-old whose drinking water contains 0.5 ppm fluoride

Rx:	Sodium fluoride tablets 0.5 mg fluoride/tablet (1.1 mg NaF/tablet)
Disp:	180 tablets
Sig:	Chew 1 tablet and swish and swallow after brushing at bedtime

tists can provide input into local pre-natal care programs so that expectant parents can be made aware of the benefits and appropriate use of fluorides.

TOPICAL FLUORIDES

In most instances, the regular use of a fluoride-containing toothpaste applied by the parent will constitute the only topical applications of fluoride for children up to age 3. Children whose teeth contain structural defects that are felt to place them at high risk to develop caries or infants who have previously experienced severe caries (i.e., nursing bottle caries) might receive additional topical applications in the form of a professionally applied or a parentally applied concentrated preparation. Irrespective of whether a toothpaste or a more concentrated form of fluoride is being applied, care should be taken to minimize the amount that is used and swallowed. Parents should place only a small dab of dentifrice on the brush and should always supervise the brushing session so that the dentifrice and saliva are expectorated.

Examples of concentrated agents for topical application in the home include a 0.5% acidulated phosphate fluoride (APF) and 0.4% stannous fluoride (SnF_2) gels. The stannous fluoride gels might be more appropriate for younger children, since a 0.4% SnF_2 preparation is only approximately one fourth as concentrated as 0.5% APF. A small amount of the gel should be brushed on the child's teeth before bedtime on a daily basis. The child should be encouraged to expectorate following the application but should not be allowed to eat or drink for approximately 30 minutes. Table 13–5 shows a sample prescription for a topical gel intended for home use.

SAFETY AND TOXICITY OF FLUORIDES

When used properly, the various forms of fluoride can enhance the oral health status of infants and children. However, as is true with many other substances, when used improperly these same agents have the potential to produce objectionable side effects. Therefore, each member of the dental profession has the responsibility to educate his or her patients regarding the appropriate storage and administration of these products.

Acute toxicity can result from the accidental ingestion of excessive amounts of fluoride. Acute fluoride toxicity usually produces manifestations that are limited to nausea and vomiting but that have on at least one occasion been associated with the death of a child. The amount of ingested fluoride necessary to produce acute symptoms is directly related to the weight of the individual; therefore, precautions should be employed in order to prevent the accidental ingestion of concentrated forms of fluoride by all children, but especially by very young children and infants. The lethal dose of fluoride for a typical 3-year-old is approximately 500 mg, and would be reduced proportionately for a younger and smaller child. In

Table 13–5 ■ Sample prescription for fluoride gel intended for home use

Three-year-old with prior history of nursing bottle caries and poor parental compliance with oral hygiene instructions

Rx:	0.4% stannous fluoride gel
Disp:	30 ml
Sig:	Brush a small amount of gel on all teeth at bedtime. Allow child to spit out remaining gel after brushing. Do not allow rinsing after gel application.

order to avoid the possibility of ingestion of large amounts of fluoride, it is recommended that no more than 120 mg of supplemental fluoride be prescribed at any one time (American Academy of Pediatric Dentistry, 1985). Likewise, prescriptions for concentrated topical fluoride preparations intended for home use (i.e., 0.5% fluoride gels, which contain 5 mg of fluoride per ml) should be limited to 30–40 ml. Fluoride mouthrinses and toothpastes contain ≤ 1 mg of fluoride per ml, and the ingestion of even moderate volumes of these agents would not be expected to cause severe symptoms, although it could produce nausea and vomiting.

Parents should be encouraged to store these and all potentially harmful substances out of the reach of small children. If excessive amounts of fluoride are ingested, vomiting should be induced as quickly as possible following the incident. This can be accomplished by administering 2 teaspoonfuls of ipecac syrup* with a few ounces of water for children less than 1 year of age or 1 tablespoonful for children 1 year of age or older. If vomiting does not occur within 20 minutes, another dose of ipecac syrup should be given. The patient should be referred to a poison control center as soon as possible, where stomach pumping may be considered. The absorption of fluoride can be delayed by administering milk or milk of magnesia, which will form complexes with the fluoride.

Repeated ingestion of lesser amounts of fluoride can result in manifestations of chronic fluoride toxicity, the most common of which is dental fluorosis. Infants and young children who cannot fully control their swallowing reflexes or who do not understand that they should expectorate products intended only for topical application may regularly swallow significant amounts of fluoride toothpaste. This amount of fluoride (approximately 0.3 mg at each brushing) may be significant in children who already receive fluoride from fluoridated water, fluoride supplements, or other dietary sources (Tinanoff, 1985). In light of concern about potential increases in the prevalence of dental fluorosis, parents should be cautioned to closely supervise and limit the amount of fluoride toothpaste used by young children. Another potential source of excessive fluoride ingestion is the inappropriate prescribing of fluoride supplements. Dentists and physicians may

be unaware that some water supplies in their area may contain varying amounts of natural fluoride or assume that the level of fluoride is relatively consistent among sources. Unless samples of drinking water are analyzed for each patient, fluoride supplements may be prescribed in instances in which they are not indicated.

Fluoride plays a major role in the prevention of dental caries in children. The dentist who assumes responsibility for the oral health of children should be knowledgeable regarding the safe and appropriate use of the various forms of fluoride that are available for this purpose. Ensuring an optimal level of dietary fluoride intake by infants and children less than 3 years of age should be a primary concern.

Diet

In Chapter 2, information was provided on the dental disease process and on the relationships among host, bacteria, and substrate. Therefore, it is important that early in the infant's life, dietary habits be established that will promote not only physical growth and development but also an environment conducive to optimal oral health.

Although there continues to be much research under way to determine the potential of various foods in promoting dental disease, evidence currently available would suggest that solubility and adhesiveness of foods are very important. Foods that stick to the teeth and tissues for long periods, as well as dissolve slowly, are more likely to produce acid, which will lower the pH of the oral environment. This drop in pH (Stephan, 1940) below 5.5 provides an environment for bacterial growth and decalcification of enamel.

Initially, the infant's diet is primarily milk, either from the breast, the bottle, or both. When comparing their acidogenic and enamel dissolution potentials, it is seen that human milk causes a greater fall in plaque pH than bovine milk. Bovine milk has a higher calcium, phosphorus and protein content than human milk, while containing 4% lactose as compared to 7% in human milk (Rugg-Gunn et al, 1985).

Therefore, both human and bovine milk have the potential for caries initiation and when inappropriately provided to the infants without daily oral care can lead to nursing caries. Infants should never be given a bottle containing milk or other sweet beverages as a pacifier to be used

---

* Eli Lilly and Co, Indianapolis, IN.

during the day or at naptime or bedtime. If a nap or bedtime bottle is customary, the infant should be held by the parent while feeding from the bottle. When finished, the infant should be placed in the bed without the bottle. If there is a need for additional sucking, a pacifier or exerciser is preferable to the bottle. If parents continue to insist on using a bedtime bottle, the contents should be limited to water.

Feeding by breast is popular in both the United States and Europe, especially during the months following birth. As earlier mentioned, because of its composition breast milk can produce acid and cause enamel demineralization. In addition, infants breast fed truly on demand may suckle 10–40 times in a 24 hour period. Nevertheless, many professionals feel that the benefits of breast feeding outweigh any harmful effects. The dentist should advise mothers who breast feed on demand, after the infants' teeth erupt, to provide frequent oral hygiene for the infant and to verify the systemic fluoride intake to ensure an optimal preventive environment.

Although surveys report that most infants in the United States are fed beikost (foods other than milk or formula fed to infants) by 2 months of age, pediatric nutritionalists recommend that the infant's total nutritional needs be supplied from milk or a formula to 5–6 months of age. At 5–6 months, iron-fortified dry cereal is recommended, followed by one or two new (commercially or home-prepared) foods each week. Sound eating habits established during infancy will assist in the continuation of sound eating habits later in life. Making an infant drain the last drop from the bottle or finish the last spoonful in the dish is not recommended. Forcing infants to eat, when there is an indication of willingness to stop, may contribute to overeating, frequent snacking, and obesity in later life (Fomon et al, 1979).

With the eruption of posterior teeth and sitting in the high chair for meals, infants are usually introduced to a variety of foods. Parents should be advised of appropriate snack foods that are not only nutritious but also safe for teeth. Finger foods — at first soft fruits and vegetables, cereals (without sugar coatings), gelatin cubes, salt-free crackers, and cheeses — are all acceptable and should be introduced as the infant develops chewing patterns and swallowing reflexes to handle these new foods. Foods with a high percentage of their content as carbohydrates should be avoided, along with foods that stick to the teeth and are slow to dissolve.

Natural fruit juices and artificially fortified fruit juices are frequently introduced to the infant. Pediatricians recommend that juices not be given to the infant in a bottle. Fruit juices should be fed only by cup. Habitual and prolonged use of juice in the bottle can lead to nursing caries.

It should also be noted by the dentist that many medications commonly prescribed to children are sweetened to enhance the child's acceptance of them. For long term use, these medications can be detrimental dentally. Also, certain pediatric drugs promote a relative xerostomia, which is also potentially bad for dental health and may indicate that more rigid home care be initiated.

Home Care

The initiation of a program to ensure an optimal environment for oral health begins in infancy. The responsibility for this program is entirely the parents', with the information and guidance coming from the dentist and his or her staff. The preventive program includes many facets — dietary management, optimal systemic fluorides, removal of plaque from the teeth, and gum massage. All are important, but probably plaque removal and gum massage in the infant and young child are most often neglected and misunderstood.

Parents frequently report that they do not brush their child's teeth because "they may hurt the tooth" or "my baby hates it" or "all she does is eat the toothpaste." From these remarks, it is obvious that parents have not been instructed in this home care procedure and therefore are having difficulty, leading to frustration.

Studies have confirmed that the bacteria for dental disease are present at the eruption of the primary teeth (Edwardson and Mejare, 1978). These bacteria, along with the infant's diet, promote the development of plaque and the subsequent production of acid. This environment around the teeth is conducive to demineralization of enamel and eventually cavitation. In addition, the gingivae are subjected to daily insult from the products of bacterial metabolism, leading to marginal gingivitis.

Daily removal of plaque and massaging of the gums will ensure sound enamel and healthy gingivae. Early initiation of plaque removal will help to establish a lifelong habit of oral care. A disease free mouth will bring happiness and satisfaction not only to the parents and children

but also to the dental team who provided the information, instructions, and reinforcement.

Once the parents have been informed of the dental disease process and have been charged with the responsibility to clean the teeth and massage the gums daily, a location to perform the procedure should be selected. Devices for plaque removal should be suggested, the pros and cons of dentifrices explained, positioning of the infant demonstrated, and a technique described. Parents should be warned to avoid the bathroom as a place to practice hygiene procedures because it is usually crowded and filled with sharp-cornered fixtures. Initially, oral hygiene in the infant will probably be best performed wherever the parent changes the child's diapers. A changing table is a convenient height and usually has appropriate lighting. As the infant grows, the knee-to-knee position (see Fig. 12-1) will probably be useful. When holding or rocking an infant, the parent should develop a habit of inspecting the mouth before the teeth erupt. Some dentists have suggested using a wet gauze pad to wipe off the gums. A small soft-bristled brush can also be used.

Once teeth have erupted, a soft-bristled wet brush can be gently wiped over the teeth. As more teeth erupt, more wiping of the teeth will be needed. When a number of teeth have erupted, a more thorough and systematic routine should be established, making sure that all surfaces of the teeth are cleaned, both in the upper and lower jaw and especially the area around the gum line. At this time, the infant will become stronger and may even object to this activity. The parent should be advised to be persistent. With time, the tooth cleaning activity will become tolerable and acceptable to the child.

Finding an appropriate time for cleaning is important. A tired infant along with exhausted parents does not produce a favorable environment for a positive experience. Developmentally, an infant is not prepared to accept or understand the activity. Games must be developed; music and singing used; the parents must create a positive experience. With time, the infant may even become less tolerant of the procedure. This is not a reason to give up the daily activity of oral hygiene.

A thorough cleaning before bed is recommended. Usually, the infant will have a bath. The cleaning can immediately follow, along with any other personal hygiene procedures. Toward the end of the second year of life, the child will be very mobile, actively involved in play and other "grownup" activities. Parents must remember to save time at the end of a busy day for oral care. Although the 24-month-old will want to clean his own teeth, parents need to understand that fine motor activity of the child remains very poorly developed. Supervision and going over missed areas is the responsibility of the parent and will be needed to some degree for years to come.

Toothbrushes are available in many shapes, colors, sizes, and designs. Soft, rounded, bristled nylon brushes are recommended. The size of the head, angle of the head to the handle, and size and shape of the handle will all be dependent on the infant and parent. A toothbrush with a design that works best in their hands and that can get the cleaning and massaging completed is the brush to use. Mechanical and novelty brushes are also available. Some dentists have found them to be motivational. Unfortunately, a poor record for longevity has been associated with these brushes by some clinicians.

It has been shown that infants cannot effectively expectorate. Therefore, dentifrices with fluoride should be used sparingly, if at all. Fluoride from the dentifrice can appreciatively increase the total fluoride intake. If a fluoride dentifrice is used, a very small amount should be placed on the brush and the cleaning should be completely performed or supervised by the parent.

Usually, spacing exists in the primary dentition. Therefore, flossing is not necessary. At this age (0–3), the importance of a good cleaning and massaging by brush should be emphasized. With growth and development and subsequent changes in the alignment of the teeth, flossing will be introduced.

Positioning for visibility and control is very important. Whether the parent uses the changing table, a bed top, a counter top, or the knee-to-knee position, appropriate stabilization; propping of the mouth; and reflection of the lips, tongue, or cheek are important for a thorough and pleasant hygiene experience.

REFERENCES

American Academy of Pediatric Dentistry: Protocol for fluoride therapy. Pediatr Dent 7:338–339, 1985.

American Dental Association Council on Dental Therapeutics. *In* Accepted Dental Therapeutics, 37th ed. Chicago, American Dental Association, 1979.

Bowden BD: A longitudinal study of the effects of digit and dummy-sucking. Am J Orthodont 52:887–900, 1966.

Carpenter, JV: The relationship betwen teething and systemic disturbances. J Dent Child 45:381–384, 1978.

Driscoll W: The use of fluoride tablets for the prevention of dental caries. *In* Forrester D, Schultz E (eds): International Workshop on Fluorides and Dental Caries Reductions. Baltimore, University of Maryland, 1974, p 25–96.

Edwardsson S, Mejare B: *Streptococcus milleri* (Guthof) and *Streptococcus mutans* in the mouths of infants before and after tooth eruption. Archs Oral Biol 23:811–814, 1978.

Fomon S, Filer LH, Anderson T, Ziegler E: Recommendations for feeding normal infants. Pediatrics 63:52–59, 1979.

Food and Drug Administration: Statements of general policy or interpretation, oral prenatal drugs containing fluoride for human use. Federal Register, October 20, 1966.

Glenn F: Immunity conveyed by a sodium fluoride supplement during pregnancy. J Dent Child 44:391–351, 1977.

Hennon DK, Stookey GK, Muhler JC: The clinical anticariogenic effectiveness of supplementary fluoride-vitamin preparation — results at the end of three years. J Dent Child 33:3–11, 1966.

Honig JJ: Teething — are today's pediatricians using yesterday's notions? J Pediatr 87:415–417, 1975.

Kula K, Wei SHY: Fluoride Supplements and Dietary Sources of Fluorides. Philadelphia, Lea and Febiger, 1985, pp 54–74.

Larsson E: Dummy and finger sucking habits with special attention to their significance for facial growth and occlusion. Swed Dent J 1:23–33, 1978.

National Caries Program, National Institute of Dental Research: Summary of Findings. *In* The Prevalence of Dental Caries in United States Children — 1979–1980. NIH Publication No. 82-2245; December, 1981, pp 5–8.

Rugg-Gunn AJ, Roberts GJ, Wright WG: Effect of human milk on plaque pH in situ and enamel dissolution in vitro compared with bovine milk, lactose and sucrose. Caries Res 19:327–334, 1985.

Stephan RM: Changes in the hydrogen ion concentration on tooth surfaces and in carious lesions. JADA 27:718–723, 1940.

Tinanoff N: Comment on "Urinary excretion of fluoride following ingestion of MFP toothpastes by infants ages two to six years." Pediatr Dent 7:345, 1985.

U.S. Department of Health, Education, and Welfare: Evaluatory Surveys of Long-Term Fluoridation Show Improved Dental Health. Atlanta, USPHS Publication No. 84-22647, March, 1979.

U.S. Department of Health and Human Services: Fluoridation Census 1980. Atlanta, Centers for Disease Control, 1984.

NON-NUTRITIVE SUCKING

John R. Christensen □ Henry W. Fields

Questions often arise concerning infants and non-nutritive sucking. Non-nutritive sucking consists of sucking fingers, pacifiers, or other objects.

Non-nutritive sucking is considered a normal part of fetal and neonatal development. As early as 13–16 weeks *in utero,* the fetus has started sucking and swallowing movements. Respiratory-like movements also begin during this stage. These fetal movements are considered to be important precursors for the life-sustaining requirements of respiration and deglutition.

Non-nutritive sucking is intimately related with two reflexes present in the infant at birth. The rooting reflex is the movement of the infant's head and tongue toward an object touching its cheek. The object is usually the mother's breast but may also be a finger or pacifier. The rooting reflex disappears in normal infants around 7 months of age. The sucking reflex expresses milk from the nipple and remains intact until 12 months of age. The disappearance of the sucking reflex does not mean the infant can

not suckle; at this stage of development, the infant has learned to feed and does not need the reflex to obtain nourishment.

During suckling, the infant will place the tongue beneath the nipple, in contact with the lower lip, and swallow with the jaws apart and the lips together. This is termed the infantile swallow (Fig. 13–1). In contrast, the adult swallow is characterized by swallowing with the teeth together, the tongue tip against the palate, and the lips relaxed (Fig. 13–2). The change from an infantile to adult swallow is gradual. As the diet of the infant changes from liquid to solid foods, there is increased activity of the muscles of mastication and the primary molars are brought into occlusion. This transitional swallow is commonly seen in children 3–10 years of age, and lip contraction and tongue to lower lip posture may or may not be present. The full adult swallow can be observed as early as 3–4 years of age and is usually present by age 9 or 10.

To summarize, non-nutritive sucking in infants is nearly universal and is considered nor-

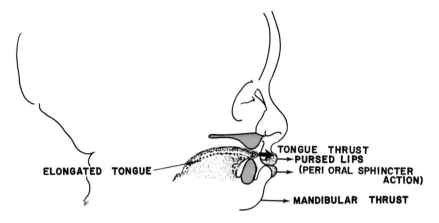

Figure 13 – 1 ■ The infantile swallow is performed with the lips together, the tongue touching the lower lip, and the jaws apart. (From Graber TM: Orthodontics, Principles and Practice, 3rd ed. Philadelphia, WB Saunders Co, 1972, p 167.)

mal. The point at which non-nutritive sucking becomes a habit and is not considered normal is unclear. Numerous studies on the prevalence of thumb and digit sucking indicate that a large majority of newborns suck their digits but that the percentage consistently drops with increasing age. These studies indicate that children spontaneously discontinue non-nutritive sucking sometime between 2 and 4 years of age (Traisman and Traisman, 1958; Nowak et al, 1986).

A variety of non-nutritive sucking habits exist, but thumb, digit, and pacifier sucking are most common (Fig. 13–3). Pacifier habits are dependent on the cultural background and may be encouraged in one setting and not in another—children usually have little choice in the matter. Children often combine a non-nutritive habit with another repetitive activity. For example, they may suck a thumb while carrying a personal blanket, stuffed toy, or favorite doll. Other children play with their hair or rub an article of clothing. In addition, certain situations and times of day influence the habit. Tired children are more likely to suck their thumb, as are children in new or threatening environments.

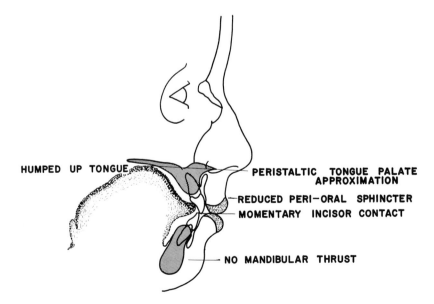

Figure 13 – 2 ■ The adult swallow is performed with the lips relaxed, the tongue against the palate, and the teeth and jaws together. (From Graber TM: Orthodontics, Principles and Practice, 3rd ed. Philadelphia, WB Saunders Co, 1972, p 168.)

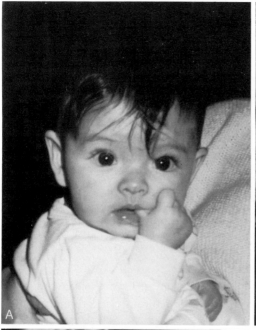

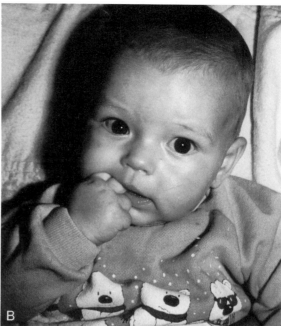

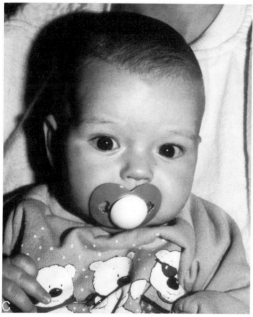

Figure 13–3 ■ Non-nutritive sucking in infants may occur as thumb sucking (A), digit sucking (B), or pacifier sucking (C). The child may engage in one or all three of the habits at one or various stages of development.

The effects of non-nutritive sucking on the developing dentition are minor in the child under 3 years of age and are usually limited to changes in incisor position. Some upper incisors become tipped toward the lips, whereas others are prevented from erupting. There is some controversy, however, concerning the influence one habit has on the dentition compared with another. At this time, there seems to be no significant difference between digit and pacifier habits in terms of their effects on the dentition.

If parents choose to have their child use a pacifier, some precautions should be taken to ensure their child's safety. The pacifier should never be attached to a ribbon or string around the child's neck because the string may get caught or tangled and cause serious injury or death by strangulation. The United States Consumer Products Safety Commission requires that pacifiers

1. Be of sturdy, one piece construction with

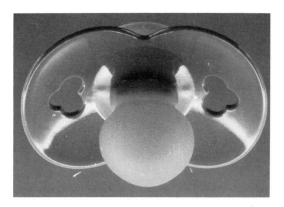

Figure 13–4 ■ This pacifier conforms to the United States Consumer Products Safety Commission standards that require pacifiers to be of sturdy, one piece construction and to have easily grasped handles, inseparable nipples and mouth guards, and mouth guards with two ventilating holes and adequate diameter to prevent aspiration.

material that is non-toxic, flexible, and firm but not brittle

2. Have easily grasped handles

3. Have inseparable nipples and mouth guards

4. Have mouth guards of adequate diameter to prevent aspiration and two ventilating holes

5. Have a label warning against tying the pacifier around the infant's neck (Fig. 13–4)

Additionally, parents should be encouraged to keep the pacifier clean, replace it when worn, and never place honey, sugar, or any sweet syrup on the nipple to encourage sucking.

Manufacturers have been quick to develop nipples and pacifiers that "closely resemble the mother's breast." These manufacturers maintain that because the pacifier resembles the breast, it is more natural and therefore best for the infant's growth and development. No long term controlled studies are available to support these claims.

In this age group, active intervention to discourage non-nutritive sucking is contraindicated. A period of watchful waiting is ordinarily successful because the majority of children spontaneously abandon the habit between the ages of 2 and 4. In a large percentage of cases, any deleterious tooth movement resulting from the habit will tend to resolve if the activity is discontinued prior to eruption of the permanent teeth. Therefore, treatment is usually best deferred until the late primary or early mixed dentition stage and will be discussed in the next chapter.

REFERENCES

Nowak A, Bishara S, Lancial L, Heckert A: Changes in nutritive and non-nutritive sucking habits: Birth to two years. J Dent Res 65:(Special Issue: Abstract 1525), 1986.

Traisman AS, Traisman H: Thumb and finger sucking: A study of 2,650 infants and children. J Pediat 52:566–577, 1958.

chapter *14*

Introduction to dental trauma: managing traumatic injuries in the primary dentition

Dennis J. McTigue

An injury to the teeth of a young child can have serious and long-term consequences, leading to their discoloration, malformation, or possible loss. The emotional impact of such an injury can be far reaching. It is therefore important that the dentist treating children is

1. Knowledgeable in the techniques for managing traumatic injuries
2. Readily available during and after office hours to provide treatment

If either of the above conditions cannot be met, the child suffering a dental injury should immediately be referred to a specialist.

The purpose of this chapter is to provide a straightforward approach to managing dental injuries in the primary dentition. Techniques for diagnosis, treatment, and follow-up care are described. Fundamental issues covered in this chapter, such as classification of injuries, history, examination, and pathologic sequelae of trauma, pertain to both the primary and permanent dentitions. Chapter 33 will focus on treating injuries to young permanent teeth and will refer to this chapter for the information just noted. The principles gleaned from both chapters should enable the dentist to manage the great majority of dental injuries encountered in children.

Etiology and Epidemiology of Trauma in the Primary Dentition

Most injuries to primary teeth occur at 1½–2½ years of age, the toddler stage. As children begin to walk, they frequently fall forward, landing on their hands and knees. Lack of coordination at this stage of development prevents them from shielding the blow from furniture and other objects they might encounter when falling. Coffee tables are most commonly the culprits, and parents are well advised to remove them from the home until toddlers are walking more confidently. Falls from highchairs and strollers are also frequent causes of dental injury.

The teeth most frequently injured in the primary dentition are the maxillary central incisors. Children with protruding incisors, as in developing Class II malocclusions, are two to three times more likely to suffer dental trauma than children with normal incisal overjets.

Another major cause of dental injuries in young children is automobile accidents. Unrestrained children who are seated or standing often hit the dashboard or windshield when the car is stopped suddenly. Dentists in many states have supported mandatory child restraint laws in automobiles, and it is hoped that the trend for universal adoption of these laws will decrease the incidence of all trauma to children in automobile accidents (Jones et al, 1986).

Children with chronic seizure disorders experience an increased incidence of dental trauma. Frequently, these high-risk children will wear protective head gear, and the fabrication of custom mouth guards for them is indicated (see Chapter 39).

Another very serious cause of dental injuries to young children is child abuse. Often overlooked by the dental profession, up to 50% of abused children suffer injuries to the head and neck. Cardinal signs of abuse are injuries in various stages of healing, tears of labial frenums, repeated injuries, and injuries whose clinical presentation is not consistent with the history presented by the parent (Needleman, 1986). Battered children frequently lie to protect their parents or from fear of retaliation. Dentists are required by law to report cases of suspected child abuse (see Chapter 1 for more specific details).

In the primary dentition, teeth are more frequently displaced, or luxated, than they are fractured. This is because the alveolar bone in a young child has large marrow spaces and is relatively pliable. It yields to blows to the primary teeth, allowing these teeth to be moved, rather than holding them firmly and thus causing fractures.

Classification of Injuries to Teeth

Tooth fractures may involve the crown, root, or both. Fractures of the crown may be limited to the enamel, may involve the dentin, or may include the pulp (Fig. 14–1). Injury to the pulp is the most complicated and demanding to treat.

As just mentioned, the most common types of injuries to primary teeth are luxation (displacement) injuries. These injuries damage supporting structures of the teeth, which include the periodontal ligament (PDL) and the alveolar bone (Fig. 14–1). The PDL is the physiologic "hammock" that supports the tooth in its socket. Maintaining its vitality is the primary objective in the treatment of all luxation injuries. Several types of luxation injuries occur (Andreasen, 1981).

1. Concussion: The tooth is not mobile and is not displaced. The PDL absorbs the injury and is inflamed, which leaves the tooth tender to biting pressure and percussion.

2. Mobility: The tooth is loosened but is not displaced from its socket.

3. Intrusion: The tooth is driven into its socket. This compresses the PDL and com-

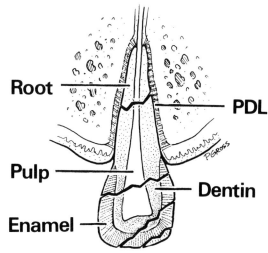

Figure 14–1 ■ Classification of tooth injuries. Tooth fractures may involve enamel, dentin, or pulp and may occur in the crown or the root.

monly causes a crushing fracture of the alveolar socket.

4. Extrusion: This is a central dislocation of the tooth from its socket (Fig. 14–2A). The PDL is usually torn in this injury.

5. Lateral luxation: The tooth is displaced in a labial, lingual, or lateral direction. The PDL is usually torn, and fractures of the supporting alveolus may occur (Fig. 14–2B).

6. Avulsion: The tooth is completely displaced from the alveolus. The PDL is severed, and fractures of the alveolus may occur (Fig. 14–2C).

History

Obtaining an adequate medical and dental history is essential to proper diagnosis and treatment. The medical history should already be on record if the child suffering an injury is brought to his or her regular dentist. Fre-

quently, however, a parent will take an injured child to the closest dentist or to one known to treat children. Thus, with the confusion of a young injured child entering the office for possibly the first time and disrupting the day's schedule, the potential to forget to gather important historical information is great. The use of a trauma assessment form to help record data and organize the management of care is highly recommended (Fig. 14–3).

MEDICAL HISTORY

Routine data on the patient's general health should be obtained. Historical information particularly relevant to the dental injury includes the following:

1. Cardiac disease, which would necessitate prophylaxis against subacute bacterial endocarditis

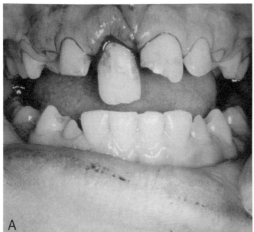

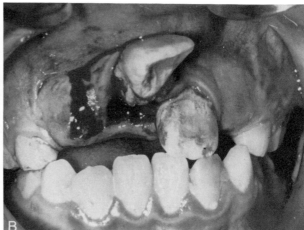

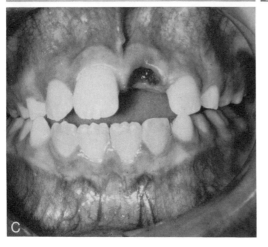

Figure 14–2 ■ A, Extruded tooth. B, Laterally luxated tooth. C, Avulsion injury.

LOUISIANA STATE UNIVERSITY
SCHOOL of DENTISTRY
DEPARTMENT of PEDIATRIC DENTISTRY

Child's Name _____   Student _____

Age _____ Sex _____ Race _____   Faculty _____

Place of Injury _____   Chart No. _____   Date_____

Date of Injury _____

Time of Injury _____

Time Elapsed Since Injury _____

HISTORY

Chief Complaint _____   Previous Trauma _____

Past Medical History _____

Past Dental History _____

How Injury Occurred _____

Tetanus Protection: ☐ No   Yes☐   Date of Last Booster _____

EXTRAORAL ASSESSMENT

CNS Status

☐ Unconsciousness   ☐ Amnesia

☐ Unequal Pupil Size   ☐ Headache

☐ Fixed Pupils   ☐ Nausea

☐ CSF from Ears   ☐ Disorientation

☐ CSF from Nose   ☐ Loss of Smell

☐ Nystagmus   ☐ Seizure

☐ Vertigo

Describe _____

Hard Tissue

☐ Cranial Fracture   ☐ Zygoma Fracture

☐ Mandibular Fracture   ☐ Infection

☐ Maxillary Fracture

Describe _____

Soft Tissue

☐ Laceration   ☐ Abrasion

☐ Contusions   ☐ Infection

☐ Swelling   ☐ Embedded Maternal

Describe _____

INTRAORAL ASSESSMENT

Hard Tissue

☐ Alveolar Fracture   ☐ Palatal Fracture

Describe _____

Soft Tissue

☐ Lips   ☐ Frenum

☐ Buccal Mucosa   ☐ Tongue

☐ Gingiva   ☐ Palate ☐

Describe _____

Dental Occlusion

Molar _____   Cuspid _____

Overjet _____ mm   Overbite _____ %

Openbite _____   Crossbite _____

Classification deviation induced by trauma _____

Describe _____

RADIOGRAPHS

☐ Periapical   ☐ Occlusal

☐ Lateral Anterior   ☐ Panorex

Other _____

Pathology _____

Figure 14–3 ■ Trauma assessment form.

Illustration continued on opposite page

2. Bleeding disorders
3. Allergies to medications
4. Seizure disorders
5. Medications
6. Status of tetanus prophylaxis

The issue of tetanus protection is particularly important when a child has suffered a dirty wound, that is, a deep laceration or intrusion in which soil is embedded in the tissues. Children acquire active immunity through a series of injections of heat-denatured tetanus toxoid in their first 18 months of life. These are normally administered as part of the DPT (diphtheria-pertussis-tetanus) immunizations. Most children are then required to receive a booster when they enter school at approximately age 6. Boosters should be repeated every 10 years unless the child suffers a dirty wound as just described. A booster is then indicated if the child has not received one in the last 5 years (Rothstein and Baker, 1978). Increasing reports indicate that children in the United States are not receiving their childhood immunizations appropriately. If there is any question about the adequacy of a child's tetanus protection, the

DENTAL FINDINGS

Fracture	Class I	Class II	Class III	Class IV

Draw Injury

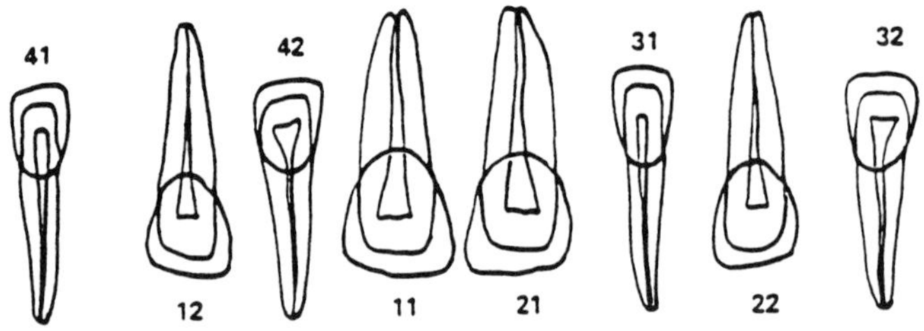

Involved Teeth _____

Tooth Response — Pulp and PDL

Tooth No.				
Exposure				
Hemorrhage				
Heat				
Cold				
Contamination				
Percussion				
Mobility				
Vitalometer				

Displacement

☐ Intrusion ☐ Subluxation

☐ Extrusion ☐ Lateral luxation

☐ Avulsion

Color

☐ Normal ☐ Dark ☐ Light

SUMMARY and DIAGNOSIS

Crown _____

Pulp _____

Root _____

Periapical Tissue _____

Aleolar Process _____

Root Displacement _____

Restoration _____

Fragments _____

TREATMENT

Soft Tissues _____

Pulp _____

Restoration _____

Splinting _____

Medication _____

Recall Follow-up

☐ 2 weeks ☐ 3 weeks ☐ 6 weeks

☐ 3 months ☐ 6 months

Other _____

Figure 14–3 ■ *Continued*

child's physician should immediately be consulted.

HISTORY OF THE DENTAL INJURY

Three important questions are asked in gathering the dental history: when, where, and how did the accident occur? The time elapsed since the injury plays a major role in determining the type of treatment to be provided. The dentist should also determine whether the tooth had been injured previously or whether the injury had first been treated elsewhere.

Where the injury occurred sheds light on its severity. Did the toddler slip and hit the coffee table in the living room or did she fall off her parent's bicycle in the park? This information can help determine the need for tetanus prophylaxis as well as signal a need to rule out more serious injury to the child.

How the accident occurred obviously provides the dentist with the most information regarding severity. Serious head injuries should

be ruled out by asking if the child lost consciousness, has vomited, or is disoriented as a result of the accident. Positive findings indicate potential central nervous system injury, and medical consultation should be immediately obtained (Croll et al, 1980). As previously discussed, the possibility of child abuse can also be ruled out through a careful dental history.

The direction of force to the teeth should be determined. A blow to the underside of the chin frequently causes posterior tooth crown fractures and, sometimes, mandibular symphysis fractures (see Fig. 33–7). These injuries have also been correlated with cervical spine fractures (Bertolami and Kaban, 1982).

Directing attention to the specific teeth involved, the dentist should ask the child if there is spontaneous pain from any teeth. Positive findings here may indicate pulp inflammation that is due to a fractured crown or injuries to the supporting structures such as extravasation of blood into the PDL. Does the child experience a thermal change with sweet or sour foods? If so, dentin or the pulp may be exposed. Are the teeth tender to touch or tender while chewing? Does the child note a change in his occlusion? These findings may indicate a luxation injury or an alveolar fracture.

Clinical Examination

Once the medical and dental histories are complete, the dentist is ready to begin the clinical examination. It is very tempting to focus immediately on a fractured or displaced tooth and thus miss other important injuries. A disciplined approach to a complete clinical examination should be followed in diagnosing every traumatic injury.

EXTRAORAL EXAMINATION

The facial skeleton should be palpated to determine discontinuities of facial bones. Extraoral wounds and bruises should be recorded. The temporomandibular joints should be palpated, and any swelling, clicking, or crepitus should be noted. Mandibular function in all excursive movements should be checked. Any stiffness or pain in the child's neck necessitates immediate referral to a physician to rule out cervical spine injury.

INTRAORAL EXAMINATION

All soft tissues should be examined, and any injuries should be recorded. The presence of foreign matter in lacerations of the lips and cheeks, such as tooth fragments or soil, should be identified. Removal at the initial appointment will eliminate chronic infection and disfiguring fibrosis.

Each tooth in the mouth should be examined for fracture, pulp exposure, and dislocation. In some crown fractures, only a very thin layer of dentin remains over the pulp, so that the pulp's outline can be seen as a pink tinge on the dentin. The dentist should be very careful not to perforate this dentin with an instrument.

Displacement of teeth should be noted, as well as horizontal and vertical tooth mobility. Mobility may be difficult to evaluate clinically in a primary tooth, as it increases with normal root resorption. Reaction to palpation and percussion of teeth is recorded.

Pulpal vitality testing is not routinely performed in the primary dentition. This is because primary teeth do not respond to such tests reliably and because the test requires a relaxed and cooperative patient objectively reporting reactions. Many young children lack the ability to report their reactions to pulpal testing objectively.

RADIOGRAPHIC EXAMINATION

Indications for radiographs ■ Radiographs are an important part of the diagnosis and treatment of dental injuries. They allow the clinician to detect root fractures, extent of root development, size of pulp chambers, periapical radiolucencies, resorptions, the degree of displacement of teeth, position of unerupted teeth, jaw fractures, and the presence of tooth fragments and other foreign bodies in soft tissues. Although some radiographs will show negative findings at the initial appointment, they are nonetheless important as baseline documentation. Subsequent radiographic evidence can thus be compared with the initial films.

Radiographic techniques ■ There is no "standard series" of radiographs for dental injuries. All films taken should clearly show the apical areas of traumatized teeth (see Chapters 17 and 29). In cases in which root fractures are suspected, a second or third radiograph should be made from slightly different angles both

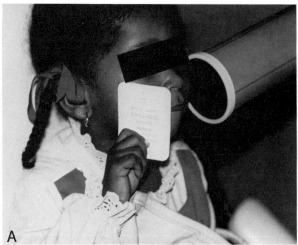

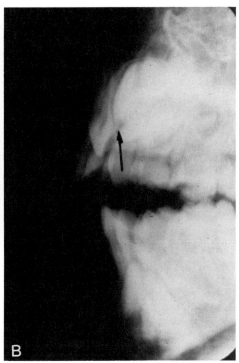

Figure 14-4 ■ *A*, Positioning a child for a lateral anterior radiograph. *B*, Radiograph shows an intruded primary incisor contacting the developing permanent incisor that will succeed it *(arrow)*.

vertically and horizontally to verify the location and extent of the fracture.

A very useful film for planning treatment of intruded primary incisors is the lateral anterior view (Fig. 14–4). As will be discussed in the section on treatment, it is essential to know the precise position of the intruded primary tooth relative to its succeeding incisor. An excellent view can be obtained if the child or parent holds a 3 × 5 inch intraoral film next to the child's cheek and perpendicular to the radiographic beam. For this view, the exposure time for a normal periapical radiograph is doubled.

To determine the presence of foreign bodies such as tooth fragments in the lips or tongue, one fourth of the normal exposure time is utilized. The film is placed beneath the tissue to be examined, and the radiograph is exposed (Fig. 14–5).

Timing of follow-up radiographs ■ As noted previously, many pathologic changes are not immediately apparent in radiographs. After

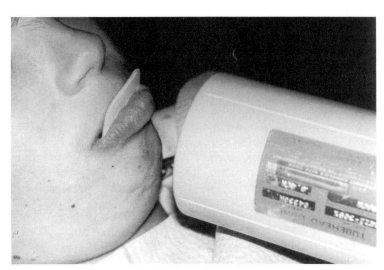

Figure 14-5 ■ Positioning film to detect presence of tooth fragments in the lip.

approximately 3 weeks, periapical radiolucencies that are due to pulpal necrosis can be detected. Additionally, inflammatory root resorption can be evident at this time. After approximately 6–7 weeks, replacement resorption, or ankylosis, can be seen. Thus, there is adequate rationale to plan postoperative radiographs at 1 month and 2 months following the injury. In the absence of any clinical signs or symptoms, such as development of a fistula, mobility, discoloration, or pain, additional films are not indicated until 6 months after the injury. If changes are to appear radiographically, they will usually do so by this time.

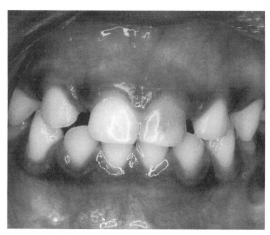

Figure 14–6 ■ Discolored primary central incisor caused by pulpal hemorrhage.

Pathologic Sequelae of Traumatized Teeth

Traumatized teeth are at substantial risk for devitalization, owing to their lack of collateral circulation. The thin band of neurovascular pulp tissue entering at the root apex can easily be severed by relatively minor blows. McDonald and Avery in 1983 outlined a number of potential sequelae to traumatized teeth, as follows.

PULPAL HYPEREMIA

The pulp's initial response to trauma is hyperemia. Capillaries in the tooth become congested, a condition that can be clinically apparent upon transillumination of the crown with a bright light. Additionally, hyperemic teeth are tender to percussion. The hyperemia may be totally reversible or it may be severe, causing stagnation of the vessels at the apex and ischemic necrosis of the pulp.

PULPAL HEMORRHAGE

As a result of hyperemia, the capillaries in the pulp occasionally hemorrhage, leaving blood pigments deposited in the dentinal tubules (Fig. 14–6). In mild cases, the blood is resorbed and very little discoloration occurs or that which is present becomes lighter in several weeks. In more severe cases, the discoloration persists for the life of the tooth.

From a diagnostic standpoint, discoloration of *primary teeth* does not necessarily mean that the tooth is non-vital, particularly when the discoloration occurs within 1 or 2 days after the injury. Color changes that occur weeks or months after the injury are more indicative of a necrotic pulp. Nevertheless, *in the primary dentition, color change alone does not indicate pulp therapy or extraction of the tooth.* Additional signs and symptoms of necrosis, such as mobility, radiographic radiolucency, or pain, must be evident before further treatment is indicated.

CALCIFIC METAMORPHOSIS

Calcific metamorphosis is a condition wherein the pulp chamber and canal are gradually obliterated by progressive deposition of dentin (Figs. 14–7A and 14–8B). This is not a normal pulpal reaction, but it represents a pathologic pulpal response to trauma. Ninety per cent of primary teeth that have undergone calcific metamorphosis resorb normally (Jacobson and Sagnes, 1978), and thus treatment in the primary dentition is usually not indicated. These teeth frequently appear somewhat yellowish in color.

PULPAL NECROSIS

As mentioned previously, a relatively minor blow to the tooth can sever the neurovascular bundle. In the absence of any collateral circulation, the pulp becomes necrotic. Necrosis also occurs when hyperemia is severe enough to strangulate the apical vessels. Periapical radiolucencies indicative of a granuloma or cyst are frequently evident radiographically in necrotic anterior teeth (Fig. 14–7A). Additionally, a pa-

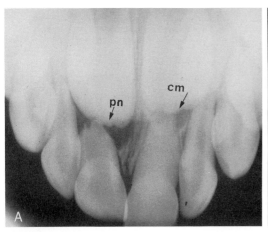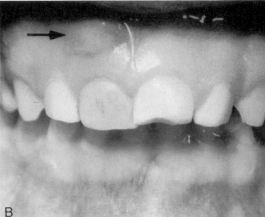

Figure 14-7 ■ *A,* Calcific metamorphosis (cm) in the left primary central incisor and pulp necrosis (pn) in the right primary central incisor. *B,* In the same patient, a parulis is present at the apical level of the necrotic right central incisor *(arrow).*

rulis is often clinically evident at the level of the involved tooth's root apex (Fig. 14–7B).

Some clinicians treat necrotic primary anterior teeth with a pulpectomy technique similar to that used in permanent teeth. A resorbable paste of zinc oxide and eugenol is packed into the thoroughly cleansed canal (see Chapter 20). Owing to the potential for damage to the developing permanent tooth bud, however, many clinicians choose to extract these teeth.

INFLAMMATORY RESORPTION

Inflammatory resorption can occur either on the external root surface or internally in the pulp chamber or canal (Fig. 14–8). It occurs subsequent to luxation injuries and is related to a necrotic pulp and an inflamed PDL. It can progress very rapidly, destroying a tooth within months. Clinicians who choose to treat this condition when it occurs in the primary denti-

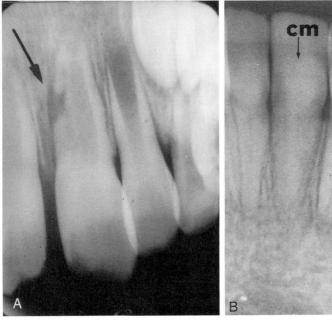

Figure 14-8 ■ *A,* External inflammatory resorption *(arrow). B,* Internal inflammatory resorption (ir) of the lateral incisor; calcific metamorphosis (cm) of the permanent central incisor. *(B* from McTigue, DJ: Management of orofacial trauma in children. Pediatr Ann *14*(2):125–129, 1985.)

tion use resorbable zinc oxide paste as an endodontic filling material.

REPLACEMENT RESORPTION

Replacement resorption, also known as ankylosis, results after irreversible injury to the periodontal ligament. Alveolar bone directly contacts and becomes fused with the root surface. As the alveolar bone undergoes its normal physiologic osteoclastic and osteoblastic activity, the root is resorbed (replaced with bone) (see Fig. 33–8). Ankylosed primary teeth should be extracted if they cause a delay in or ectopic eruption of a developing permanent tooth.

INJURIES TO DEVELOPING PERMANENT TEETH

The most damaging sequelae of injuries to primary teeth are their effect on the unerupted developing permanent teeth. Anatomically, the permanent anterior teeth develop in close proximity to the apices of primary incisors (Fig. 14–4B). Thus, periapical pathology that is due to necrotic pulps, intrusion injuries, or over-instrumentation of primary root canals can irreversibly damage the permanent teeth. If the injury occurs during the development of the permanent tooth crown, enamel hypoplasia or hypocalcification may occur (Fig. 14–9). These injuries can also alter the path of the developing permanent tooth crown, causing root dilaceration or ectopic eruption. For these reasons, the clinician should plan treatment for injuries to primary teeth with the ultimate objective of minimizing any damage to the succeeding permanent teeth.

Treatment of Traumatic Injuries to the Primary Dentition

No injury to the primary teeth should be considered insignificant. A complete diagnostic work-up as described in this chapter should precede all treatment. Even a blow that causes little if any obvious injury to a tooth can lead to pulp necrosis as a result of the severance of the neurovascular bundle at the apex. Any such injury threatens the developing permanent tooth bud; thus, diagnostic follow-up examina-

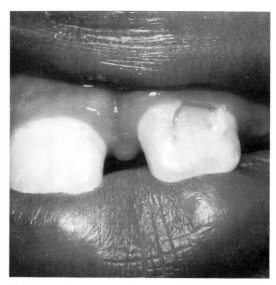

Figure 14–9 ■ Hypoplasia of the maxillary left permanent central incisor as a result of intrusion of a primary incisor.

tions after treatment should occur for all injuries to primary teeth.

TRAUMA TO TEETH

Enamel fractures ■ In small fractures, rough enamel margins can be disked, and no restoration may be necessary. In larger enamel fractures, the tooth can be restored using an acid-etch–composite resin technique (see Chapter 19).

Enamel and dentin fractures ■ Exposed dentin should be covered with calcium hydroxide to prevent insult to the pulp. An acid resistant calcium hydroxide paste is recommended. The tooth is then restored with an acid-etch–composite resin technique. If immediate restoration is not possible, a temporary restoration can be placed, using an orthodontic band cemented with polycarboxylate cement.

Fractures involving the pulp ■ These injuries are rare in the primary dentition. Their treatment depends upon the vitality of the pulpal tissue. A formocresol pulpotomy is completed if the injury has occurred in the last several hours and if the pulp tissue in the canal is judged to be vital (see Chapter 20). If the tissue in the root canal is not vital, a pulpectomy with zinc oxide and eugenol or extraction is indicated. Three fourths of the root formation must be present to consider a pulpectomy, and the canals should be instrumented 1–2 mm short

of the apex. In the primary dentition, a direct pulp cap is not indicated for a crown fracture that exposes the pulp.

Final restoration of the tooth depends upon the amount of tooth structure remaining. A composite resin crown utilizing a celluloid crown matrix is preferred by most clinicians (see Chapter 19). A stainless steel crown with a composite facing is an alternative if little crown structure remains. An orthodontic band cemented with polycarboxylate cement is again an acceptable temporary restoration.

Posterior crown fractures ■ Fractures of posterior primary crowns usually occur as a result of indirect blows, that is, those that occur to the underside of the chin. Therapy in these cases follows the same principles just described. The only difference is that the final restoration will have to be a stainless steel crown in most instances. This is because the fracture involves cusps and other stress-bearing areas, which cannot be restored using composite resin materials currently available.

Root fractures ■ Management of root fractures in primary teeth depends upon the level of the fracture. The best prognosis is for fractures in the apical one third of the root. Most of these teeth maintain their vitality and are minimally mobile. The tooth, including the apical fragment, should resorb normally and should be monitored periodically with radiographs.

Fractures that occur in the middle or cervical thirds of the root indicate extraction. A *gentle* attempt should be made to dislodge the apical root fragment. If it cannot be easily extracted, it should be left and monitored with radiographs. The clinician should make every attempt to avoid disrupting the developing permanent tooth bud.

TRAUMA TO SUPPORTING STRUCTURES

Concussion ■ These injuries will be evident clinically because the teeth are tender to percussion or to biting pressure. If the child complains of pain, the tooth can be gently taken out of occlusion. Follow-up examination is important.

Mobility ■ Increased mobility is a very common reaction of primary teeth to trauma. The child should be instructed to avoid eating with the involved teeth, and follow-up examination should occur in 1 month. No splint should be placed. Prognosis in these cases is usually good.

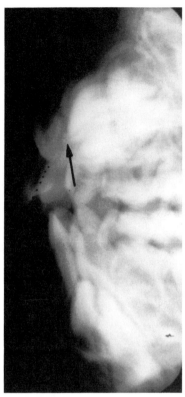

Figure 14–10 ■ An intruded primary incisor not contacting the developing permanent tooth bud (*arrow*) is allowed to re-erupt spontaneously.

Intrusion injuries ■ The intrusion of a primary incisor is potentially one of the most dangerous injuries to the developing tooth bud. A lateral anterior radiograph (described earlier in the chapter) should be taken. If the intruded incisor is contacting the permanent tooth bud (see Fig. 14–4B), the primary tooth should be extracted. If it does not contact the tooth bud but is directed more labially (Fig. 14–10), it should be allowed to re-erupt. Ninety per cent of these teeth re-erupt in 2–6 months, although many develop calcific metamorphosis. Again, calcific metamorphosis is not treated in primary teeth, as the great majority of these cases will resorb normally. Follow-up examination should occur each month until the tooth is completely re-erupted. Post-treatment examinations should then occur every 3 months. Extraction of the tooth is indicated if a fistula or a periapical radiolucency develops.

Extrusion and lateral luxation injuries ■ In these injuries, serious damage to the PDL usually occurs (Fig. 14–11). Some clinicians recommend splinting with sutures until periodontal ligament attachment occurs (approxi-

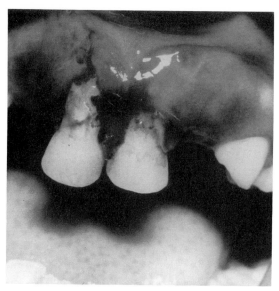

Figure 14–11 ■ Lateral luxation of maxillary primary central incisors.

mately 2 weeks). The author recommends extraction of these teeth, however, because of the potential for aspiration of mobile teeth in young children and because of the potential for subsequent damage to developing permanent tooth buds.

Avulsion injuries ■ Primary teeth that have been avulsed should not be re-implanted. The maxillary anterior region is at low risk for space loss unless the avulsion occurs prior to eruption of the permanent canines. Either fixed or removable appliances can be fabricated to satisfy parental concerns for esthetics (see Chapter 19), and the risk of injuring developing tooth buds is reduced. However, parents should be informed that the permanent teeth may have been injured when the primary teeth were avulsed. Permanent teeth may be delayed in eruption by 1–2 years when the primary teeth that they succeed are lost prematurely. This may be due to the development of fibrotic scar tissue in the path of the erupting teeth.

REFERENCES

Andreasen JO: Traumatic Injuries of the Teeth, 2nd ed. Philadelphia, WB Saunders Co, 1981, p 151.

Bertolami CN, Kaban LB: Chin trauma: A clue to associated mandibular and cervical spine injury. Oral Surg 53:122, 1982.

Croll TP, Brooks EB, Schut L, Laurent JP: Rapid neurologic assessment and initial management for the patient with traumatic dental injuries. JADA 100:530, 1980.

Jacobsen I, Sangnes G: Traumatized primary anterior teeth: Prognosis related to calcific reactions in the pulp cavity. Acta Odontol Scand 36:199, 1978.

Jones JE, Stroup KB, Alley C, Bull MJ: Infant and child passenger restraint systems: The role of pediatric dentistry. Pediatr Dent 8:109, 1986.

McDonald RE, Avery DR: Dentistry for the Child and Adolescent, 4th ed. St. Louis, CV Mosby Co, 1983, p 447.

Needleman HL: Orofacial trauma in child abuse: Types, prevalence, management, and the dental profession's involvement. Pediatr Dent 8:71, 1986.

Rothstein RJ, Baker FJ: Tetanus: Prevention and treatment. JAMA 240:675, 1978.

chapter *15*

Congenital genetic disorders and syndromes

James Bartley

Dentists treat patients with a variety of health problems. Some of these problems are of genetic origin, and manifest themselves very early in life. By becoming familiar with these disorders and syndromes, the dentist will readily identify and treat abnormalities and in addition have the opportunity to enter the patient into a program of genetic health care services.

The initial step in providing genetic health care services is recognition of a genetic health problem or congenital malformation. Any one of the following features should alert the dentist to refer the patient and his or her family into a unified program of genetic health care services, which includes the participation of pediatric dentists, geneticists, pediatricians, and other health care providers. Developmental delay or mental retardation is the most common feature found in genetic syndromes or teratogenic disorders. If a child cannot follow the usual verbal instructions that other children his age follow, a more thorough evaluation is indicated. A child with an unusual facial appearance should spark an inquiry about how many other family members also have similar facial features. In many instances, the facial features are the primary cause for the child's dental

problem. A small mandible (micrognathia) leads to overbite; a flat maxilla leads to deepbite. Other features that should also arouse suspicion of a genetic syndrome are absent or decreased facial expression, limitation of opening the mouth, small or abnormally formed ears, or unusually shaped nose. Within the mouth, microform cleft lip, cleft palate, bifid uvula, multiple frenula, hamartoma of the tongue, bifid tongue, large tongue, or small tongue should alert the primary dentist to question the possibility of a genetic syndrome or congenital malformation. Abnormalities of tooth number, size, shape, structure, or form should also be a signpost of a possible genetic disorder.

The goal of this program is to minimize the burdens that genetic disorders and birth defects impose on patients, families, and the community. These burdens include fear and anxiety, pain and suffering, disproportionate consumption of health care resources, and loss of productivity. Genetic health care services are designed to alleviate fear and anxiety, improve the health of affected individuals, increase productivity of affected individuals, and where possible prevent people from being affected with these conditions.

Mendelian Genetic Inheritance

Gene mutations cause the clinical features that characterize each of the mendelian disorders. A mutation causes a small change in a gene. These changes cannot be visualized by karyotyping (photomicroscopic chromosome analysis). Geneticists delineate the pattern of inheritance of disorders only through the evaluation of family pedigrees. Nine hundred and thirty four autosomal dominant disorders, 588 autosomal disorders, and 115 X-linked disorders have been identified in humans (McKusick, 1986).

The position of a gene on a chromosome is referred to as a *locus.* The paternal chromosome (paternal homologue) and the maternal chromosome (maternal homologue) in a chromosome pair have the same sequence of loci. *Alleles* are alternative forms of a gene that occupy a specific locus. Most alleles do not cause illness. However, those abnormal alleles that cause disease have been the impedus for the evolution of medical genetics. An abnormal allele that causes a disorder, if it is present on only one homologue, produces an autosomal dominant disorder. If the abnormal allele is at the locus on the X chromosome, it causes an X-linked disorder. An abnormal allele that causes a disorder only if it is present on both autosomal homologues produces an autosomal recessive disorder.

Autosomal Dominant Inheritance (Tables 15–1 to 15–3)

An autosomal dominant disorder, such as Van der Woude syndrome, Stickler syndrome, cleidocranial dysostosis, or Crouzon syndrome, has an abnormal allele at one locus and a normal allele at the other locus. Clinical manifestations of autosomal disorders are quite variable, such as cleft lip, cleft palate, or lip pits in Van der Woude syndrome. The presence of any characteristic of an autosomal dominant disorder is called *penetrance* of the gene causing the disorder. *Variable expression* means that a penetrant gene may display different manifestations. For example, lip pits are a mild expression of Van der Woude syndrome, whereas cleft lip and cleft palate are severe expressions of the Van der Woude syndrome. Transmission of an

Table 15–1 ■ Autosomal dominant syndromes associated with cleft palate or bifid uvula without cleft lip

Apert
Cleidocranial dysostosis
Hay-Wells
Kneist
Shprintzen
Spondyloepiphyseal dysplasia congenita
Stickler
Treacher Collins

autosomal dominant disorder within a family is vertical through the pedigree (Fig. 15–1). Each child of an individual with an autosomal dominant disorder has a 1 in 2 chance of inheriting the disorder. The risk is the same for each child regardless of the number of siblings who inherit the disorder. Parents and other family members who are at risk for inheriting the autosomal dominant disorder must be evaluated.

X-linked Inheritance

(Tables 15–4 to 15–6)

X-linked disorders usually are present only in males. Clinical features tend to be similar in all males who have a specific X-linked disorder. For example, males with X-linked hypohidrotic ectodermal dysplasia have very similar characteristics.

Table 15–2 ■ Autosomal dominant syndromes associated with cleft lip with or without cleft palate

Ectrodactyly–ectodermal dysplasia–clefting
Hay-Wells
Oculodentodigital
Opitz
Opitz-Frias
Popliteal web
Rapp-Hodgkin ectodermal dysplasia
Shprintzen
Van der Woude
Waardenburg

Table 15 – 3 ■ Autosomal dominant syndromes associated with anomalies of dentition

Basal cell nevus	Hypohidrotic ectodermal dysplasia
Cleidocranial dysostosis	Oculodentodigital
Crouzon	Osteogenesis imperfecta
Dentinogenesis imperfecta	Pachyonychia
Ectrodactyly – ectodermal dysplasia – clefting	Rieger
Gardner	Robinow
Hallermann-Streiff	Tricho-dento-osseous
Hay-Wells	Van der Woude

Females who are carriers of X-linked disorders usually have fewer and less severe manifestations of the disorder than do the males. However, if through lyonization (the normal process in which in early embryogenesis one of the two X chromosomes in a female is inactivated), a female's normal X chromosome is inactivated in a large proportion of her cells, she will have clinical manifestations that are severe as those seen in males. The inheritance pattern of an X-linked disorder is vertical in a family pedigree (Fig. 15 – 2). If a male with an X-linked disorder has children, none of his sons will have the disorder because each son will inherit the father's Y chromosome. Each of his daughters will be a carrier. A woman who is a carrier of an X-linked disorder has a 1 in 2 chance that each of her sons will have the disorder and a 1 in 2 chance that each of her daughters will be a carrier. If a family decides not to have the sex of the fetus determined through amniocentesis and karyotyping, the risk is 1 in 4 that each child will inherit the X-linked disorder.

Table 15 – 4 ■ X-linked syndromes associated with cleft palate or bifid uvula without cleft lip

Oral-facial-digital
Oto-palato-digital

Some X-linked disorders, such as incontinentia pigmenta, are referred to as X-linked lethal disorders. Many more females than males are live-born with incontinentia pigmenta. The explanation for this ratio is the hypothesis that in females the presence of a normal allele on one X chromosome is necessary for the gestational survival of the female fetus. The male fetus who has only the abnormal allele is spontaneously aborted during gestation.

Table 15 – 5 ■ X-linked syndromes associated with cleft lip with or without cleft palate

Oral-facial-digital

Table 15 – 6 ■ X-linked syndromes associated with anomalies of dentition

Aarskog
Albright hereditary osteodystrophy
Goltz
Hypophosphatemic rickets
Hypohidrotic ectodermal dysplasia
Incontinentia pigmenti
Oral-facial-digital
Oto-palato-digital

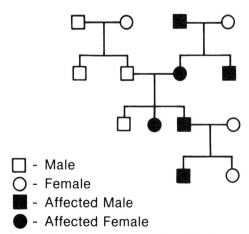

□ - Male
○ - Female
■ - Affected Male
● - Affected Female

Figure 15 – 1 ■ Autosomal dominant inheritance.

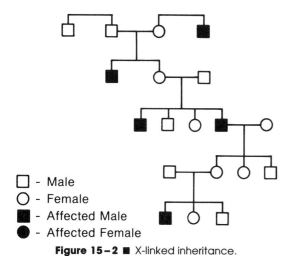

- □ - Male
- ○ - Female
- ■ - Affected Male
- ● - Affected Female

Figure 15-2 ■ X-linked inheritance.

Autosomal Recessive Inheritance

(Tables 15–7 to 15–9)

In autosomal recessive disorders, both alleles are abnormal in an affected person (homozygote). Carriers are asymptomatic. Parents are usually identified as carriers (heterozygote) only after they have a child with a recognized autosomal disorder (Fig. 15–3). Once parents are identified as carriers for a specific autosomal recessive disorder, they have a 1 in 4 chance that each of their children will have the disorder. Marriage between close relatives (consanguineous matings) increases the risk, relative to the risk of the general population, for producing children with autosomal recessive disorders because relatives share genes in common.

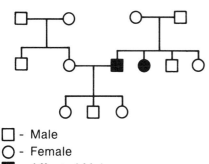

- □ - Male
- ○ - Female
- ■ - Affected Male
- ● - Affected Female

Figure 15-3 ■ Autosomal recessive inheritance.

Table 15-7 ■ Autosomal recessive syndromes associated with cleft palate or bifid uvula without cleft lip
Cerebro-costo-mandibular
Dubowitz
Meckel-Gruber

Some clinical disorders may be inherited in more than one manner. Hypohidrotic ectodermal dysplasia may be inherited as an X-linked, an autosomal recessive, or an autosomal dominant disorder. The clinical features alone in a child with hypohidrotic ectodermal dysplasia will not identify the specific inheritance pattern. All family members must be carefully evaluated to achieve an accurate diagnosis.

Multifactorial Disorders

Many of the more frequent congenital malformations and common health problems are inherited in a multifactorial manner. These disorders, such as cleft lip and palate, cleft palate, congenital heart disease, neural tube defects (spina bifida), and diabetes mellitus, occur more frequently within families than within the general population. These conditions have been referred to as polygenic, but multifactorial inheritance is a better term because it encompasses the concept of both multiple gene effects and multiple environmental effects. The inheritance pattern for multifactorial disorders does not follow the monogenic pattern, nor is the recurrence risk within a family as great as it is for any of the mendelian inherited disorders. In general, the recurrence risk for siblings of an affected individual or for the children of an affected individual who has a multifactorial disorder is 2–5%.

Table 15-8 ■ Autosomal recessive syndromes associated with cleft lip with or without cleft palate
Meckel-Gruber
Mohr
Robert's

Table 15–9 ■ Autosomal recessive syndromes associated with anomalies of dentition

Dyskeratosis congenita	Maroteaux-Lamy pyknodysostosis
Dubowitz	Morquio
Ellis–van Creveld	Osteogenesis imperfecta
Hurler	Sanfilippo
Hypohidrotic ectodermal dysplasia	Weill-Marchesani
Johanson-Blizzard	

Chromosomal Disorders

(Tables 15–10 to 15–12)

A chromosomal disorder is a microscopically visible chromosome abnormality. Three general types of chromosome abnormalities are recognized: aneuploidy, structural rearrangements, and mosaicism. Aneuploidy implies more or less than the normal diploid number (46) of chromosomes. Out of 46 chromosomes, 22 pairs are autosomes and there are 2 sex chromosomes. Non-disjunction of one or more pairs of chromosomes during gametogenesis leads to a gamete that does not have the haploid number of chromosomes (22 autosomes and 1 sex chromosome). If this gamete is fertilized, the embryo will have either too many or too few chromosomes. Aneuploidy occurs in approximately 1 in 200 live-born children. Down's syndrome (47 XY + 21 or 47 XX + 21) is the most common autosomal trisomy (Fig. 15–4). The extra chromosome 21 causes specific physical characteristics. The Kleinfelter syndrome (47 XXY), the X–double-Y syndrome (47 XYY), and the triple-X syndrome (47 XXX) are common aneuploidies of the sex chromosomes.

Table 15–10 ■ Chromosomal syndromes associated with cleft palate or bifid uvula without cleft lip

4p–
5p–
9p–
18q–
Triploidy
Trisomy 13
Trisomy 18
XXXXY

Table 15–11 ■ Chromosomal syndromes associated with cleft lip with or without cleft palate

4p–
5p–
Triploidy
Trisomy 4p
Trisomy 9p
Trisomy 9 mosaic
Trisomy 13
Trisomy 18

There are two types of structural rearrangements of chromosomes. Rearrangements occur (1) within a single chromosome (paracentric or pericentric inversions) or (2) between non-homologous chromosomes (translocations). If the rearrangement preserves the normal amount of chromosomal material, the individual will be normal. If, however, there is an abnormal amount of autosomal material (duplication, deletion, or unbalanced translocation), the individual will have malformations and mental retardation. Cytogeneticists have developed a special nomenclature for describing chromosome abnormalities. For example, a deletion of the terminal segment of the short arm of the number four chromosome is written 4p– (– indicates minus).

Table 15–12 ■ Chromosomal syndromes associated with anomalies of dentition

Trisomy 4p–
Trisomy 20p
Trisomy 21
XXY

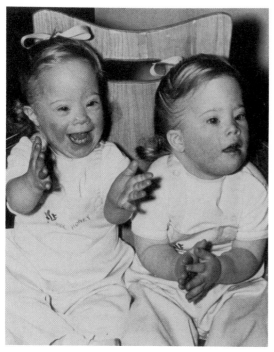

Figure 15–4 ■ Facial characteristics of siblings with Down's syndrome.

Mosaicism is the presence of an unequal number of chromosomes in two or more cell lines within an individual. This occurs during early embryogenesis and results from unequal mitotic separation of chromosomes. The proportion of one cell type relative to the other will vary from tissue to tissue, depending on when the mitotic error occurred and where the cell was located within the embryo. Twenty-five per cent of patients with Turner's syndrome (45 XO) are mosaic (45 XO, 46 XX). A karyotype (photomicroscopic chromosome analysis) is usually taken from blood lymphocytes. Other tissues may be used. Buccal smear analysis of sex chromatin has been used to evaluate patients with sexual ambiguity or Turner's syndrome. However, the test has major limitations because it does not detect structural rearrangement of the X chromosome, X chromosome mosaicism, or multiplicity of the Y chromosome.

BIBLIOGRAPHY

McKusick VA: Mendelian Inheritance in Man, Catalogs of Autosomal Dominant, Autosomal Recessive, and X-linked Phenotypes, 7th ed. Baltimore and London, The Johns Hopkins University Press, 1986.

Smith DW: Recognizable Patterns of Human Malformation, Genetic, Embryologic and Clinical Aspects, 3rd ed. Vol. VII in the Series Major Problems in Clinical Pediatrics, Philadelphia, WB Saunders Company, 1982.

Stewart RE, and Prescott GH: Oral Facial Genetics, Saint Louis, CV Mosby Company, 1976.

SUMMARY FOR SECTION I

Dentists who have been routinely seeing normal children as infants and having the youngsters recalled before their third birthday have noted that it is very rare for children at age 3 to display fears of a dental appointment. This finding is cited as another one of the benefits of these early evaluation appointments. The education of the parents of infants in home care, nutrition, and feeding techniques that attend this movement to see children before their third birthday is also a bonus because it is harder to change a diet at age 3 than it is to adopt a good one a year or two earlier.

Unquestionably, dentistry can be important to this age group. Those children who are on an appropriate fluoride supplementation regimen who would not have been otherwise are definitely benefited. Those who ceased a possibly detrimental nursing habit because of the dentist's urgings also benefit. Also, those children who saw significant improvements in their diet and home care by their parents will, as a group, experience better dental health than would a similar group who did not have any professional intervention before age 3–4 and because of this did not benefit from those aforementioned circumstances.

Today's contemporary dentist who treats children must be prevention oriented. With allegiance to prevention, it only makes sense that a child be seen during infancy. The modest amount of time and the small fee associated with this examination are certainly justified in the long run. The dentist who is concerned with the health of a mother's infant will certainly be the dentist of choice the next time that mother seeks dental care for her child and probably for future siblings of that child. Involvement in pre-natal classes and with the medical community that sees children in one's community is also encouraged. No longer can the dental welfare of the infant and young child be a situation of just intellectual intrigue. The infant and young child must be integrated into professional supervision.

In summary, the ultimate responsibility of the dentist to the age group from conception to three years is to deliver the child to his third birthday as caries free and gingivally healthy as possible, with effective home care techniques being practiced by the parents. This includes a dietary regimen that predicts good dental health as well as the appropriate amount of bioavailable fluoride.

section II

The primary dentition years: three to six years

II

This section on the primary dentition years is the largest section of the textbook. The reason is that children between the ages of 3 and 6 have the need for almost the entire range of diagnostic, treatment, and prevention techniques available to today's dentist. The only real exceptions are the treatment of permanent teeth; certain orthodontic, diagnostic, and treatment decisions; and issues such as temporomandibular joint (TMJ) pathology, which could be pertinent at these years but usually do not manifest problems until later in life. The discussion of acid etching of teeth has been saved for Section III, The Transitional Years, although such techniques are pertinent in the primary dentition also, albeit probably not to the same degree as in the permanent dentition.

Patient management is included along with hospital dentistry in this section because the majority of patient management problems that a dentist will encounter will probably be in this age group. Along with that, the need for hospitalization of children is probably higher in this age group than in the other three groups that we have spoken about. This assumes that to some degree, with good prevention, children have escaped ravaging dental disease and the need for hospitalization for treatment before 3 years of age. It is also assumed that most children's gross dental problems are managed well before age 6. Therefore, if a child requires hospitalization for whatever reasons, this will be done before he or she gets to the transitional years.

This is also an age group in which dental needs today, when compared with those in past years, are changing or have changed dramatically. The good news is that there is the emergence of the caries free child who because of fluoride, home care, proper nutrition, and sealants does not present with any decay at all or, at most, only very modest decay. The bad news is that there are still children who for a variety of reasons need restorative care and sometimes extensive restorative care, including stainless steel crowns and pulp therapy. There are also children who have

had extractions and damaging interproximal decay who need space maintenance and, in instances, space regaining.

The oral habits acquired by children in the first three years, which often were of no concern to the parent or the clinician, become of concern now. Sometimes the possible detrimental effects of these habits are easily discernible even by the untrained eye.

In discussing the dentist's responsibility for the child during infancy and between his first and third birthdays, it was emphasized in Section I that the dentist needed to be able to diagnose the child's prevention needs and to inform and motivate the parents as to their responsibilities in making sure that the child has desirable oral health. When discussing the child between ages 3 and 6, the dentist must also address the child's prevention needs but will in many instances have to be able to manage the child in treatment sessions. Some of these treatment sessions will involve the utilization of local anesthesia, the preparation of teeth, the treatment of pulpal tissue, and sometimes the extraction of teeth. In some instances, these treatments will need to be performed with the parents away from the child and out of the operatory. Unquestionably, patient management is a demanding aspect of dentistry for children. Fortunately, dentistry has many useful child management techniques that are quite effective.

Lastly, this age group, with its skills at talking to people and relating to them, is one that many clinicians find delightful. Their efforts with these children feel unusually rewarding. Dentists who enjoy dentistry for children certainly enjoy this age group in particular.

chapter *16*

The dynamics of change

PHYSICAL CHANGES

BODY

J. R. Pinkham

By the third birthday, the average boy will be approximately 38 inches tall and will weigh about 33 pounds. The average girl will be slightly less than 38 inches (37.6 inches) tall and will weigh about one-half pound less than a boy. For the next 3 years, children will average about 5 pounds of weight gain per year and will gain about 4 inches of height per year. Boys will be on the whole during this time slightly taller and heavier than girls.

There is a strong tendency for children to maintain their comparative weight and height to other children during the preschool period. Tall or heavy children at age 2 are very likely at age 5 to be regarded as tall or heavy also. By this same comparison, children who are light or short at age 2 will likely be regarded as light or short at age 5 when compared with their peer group (Meredith, 1965).

During the preschool period, the correlation between height of the child and his height in early adulthood is moderately good (Meredith, 1965). It should be pointed out, however, that this is not an absolute correlation, particularly for some short individuals who may later, when compared with their peers, become taller. As pointed out in the discussion of the growth changes from birth to age 3, the child's developing elongation of body continues to be apparent during the preschool years. During this time, the head growth seems slow, whereas limb growth seems extremely rapid. In speed of change, trunk growth can be regarded as intermediate. The protuberant, pudgy abdomen of the toddling 2-year-old gradually disappears between ages 3 and 4.

A variety of other bodily changes take place during these critical years of development. Both the heart rate and respiration rate slow down. Conversely, blood pressure rises. At around 4 years of age, the growth of the muscular system in relation to the growth of other tissues of the body significantly changes its rate. Before age 4, the growth of the muscular system is roughly the same as the growth of the body as a whole. However, after age 4 because of the change in rate, approximately 75% of the child's acquired weight during his or her fifth year of development is the result of acquisition of muscle (Thompson, 1954).

During this preschool period of ages 3–6, it will become evident to some degree which children have natural athletic ability and which do

193

not. During these years, the cartilage in the skeletal system is increasingly being replaced by bone and all the bones of the body become more calcified and harder. This calcification predicts an increased incidence in fractured and broken bones.

REFERENCES

Meredith HV: Selected anatomic variables analyzed for interage relationships of the size-size, size-gain, and gain-gain varieties. *In* Lipsitt LP, Spiker CC (eds): Advances in Child Development and Behavior, Vol 2. New York, Academic Press, 1965, pp 221–256.

Thompson H: Physical growth. *In* Carmichael L (ed): Manual of Child Psychology, 2nd ed. New York, John Wiley, 1954, pp 292–334.

HEAD AND NECK

Jerry Walker

The growth of the head and face remains a continuous process during the period from 3–6 years of age. Figure 16–1 illustrates that the percentage of increase in facial growth versus

cranial growth becomes substantially greater around the age of 3 years (Ranly, 1980). This increased change in growth of the face over the cranium will have important effects on a child's appearance. Most children through the age of 2–2 ½ years are relatively nice-looking. A great majority of these children can be described as "cute" or "very cute." The state of being "uncute" or esthetically compromised rarely exists at this age level.

Facial diversity starts to become apparent around age 3. By growth, a child starts to modify the small pug nose associated with early infancy. In the 3- to 6-year-old, in contrast to the newborn, the face becomes larger, wider, longer, and more detailed. During this stage of life, one begins to see the effects of the eruption of permanent teeth. The alveolar ridges grow more prominent, and consequently the jaws become larger. In summary, the small nose, jaws, and mouth of the child younger than age 3 are basically always appealing. It is the details of a face that start emerging after the third birthday that decide its esthetic merit in a growing child, adolescent, and adult.

In 1978, Vann reported the results of a study reviewing cephalometric analyses of children in the primary dentition. He found no statistical differences between males and females at the .01 significance (p > .01), although differences did exist at the .05 level. The various points and planes used in this investigation can be seen in Figure 16–2. Twelve landmarks were identified for this cephalometric analysis. In compar-

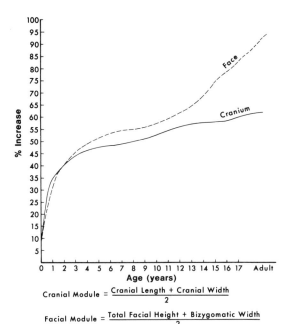

$$Cranial\ Module = \frac{Cranial\ Length + Cranial\ Width}{2}$$

$$Facial\ Module = \frac{Total\ Facial\ Height + Bizygomatic\ Width}{2}$$

Figure 16–1 ■ Comparison of cranial and facial modules (males). Increase in cranial and facial modules during growth. (From Ranly DM: A Synopsis of Craniofacial Growth. New York, Appleton-Century-Crofts, 1980. Data from Scott JH: The growth of the human face. Proc Royal Soc Med 47:5, 1954.)

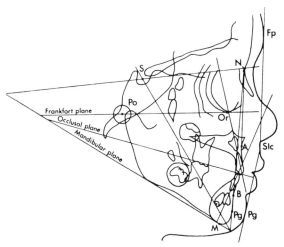

Figure 16–2 ■ Cephalometric landmarks and planes. From Vann WF, et al: A cephalometric analysis for the child in the primary dentition. J Dent Child 45:45–52, 1978.

	Vann (n=32)*	Adult**
SNA	82.9	82.0
SNB	78.1	80.0
SNPg	77.4	83.0
ANB	4.9	2.0
FNA	89.1	88.0
FNB	84.4	87.0
FNPg	85.5	88.0
IMPA	85.2	92.0
FMIA	65.9	65.0
UI-SN	92.4	104.0
UI-F	97.6	110.0
$\overline{1}$-$\underline{1}$	148.4	130.0
M	67.5	69.0
Y-axis	58.5	59.0
OCC-SN	18.8	14.5
SN-MP	35.3	32.0
FMA	29.2	25.0

*All children in this study were between their fourth and fifth birthdays.

**Generally accepted adult norms borrowed from Downs, Steiner, and Tweed.[8-10]

Figure 16–3 ■ Cephalometric angles: a comparison between preschoolers (4–5 yr) and adults. From Vann WF, et al: A cephalometric analysis for the child in the primary dentition. J Dent Child 45:45–52, 1978.

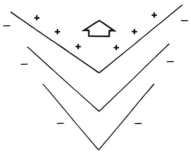

Figure 16–4 ■ An ever-enlarging V brought about by addition on the inside (in the direction of growth) and subtraction on the outside (away from the direction of growth.) (From Ranly DM: A Synopsis of Craniofacial Growth. New York, Appleton-Century-Crofts, 1980. Adapted from Enlow: The Human Face. New York, Harper and Row, 1968.)

ing 17 cephalometric norms established from a sample of 32 Caucasian children of North American ancestry with those of adults, the following conclusions can be drawn (Fig. 16–3):

● It would appear that the maxillary incisor is more flared in the young boy versus the girl.
● It would also seem that the primary incisors are more upright than the permanent incisors (in both boys and girls) (compare UI-SN and UI-F).
● The similarity between angle SNA when comparing children (89.2) and adults (82.0) supports the concept that nasion and point A move forward in relationship to sella in such a fashion that angle SNA is not different in preschool children and adults.
● When angles SNB and SNPg are compared, one sees in children angles of 78.1 degrees and 77.4 degrees in comparison with adult angles of 80.0 degrees and 83.0 degrees, while the ANB angle is greater for children at 4.9 degrees compared with 2.0 degrees in adults.

These findings suggest that mandibular growth from age 4 years to adulthood is more forward than vertical. It is evident that the central inci-

sors' angle to each other ($\overline{1}$–$\underline{1}$) is much larger for children than for adults. The similarities between SNB and SNPg in the child, 78.1 versus 77.4 degrees, suggest that the anterior point on the bony chin has not begun to express itself downward and forward from the cranial base because pogonion and point B are both nearly equal in position to Frankfurt and SN's horizontal planes. Point B will also advance downward and forward, although not to the same degree as will pogonion. This direction of growth continues through adolescence.

The "V" principle of growth was described by Enlow in 1968. This theory hypothesizes that as new bone is deposited at the inside of the "V" in the direction of growth, there is on the opposing side a resorption of bone, and therefore bone growth becomes a series of increasing "V's" (Fig. 16–4). The pattern of growth of deposition and resorption of the maxilla is illustrated by the "V" principle, using the midsagittal section of the maxilla as a shallow "V" and the palate in the floor of the nasal cavity as the opposite side of this "V," the resorptive side (Fig. 16–5). This process results in the movement of the palate away from the cranial base and in an enlargement of the nasal cavity. Other areas where the "V" principle operates in facial growth are demonstrated in Figure 16–6. The condyles, where the condylar cartilage is situated on an ever-expanding "V," and also the coronoid process grow by this principle superiorly and buccally, with the anterior portion of the ramus being continually resorbed (Ranly, 1980). By age 6, the growth of the craniofacial complex has become almost linear and will stay so until adolescence.

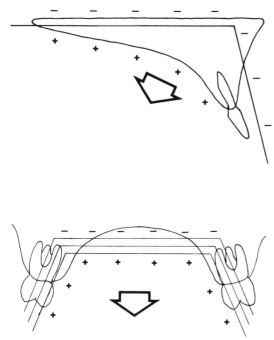

Figure 16–5 ■ *A,* Midsagittal section of the maxilla. Growth visualized as following the V principle. *B,* Cross section of the maxilla. Growth visualized as following a V, albeit somewhat modified. (From Ranly DM: A Synopsis of Craniofacial Growth. New York, Appleton-Century-Crofts, 1980. After Enlow DH and Bang S: Growth and remodeling of the human maxilla. Am J Orthod *51:*446, 1965.)

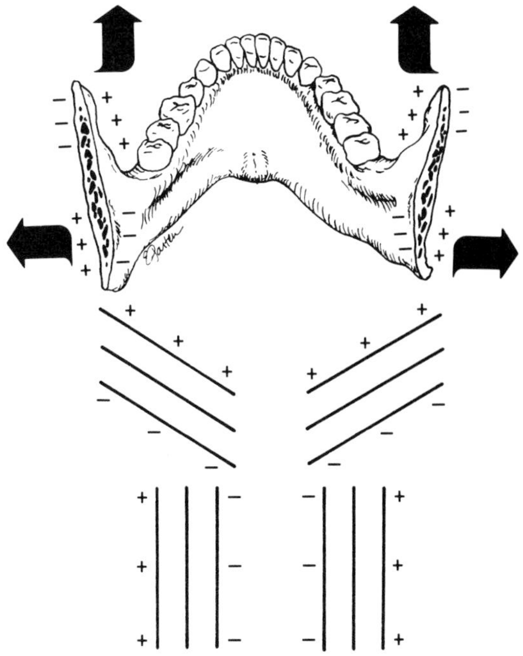

Figure 16–6 ■ Cross section through the rami and coronoid processes, illustrating how these areas of the mandible can be visualized as following the V principle. (From Ranly DM: A Synopsis of Craniofacial Growth. New York, Appleton-Century-Crofts, 1980. Adapted from Enlow DH and Harris DB: A study of the postnatal growth of the human mandible. Am J Orthod *50:*25, 1964.)

REFERENCES

Enlow DH: The Human Face. An Account of the Postnatal Growth and Development of the Craniofacial Skeleton. New York, Harper and Row, 1968.

Ranly DM: A Synopsis of Craniofacial Growth. New York, Appleton-Century-Crofts, 1980.

Vann WF, Dilley GJ, Nelson RM: A cephalometric analysis for the child in the primary dentition. J Dent Child *45:*1, 1978.

DENTAL CHANGES

C. A. Full

Table 6 of Chapter 11 presents a chronology of human dentition. This table demonstrates that the entire primary dentition has completed root development by 3 years of age. This is a relatively stable period clinically for the primary dentition, which was very active before completing its eruption by 24–36 months and root formation by age 3 years. However, this is a significant period of time for the development of the clinical crowns of the permanent denti-tion and their subsequent eruption. There will also be some root resorption of the primary incisors for most children during the last 6 months of this period.

As the permanent dentition develops, some obvious differences in morphologic appearance to the primary dentition become apparent (Fig. 16–7). Wheeler (1958) described the following essential differences:

1. The crowns of primary anterior teeth are wider mesiodistally in comparison with their cervicoincisal length than are the crowns of the permanent teeth.

2. The roots of primary anterior teeth are narrower mesiodistally. Narrow roots with wide crowns present a morphologic appearance at the cervical third of crown and root that differs markedly from the permanent anterior teeth. When the teeth are examined from the mesial or distal aspects, somewhat the same situation in the root and crown measurement at the cervix is observed. The cervical ridge of enamel at the cervical third of the crown, labially and lingually, is much more prominent in the primary teeth than in the permanent teeth.

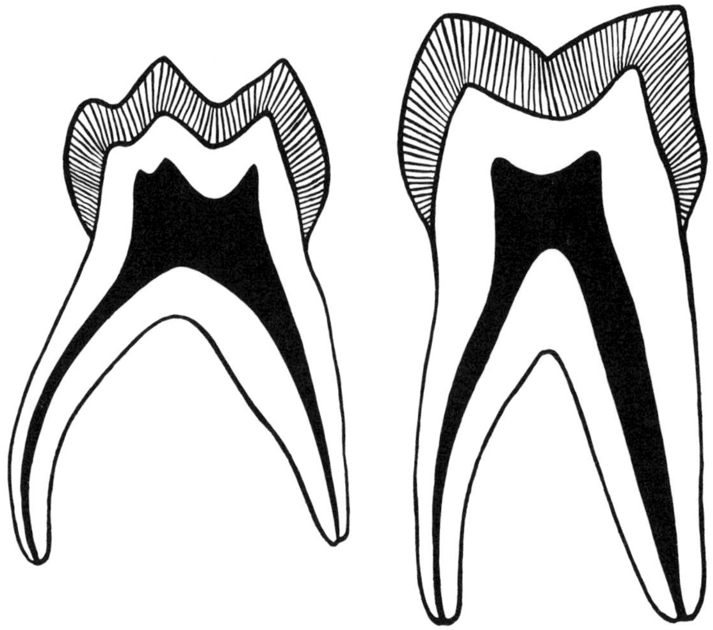

Figure 16–7 ■ Comparison of maxillary second primary and permanent molars, linguobuccal cross section. (From Finn SB: Clinical Pedodontics, 4th ed. Philadelphia, WB Saunders Co, 1973.)

3. The crowns and roots of primary molars are more slender mesiodistally at the cervical third than those of permanent molars.

4. The cervical ridge buccally on the primary molars is much more pronounced, especially on both the maxillary and mandibular first molars.

5. The roots of the primary molars are relatively more slender and longer than the roots of the permanent teeth. They also flare out more apically, extending out beyond projected outlines of the crowns. This flaring allows more room between the roots for the development of permanent tooth crowns before it is time for primary molars to lose their anchorage.

6. The buccal and lingual surfaces of primary molars are flatter above the cervical curvatures than those of permanent molars.

7. The primary teeth are usually lighter in color than the permanent teeth.

REFERENCE

Wheeler RC: Dental Anatomy and Physiology. Philadelphia, WB Saunders Co, 1958.

COGNITIVE CHANGES
J. R. Pinkham

The years between ages 3 and 6 are often referred to in our society as the preschool years, and the children are called preschoolers. Cognitively, these years represent an enormous change. The child's power of reason grows substantially. The simplistic "why" questions of the 2-year-old are replaced by more sophisticated and specific inquiries, such as "How did it get so big?" and "Where did it come from?"

In Piaget's categorization of cognitive intelligence, the years between ages 3 and 6 are called preoperational. The preoperational phase of

cognitive development begins at the end of stage six of the sensorimotor period, somewhere around 18–24 months of age, and lasts until age 6 or 7 years.

Piaget further labeled the first part of preoperational phase as preconceptual and concluded that it lasted until about age 4 years. The preconceptual phase sees the child's mind and mental prowess developing at a rapid rate. The ability of the child's mind to think symbolically with mental imagery is acquired. In the sensorimotor period, the child was restricted to actions with real objects. By the preconceptual phase, the child can play and fantasize using mental symbols.

The child in the preconceptual stage, although he is increasing his cognitive abilities almost immeasurably, must still be regarded as unsophisticated in thinking. The child still generalizes all entities. For example, a bird is *any* bird or, better yet, any bird is *a* bird. The more specific nouns like robin, quail, or heron must await a later level of development. If a child of this age masters both the word chicken and the word bird, he or she will not understand that a chicken is also a bird.

The preconceptual mind is also *centered.* Centration was defined by Piaget as the process of focusing all thought and reason of any mental problem on only one aspect of the whole of the structure and disregarding all other features. Piaget used a dramatic experiment to prove this assumption. He found that children who watched him pour water from one of two identically filled tall, thin vases into a short, wide one often asserted that the tall one has more water in it than the short one. Those children making that assertion have centered on the height of the water. Furthermore, the child's thought during these years is irreversible. The child cannot mentally pour the water back from the short vase to the tall one and see that it would be the same level as the other tall vase.

After the preconceptual stage comes a stage labeled the period of intuitive thought. This stage starts around age 4 and lasts until age 7 or 8. This is a period of sophistication of the child's abilities of grouping objects according to class, using more complex thoughts and images, and outgrowing the tendency toward centration. Late in this period, the child can begin acquiring reading and writing skills. All of this, when combined with increased vocabulary, longer attention span, control over impulses, and toleration of separation from parents, demonstrates that the child is ready for school.

EMOTIONAL CHANGES

J. R. Pinkham

As discussed in Section I, the fear status of most children regarding strangers, separation from parents, and new experience has diminished by the third birthday to the point that these youngsters can take on new social situations without emotional consequences. The process of self-control and control of emotions, such as frustration and fear, develops dramatically between age 3 and age 6 and is paralleled by an equally dramatic socialization process. During these years, a child's sense of sexual identity emerges and a certain degree of masculine and feminine qualities become adopted by the child. A sense of identity and the development of a concept of self-esteem emerge during these years.

One dramatic difference between the child from birth to age 3 and the child from age 3 to age 6 is the development of self-control. Preschool children can be taught methods of self-control, such as distracting themselves when they become impatient or when they are receiving a local anesthetic from a dentist. They can be taught to monitor their own behavior. During the preschool years, the conscience of the child develops and the child becomes capable of feeling guilty or anxious if and when he violates a moral norm.

Aggression is an important concept to understand for parents who have preschool children and for other adults who interface with preschool children. Aggression is often caused by a child's inability to exert self-control. There are two kinds of aggression. One is called instrumental, and it is designed to getting a goal such as obtaining a piece of candy that a sibling has. The other is hostile aggression, and this type is intended to cause a hurt or pain to another person. During the preschool years, the frequency of instrumental aggression should decline. Children who remain hostilely aggressive during the preschool years are children who come from families in which parents and other children are also very overtly aggressive. A parenting philosophy that is inconsistent and unclear in the enforcement of rules has also been linked with aggression in children (Mussen et al, 1984).

In summary, at the sixth birthday a child is certainly not emotionally mature, but he or she is emotionally complex. He is capable now of feeling friendship and hostility, acting out aggression, and experiencing guilt and anxiety. This is a child who is susceptible to praise and is also one who can have his feelings hurt. Much of the literature available in bookstores for this age group covers "how people feel about things." Obviously, these children can relate to the emotions other people have.

REFERENCE

Mussen PH, Conger JJ, Kagan J, Huston AC: Child Development and Personality, 6th ed. New York, Harper and Row, 1984.

SOCIAL CHANGES
J. R. Pinkham

Ages 3–6 represent a time of enormous social growth in the child. Two-years-olds, for instance, cannot for the most part play with a peer. Their play is at best separate but parallel. For example, a pair of 2-year-olds may play in the same sandbox, but there is no relationship of the project of one to the project of the other. By age 3 a child can understand turn taking, and by age 4 cooperative play is possible. By age 6, a child is capable of simple team games.

Between ages 3 and 6, a child needs to gain an understanding of his own personal identification and how he is to relate to other people, ranging from nurturing parents, siblings, peers, and authority figures. During these years, a value system will develop, self discipline will be imposed upon basic urges, and a consciousness that is capable of feeling guilt will emerge. The social transformations of the preschooler predict that his life will never be the same.

There are many theories that seek to explain reasons for the dramatic psychosocial transitions in this age group. The medical-psychoanalytical theory asserts that sexual fantasies and the guilt associated with these fantasies, which at first take the form of an unusual feeling for the parent of the opposite sex (Oedipus or Electra complexes), are the underlying reasons for personality changes. As a child seeks a way to resolve these problems, he or she is forced into identification with the parent of the same sex and adoption of a system of morality, complete with its code of values. This code of moral values has been labeled the *superego*. Behavioralists ascribe the assumption of sex appropriate roles and social values to the effects of reinforcement, both positive and negative, during this period. Social learning theories explain the changes during this period as being the product of the influences of parenting and parental be-

havior. Some theorists believe that as the child becomes conscious of the reasons behind systems of things, he is better able to recognize and be allegiant to the reasoning that underlies social order and values.

Regardless of the theoretical position one may subscribe to, it cannot be argued against the fact that the role of parents is extremely powerful in the preschooler's life. In 1983, Shonkoff pointed out that anyone observing the play of preschoolers will note that the fantasies they enact are rich in their relationship to sexual and adult values. He further noted that many parents have seen and have often been embarrassed by their children acting out realistic domestic situations that have occurred in the family's home.

There continues to be considerable debate in the literature as to where stereotypical sex roles emerge and how much they are controlled biologically or culturally. Data do exist that would suggest that boys are inherently more aggressive than girls. Conversely, preferences for activities such as active sports and playing with dolls are certainly influenced by reinforcement. It can also be argued that media such as television may in a given situation provide information that stereotypes a child's behavior and that media may have more influences than the parents in some situations.

REFERENCE

Shonkoff JP: Patterns of variation over time: Preschool. *In* Levine MD, Carey WB, Crocker AC, Gross RT (eds): Developmental-Behavioral Pediatrics. Philadelphia, WB Saunders Co, 1983, pp 97–107.

Chapter 17

Examination, diagnosis, and treatment planning

Paul Casamassimo □ John Christensen □ Henry Fields

The examination of the 3-year-old child often represents a youngster's first dental experience. For a child who has not had a dental examination previously, the new environment, new people, and the manipulations of tissues previously reserved for self and parent create stress that can be difficult or overwhelming.

An initial examination for this age child is also stressful for the dentist, who is faced with a potential behavior problem, a dental "unknown" without history or clinical baseline, and the challenge to provide both immediate and long-term planning.

The initial examination is a first experience for both dentist and patient and is the opportunity to establish a course of dental health for years to come. Of particular interest in the examination of the 3- to 6-year-old are the following:

1. Lack of an existing history
2. No clinical baseline data
3. Behavioral unknowns
4. A primary dentition occlusion with limited predictive value
5. Unknown preventive needs

All of the above need to be addressed in the evaluation of this age child, especially if this is the child's initial dental visit.

Patient Records

The nature of health care record-keeping in dentistry has evolved from an historical or financial repository to a vital working document. The bare essentials for a pediatric dental record are a health history, examination record, treatment plan, and a series of visit notes. Parental or guardian consent should be obtained and recorded at the initial visit. Adjunctive records, such as study casts and preventive and dietary forms or analyses, also should be kept with the record, if indicated. The history form should allow for updating and a summary.

The possibilities for a dental examination record for children are endless. Many practitioners opt for a standard form or use the one they employed in dental school. No clear-cut guidelines exist for choice of a pediatric dental tooth chart, but some basic requirements exist

from a medico-legal standpoint and from the standpoint of providing a developmental history. The examination record should do the following:

1. Adequately record both developmental status and existing pathosis of teeth
2. Provide a record of each examination, including recalls or periodic examinations
3. Record facial and occlusal status
4. Record oral hygiene and periodontal status

The tooth chart need not be anatomically correct, and in many cases a diagrammatic representation of teeth is of more value. It is critical that the charting system address both primary and permanent teeth so that each record of examination provides an up-to-date developmental profile. In addition to noting presence or absence of a tooth, as is done with adults, looseness of primary teeth and clinically evident eruption of teeth are noted in pediatric dental charting.

Current interest in child safety strongly suggests an initial charting of the dentition, including restorations and abnormalities, but for many children, the absence of restorations or caries may make this an academic exercise.

Periodontal probing of all teeth is not routine, but the dental chart should provide an area for noting particular problems in a numerical or graphic fashion. The nature of this notation simply requires adequate baseline data to accomplish treatment and follow-up.

Many practitioners develop individualized approaches to prevention that can be efficiently addressed on the examination record. A serial chart of oral hygiene performance or gingival scores can be helpful.

Other helpful items on the examination record are vital signs, medical alerts, behavior notes, and unusual findings. These data provide quick reference to the dentist at chairside.

The treatment plan should indicate sequence and permit notation of date of completion of individual procedures. Each visit's progress note indicates what was done and any notable occurrences.

The History

The parent or guardian is the historian for the child. The dentist needs to address both real and perceived problems. Parents may provide erroneous and unverified information simply because the information has not been tested by the health system. Two examples are reported heart murmurs and allergies. Parents may have been informed of a murmur but are unaware of its seriousness. Parents also may confuse nausea with a true allergic reaction. The dentist may be required to address these concerns directly with a physician to obtain accurate information.

A general health history form can be used to elicit a child's health background if attention is given to specific elements that relate to children. The dentist should be well versed in conditions that relate specifically to children. Table 17-1 provides a list of health items that are particularly common in the 3- to 6-year-old age group.

A short and non-contributory history was peculiar for this age group, but with the improvement in infant health practices and home care, immunization, and early intervention, it now is more common. In other situations, a long-established or past problem may have been forgotten or dismissed as unimportant. A non-contributory history should be completed by reiterating the well status of the child, especially the areas of drug allergies, surgical procedures and related problems, cardiac abnormalities, and developmental status.

The dental history should focus on being comprehensive in nature. Many parents have not thought to characterize their child's dental history, other than the eruption of the first tooth. A dental history should minimally cover past problems and care, fluoride experience, current hygiene habits, and an eruption-developmental profile. Table 17-1 addresses the essential elements of the dental history.

The history should be written and reviewed with the parent for clarification before the child is examined. A helpful technique is to use a printed general review list to obtain the history and to distill important information into a concise summary section that is readily accessible and that addresses critical items.

The Examination

The examination encompasses six major sections: behavioral assessment; general appraisal; and head and neck, facial, intraoral, and radiographic examinations.

Table 17 – 1 ■ Selected health history considerations with common findings in the 3- to 6-year-old age group

Area of Concern	Common Findings
General Health	
Allergies	Probably related to food and other environmental allergens; may have allergy to medications such as antibiotics; rash is common manifestation; false allergies often reported
Asthma	May be reported; triggering factors usually known; medications also well-known; impact of dental intervention usually not known
Bleeding	Parent may suggest excessive bruising without real problem
Blood transfusion	May have been performed at birth
Childhood infections	Immunizations will have occurred, or clear history of having had a specific illness such as measles or chickenpox
Development	Poor parental knowledge for normal children; for those with developmental delays, a good history of diagnostic procedures and status
Heart	Functional murmur may exist, or parent may have been told of a murmur
Hypertension	Usually unknown, unless child has chronic problem
Illnesses	Probable history of upper respiratory infections
Jaundice	Possible at birth
Medications	Probably takes acetaminophen (Tylenol) PRN: may have received amoxicillin or other antibiotic
Surgical procedures	Possible tonsillectomy/adenoidectomy; possible ear tubes; circumcision seldom noted as procedure
Seizures	Possible febrile; may be on seizure medication for only one seizure
Dental Health	
Bottle use	Probably considered not contributing to decay
Developmental/eruption	Knowledge may be limited to eruption dates of first teeth, unless consistently very early or late
Fluoride	May know water status; possible vitamin with fluoride supplementation
Habits (thumbsucking)	Will be well known to parent if present
Home care	Usually confined to toothbrushing; may be largely left to child
Previous care	Possibly none; no dentist or care rendered
Reaction to care (behavior)	Possibly none; likely poor or tentative
Trauma to teeth	Possible, but usually left untreated unless serious

This table suggests usual or common responses to questions put to parents of this age group for the average child, but it does not suggest a norm or most frequent response for all children.

BEHAVIORAL ASSESSMENT

A complete behavioral assessment is discussed in Chapter 21 of this section of the text. The general appraisal and chairside examination provide two opportunities to observe behavior and make an initial assessment of potential cooperativeness.

GENERAL APPRAISAL

The general appraisal addresses physical and behavioral status. The classic areas of this component include gait, stature, and presence of gross signs and symptoms of disease. The normal 3- to 6-year-old is ambulatory, well coordinated in basic tasks, engaging, and should ap-

Table 17–2 ■ Selected developmental characteristics of the 3- to 6-year-old

3-Year-Old	4-Year-Old	5-Year-Old
Intellectual Development		
Gives first and last name	Recognizes colors	Names 4 colors
Counts 3 objects	Counts 4 objects	Counts 10 objects
States own age and sex	Tells a story	Asks about the meaning of words
Gross/Fine Motor Skills		
Puts on shoes	Dresses without supervision	Dresses and undresses
Pedals tricycle	Balances on one foot	Hops on one foot
Copies a circle	Copies cross and square	Draws a triangle
Psychological		
The 3- to 6-year-old is in the *phallic* stage of development. During this period, the child undergoes *oedipal* conflicts, which may lead to opposite sex parental preference. The child may exhibit some aggression to siblings. By age 6, the child may be ready to surrender some dependency toward parents.		
Dental Implications		
Needs maternal presence, especially during stress	May be difficult and aggressive	Should leave parent for treatment
Fear of separation	Responds to verbal direction	Proud of possessions
Visual fear	Auditory fear	Bodily harm fear
Physiological		
Height (75th percentile)		
Boys = 97.5 cm	Boys = 106 cm	Boys = 113 cm
Girls = 97 cm	Girls = 104.5 cm	Girls = 111.5 cm
(Growth rate for this period is approximately 6–8 cm/year.)		
Weight (75th percentile)		
Boys = 15.5 kg	Boys = 18 kg	Boys = 20 kg
Girls = 15.5 kg	Girls = 17.5 kg	Girls = 19.5 kg
(Growth rate for this period is approximately 2 kg/year.)		
Pulse (90th percentile)		
105/min	100/min	100/min
Respiration (90th percentile)		
30/min	28/min	26/min
Blood pressure		
100/60	100/60	100/60

pear physically healthy. Table 17–2 lists physical and behavioral milestones for the 3- to 6-year-old. The dentist should incorporate these markers mentally into a profile for evaluation of the child. The general appraisal of the child should be accomplished in the waiting room, if possible, to allow time for observation and clarification of abnormal findings with the parent. This period also permits time to determine and prepare for behavioral problems.

The role of vital signs in the general appraisal is two-fold. The first is to identify abnormalities. The second is the medico-legal role of providing baseline health data for emergency situations. Vital signs may be distorted if the child is upset or anxious. The taking of vital signs of blood pressure, pulse, and respiration may be put off until the child has become accustomed to the environment, but these data must be obtained before any drugs are administered.

Weight should also be obtained and recorded in a conspicuous location on the chart to be available in an emergency. Height should also be recorded, which together with weight, serves as an index of physical development.

THE HEAD AND NECK EXAMINATION

Examining a 3-year-old requires attention to both clinical findings and the patient's behavior in the dental setting. Said differently, the product (dental findings) cannot be separated from the process (behavior) of the examination.

Table 17–3 outlines the elements and expectations for a thorough head and neck examination. The process begins with an orientation to what is to occur. The tell-show-do technique, which involves explanation, demonstration, and finally completion of a step, is a must in the

Table 17 – 3 ■ Elements of head and neck examination

Structure	Diagnostic Technique	Normal Characteristics	Selected Abnormal Findings/Possible Causes
Hair	Visualization	Quality Thickness Color	Dryness/malnutrition, ectodermal dysplasia Baldness/child abuse, self-abuse, chemotherapy Infestation/neglect
Scalp	Visualization	Skin color Dryness Ulceration	Scaling/dermatitis Sores/abuse, infection, neglect
Ears	Visualization Palpation Assessment of hearing	Intact and normally formed external ear and auditory canal Gross normal hearing	Malformed ears and canals/genetic malformation syndrome (e.g., Treacher Collins) Conductive and neurologic hearing loss/trauma, developmental disability
Eyes	Visualization Assessment of vision	Position and orientation in face Movement of eyes Vision Reaction to light	Variation in separation and orientation/genetic malformation syndromes Cranial nerve damage/trauma, developmental disability
Nose	Visualization	Normal size, shape, function, and location	Malposition/genetic malformation syndrome (e.g., median facial cleft) Misshapen/ectodermal dysplasia, congenital syphilis, achondroplasia Discharge/upper respiratory infection, asthma, allergy Poor smell/upper respiratory infection (URI), cranial nerve damage
Lip	Visualization Assessment of function	Speech, closure Integrity Absence of lesions	Poor closure/lip incompetence Clefting/genetic clefting syndrome Asymmetry/Bell's palsy or cranial nerve damage Ulceration/herpes infection
Temporomandibular joint	Visualization Palpation Auscultation	Symmetry in function Smooth movement Absence of pain Range of motion	Deviation/trauma Crepitus, pain/TMJ disorder Limitation/arthritis, trauma
Skin	Visualization	Color Tone Moisture Absence of lesions	Edema/cellulitis, renal disorder Redness/allergic response Dryness/dehydration, ectodermal dysplasia Ulceration/infectious disease, abuse
Neck Lymph nodes	Palpation	Normal size, mobility	Increased size/infection, neoplasia Fixation/neoplasia
Thyroid	Palpation	Normal size	Increased size/goiter, tumor

Table continued on following page

Table 17-3 ■ Elements of head and neck examination *Continued*

Structure	Diagnostic Technique	Normal Characteristics	Selected Abnormal Findings/Possible Causes
Oral Cavity			
Palates	Visualization Palpation Assessment of function	Integrity Absence of lesion Normal function	Cleft/genetic syndrome Ulceration/herpes, mononucleosis, or other infection, abuse Petechiae/sexual abuse Deviation/cranial nerve damage
Pharynx	Visualization	Normal color Normal size of tonsils	Redness/URI, tonsillitis
Tongue	Visualization Palpation Assessment of function	Normal color Range of motion Absence of lesions	Redness/glossitis Ulceration/herpes, aphthous, or other infection, trauma Deviation/cranial nerve damage Limited movement/cerebral palsy
Floor of mouth	Visualization Palpation	Salivary function Absence of swelling Absence of lesions	Swelling/mucocoele, sialolith Ulceration/aphthous ulceration or other infection, abuse
Buccal mucosa	Visualization Palpation	Absence of lesions Absence of swelling Salivary function	Ulceration/cheek bite, abuse Swelling/salivary gland infection, mumps
Teeth	Visualization Palpation Percussion	Normal development Morphologic appearance Occlusion Color Integrity Mobility Hygiene	Absence/delayed eruption/ congenital absence, genetic syndromes Extra teeth/supernumerary, cleidocranial dysplasia Abnormal morphologic appearance/micro-, macrodontia, fusion Abnormal color/amelo-, dentinogenesis imperfecta, staining, pulpal necrosis, caries Fracture/trauma, abuse, caries Mobility/periapical infection, trauma, bone loss conditions, exfoliation Malposition/malocclusion, trauma Pain/periapical involvement

diagnostic process. It begins with discussion in the reception area and reiteration prior to having the child take a seat in the dental chair. What will take place at each step in the examination should be described by the dentist. Acknowledgment by the child—positive or negative—should be elicited. Children should be warned and supported prior to positional changes or intraoral manipulation. The examination provides a non-threatening environment for development of behavioral agreements between dentist and child.

Parental presence is always a matter of controversy. Initial parental involvement may be encouraged to allow a transition into a more direct dentist-child relationship. This is more important for those children under 3 years of age, but it is less so for children near school age. Each child reacts differently to a parent in the operatory, and the dentist must assess the benefit of that presence on the developing relationship he or she has with that child.

The examination must involve evaluation of the head and neck. Palpation to identify enlarged and fixed lymph nodes or other swellings is critical. Many children of this age have swollen nodes, but they are usually movable and confined to the lower face and jaws and indicative of minor infections. Nodes in the clavicular region and occipital areas are more rare and may indicate more serious ailments.

Critical to a thorough examination is evalua-

tion of form and function. The cranial nerves and speech should be evaluated. A complete cranial nerve examination need not be performed, however, because careful observation of sensory and motor function and the child's responses can describe nerve status to a large degree. Normal conversation can be used to identify gross speech pathosis. While palpating the craniofacial structures, the dentist should talk with the child and observe responses.

Verbal responses also serve as behavioral signals of the child's adaptation. A child's cooperation, non-verbal communication, and physiologic responses will often suggest deteriorating behavior. The examination setting is non-threatening, so it provides a good opportunity to develop cooperation.

The manual examination should address physical variations as well as strength and mobility of structures. The visual aspect of the process should address color changes, asymmetry, and physiologic responses such as sweating or dryness.

FACIAL EXAMINATION

A systematic facial examination should be undertaken to ensure that the evaluation is complete and that relevant information is not omitted. A systematic facial examination is one portion of a complete orthodontic evaluation that describes skeletal and dental relationships in three spacial planes — anteroposterior, vertical, and transverse.

First, the facial profile is evaluated in the anteroposterior and vertical planes of space. An assumption is made that the soft tissue profile reflects the underlying skeletal relationship. To begin the examination, the child should be seated in an upright position, looking at a distant point. Three points on the face are identified: the bridge of the nose, the base of the upper lip, and the chin. Line segments connecting these points form an angle that describes the profile as straight, convex, or concave. A well-balanced profile in this age group is slightly convex. If the profile is excessively convex or concave, the clinician should try to determine which skeletal or dental component is contributing to the problem. This can be accomplished by extending a vertical reference line from the bridge of the nose and noting where other soft tissue points are located relative to the reference line. If the maxilla is properly oriented relative to other skeletal structures, the base of the upper lip will be on or slightly anterior to the vertical line. The soft tissue chin will be on or slightly behind the reference line if the mandible is of proper size and in the correct position. If the maxilla is positioned significantly in front of the vertical reference line, the patient is said to exhibit maxillary protrusion. If the maxilla is behind the line, the patient exhibits maxillary retrusion. The position of the mandible is described in the same way.

A well-balanced profile in the anteroposterior dimension has an underlying skeletal relationship that is labeled Class I (Fig. 17–1A). This terminology is used because most Class I skeletal relationships also have Angle Class I dental relationships. When the maxilla is positioned in front of the line or the mandible is positioned behind the line, the profile is described as convex and the skeletal relationship is Class II (Fig. 17–1B). Class II skeletal relationships are rarely caused by one jaw alone but are often the result of some combination of maxillary protrusion and mandibular retrusion. If the maxilla is positioned behind the line or the mandible is positioned in front of the line, the profile is described as concave and the patient has a Class III skeletal relationship (Fig. 17–1C). Again, both jaws usually contribute to the skeletal dysplasia. Class II and III skeletal relationships usually have Angle Class II and III dental relationships, respectively. The Angle dental classification will be described in a following section.

Some caution must be exercised because soft tissues do not always accurately reflect the underlying hard tissue relationships. Research has shown that the 3- to 6-year-old age group is especially difficult to classify accurately from a profile analysis (Fields and Vann, 1979). In addition, vertical facial relationships influence the anteroposterior relationships. This interaction between the horizontal and vertical planes of space and its effect on the profile will be discussed shortly.

The clinician should evaluate the anteroposterior position of the lips and teeth. Incisor position is reflected in lip contour and posture. Lip posture is assessed by drawing a line from the tip of the nose to the soft tissue chin. The lips normally lie slightly behind this line; however, in the 3- to 6-year-old child, the lower lip is 1 mm anterior to the line (Fig. 17–2). Two facts must be kept in mind. First, lip protrusion is characteristic of different racial groups, and lips that are considered protrusive in one group may not be considered protrusive in another. For example, blacks and Asians tend to have more lip protrusion than Northern Europeans. Second, the lips are evaluated in the context of the nose and chin. A large nose and chin can accommo-

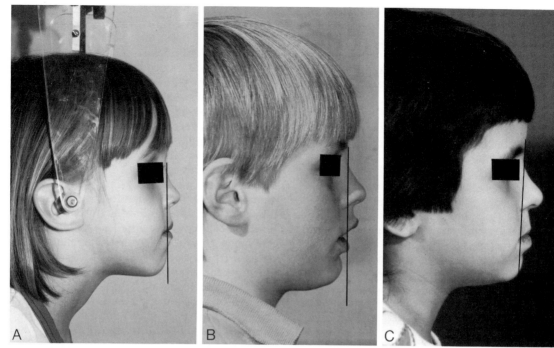

Figure 17–1 ■ *A,* A Class I skeletal relationship is characterized by a well-balanced profile in the anteroposterior dimension. The base of the upper lip (maxilla) should touch or be slightly anterior to a vertical reference line. The soft tissue chin (mandible) should touch or be slightly posterior to the reference line. *B,* A Class II skeletal relationship is characterized by a convex profile. The maxilla is positioned in front of the reference line, or the mandible is positioned behind the line. *C,* A Class III skeletal relationship is characterized by a concave profile. The maxilla is positioned behind the reference line, or the mandible is positioned in front of the line.

date more protrusive lips, whereas a small nose and chin requires less protrusive lips to be proportional.

Vertical facial proportions are also assessed during the profile analysis. Proportionality is judged by dividing the face into thirds, the first extending from approximately the hair line to the bridge of the nose, the second from the bridge of the nose to the base of the upper lip, and the third from the base of the upper lip to the bottom of the chin (Fig. 17–3*A*). These thirds are usually equal. Vertical facial height can also be evaluated by comparing the mandibular plane, a line tangent to the lower border of the mandible, to a horizontal reference line. Vertical problems tend to manifest themselves below the palate in the lower third of the face (Fields et al, 1984). The short face individual tends to have a lower facial third that is proportionately smaller than the other thirds and that has a small or flat mandibular plane angle (Fig. 17–3*B*). The long face patient has a lower facial third that is proportionately larger than the other thirds and a steep or high mandibular plane angle (Fig. 17–3*C*).

There is an interaction between the anteroposterior and vertical dimensions. To illustrate this interaction, imagine a patient with an ab-

normally large mandible or a skeletal Class III relationship. The size of the mandible will be perceived differently, depending on the patient's vertical proportions. A short vertical dimension will cause the patient to appear more concave because the mandible has rotated upward and forward (Fig. 17–4*A*). If an individual has normal vertical proportions, the profile will still be concave but not nearly so exaggerated (Fig. 17–4*B*). Finally, an individual with a long lower face will appear to have a straight or slightly convex profile because the mandible has rotated downward and backward, which in effect hides the large mandible by making it more retrusive (Fig. 17–4*C*).

Transverse facial dimensions are examined to rule out facial asymmetry. Facial symmetry is best evaluated with the patient reclined in the dental chair and the dentist seated in the 12 o'clock position (Fig. 17–5). Hair is pulled away from the face, and a piece of dental floss is stretched down the middle of the upper face to aid in judging lower face symmetry. All faces show a minor degree of asymmetry, but marked asymmetry is not normal (Fig. 17–6). Asymmetry is usually manifested in the lower facial third, whereas upper facial asymmetry is extremely rare. In this age group, a deviation of

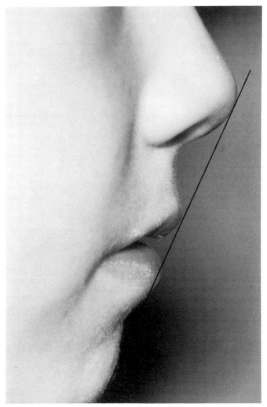

Figure 17–2 ■ The anteroposterior position of the lips is determined by drawing a line from the tip of the nose to the soft tissue chin. The upper lip should normally lie slightly behind the line, while the lower lip should lie slightly in front of this line in the 3- to 6-year-old child.

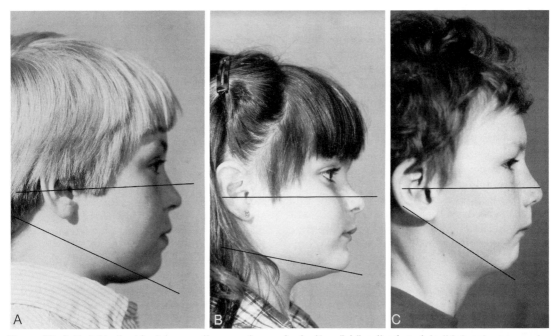

Figure 17–3 ■ *A,* Vertical facial proportions can be evaluated by dividing the face into thirds or by comparing the mandibular plane with a horizontal reference line. In a well-proportioned face, the facial thirds are equal in size. *B,* A child with short vertical facial dimensions has a proportionately smaller lower facial third and a flat mandibular plane. *C,* A child with long vertical facial dimensions has a proportionately larger lower facial third and a steep mandibular plane.

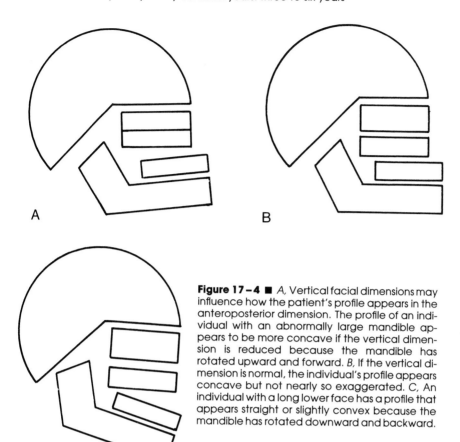

Figure 17–4 ■ A, Vertical facial dimensions may influence how the patient's profile appears in the anteroposterior dimension. The profile of an individual with an abnormally large mandible appears to be more concave if the vertical dimension is reduced because the mandible has rotated upward and forward. B, If the vertical dimension is normal, the individual's profile appears concave but not nearly so exaggerated. C, An individual with a long lower face has a profile that appears straight or slightly convex because the mandible has rotated downward and backward.

the midpoint of the mandible to one side or another may be due to true asymmetry, but it is most often indicative of a posterior crossbite and mandibular shift, two findings that are discussed later in the chapter. During the evaluation of the transverse dimension, the dental midline of each arch should be checked and compared with the midsagittal plane. The dental midlines should also be checked with one another in centric relation and centric occlusion. Deviations or asymmetric positioning of the eyes, ears, or nose may be symptoms of a cranial synostosis or an undiagnosed syndrome. A child with these findings should be referred to appropriate professionals for a complete evaluation.

INTRAORAL EXAMINATION

The armamentarium for the intraoral examination includes mirror, explorer, gauze, and periodontal probe, if needed. Additional materials are disclosing solution, dental floss, toothbrush, and scaler. Gloves should be worn for all clinical care, especially for new patients. This protection is as much for the young child as it is for the dentist.

The intraoral examination begins with an excursion around the oral cavity, noting general architecture and function. The fingers should be used to identify soft tissue abnormalities before instruments are placed in the mouth. Children in this age group will often permit oral inspection with "just fingers," and the dentist can use this as a springboard to obtain cooperation for use of mirror and explorer. The mirror should be the first instrument introduced. This is usually readily accepted by the child, owing to its familiarity.

Young children are sometimes uncooperative. A decision must be made to manage behavior early. Parental assistance can be used to obtain an examination of the oral cavity. Use of physical restraint by the dentist without parental consent is risky and is not advisable.

An important portion of the intraoral examination is directed toward the teeth. Each of the 20 primary teeth should be explored, per-

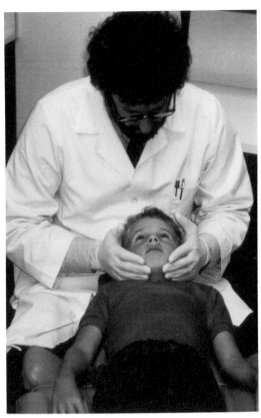

Figure 17–5 ■ Facial symmetry is best judged with the patient reclined and the dentist seated in the 12 o'clock position.

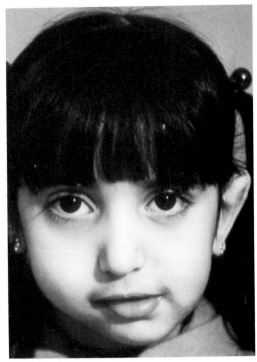

Figure 17–6 ■ This patient exhibits marked asymmetry that is a result of a congenital fusion of the left condyle and coronoid process to the temporal bone.

cussed, and visually scrutinized. Selective periodontal probing may be performed, but the yield is likely minimal as a result of the infrequency of irreversible attachment loss in the primary dentition.

Occlusal Evaluation

Another portion of the intraoral examination is the systematic analysis of the occlusion in three spatial planes. In addition, each dental arch is analyzed individually to describe arch form and symmetry, spacing and crowding, and the presence or absence of teeth. Arch analysis is best performed on diagnostic study models; however, diagnostic casts are usually not indicated in this age group unless there is some need to clarify findings or if tooth movement is contemplated.

If diagnostic casts are necessary, an appropriate impression tray must be chosen. Properly fitted trays will seat comfortably into the mouth and will extend far enough posteriorly to cover the most distal tooth and either the maxillary

tuberosity or the mandibular retromolar pad. The trays should be of a non-perforated variety that will hold the impression material in the tray and express the excess material into the vestibule. Expression of the excess material into the vestibule is desirable because it displaces the soft tissues, which allows the dentoalveolar morphology to be clearly viewed on the cast. The trays can also be lined with wax that will aid in tissue displacement and make seating the tray into position more comfortable (Fig. 17–7A). After the appropriate tray has been selected, the alginate is mixed and placed in one tray. For either arch, the tray should be rotated laterally into the mouth and seated first, posteriorly against the palate or the retromolar pad (Fig. 17–7B). This technique limits the posterior flow of alginate. The tray is then rotated and seated over the anterior teeth, which causes the excess impression material to flow out around the sides and front of the tray (Fig. 17–7C). Finally, the tray is held in place until the alginate has set. After the upper and lower impressions are made, a wax bite is made by placing a softened piece of baseplate wax between the teeth and having the patient close in centric occlusion. The wax is cooled with air and serves to orient the casts properly during trimming.

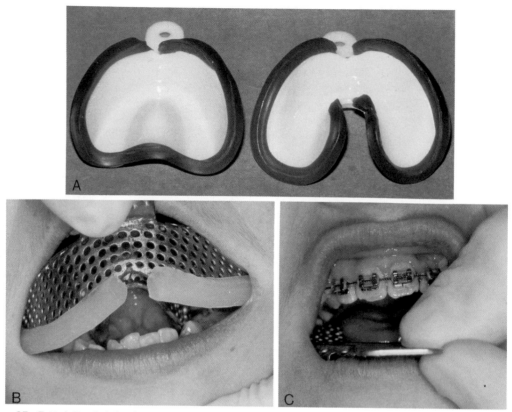

Figure 17 – 7 ■ *A,* The first step in making diagnostic casts is to select impression trays of appropriate size and line the trays with wax. The wax aids in tissue displacement and makes seating the tray more comfortable. *B,* The tray should be rotated laterally into the mouth and should be seated first in the posterior area. *C,* The tray is then seated anteriorly, causing the impression material to flow out the sides and front of the tray.

Impressions should be poured quickly in white plaster because the alginate will dehydrate and distort if it is left sitting for more than a few minutes. The plaster is vibrated into the impression and flowed from one tooth to another to prevent air entrapment, which results in holes in the models. Separate plaster bases are poured and the impressions inverted on the bases when the plaster is partially set (Fig. 17–8A). After the plaster has set, the trays are separated carefully from the casts to prevent breaking the teeth. The maxillary cast is trimmed so that the top of the base is parallel to the occlusal plane. The back of the upper cast is trimmed perpendicular to its top and the midpalatal raphe. The maxillary and mandibular casts are occluded, and the back of the mandibular base is trimmed parallel to the top of the maxillary cast. Finally, the sides of the casts are trimmed in a symmetrical manner, which allows the clinician to judge arch symmetry (Fig. 17–8B).

Alignment

Dental arches can be categorized as having either a U-shaped or V-shaped form. The mandibular arch is normally U-shaped, whereas the maxillary arch can be either shape. The dental arch should be symmetrical in the anteroposterior and transverse dimensions. Individual teeth are compared with their antimeres to determine if there is anteroposterior and transverse symmetry (Fig. 17–9).

The ideal arch in the primary dentition has spacing between the teeth. Two types of spaces are identified. The first type, primate space, is located mesial to the maxillary canine and distal to the mandibular canine. Developmental space is the space present between the remaining teeth (Fig. 17–10). Anterior spacing is desirable in the primary dentition because the permanent incisors are larger than their primary precursors. Although the presence of primate

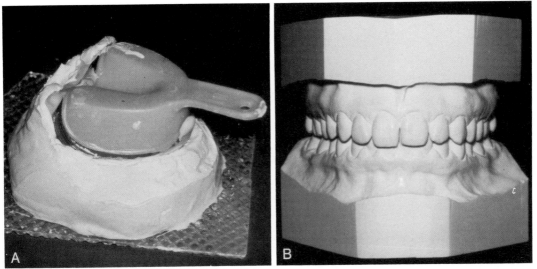

Figure 17–8 ■ *A,* The impressions should be quickly poured in white plaster and inverted on separate plaster bases after the plaster has partially set. *B,* After the plaster has set, the casts are separated from the impressions and are trimmed in a symmetrical manner to allow the dentist to judge arch symmetry.

and developmental spacing does not ensure that the permanent dentition will erupt without crowding, these spaces usually alleviate some crowding. Crowding or overlapped teeth in the primary dentition may occur, although it is rare. True crowding in the primary dentition almost always guarantees a crowded permanent dentition. Crowding of isolated teeth, however, is sometimes indicative of a sucking habit. Teeth can be tipped lingually into a crowded position as a result of constant pressure from a finger (active digit habit). This is most evident in the lower incisor region (Fig. 17–11).

Although it seems elementary, the clinician should carefully count the number of teeth in the mouth. Children in this age group should have all their primary teeth present at this time. Those with delayed dental eruption may have either a very slow but normal sequence of eruption or some isolated eruption problem. To distinguish the two, the eruption sequence of the child is compared with the normal sequence of eruption and the eruption pattern on the right side is compared with that on the left. If the sequence seems to be appropriate, dental development is probably slow. If, however, the patient's eruption pattern deviates from the normal sequence and there are differences between contralateral sides of the mouth, further investigation is warranted to determine if

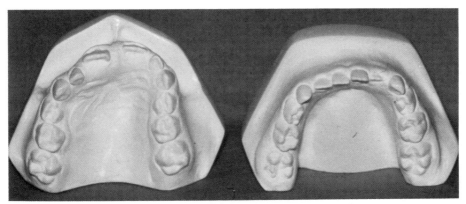

Figure 17–9 ■ These casts illustrate marked dental arch asymmetry in both the anteroposterior and transverse dimensions. Asymmetry of this magnitude is not normal.

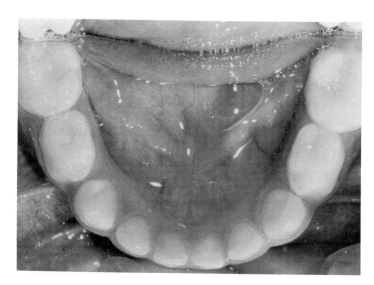

Figure 17–10 ■ This arch shows both primate spacing (distal to the canine in the mandibular arch) and developmental spacing (space between the remaining teeth).

teeth are missing or are impeded from erupting. The maxillary lateral incisor is the most common missing tooth in the primary dentition (Valachovic and Lurie, 1980).

Counting teeth will also reveal the presence of supernumerary or extra teeth. Approximately 0.3 per cent of children have supernumerary teeth in the primary dentition. The prevalence of fused and geminated teeth is approximately 0.1 to 0.5 percent (Valachovic and Lurie, 1980). Fusion of two primary teeth usually can be distinguished from gemination without the aid of radiographs by counting the number of teeth. There should be nine teeth in the arch, one of which is very large, rather than the normal number of ten if two primary teeth have fused. If gemination has occurred, there should be ten teeth in the arch and one will be very large. A radiograph may be necessary to confirm the preliminary diagnosis of fusion or gemination. Fused primary teeth will show two distinct and independent pulp chambers and canals with union of the dentin. Geminated primary teeth show two crowns and two pulp chambers connected to a single root and pulp canal.

Anteroposterior Dimension

After the maxillary and mandibular arches have been examined for symmetry, spacing, and tooth number, the two arches are examined together. In the anteroposterior dimension, primary molar and canine relationships are determined and compared with the skeletal classification. In the primary dentition, molars are termed flush terminal plane, mesial step, or distal step (Fig. 17–12). Primary canines are classified as Class I, Class II, Class III, or end-to-

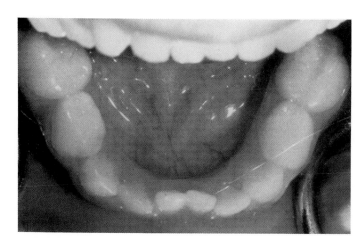

Figure 17–11 ■ An active digit habit has caused the mandibular central incisors to tip lingually in this child, which also caused the arch to appear more crowded.

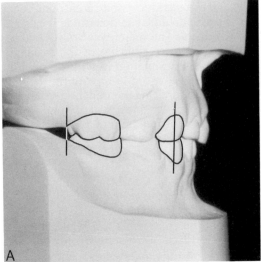
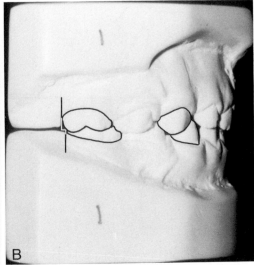
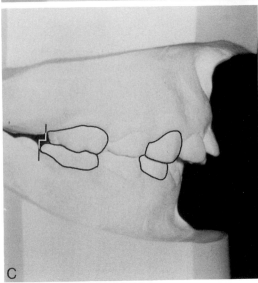

Figure 17–12 ■ *A,* In the primary dentition, the occlusion is classified according to the relationship of the mandibular second molars and canines to the maxillary second molars and canines. In this example, the distal surface of the mandibular second molar is flush with the distal surface of the maxillary second molar. This primary molar relationship is termed flush terminal plane. The long axis of the mandibular canine is coincident with the long axis of the maxillary canine. This is described as an end-to-end canine relationship. *B,* In this example, the distal surface of the mandibular molar is mesial to the distal surface of the maxillary molar. This primary molar relationship is termed mesial step. The maxillary canine is positioned in the embrasure between the mandibular canine and first molar. This is described as a Class I canine relationship. *C,* In this example, the distal surface of the mandibular molar is distal to the distal surface of the maxillary molar. This primary molar relationship is termed distal step. The maxillary canine is positioned in the embrasure between the mandibular canine and lateral incisor. This is described as a Class II canine relationship.

end. These dental classifications generally reflect the skeletal classification.

Primary molar relationships as described by the distal surfaces of the primary second molar are worthy of attention not only because they describe the relationship of the primary mandibular teeth to the primary maxillary teeth, but also because these surfaces guide the permanent molars into occlusion and determine permanent molar relationships. Documenting primary molar relationships also allows one to follow the effects of growth or treatment.

Overjet, the horizontal overlap of the maxillary and mandibular incisors, is measured in mm (Fig. 17–13). It may be more meaningful to describe overjet in terms of ideal, excessive, or deficient rather than as a millimetric measure. Incisor position should be described as normal; protrusive, if flared outward; or retrusive, if excessively upright.

Transverse Relationship

The transverse relationship of the arches is examined for midline discrepancies and posterior crossbites. The midline of each arch is compared with the other and with the midsagittal plane. A large midline discrepancy is unusual in the early primary dentition, and the clinician should be suspicious of a mandibular shift. The presence of a mandibular shift is often indicative of a posterior crossbite.

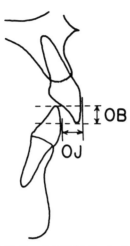

Figure 17 – 13 ■ Overjet (OJ) is the horizontal overlap of the maxillary and mandibular central incisors and is measured from the most anterior point on the facial surfaces of the incisors. Overbite (OB) is the vertical overlap of the incisors and is measured from the incisal edge of one incisor to the other. Overbite can be recorded in mm or as a percentage overlap of the total length of the mandibular incisor.

If a posterior crossbite is encountered, the clinician should try to determine the cause of the crossbite. The majority of posterior crossbites are due to constriction of the maxillary arch. This is one situation in which diagnostic casts are helpful to aid in or confirm the diagnosis. After the arch at fault is identified, an attempt is made to determine if the crossbite is bilateral or unilateral. If models are available, they can be measured to see if teeth are equidistant from the midpalatal raphe. If models are not available, the determination must be made clinically. The first step is to guide the mandible into centric relation. If teeth are in crossbite on both sides of the arch when the mandible is in centric relation, the child exhibits a bilateral crossbite. If the teeth are in crossbite on only one side of the arch with the mandible in centric relation, the crossbite is unilateral (Fig. 17 – 14). It is important to check the child with the mandible in centric relation because a bilateral crossbite will appear to be unilateral if the mandible is shifted into maximum intercuspation (Fig. 17 – 15). The child shifts the jaw because the teeth do not fit

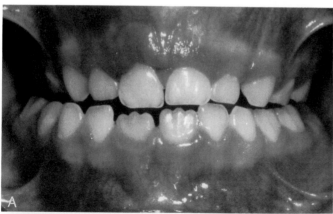

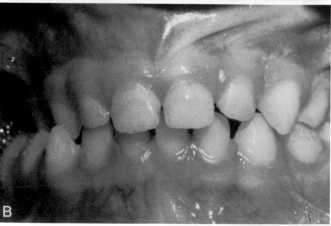

Figure 17 – 14 ■ *A*, This patient exhibits a bilateral posterior crossbite when positioned in centric relation. *B*, This patient exhibits a unilateral posterior crossbite when positioned in centric relation. The distinction between bilateral and unilateral crossbite in centric relation is important because treatment considerations are different for each type of crossbite.

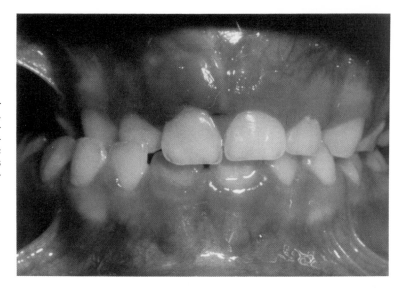

Figure 17–15 ■ The same patient pictured in Figure 17–14A, with the teeth in centric occlusion. This emphasizes the importance of determining centric relation occlusion because it is the basis for most treatment decisions.

well together and the bite is uncomfortable. A true unilateral crossbite that is due to a unilateral maxillary constriction in the primary dentition is rare but can occur.

Vertical Dimension

Overbite, the vertical overlap of the primary incisors, is measured and recorded in mm or as a percentage of the total length of the mandibular incisor (see Fig. 17–13). Deepbite is the complete or nearly complete overlap of the primary incisors. Anterior open bite, the absence of vertical overlap, is usually indicative of a sucking habit in this age group (Fig. 17–16). If the patient and parent deny the existence of a sucking habit, further investigation into the cause of open bite is needed. Skeletal malocclusion, condylar fracture, and degenerative diseases such as juvenile rheumatoid arthritis may account for the open bite and should be investigated. Overbite is approximately 2 mm in the primary dentition.

Ankylosis, the fusion of tooth to bone, is rather common in the primary dentition (Fig. 17–17). Although an ankylosed tooth cannot erupt further, the unaffected adjacent teeth will continue to erupt. This creates the illusion of the ankylosed tooth submerging into the bone. The prevalence of ankylosed teeth is between 7 and 14% in the primary dentition (Brearly and McKibben, 1973; Kurol and Koch, 1985). In addition, 50% of the patients with an ankylosed tooth will exhibit more than one ankylosis. The following is a list of the most commonly anky-

losed teeth in the primary dentition (Brearly and McKibben, 1973):

1. Mandibular primary first molar
2. Mandibular primary second molar
3. Maxillary primary first molar
4. Maxillary primary second molar

A number of eruption and exfoliation problems have been blamed on ankylosed teeth. However, longitudinal studies indicate that ankylosed primary teeth exfoliate normally and

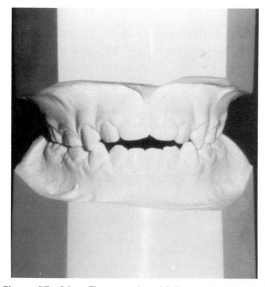

Figure 17–16 ■ These casts exhibit an anterior open bite, the absence of vertical overlap. Anterior open bite is most commonly caused by a sucking habit in this age group.

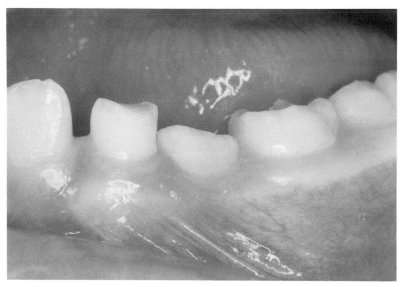

Figure 17-17 ■ Ankylosis, the fusion of tooth to bone, is common in the primary dentition. This patient has an ankylosed primary mandibular first molar that is below the plane of occlusion.

allow normal eruption of succedaneous teeth (Messer and Cline, 1980; Kurol and Koch, 1985). An ankylosed tooth should not be removed routinely unless a large marginal ridge discrepancy develops between it and the unaffected adjacent teeth. If a marginal ridge discrepancy develops, the adjacent teeth may tip into the space occupied by the ankylosed tooth and cause space loss.

RADIOGRAPHIC EVALUATION

The dentist will require radiographs to make a thorough diagnosis or problem list in the 3- to 6-year-old child.

Children in this age range may have difficulty cooperating with the radiographic procedures, in which case radiographic examination should be deferred until behavior improves or can be managed. Introduction of the child to

intraoral radiography can be done by use of the following:

1. Tell-show-do introduction, using a camera analogy. It helps to do a dry run and to show an unexposed packet of film and an exposed radiograph to explain the process. By positioning the film and x-ray machine, the dentist will also determine if a child will sit for an exposure, to prevent unproductive irradiation.

2. Matching film size to comfort. Many children have difficulty with the film impinging on the lingual surface of the mandible. In some cases, bending the anterior corners will help. Another technique is to place the film vertically to minimize anteroposterior size (Fig. 17-18).

3. Use of the least difficult procedures to acquaint the child. Anterior occlusal films are usually easiest.

4. Being sure that all settings are made on the machine and that the apparatus is positioned

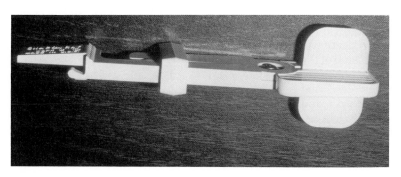

Figure 17-18 ■ Decreasing anteroposterior size by rotating a 0-size film 90 degrees. Care must be taken to obtain views of all contacting posterior tooth surfaces.

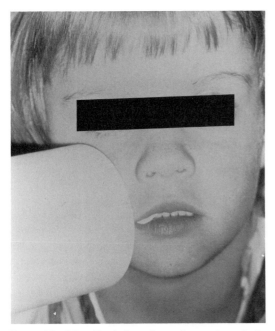

Figure 17 – 19 ■ Technique for radiograph posterior bitewing (No. 0 film). *Vertical angulation:* + 10. *Horizontal angulation:* Face of cone is parallel to film packet, with beam directed to open embrasures. *Film placement:* Film packet with bitewing tab is placed lingual to teeth, and child bites on tab. Film should be placed to get view of distal surfaces of canines anteriorly. Child should smile to show teeth, which helps to orient beam to prevent overlap.

A-Ray* has been used for film positioning in this age group with great success, owing to its small size and light weight. Other positioning instruments can be used, but some thought should be given to the size and weight of the instrument that must be placed intraorally. The patient should be adequately protected from unnecessary radiation. A lead apron and collar is necessary to provide thyroid and gonadal protection. A 16-inch or long cone will further reduce skin exposure. Prior to exposure of the radiographs, the ability of the child to cooperate must be assessed to prevent wasted film. When parents are used to stabilize films, they must be adequately shielded, pregnancy must be ruled out, and the parent must demonstrate the ability to stabilize the film and patient before exposure.

A concerned parent should ask about frequency of films. The American Academy of Pediatric Dentistry (1985) advises radiographic exposure at a rate necessary to maximize detection of abnormalities yet minimize exposure to ionizing radiation. Table 17 – 4 addresses selection criteria for pediatric radiographs in the 3- to 6-year-old. All radiographs should be made only after a clinical examination and history.

Diagnosis and Treatment Planning for Non-orthodontic Problems

The process of diagnosis of disease is a complicated one, based on clinical, historical, and supportive data. A problem list may be preferable to a series of diagnoses, since the list presumes that treatment will be done. A synthesis of all data is required. The practical portions of the process are to consider the following:

1. Existence of abnormal state
2. Determination of cause
3. Alternatives or options to correct the problem
4. Anticipated benefits, immediate and long-term
5. Problems or requirements for accomplishment of treatment

A primary consideration is denoting an abnormal state, such as caries or a non-vital pulp. A problem list helps separate those abnormali-

before positioning the film. Some children can hold a film for only a short period, owing to gagging or short attention span.

For the primary dentition, no radiographs are indicated when all proximal surfaces can be visualized and clinically examined. When the proximal surfaces cannot be visualized and clinically examined, bitewing radiographs are indicated to determine the presence of interproximal caries (Fig. 17 – 19). Other projections are indicated in the following circumstances: history of pain, swelling, trauma, mobility of teeth, unexplained bleeding, disrupted eruption pattern, or deep carious lesions. These views include the maxillary (Fig. 17 – 20*A*) and mandibular periapical (Fig. 17 – 20*B*) and the maxillary (Fig. 17 – 20*C*) and mandibular occlusal (Fig. 17 – 20*D*). An occlusal size film can be used to obtain a lateral jaw radiograph in this age child. The lateral jaw film can be made by having the child hold the film or lie on his side, as shown in Figure 17 – 21. Pediatric (0-size) films should be used, with the exception of the occlusal films, which are No. 2 size. The Snap-

---

* Rinn Corporation, Elgin, IL.

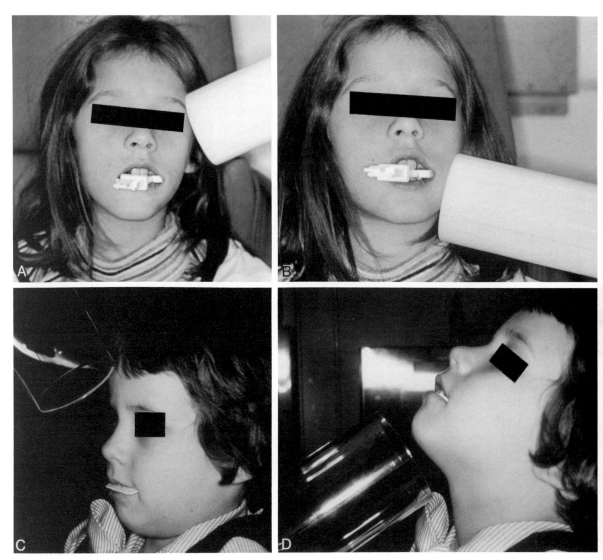

Figure 17–20 ■ Techniques for supplementary diagnostic radiographs.

A, Maxillary periapical (No. 0 film). *Vertical angulation:* Beam is at right angle to film; starting angle of +30. *Horizontal angulation:* Face of cone is parallel to facial surface of teeth. *Film placement:* With film in jaw of holder, holder is placed between maxillary and mandibular teeth with dimpled surface of film against lingual surfaces of teeth. Child bites on larger sides of jaws.

B, Mandibular periapical (No. 0 film). *Vertical angulation:* Beam is at right angle to film; starting angle of −5. *Horizontal angulation:* Face of cone is parallel to facial surface of teeth. *Film placement:* With film in jaws of holder, holder is placed between maxillary and mandibular teeth, with dimpled surface of film against lingual surfaces of teeth. Child bites on larger side of jaws.

C, Maxillary occlusal (No. 2 film). *Vertical angulation:* +60, with beam directed down. *Horizontal angulation:* Beam is directed along midsagittal plane. *Film placement:* Film packet is placed between maxillary and mandibular teeth so that it is parallel to floor. Film is oriented so that the long dimension extends right and left. The child bites gently on the film while seated upright.

D, Mandibular occlusal (No. 2 film). *Vertical angulation:* −15, with beam directed up. *Horizontal angulation:* Beam is directed along midsagittal plane. *Film placement:* Film packet is placed between maxillary and mandibular teeth, and child is instructed to bite gently on the film. Patient is reclined so that the chin is extended. Bisecting angle technique is used.

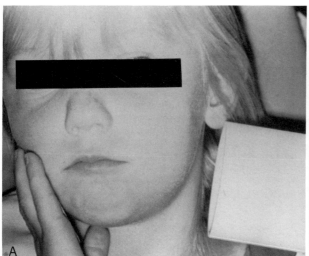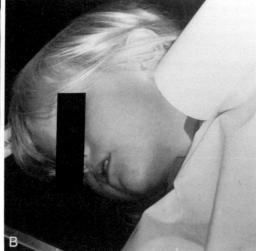

Figure 17–21 ■ Lateral jaw techniques. *A,* Child is seated upright with head tilted approximately 20 degrees. Film packet is held or taped across area to be exposed. Beam is directed from side opposite film through the tissues at about − 10 degrees. The central beam is directed perpendicular to the film and is aimed at the center of the film. *B,* This technique can be used for an active child or a patient with cerebral palsy. The dental chair is reclined, and the patient lies on side with head tilted. Pillows can be used to stabilize the body and head. The film is placed between the child and chair, and beam angulation is adjusted accordingly.

Table 17–4 ■ **Selection criteria and guidelines for pediatric radiographs in the 3- to 6-year-old**

Projection	Criteria	Frequency
Posterior bitewing	Proximal surfaces of posterior teeth cannot be examined clinically Child is cooperative	*At initial examination* if contacts closed *Semi-annually* if interproximal surfaces have been restored, until child demonstrates low risk* or is caries free; also semi-annually if child is at high risk* *Annually* to 18-month interval if child caries free at initial bitewing examination
Posterior periapical	Suspected pathosis Confirmed pathosis Child is cooperative	As needed to diagnose and monitor treatment or patient condition
Anterior occlusal	Suspected pathosis Confirmed pathosis Child is cooperative	Same as above

* High risk for dental caries may be associated with (1) poor oral hygiene, (2) fluoride deficiency, (3) prolonged or inappropriate nursing, (4) high carbohydrate diet, (5) poor family dental health, (6) developmental enamel defects, (7) developmental disability or acute medical problem, or (8) genetic abnormality.

Excerpted from conference proceedings: Radiation Exposure in Pediatric Dentistry, April 22–25, 1981, Cincinnati, Ohio, *Pediatr Dent 3*(Special Issue 2):462, 1981.

ties that are in need of treatment from those that are simply identified. For example, a carious primary molar in a 6-year-old is a problem; a loose carious mandibular incisor may not be if it is about to exfoliate. The cause of the abnormality is critical to determine short- and long-term treatment. A manageable cause will most often result in both short- and long-term success. Caries is a largely environmental condition that can be managed with great likelihood of success in both the short- and long-term. On the other hand, dentinogenesis imperfecta is genetic, and has a guarded and limited prognosis.

For most patients, no single treatment plan is ideal. A variety of alternatives must be considered, based on health, parental finances, cooperation, and the anticipated benefits from the treatment. These issues are shared by dentist and parent. For example, extraction of decayed primary teeth may be preferred to restoration if there is likelihood of unsuccessful pulpal therapy. Another example is the choice of a stainless steel crown rather than a three-surface amalgam restoration in a decay-prone individual, since fewer surfaces are left open to recurrent decay.

Finally, a frank assessment of cooperation and involvement in treatment by the family must be considered. Dental treatment is necessarily a cooperative effort, with success resting on both personal and professional maintenance. The behavioral plan is critical to the success of the treatment plan in general. For the 3- to 6-year-old child, the methods of behavior management must be included in the treatment plan. The sequencing of behavior management, obtaining consent for medication, and reasonable alternatives to recommended procedures should be covered in discussion of the behavioral plan.

REFERENCES

American Academy of Pediatric Dentistry: Oral Health Policies. Dental Radiographs in Children. Chicago, American Academy of Pediatric Dentistry, 1985.

Brearly JL, McKibben DH: Ankylosis of primary molar teeth: Parts I and II. ASDC J Dent Child 40:54–63, 1973.

Fields HW, Vann WF: Prediction of dental and skeletal relationships from facial profiles in preschool children. Pediatr Dent 1:7–15, 1979.

Fields HW, Proffit WR, Nixon WL, Phillips CL, Stanek E: Facial pattern differences in long-faced children and adults. Am J Orthod 85:217–223, 1984.

Kurol J, Koch G: The effect of extraction on intraoccluded deciduous molars: A longitudinal study. Am J Orthod 87:46–55, 1985.

Messer LB, Cline JT: Ankylosed primary molars: Results and treatment recommendations from an eight-year longitudinal study. Pediatr Dent 2:37–47, 1980.

University of Texas Dental School at San Antonio: Pediatric Dentistry Radiography. Early Eruptive Stage (5 years and under). San Antonio, University of Texas Dental School at San Antonio, 1987.

Valachovic RW, Lurie AG: Risk-benefit considerations in pedodontic radiology. Pediatr Dent 2:128–146, 1980.

White SC: Radiation exposure in pediatric dentistry: Current standards in pedodontic radiology with suggestions for alternatives. Pediatr Dent 3:441–447, 1982.

chapter 18

Prevention of dental disease

Arthur Nowak □ James Crall

With the complete eruption of all the primary teeth, the preschool child enters a relatively short period of stabilization in preparation for the loss of the first primary teeth and the lengthy process of eruption of the permanent teeth. Historically, preschoolers have their first dental examination during this period. Instructions are provided on appropriate oral hygiene techniques. Adjustments are made for optimal systemic fluoride supplementation if the child is not living in a fluoridated community.

Dietary management can now become a problem. This is the period of developing favorite foods and dislikes for other foods. The effect of commercials, both from television, radio, and the press, begins to take its toll. Children are frequently sent off to a preschool educational environment for a quasi-educational experience, a babysitting service, or a true preschool developmental experience. These lifestyle changes predict meals prepared by surrogate parents, lunches packed by parents to be consumed later, and snacks provided by peers or care providers; therefore, the control of the quality and quantity of these meals is sometimes greatly sacrificed.

With the end of the day in sight and the "I want to watch just one more TV program" routine common, the daily supervised oral hygiene regimen is sacrificed for the quick 30-second unsupervised brushing. Additionally, it is amazing how quickly parents assume that 4-year-olds can be responsible for their own oral hygiene when they cannot even comb their hair or clearly print their name.

Fluoride Administration

DIETARY FLUORIDE SUPPLEMENTATION

Steps to ensure an optimal dietary intake of fluoride should continue to be a primary concern for children 3–6 years of age. For children who do not have access to fluoridated drinking water, this means continuing to provide adequate fluoride supplementation. By age 3, most

children will be able to chew and swallow tablets. Therefore, prescriptions for supplemental fluoride should be changed accordingly to reflect this change in developmental status. The recommended supplemental fluoride dosage schedule also requires an increase in the amount of fluoride that is prescribed once a child has reached 3 years of age. The recommended daily dosage of supplemental fluoride for children aged 3–14 is 1.0 mg fluoride for children whose drinking water contains less than 0.3 ppm fluoride and 0.5 mg fluoride for children whose water contains between 0.3 and 0.7 ppm fluoride. Children whose drinking water contains more than 0.7 ppm fluoride do not require any supplementation. Although the potential for producing esthetically objectionable dental fluorosis will have diminished in this age group as a result of substantial crown formation of the anterior teeth, the practice of analyzing samples of each child's drinking water prior to prescribing supplemental fluoride should continue to be followed.

Because parental compliance continues to play a key role in determining the effectiveness of these supplements, efforts to reinforce parental motivation should be provided. One method of assessing parental compliance is to monitor the necessity to rewrite supplemental fluoride prescriptions at recall visits. The dosage and amount of fluoride prescribed should be noted in each patient's record whenever a prescription is written. Parents who indicate no need for an additional prescription when the patient's record suggests that the previously prescribed amount of supplement should have been consumed should be questioned as to the number of tablets remaining. A large existing supply would suggest poor compliance during the period prior to the recall visit.

TOPICAL FLUORIDE THERAPY

Topical fluorides play an increasing role in the 3- to 6-year-old group. The child's ability to use fluoride dentifrices increases throughout this period, although restraint should continue to be exercised in terms of the amount of toothpaste used at each brushing. Professional topical applications are often initiated during this interval. One mode of topical application that is generally not recommended for the younger members of this age group is the use of fluoride mouthrinses, since most preschoolers are unable to avoid swallowing these solutions.

PROFESSIONAL APPLICATIONS OF FLUORIDE

Topical applications of highly concentrated forms of fluoride have been provided in dental offices for over 40 years. The most commonly used agents have included 8–10% solutions of stannous fluoride, as well as 2% sodium fluoride and 1.23% acidulated phosphate fluoride (APF), the latter two being available in both solution and gel formulations. Numerous studies conducted prior to 1980 reported caries reductions averaging approximately 30% for these agents (Ripa, 1982; Brudevold and Naujoks, 1978). However, several more recent studies, including a large-scale national demonstration program, have shown reductions of less than 15% and savings, in terms of the actual number of tooth surfaces saved from becoming carious by semi-annual applications of these agents, that were much less than in earlier trials (Bell et al, 1984; Wefel, 1985).

Indications for Professional Topical Fluoride Applications

The questions of for whom and when topical applications of fluoride should be provided in the dental office are the source of some controversy. One school of thought invokes the argument that professional fluoride applications are a primary preventive measure and should be provided to all children in order to minimize the potential for developing new carious lesions. This argument would seem to have some merit in the absence of methods for predicting whether an individual patient is likely to develop caries. Advocates of this philosophy tend to focus only on the potential benefits that might be achieved from topical fluoride applications while ignoring the costs associated with providing the service.

Other professionals feel that the decision to provide topical fluoride therapy should be made on the basis of those factors that have been shown to be associated with the risk of developing caries at the level of groups of individuals (i.e., access to fluoridated drinking water, use of other forms of topical fluoride, degree of spacing between teeth, etc.). Their approach would be to consider the likelihood that each individual will develop disease, based upon these factors, and then recommend professional topical fluoride therapy for those who are deemed to be at significant risk to develop caries. Proponents of this philosophy tend to give consideration to the costs associated with

providing the preventive service as well as to the potential benefits to be gained.

The validity of the second approach obviously depends upon the degree of accuracy with which one is able to predict which individuals are more likely to develop caries at some future point in time. Several approaches aimed at differentiating high risk and low risk patients are currently being developed and evaluated. As methods of caries prediction for individuals are refined over time, the argument for individualizing preventive treatments is likely to become increasingly more compelling.

Cost-Benefit Considerations

In a private practice setting, the patients' willingness to pay for different forms of treatment usually is an important factor in determining which types of services are provided. In the case of public programs or private third-party payers, the decision to provide reimbursement for various services may be based on a more formal analysis of the relationship between the costs and benefits associated with those services. The ratio of costs to benefits has historically been higher for topical fluoride applications provided in dental offices than for other types of preventive services or for the same services provided in other settings. Consequently, professional topical fluoride treatments have not been justifiable as a public health measure because of their unfavorable cost-to-benefit ratio.

The recently documented changes in caries levels and patterns of decay in U.S. children have pushed these ratios even higher. Specifically, two recent large-scale studies (Bell et al in 1984 and the National Caries Program in 1981) have reported that a substantial proportion of U.S. school age children are caries free and that a relatively small percentage of children account for a large percentage of all decay. In addition to the overall decline in the level of caries, there has been a decrease in the proportion of smooth surface caries and a corresponding increase in the proportion of pit and fissure caries. The combination of these factors seems to have been associated with a reduction in the effectiveness of concentrated topical fluoride therapy in terms of the actual number of surfaces saved from becoming carious during a given period of time (Bell et al, 1984).

Changes of this nature have led some investigators to call for a re-examination of the manner in which various preventive measures are provided. In an era when increased attention is being focused on measures for controlling all types of health care costs, some professionals have proposed that consideration be given to making preventive dental services more cost-effective. One means of improving the cost-to-benefit ratio of topical fluoride therapy would be to provide these procedures in settings other than dental offices, using self-application techniques (i.e., at school or in the home). Another previously mentioned method that also would apply to preventive services provided in dental offices would be to identify patients who are more likely to develop caries and to target preventive services to those individuals.

One factor that has repeatedly been demonstrated to be associated with a reduction in both the risk of developing caries and the relative effectiveness of topical fluoride therapy is the availability of drinking water containing fluoride. Studies have shown that topical fluorides are considerably less effective in reducing the incidence of decay in fluoridated areas compared with non-fluoridated areas (Bell et al, 1984; Wei, 1974). Therefore, the cost of preventing a carious lesion in a fluoridated area via professional topical fluoride therapy is significantly greater than the cost of preventing a lesion in a non-fluoridated area. From a cost-benefit perspective, this suggests that in fluoridated areas topical fluoride treatments should be reserved for those patients with a history of moderate to high caries increments or who belong to proven high risk categories. Those patients who do not seem to be particularly prone to developing caries, especially smooth surface decay, would probably benefit more from other forms of prevention, such as occlusal sealants.

The question of which preventive services are to be provided for a particular child in the dental office remains a private matter between the dentist and the patient (or the parents or guardian in the case of a child). Thus, the final decision regarding the costs and benefits of professional preventive services must be made by the child's parent. However, the influence of third-party coverage for different types of services can have a significant influence on this decision and ultimately on the care that the child receives.

Need for Prophylaxis Prior to Topical Fluoride Treatment

Another issue related to the effectiveness of professional topical fluoride therapy, which also has implications for lowering the cost-to-

benefit ratio, concerns the need for the prophylaxis that has traditionally been provided prior to fluoride application. Research in both laboratory and clinical settings has shown that the ability of a variety of topical fluoride agents to penetrate through dental plaque and to deposit fluoride in enamel is not significantly reduced by the presence of an organic layer on the tooth surface (Klimek et al, 1982; Tinanoff et al, 1974; Joyston-Bechal et al, 1976). This concept has been tested further in a 3-year clinical study, which demonstrated that the ability of a professionally administered APF gel treatment to prevent caries was not influenced by whether a prior prophylaxis had been performed (Ripa et al, 1984).

It has been pointed out that elimination of the prophylaxis could significantly reduce the labor cost of delivering topical fluoride treatments (Heifertz, 1978). The practical implications of these findings in terms of a dental office are (1) that the decision to provide a thorough prophylaxis, less rigorous cleaning (i.e., toothbrushing prior to fluoride treatment), or no prior cleaning can be made on an individual basis, depending upon the condition of the patient; and (2) that several children could be treated simultaneously, thereby reducing the time and cost of the procedure (Ripa, 1982).

Some individuals insist that the prophylaxis is an excellent way to introduce children to the sensations associated with the use of a handpiece in the mouth. Although this may be true, the practitioner should realize that elimination of this step would not appear to adversely affect the caries protection provided by topical fluoride therapy in most cases.

Methods of Application

The most popular professional topical fluoride agents in use today are APF and sodium fluoride. APF was developed as a solution containing 1.23% fluoride at pH 3.2 (Wefel, 1985). Several new products containing lower fluoride concentrations and at higher pH have been developed and marketed in recent years. Many of these products have not been tested in clinical trials, as were the original formulations. Therefore, the effectiveness of these agents remains unproved in many instances.

Applications of APF or sodium fluoride are usually provided to patients on a semi-annual basis in disposable polystyrene trays using a gel as a vehicle. The recommended application time for both APF and sodium fluoride is 4 minutes. Although gels are favored over solutions because of their ease of application, there is some evidence that the gels may not reach into caries-susceptible interproximal areas (Goodman, 1983), prompting some investigators to recommend that the gel be carried into the interproximal sites via dental floss following topical fluoride application (Wefel, 1985).

The advantages of the gel-tray system include (1) generally good patient acceptance; (2) a relatively long shelf life of the agents; (3) control over the areas to which fluoride is applied; and (4) minimization of personnel time, since the application process usually involves treating both arches simultaneously and requires very little patient supervision, thereby freeing personnel to perform other tasks. Occasionally, a child will not be able to tolerate the use of two trays at once. In these instances, each arch may have to be treated separately.

The usual procedure involves (1) dispensing approximately 5 cc of gel into each tray (care should be taken not to overfill the trays), (2) drying the teeth in the maxillary and mandibular arches with a gauze or stream of air prior to placement of the trays, (3) inserting the trays and checking for proper coverage, (4) placing a saliva ejector, and (5) asking the child to bite down and close his or her lips around the saliva ejector. The saliva ejector should always be used during topical fluoride applications, using trays to minimize the swallowing of these highly concentrated agents. Following the topical application, the saliva ejector should be used to remove any excess fluoride that may have remained.

Considerations for Special Patients

As with any age group, certain children will require special consideration with respect to their needs for fluoride therapy or the manner in which this therapy must be provided. Specifically, alternative approaches should be available for children with developmental disabilities or medical conditions that either place them at higher risk to develop caries or limit their ability to obtain fluoride in the usual manner.

For example, patients with cerebral palsy may find it difficult to tolerate trays for topical fluoride applications. Topical fluorides may have to be applied with a brush or cotton swab for these individuals. Children being treated with irradiation or chemotherapy often experience ulcerative degeneration of their soft tissues, causing them to become extremely sensitive to preparations having a low pH (i.e., APF) or to certain flavoring agents. A dilute, neutral,

non-irritating formulation should be provided for these patients. Children with chronic renal failure may experience elevated serum fluoride levels for prolonged periods following ingestion of concentrated fluoride preparations as a result of their kidney impairment. Because children with chronic renal failure also have been noted to have a lower caries experience than matched controls, systemic or professional topical fluorides are not recommended for these individuals (Crall and Nowak, 1985). These are but a few of the many types of patients who require modification of usual preventive practices. The National Foundation of Dentistry for the Handicapped has prepared a manual that outlines recommendations for conventional as well as alternative preventive regimens for individuals with handicapping conditions (A Guide to the Use of Fluorides, 1981).

Dietary Management

A number of factors begin to emerge during the preschool period that can have a profound effect on the growth and development of a child as well as on his or her dental health. Following the large gains in growth during the first 3 years of life, the preschool child's rate of growth slows markedly. Therefore, caloric requirements need to be reduced accordingly, but a balanced diet need not be sacrificed.

It is becoming common for both parents to be employed once the child reaches 3 years of age. Therefore, the management and control of diet, enjoyed during the first 3 years of life, can become threatened. With preschoolers sent off to the sitter, grandparents, or schools, children become introduced to new environments, food selections, and management styles. It is no wonder that they become confused, begin to question routine dietary practices, and may even stop eating foods that were once their favorite.

By this time, the effect of television begins to be felt. The preschooler may be exposed to 2 – 8 (or more) hours of television on any one day. Advertisements during this period are many, and unfortunately most of these are for food items, all of which the preschooler seems to want when accompanying the parents to the market to do the weekly shopping (Galst and White, 1976).

Fortunately during this period, children are still willing to try new foods. Parents need to experiment not only with new foods but also with the preparation of those foods. In addi-

tion, the presentation of the foods is most important. Appropriate amounts of a variety of colorful foods will go a long way in increasing the overall consumption at meal time.

Although preschoolers seem to be always busy, there is an increasing amount of idle time because of the decreasing willingness to take a morning or afternoon nap. With more time available, reinforcement from the comments on television, and the encouragement of peers, snacking increases during this period. Appropriate snacking is encouraged. It is only when snacks are restricted to foods heavy with salt and fats or refined carbohydrates of the consistency that would adhere to the teeth and oral tissues or dissolve slowly will there be a problem. Parents, teachers, and caretakers must be educated and directed by dentists on the kinds of snacks best for their children. On special occasions (e.g., birthday parties, Halloween, or Valentine's Day), a special treat of sweets can be suggested. At all other times, snacks should be selected from a list of foods that have been shown to be "friendly to teeth."

Fortunately, preschoolers are also highly impressionable and can be influenced greatly by experiences within the family. Therefore, mealtimes are important "classrooms" for them to learn and observe the feeding practices of older siblings and their parents. A friendly, congenial atmosphere at mealtime without the threats of "you better eat all your food or no dessert" or badgering from siblings will go a long way in establishing positive dietary practices.

It is because of these factors that the dentist may have a difficult time encouraging parents to modify dietary practices when these practices are implicated in dental disease. Although many approaches are available to the dental team, no one approach will ensure success in every case. The approach used must be individualized to the personalities involved, the willingness of the family to learn, and the specific dental problems encountered.

Although many studies on the effect of diet and dietary practices on dental disease have been and continue to be conducted, there continues to be considerable reluctance as well as controversy on the approach to be used by the dental team.

Although historically sucrose has been implicated as the major carbohydrate necessary for acid production, it is now known that other simple carbohydrates can produce acid — corn sweeteners, commonly used in processed and convenience foods; fructose and glucose, occuring naturally in honey; fruits; and vegeta-

bles. Therefore, it is no longer a simple matter of recommending that one reduce the sucrose intake. Over the years, sucrose has appreciably been replaced in the food industry with fructose and other sweeteners.

The critical factor that remains is the ability of the food to produce acid and lower the pH in and around the tooth in the presence of plaque.

Table 18 – 1 ■ Foods that cause the pH of interproximal plaque to fall below 5.5

Apples, dried

Apples, fresh

Apple drink

Apricots, dried

Bananas

Beans, baked

Beans, green canned

White bread

Whole wheat bread

Caramels

Cooked carrots

Cereals, both pre-sweetened and regular

Chocolate milk

Cola

Crackers, soda

Cream cheese

Doughnuts

Gelatin-flavored dessert

Grapes

Milk, whole

Milk, 2%

Oatmeal

Oranges

Orange juice

Pasta

Peanut butter

Potato, boiled

Potato chips

Raisins

Rice

Sponge cake, cream filled

Tomato, fresh

Wheat flakes

Many foods have been tested and found to lower the pH to 5.5 or less (Table 18–1) (Schachtele and Jensen, 1984).

Other critical factors are the ability of the food to adhere to the teeth, the rate at which the food dissolves, the ability of the food to stimulate saliva production, and the ability of the food to be able to buffer the production of acid. It has been suggested by Schachtele in 1982 that a food with low cariogenic potential would have the following:

1. Relatively high protein content
2. Moderate fat content to facilitate oral clearance
3. Minimal concentration of fermentable carbohydrates
4. Strong buffering capacity
5. High mineral content, especially of calcium and phosphorus
6. pH greater than 6.0
7. Ability to stimulate saliva flow

Although foods have been identified with the above characteristics, it continues to be difficult to assist parents in the selection of a diet and dietary practices best for an individual family.

Dietary Counseling

Although the dental profession recognizes the role of good nutrition and appropriate dietary practices in achieving and maintaining good oral health, the execution of the process has been difficult to promote. Fortunately, in recent years the dental profession has been greatly assisted by the popularity of the promotion of physical fitness, dietary practices, and professional health supervision. Parents appear to be more aware, they are willing to listen, and many are even ready to make some changes. How can the dentist and his or her staff assist?

For the preschool child with no dental disease present, the approach would be quite different than for the preschool child with disease present. With all children during the initial parental interview, the dentist should ask parents or guardians the following questions to develop a baseline for further dietary assessments:

1. What was the child's age when he or she was weaned from the breast or bottle?
2. If the child was on the breast or bottle after 1 year of age, what was the frequency and duration of use?
3. When were solids introduced?

4. Were baby foods commercially prepared or homemade?

5. How many meals are served presently? Does the family eat together?

6. Who selects the menu and prepares the food?

7. Are snacks provided? At home, nursery school, or the babysitter's house, do you as a parent choose the meals and snacks? If you do not, do you know what these meals and snacks are?

8. Is your child a good eater — enjoy a balanced diet? If he is not, what are his problem areas?

9. Do you have any grandparents living at home? Or does the child spend appreciable time at the grandparents home?

10. Are there any religious or ethnic preferences that would limit dietary choices?

11. Where does the water used for drinking and preparation of foods come from?

12. What is your child's daily liquid intake? How much of that liquid is made from drinking water in your community?

If the child has a disability, additional questions are indicated:

1. Which dietary practices are modified because of the child's disability?

2. Are there additional nutritional requirements because of the disability?

3. Does the child feed himself, or does he require assistance?

4. Which medications are taken by mouth and how often?

5. Does the child have difficulty with chewing and swallowing?

6. Does your child hold (ruminate) food in his or her mouth for long periods; does your child regurgitate his food?

From these questions, a dentist should have basic background information on the nutritional requirements and dietary practices of the patient and his or her family.

For the preschool child with no dental disease present who has a family practicing sound dietary management, a word of positive reinforcement from the dentist is indicated to the child and parents. Dietary histories and counseling would seem to be counterproductive in this situation.

For preschool children with caries or who appear to be at high risk to caries, further assessment by the dentist is indicated. A dietary history should be obtained by either a 24 hour recall of foods eaten or keeping a record for 3 – 7 days. Although the reliability of dietary histories is often questioned, with a spirit of trust and respect between dentist and parent much can be learned. However, attempts to embarrass or reprimand the parents should be avoided.

Many dietary history forms are available commercially or can be easily made. Parents need to be instructed on how to complete the history, making sure to list all foods at each meal, the amounts eaten by the child, the types and quantities of food consumed between meals, and the liquid intake. Dietary and vitamin supplements as well as oral medications should also be listed.

Although the primary purpose of the dietary assessment in the dental office is to identify patterns that are or will be potentially deleterious to oral health, the dentist should be aware of dietary intakes and patterns that may also greatly influence overall growth and development. When problems are noted in this area, the parents should be referred to their primary health provider for further assessment and counseling.

With the dietary history available, the dentist can, alone or in conjunction with the parent, review the following findings:

1. How many times a day does the child eat?

2. Are food selections diversified; are the meals well balanced?

3. Are the four basic food groups being satisfied daily?

4. What is the frequency of snacking?

5. Are foods high in carbohydrates (refined) frequently consumed? Are they eaten during meals, after meals, or between meals?

6. Are snack foods of the kind that will dissolve slowly or adhere to the teeth?

Once these areas have been identified, the recommendations can be offered. Sweeping modifications of the family diet and dietary practices will be met with resentment, poor compliance to change, and negative results. It is recommended that the dentist select one area and make a recommendation for change, then wait a few weeks and evaluate the results. If the results are positive, another area can be modified; thereby, the dentist builds upon successes.

Follow-up histories are indicated, depending on the oral health status. Dietary counseling is only a part of a comprehensive preventive program, although at times it is the most obvious area in need of adjustment. It can also be the most difficult area to obtain success.

Home Care

With the changes in the child's knowledge base, socialization, and maturation during this period, it would appear that daily home care should become less difficult. Unfortunately, that usually is not the case. Parents tend to assume that children can be more independent than they actually are able to be. Parents also assume too early that their child's motor coordination has progressed to the point at which manipulation of the brush and floss is within reach. Meanwhile, children increasingly want independence. They like to go to the bathroom themselves; they don't need help from Mom and Dad.

A negotiated settlement has to be reached. For example, after meals children can *brush* their teeth with minimal, if any, supervision. At bedtime, the parents will *clean* the teeth and massage the gums. Parents and children working together as a team, each with their identified responsibilities, can help to develop a program of success that can be further monitored and modified by the dentist.

During this period, all the primary teeth should be present. Spaces that were visible earlier may begin to close. Cleaning of the mouth includes brushing the teeth and cleaning the areas of the tooth where the gingivae touch the teeth. This is a fine motor activity, which most 3- to 6-year-olds cannot completely perform without assistance. In addition, the lingual surfaces of the mandibular posterior teeth and the buccal surfaces of the maxillary posterior teeth are the most difficult to reach and to see if all the plaque has been removed.

As spaces close, the use of dental floss is indicated. Generally, 3- to 6-year-olds will be unable to floss. Parents will be responsible for this activity. A commercially available floss holder will greatly assist. Care should be taken not to snap the floss into the interproximal gingiva, causing injury.

Visibility and accessibility can be greatly enhanced by positioning. Although most preschoolers will want to stand at the sink, it is a very difficult position for parents to assist comfortably. Placing the child in a supine position periodically, so that visibility is improved, is recommended. A wet, soft-bristled brush will clean the teeth and massage the gums. Once the cleaning is completed, the child can be directed to the bathroom for additional brushing, with a dentifrice added to the brush.

A fluoride-containing dentifrice is recommended but should be used with supervision. A small amount of dentifrice should be wiped on the brush and the child instructed to expectorate when cleaning is completed. Large amounts of dentifrice are not indicated. Studies have shown that 3- to 6-year-olds swallow large amounts of dentifrice, which may cause fluorosis (Barnhart et al, 1974).

Good hygiene practices would suggest that mouth care be performed after meals. Children should establish this habit early in life. When children are unable to brush, a thorough swishing of the mouth with water is recommended. At bedtime, the mouth care is especially important because of the reduction of saliva production at nighttime with an increase in acid production. Therefore, it is important that parental supervision and assistance be provided. Toward the end of this developmental period, the preschool child will begin to lose teeth. The areas of exfoliation may be painful, and the gingivae may swell and be uncomfortable. During these times, the parent must assist the child daily to maintain the habits earlier established and to eliminate additional inflammation around exfoliating teeth.

Children with disabilities may require additional assistance. Depending on the disability and its severity, various positioning methods may be helpful to increase visibility into the mouth and to reduce excessive movements. Mouth props will help to keep the mouth open for thorough cleaning. Brushes can be modified to increase handle size for improving grip. Minimal dentifrice should be used, to reduce the potential for gagging.

REFERENCES

A Guide to the Use of Fluorides. Denver, National Foundation of Dentistry for the Handicapped, 1981.

Barnhart WE, Hilles HL, Leonard GJ, Michaels SE: Dentifrice usage and ingestion among four age groups. J Dent Res 53:1317, 1974.

Bell RM, Klein SO, Bohannan HM, III, et al: Analysis of DMFS increments. *In* Treatment Effects in the National Preventive Dentistry Demonstration Program. Santa Monica, Rand Corporation, 1984, pp 19–41.

Brudevold F, Naujoks R: Caries-preventive fluoride treatment of the individual. Caries Res 12(Suppl 1):52–64, 1978.

Crall JJ, Nowak AJ: Clinical uses of fluoride for the special patient. *In* Wei SHY (ed): Clinical Uses of Fluorides. Philadelphia, Lea and Febiger, 1985, pp 193–201.

Galst JP, White MA: The unhealthy persuaders. The reinforcing value of television and children's purchase influencing attempts at the supermarket. Child Develop 47:1089–1096, 1976.

Goodman SD: An in vitro model to assess the interproximal coverage and fluoride uptake following topical fluoride application. M.S. Thesis, University of Iowa, 1983.

Heifetz SB: Cost effectiveness of topically applied fluorides. *In* Burt B (ed): The Relative Efficiency of Methods of Caries Prevention in Dental Public Health. Ann Arbor, University of Michigan Press, 1978, pp 69–104.

Joyston-Bechal S, Duckworth R, Braden M: The effect of artificially produced pellicle and plaque on the uptake of 18F by human enamel in vitro. Arch Oral Biol 21:73–78, 1976.

Klimek J, Hellwig E, Ahrens G: Fluoride taken up by plaque, by the underlying enamel and by clean enamel from three compounds in vitro. Caries Res 16:156–161, 1982.

National Caries Program, National Institute of Dental Research: Summary of findings. *In* The Prevalence of Dental Caries in United States Children, 1979–1980. NIH Publication No. 82-2245, December, 1981, pp 5–8.

Ripa LW: Professionally (operator) applied topical fluoride therapy: A critique. Clin Prev Dent 4:3–10, 1982.

Ripa LW, Leske GS, Sposato A, Varma A: Effect of prior toothcleaning on bi-annual professional acidulated phosphate fluoride topical fluoride gel-tray treatments: Results after three years. Caries Res 18:457–464, 1984.

Schachtele CF: Changing perspectives on the role of diet in dental caries formation. Nutrition News 45:13–15, 1982.

Schachtele CF, Jensen ME: Can foods be ranked according to their cariogenic potential? *In* Guggenheim B (ed): Cariology Today. Basel, Karger, 1984, pp 136–146.

Tinanoff N, Wei SHY, Parkins FM: Effect of a pumice prophylaxis on fluoride uptake in tooth enamel. JADA 88:385–389, 1974.

Wefel JS: Critical assessment of professional application of topical fluorides. *In* Wei SHY (ed): Clinical Uses of Fluorides. Philadelphia, Lea and Febiger, 1985, p 20.

Wei SHY: The potential benefits to be derived from topical fluorides in fluoridated communities. *In* Forrester DJ, Schultz EM, Jr (eds): International Workshop on Fluorides and Dental Caries Prevention. Baltimore, University of Maryland, 1974.

Restorative dentistry for the primary dentition

William F. Waggoner

Restorative dentistry in the primary dentition is based on time-tested principles and preparations. In 1924, G. V. Black outlined several steps for the preparation of carious permanent teeth to receive a restoration. These steps have been adapted, though slightly modified, for the restoration of primary teeth. Restorative techniques for the primary dentition have remained relatively consistent for many years (Fig. 19 – 1). However, there has been a shift toward more conservative preparations and restorations, an increase in the use of composite resins and bonding systems, and a continued improvement in dental materials. All of these make pediatric restorative dentistry a dynamic combination of ever-improving materials and tried and true techniques.

Common Dental Materials in Pediatric Restorative Dentistry

All of the dental materials that are used in pediatric dentistry, with the possible exception of stainless steel crowns, are used frequently in adult restorative dentistry. The most frequently utilized materials and their clinical considerations for pediatric dentistry are summarized in Tables 19 – 1 and 19 – 2. The reader is referred to a dental materials text for a more exhaustive review of any of the listed materials (Craig, 1980; Phillips, 1982).

Table 19 – 1 ■ Commonly used biomaterials in pediatric dentistry

Materials	Types Available	Composition	Clinical Considerations
Varnish	—	Natural gums such as copal, dissolved in an organic solvent	Two coats applied to amalgam cavity preparations Applied to vital teeth prior to use of zinc phosphate cement Not placed under composite resins
Intermediary bases	*Calcium hydroxide Zinc oxide/eugenol	Thin pastes of calcium hydroxide or zinc oxide and eugenol suspended in resins	Placed on small areas of cavity preparation deeper than ideal depth Placed on exposed dentin of preparations undergoing acid etching Used for direct pulp capping of permanent teeth Must not be left on enamel of preparations
Amalgam	Lathe-cut Spherical *Admixed *Unicompositional	Silver (40–74%) Tin (25–30%) Copper (2–30%) Zinc (0–2%) Mercury (0–3%)	A high copper (>6%) admixed or unicompositional, precapsulated alloy is recommended for restoration of pit and fissure and inter-proximal caries in posterior teeth
Stainless steel crowns	Straight sides *Precontoured *Pretrimmed	Iron (65–73%) Chromium (17–20%) Nickel (8–13%) Manganese, silicon, and carbon (<2%)	Restoration of badly broken down teeth, usually posterior Must be well trimmed, contoured, polished, and cemented to ensure optimum gingival health
Filled composite resin	(Based on filler size) Traditional, 5–30 μm *Microfill, .04–1 μm *Hybrids, .04–100 μm (*Available as auto-cure or visible light activated)	Dimethacrylate (BIS-GMA) resin or urethane matrix with filler particles of quartz, silicates, or glass	Esthetic restoration of anterior teeth Available for use in Class I, II restorations in posterior teeth Microfills provide most polishable surface and excel-lent esthetics Hybrids demonstrate least shrinkage and wear and have good polishability and esthetics Visible light activation provides better polymerization control, better color stability, and less porosity than auto-polymerized resins
Cements	*Zinc phosphate	Zinc oxide and phosphoric acid	Primary use is cementation of stainless steel crowns
	*Polycarboxylate	Zinc oxide and polycarboxylic acid	May be used as a base Glass ionomer may be used
	*Glass ionomer	Silicate glass containing Ca, Al, F, Polycarboxylic acid	as a liner for resins
	*Reinforced zinc oxide and eugenol	Zinc oxide reinforced with EBA or alumina or polymer, eugenol	Reinforced zinc oxide and eugenol most frequently used for obliterating primary pulp chambers following pulpot-omy
	Zinc silicophosphate	Zinc oxide and silicate phosphoric acid	
	Zinc oxide and eugenol	Zinc oxide, eugenol	

* Denotes types most frequently used.

Table 19–2 ■ Comparison of dental cements

Cement	Composition	Working Time	Setting Time	Compressive Strength	Bond Strength to Dentin	Release of Fluoride	Pulpal Response	Removal of Excess
Ideal	—	Medium	Short-medium	Very high	High	Yes	None	Easy
Zinc phosphate	Zinc oxide and phosphoric acid	Medium	Medium	Medium	None	No	Low-medium	Easy
Polycarboxylate	Zinc oxide Polycarboxylic acid	Short	Short	Low-medium	Low-medium	No	None	Medium-difficult
Glass ionomer	Silicate glass containing Ca, Al, F Polycarboxylic Acid	Short-medium	Short	High	Medium	Yes	Low	Moderate
Zinc silicophosphate	Zinc oxide and silicate Phosphoric Acid	Medium	Medium	High	None	Yes	Medium	Easy
Zinc oxide and eugenol	Zinc oxide Eugenol	Long	Medium	Low-medium	None	No	None	Easy
Reinforced zinc oxide and eugenol	Zinc oxide reinforced with EBA or alumina or polymer Eugenol	Long	Medium-long	Low-medium	None	No	None	Easy

Adapted from Farah JW, Powers JM: Rating permanent cements. Dental Advisor 2(1):3, 1985.

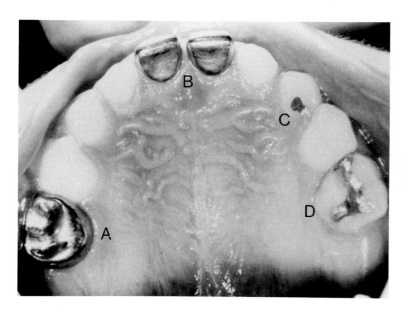

Figure 19–1 ■ Restored primary dentition demonstrating stainless steel crown (A), open-face steel crowns (B), Class III amalgam (C), and Class II amalgam (D).

Instrumentation

Nearly all instrumentation for restorative procedures is carried out with the high speed air turbine handpiece (100,000–300,000 rpm) with coolant. The coolant may be water spray or air alone. Research indicates that either coolant may be utilized without creating irreversible pulpal damage (Bhaskar and Lilly, 1965; Bouschor and Matthews, 1966). A water spray is always recommended when removing old amalgam restorations or using diamond burs. Regardless of the coolant used, intermittent cutting at intervals of a few seconds with light, brushing strokes should be used to prevent excessive heat generations. Protective eyewear should always be worn when using the high speed air turbine handpiece.

The slow speed handpiece (500–15,000 rpm) is most frequently used for caries removal and for polishing and finishing procedures. As with high speed instrumentation, light pressure and brushing strokes should be used when using the slow speed handpiece. Hand instrumentation is minimal in most operative preparations in the primary dentition. It is usually limited to final caries removal or planing of enamel walls.

Anatomic Considerations of Primary Teeth

Although some primary teeth show resemblance to their permanent successors, they are not miniature permanent teeth. Several anatomic differences must be distinguished before restorative procedures are begun.

1. Primary teeth have thinner enamel and dentin thickness than permanent teeth.
2. The pulps of primary teeth are larger in relation to crown size than permanent pulps.
3. The pulp horns of primary teeth are closer to the outer surface of the tooth than permanent pulps. The mesio-buccal pulp horn is the largest.
4. In primary teeth, the enamel rods of the gingival third of the crown extend in an occlusal direction from the dentino-enamel junction. This is in contrast to the permanent dentition in which the rods extend in a cervical direction.
5. Primary teeth demonstrate greater constriction of the crown in the cervical region than permanent teeth.
6. Primary teeth have broad, flat proximal contact areas.
7. Much of the enamel surface of primary teeth is covered with a prismless layer of enamel.

Use of the Rubber Dam in Pediatric Restorative Dentistry

The use of the rubber dam is indispensable in pediatric restorative dentistry. Numerous advantages have been listed for its use, all allowing for provision of the highest quality of care.

1. Better access and visualization is gained by retracting soft tissues and providing a dark contrasting background to the teeth.

2. Moisture control is superior to other forms of isolation.

3. The safety of the child is improved by preventing aspiration or swallowing of foreign bodies and by protecting the soft tissues.

4. Placement generally results in a decreased operating time.

5. Many children tend to become more quiet and relaxed with a rubber dam in place. The dam seems to act as a separating barrier, so that movements in and out of the oral cavity are perceived by the child as being less invasive than without the dam in place.

6. With a rubber dam in place, a child becomes primarily a nasal breather, thereby enhancing the administration of nitrous oxide.

Most all pediatric restorative procedures should be completed with the rubber dam in place. The few instances in which it would not be used include (1) a child with an upper respiratory infection, congested nasal passages, or other nasal obstruction; (2) the presence of some fixed orthodontic appliances; and (3) a very recently erupted tooth that will not retain a clamp.

PREPARING FOR PLACEMENT OF THE RUBBER DAM

A 5 X 5 inch medium gauge dark rubber dam is best suited for use in children. The holes should be punched so that the rubber dam is centered horizontally on the face and the upper lip is covered by the upper border of the dam, but the dam does not cover the nostrils. One method of proper hole placement is seen in Figure 19–2A. Figure 19–2B demonstrates proper hole size selection for different teeth.

Punch the minimum number of holes necessary for good isolation of all tooth surfaces to be restored. For single Class I or V restorations, only the tooth being restored need be isolated. If interproximal lesions are being restored, at least one tooth anterior and one tooth posterior to the tooth being restored should be isolated.

Proper clamp selection is one of the most critical aspects of good rubber dam application. Table 19–3 lists the most frequently used

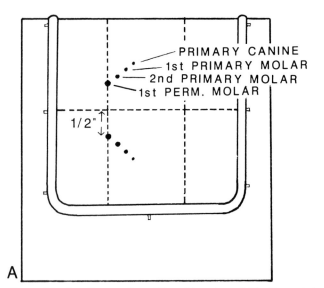

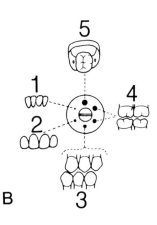

Figure 19–2 ■ Preparation of the rubber dam. A, The Young's frame is applied to the rubber dam. The upper limit of the frame coincides with the upper edge of the rubber dam material. The dam is divided vertically into thirds, and the area inside the frame is divided in half horizontally. The holes for each tooth are placed as indicated, at a 45 degree angle 3–4 mm apart. B, The rubber dam punch table with corresponding teeth and hole sizes. *B* reprinted by permission of the publisher from, The DAE Project, *Instructional Materials for the Dental Health Professions: Rubber Dam.* (NY, Teachers College Press, © 1982, Teachers College, Columbia University. All rights reserved.) p. 42.

Table 19–3 ■ Common rubber dam clamps for pediatric restorative dentistry

Teeth	Clamp No.
Partially erupted permanent molars	14A, 8A*—Ivory†
Fully erupted permanent molars	14, 8—Ivory
Second primary molars	3—Ivory 26, 27—SS White‡
First primary molars/bicuspids/permanent canines	2, 2A—Ivory
Primary incisors and canines	0—Ivory

* "A" clamps have jaws angled gingivally to seat below subgingival heights of contour.
† Ivory Co, Inc, Philadelphia, PA.
‡ SS White, Philadelphia, PA.

clamps and their areas of utilization. Incisors usually require ligation with dental floss for stabilization instead of a clamp. After selecting an appropriate clamp, place a 12–18 inch piece of dental floss on the bow of the clamp as a safety (Figure 19–3). This is necessary for easy retrieval of the clamp in the event that it is dislodged from the tooth.

Before trying the clamp onto the tooth, floss the contacts through which the rubber dam will be taken. If floss is unable to pass through the contact because of defective restorations or other reasons, modification of the contacts or rubber dam will be necessary before placement. Next, using the rubber dam forceps, try the selected clamp on the tooth. Place the clamp on the tooth, seating from lingual to buccal. Be certain that the jaws of the clamp are placed below the height of contour and are not impinging on the gingival tissues. After seating the clamp, remove the forceps and place a finger on the buccal and lingual jaws of the clamp and apply gingival pressure to ensure that the clamp is

stable and has been seated as far gingivally as possible.

PLACEMENT OF THE RUBBER DAM

The punched rubber dam should be lightly stretched onto the rubber dam frame. This will hold the corners of the dam out of the line of vision during placement. If the material is stretched too tightly, there will be too much tension and the clamp may be dislodged when the material is stretched over the bow. Next, instruct the child to open the mouth widely, and with the index fingers, stretch the most posterior hole of the rubber dam over the bow and wings of the clamp. Sometimes when isolating the most posterior maxillary molars, the bow of the clamp rests very close to the anterior border of the ramus when the mouth is opened wide. This makes slipping the dam material over the bow difficult, but by simply asking the child to close the mouth slightly, the ramus will move posteriorly and allow the material to slide between the bow and the ramus.

If needed, adjust the tension of the rubber dam on the frame. Next, stabilize the rubber dam around the most anterior tooth. This may be done by placing a wooden wedge interproximally, by stretching a small piece of rubber dam through the contact or by ligating with dental floss. To ligate, place floss (12–18 inches) around the cervical of the tooth and have the dental assistant hold the floss gingivally on the lingual with a blunt instrument. Draw the floss tightly around the tooth from the buccal and tie a surgical knot below the cervical bulge. Leave the ends of the ligature tie long. After anterior stabilization, all other teeth can be isolated that have been included in the dam.

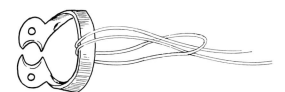

Figure 19–3 ■ A floss safety through the bow of the rubber dam clamp allows for easy retrieval of the clamp, should it become dislodged from the tooth. Reprinted by permission of the publisher from, The DAE Project, *Instructional Materials for the Dental Health Professions: Rubber Dam.* (NY, Teachers College Press, © 1982, Teachers College, Columbia University. All rights reserved.) p. 66.

A blunt instrument (plastic instrument No. 7) can be used to invert the rubber dam.

REMOVING THE RUBBER DAM

First, rinse away all debris and cut and remove any ligatures used for stabilization. Next, stretch the rubber dam so that the dam's interproximal septa may be cut with a pair of scissors. The clamp, frame, and dam are then removed as a unit with the rubber dam forceps. Inspect the dam and the mouth to see that no small pieces of dam material have been left interproximally. Gently massage the tissue around the previously clamped tooth, and rinse and evacuate the oral cavity.

Restoration of Primary Molars

The anatomy of the primary molars, with their fissured occlusal surfaces and broad, flat interproximal contact areas, makes them the most caries susceptible primary teeth. The importance of primary molars in mastication and as maintainers of space for the succedaneous teeth, coupled with the development of suitable economic restorative materials, has shaped a philosophy of restoring and conserving primary molars. Stainless steel crowns, amalgam, and, most recently, composite resin are the materials utilized in the restoration of primary molars.

CLASS I AMALGAM RESTORATIONS

General Considerations

The outline form for Class I restorations in primary molars can be seen in Figure 19–4. The outline form should include all retentive fissures and carious areas but should be as conservative as possible. Ideal pulpal floor depth is 0.5 mm into dentin (approximately 1.5 mm from the enamel surface). The length of the cutting end of the No. 330 bur is 1.5 mm, so this becomes a good tool for gauging cavity depth. The cavosurface margin should be placed out of stress-bearing areas, with no bevel. To help prevent stress concentration, the outline form should be composed of smooth, flowing arcs and curves, and all internal angles should be rounded slightly. When a dovetail is placed in

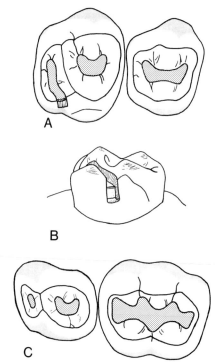

Figure 19–4 ■ Class I cavity preparations. *A*, Maxillary right second and first primary molars (occlusal view). *B*, Maxillary second primary molar, lingual view of distolingual groove preparation. *C*, Mandibular right first and second primary molars (occlusal view).

the second primary molars, its bucco-lingual width should be greater than the width of the isthmus to produce a locking form to provide resistance against occlusal torque, which may displace the restoration mesially or distally. The isthmus should be one third of the intercuspal width, and the bucco-lingual walls should converge slightly in an occlusal direction. The mesial and distal walls should flare at the marginal ridge so as not to undercut ridges. Oblique ridges should not be crossed unless they are undermined with caries or are deeply fissured. Primary second molars often exhibit buccal developmental pits. When carious, these should be restored with a small teardrop or ovoid-shaped restoration, including all the adjacent susceptible pits and fissures.

Steps of Preparation and Restoration of Class I Amalgam Restorations

1. Administer appropriate anesthesia and place the rubber dam.
2. Using a No. 330 bur in the high speed turbine handpiece, penetrate into the tooth par-

allel to its long axis in the central pit region and extend into all susceptible fissures and pits to a depth 0.5 mm into dentin.

3. Remove all carious dentin. Utilize a large, round bur in the slow speed handpiece or a sharp spoon excavator.

4. Smooth the enamel walls, and refine the final outline form with the No. 330 bur.

5. Rinse and dry the preparation, and inspect for (1) caries removal, (2) sharp cavosurface margins, and (3) removal of all unsupported enamel.

6. Place pulp protection as needed. Calcium hydroxide should be placed in the portions of the preparation that are significantly deeper than ideal. Bases other than calcium hydroxide are rarely placed in primary teeth.

7. Place cavity varnish, air dry, and then place a second coat.

8. Triturate the amalgam, and place one carrier load of amalgam into the preparation.

9. Using a small condenser, immediately begin condensation of the amalgam into the preparation, condensing small overlapping increments with a firm pressure until the cavity is slightly overfilled.

10. Following condensation, carving of most of the newer alloys can begin almost immediately. A small cleoid-discoid carver works very well for carving primary restorations. Always keep part of the carving edge of the instrument on tooth structure so that overcarving of the cavosurface margin does not occur. Remove all amalgam flash from cavosurface margins. Keep the carved anatomy shallow. Placing deep anatomy in primary teeth (i.e., grooves) can weaken the restoration by creating a thin shelf of amalgam at the cavosurface margin and also by reducing the bulk of amalgam in the central stress bearing areas, both leading to fracture.

11. Burnish the carved amalgam when the amalgam has begun its initial set and resists deformation. Burnishing is done with a small, round burnisher, which is lightly rubbed across the carved amalgam surface to produce a satin-like appearance. Besides smoothing, burnishing creates a substructure with fewer voids and reduces finishing time.

12. A wet cotton pellet can be wiped across the burnished amalgam for a final smoothing (optional).

13. Remove the rubber dam, and check the occlusion. Children must be cautioned before the rubber dam is completely removed that they must not close their teeth into occlusion until instructed to do so. With articulating paper,

check the restoration for occlusal irregularities, instructing the child to close gently. Make necessary adjustments with the carver.

14. Rinse the oral cavity, and massage the soft tissue around the previously clamped tooth.

Common Errors with Class I Amalgam Restorations

Some frequent errors made in Class I amalgam restorations are (1) not including all susceptible fissures, (2) preparing the cavity too deep, (3) undercutting the marginal ridges, (4) carving the anatomy of the amalgam too deep, and (5) not removing amalgam flash from cavosurface margins.

CLASS II AMALGAM RESTORATIONS

General Considerations

The outline form for several Class II amalgam preparations can be seen in Figure 19–5. The guidelines given for the Class I preparation should be followed during the preparation of the occlusal portion of the Class II preparation, and, additionally, there are several recommendations for the proximal box preparation. The proximal box should be broader at the cervical than at the occlusal. The buccal, lingual, and gingival walls should all break contact with the adjacent tooth, just enough to allow the tip of an explorer to pass. The buccal and lingual walls should create a 90 degree angle with the enamel. The gingival wall should be flat, not bevelled, and all unsupported enamel should be removed. Ideally, the axial wall of the proximal box should be 0.5 mm into dentin and should follow the same contour as the outer proximal contour of the tooth. The axio-pulpal line angle should be rounded, and no buccal or lingual retentive grooves should be placed. The mesio-distal width of the gingival seat should be 1 mm, which is approximately equal to the width of a No. 330 bur.

Matrix Application

Matrices must be placed for interproximal restorations to aid in restoring normal contour and normal contact areas and to prevent extrusion of restorative materials into gingival tissues. Three types of matrix bands are available for use in pediatric dentistry.

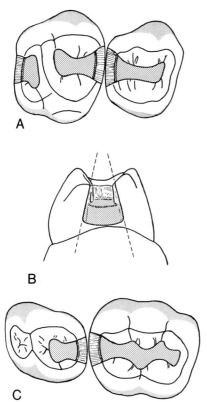

Figure 19-5 ■ Class II cavity preparations. *A,* Maxillary right second and first primary molars (occlusal view). *B,* Mandibular second primary molar (proximal view)—note occlusal convergence of proximal walls. *C,* Mandibular right first and second primary molars (occlusal view).

1. T-band: allows for multiple matrices; no special equipment is needed
2. Tofflemeire matrix: used infrequently because it does not fit primary tooth contour well and is difficult to place as multiple matrices
3. Spot welded matrix: allows for multiple matrix placement; a spot welder is required at chairside

T-bands are available in different sizes, contours, and materials. A straight, narrow, brass T-band will work in almost all pediatric restorative procedures. The T-band matrix (Fig. 19-6) is formed by folding the band back on itself in the form of a circle and by folding over the extension wings of the T to make an adjustable loop. The band is contoured and positioned onto the tooth with the folded extension wings on the buccal surface. The free end of the band is drawn mesially to pull the band snugly against the tooth. The extension folds are then grasped firmly with a pair of Howe No. 110 pliers and removed from the tooth. The band

should then be tightened an additional 0.5–1.0 mm, and the free end should be bent back over the vertical folds and cut with scissors to a length of 5–6 mm. The band is then reseated onto the tooth and wedged. It must fit below the gingival margin of the preparation and must also be at least 1 mm higher than the marginal ridge of the adjacent tooth.

Removal of the T-band is accomplished by opening the extension wings with an explorer or spoon excavator and allowing the band to open. Scissors are then used to cut one end of the band close to the restored proximal surface, and the band is then drawn buccally or lingually through the contact.

Steps of Preparation and Restoration for Class II Amalgam Restorations

1. Administer appropriate anesthesia, and place the rubber dam.

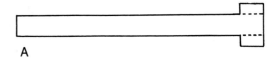

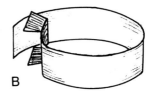

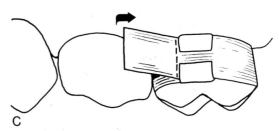

Figure 19-6 ■ *A,* The T-band matrix. *B,* The T-band is formed into a circle, and the extension wings are folded down to secure the band. *C,* The T-band is adapted to fit the tooth tightly and is trimmed with scissors, and the free end is bent back.

2. Place a wooden wedge in the interproximal area being restored (optional). This acts to retract the gingival papilla during instrumentation and creates some prewedging, which will help ensure a tight proximal contact of the final restoration.

3. Using a No. 330 bur in the high speed turbine handpiece with a light, brushing motion, prepare the occlusal outline form at ideal depth.

4. To prepare the proximal box, begin by brushing the bur bucco-lingually in a pendulum motion and in a gingival direction at the dentino-enamel junction. Continue until contact is just broken between the adjacent tooth and the gingival wall. If the gingival wall is made too deep, the cervical constriction of the primary molar will create a very narrow gingival seat. The widest bucco-lingual width of the box will be at the gingival margin. Care must be taken not to damage the adjacent proximal surface.

5. Remove any remaining caries with a sharp spoon excavator or with a round bur in the slow speed handpiece.

6. Round the axio-pulpal line angle slightly. Because of the shape of the No. 330 bur, all other internal line angles will automatically be gently rounded.

7. Remove any unsupported enamel of the buccal, lingual, or gingival walls with an enamel hatchet.

8. Place a thin layer of calcium hydroxide over the deepest regions of the preparation, and apply two coats of cavity varnish.

9. Remove the wedge placed at the beginning of the treatment, and place a T-band matrix.

10. While holding the T-band in place, forcefully reinsert the wedge between the matrix band and the adjacent tooth, beneath the gingival seat of the preparation. The wedge is placed with a pair of Howe pliers or cotton forceps from the widest embrasure. The wedge should hold the band tightly against the tooth but should not push the band into the proximal box. It may be necessary to trim the wedge slightly to achieve a proper fit.

11. Triturate the amalgam, and with the amalgam carrier, add the amalgam to the preparation in single increments, beginning in the proximal box.

12. Using a small condenser, condense the amalgam into the corners of the proximal box and against the matrix band to ensure the reestablishment of a tight proximal contact. Continue filling and condensing until the entire cavity is overfilled.

13. Carving of the occlusal portion is performed with a small cleoid-discoid carver, as in Class I restorations. The marginal ridge can be carved with the tip of an explorer or with a Hollenback carver.

14. Carefully remove the wedge and the matrix band.

15. Remove excess amalgam at the buccal, lingual, and gingival margins with an explorer or Hollenback carver. Check to see that the height of the newly restored marginal ridge is approximately equal to the adjacent marginal ridge.

16. Gently floss the interproximal contact to check the tightness of the contact, to check for gingival overhang, and to remove any loose amalgam particles from the interproximal region.

17. Burnish the restoration, and use a wet cotton pellet held with the cotton pliers for final smoothing if this is needed.

18. Remove the rubber dam carefully.

19. Check the occlusion for irregularities with articulating paper, and adjust as needed.

Adjacent or Back-to-Back Class II Amalgam Restorations

Adjacent interproximal lesions are not uncommon in the primary dentition. From a time and patient management standpoint, it is desirable to restore these lesions simultaneously.

The preparations for adjacent proximal restorations are identical to those previously described. A T-band matrix is placed on each tooth and is properly wedged. Condensation of the amalgam should be done in small increments, alternately in each preparation, so that the restorations are filled simultaneously (Fig. 19–7). Condensation pressure toward the matrix will help ensure a tight interproximal contact. Carve the marginal ridges to an equal height, and carefully remove the wedge and matrix bands one at a time. Final carving is similar to that described for solitary Class II restorations.

PROBLEMS WITH AMALGAM RESTORATIONS

Most restorative problems in pediatric dentistry result from a failure to prepare and restore the teeth in a way that takes into account their

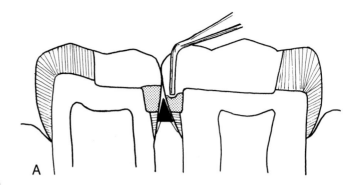

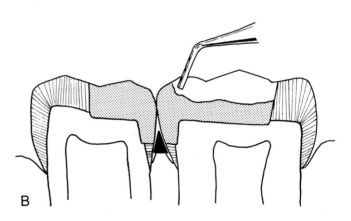

Figure 19–7 ■ "Back-to-back" amalgam preparations. *A,* After wedging, begin condensing the adjacent proximal boxes alternately. *B,* Continue condensing the amalgams alternately until both preparations are slightly overfilled.

structural characteristics and limitations (Fig. 19–8). Fracture of the isthmus of a Class II amalgam restoration is a frequent problem that usually results from insufficient bulk of amalgam in the isthmus, either because the preparation is too shallow or because the amalgam has been overcarved. A sharp axio-pulpal line and hyperocclusion of the restoration may also result in isthmus fracture. Marginal failure in the proximal box, usually owing to an excessive flare of the cavosurface margin, is another frequent problem with Class II amalgam restorations. Failure to remove all caries or to extend preparations into caries-susceptible fissures is another common reason for failure of restorations (Myers, 1977).

FINISHING OF AMALGAM RESTORATIONS

Polishing of amalgam restorations is performed to eliminate surface scratches and blemishes, which act as centers of corrosion; to remove any remaining amalgam flash not carved away; and to refine the anatomy and occlusion.

A technique with a simple armamentarium and a low potential for heat production is most desirable. Such a technique is outlined here. Polishing should be delayed for at least 24 hours following amalgam placement.

1. With a tapered green stone in the slow speed handpiece, gross contouring of the amalgam or flash removal is carried out.
2. Multiple fluted amalgam finishing burs in the slow speed handpiece brushed lightly across the restoration at high speeds will smooth and shine the surface. For primary teeth, three sizes of round finishing burs, together with a pear-shaped and flame finishing bur, will be sufficient to polish any amalgam restoration.
3. A final polish can be placed on the restoration, using a rotary bristle brush with a pumice slurry to remove small scratches, followed by a polishing agent such as tin oxide for the finish luster. Rubber abrasives may be used for final polishing, but great care should be taken not to generate excessive heat.
4. Proximally, small sandpaper disks will polish the enamel-amalgam margins. A well-

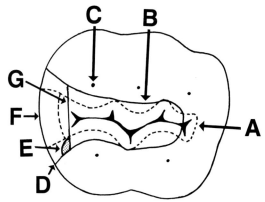

Figure 19–8 ■ Common errors with Class II cavity preparations. *A,* Failure to extend occlusal outline into all susceptible pits and fissures. *B,* Failure to follow the outline of the cusps. *C,* Isthmus cut too wide. *D,* Flare of proximal walls too great. *E,* Angle formed by the axial, buccal, and lingual walls too great. *F,* Gingival contact with adjacent tooth not broken. *G,* Axial wall not conforming to the proximal contour of the tooth, and the mesio-distal width of the gingival floor is greater than 1 mm. (From Forrester DJ, Wagner M, and Fleming J: Restorative procedures. *In* Sheldon P: Pediatric Dental Medicine. Philadelphia, Lea and Febiger, 1981.)

polished amalgam restoration should allow the explorer to pass easily from enamel to amalgam and back again.

RESIN MATERIALS IN PRIMARY MOLARS

Over the past 20 years, composite resins have periodically been suggested as esthetic replacement for Class I and Class II amalgam restorations in molars. Initial results were promising, but clinical failures began to occur after approximately 2 years, the greatest problem being occlusal wear (Leinfelder et al, 1980). Recent improvements in composite materials, such as smaller filler particles, increases in material strength, and introduction of dentin bonding agents, have lead to much improved clinical results. Resin restorations in primary molars offer the advantages of improved esthetics, elimination of mercury and galvanic shock, and low thermal conductivity. Disadvantages include an exacting technique, potential marginal leakage, postoperative sensitivity, and a tendency toward open or loose contacts (Waggoner, 1984; Leinfelder and Vann, 1982).

The American Dental Association (ADA) has recently approved some composite resins for use in posterior teeth, and there is no doubt that

several more will be approved in the future; therefore, a brief discussion of their use in primary molars is included in this section.

STEPS IN PREPARATION AND RESTORATION OF PRIMARY MOLARS WITH RESIN

The steps in preparation of a primary molar for restoration with composite resin are very similar to those followed for restoration with amalgam, with a few alterations. In a Class II resin restoration, pre-wedging of teeth is highly desirable to achieve a slight separation of teeth and consequently a tighter interproximal contact of the final restoration. All accessible enamel margins of the preparation should be bevelled at a 45 degree angle approximately 1 mm, and the enamel margins should be etched for one minute with an acid gel. A dentin-bonding agent or glass ionomer liner is placed before placement of a matrix band and the composite material.

A plastic instrument is used to pack or condense the composite into the preparation. Some composites are pre-packaged in small ampules that can be injected directly into the preparation. No more than 2 mm depth of composite should be polymerized at one time. Deep preparations will require incremental placement. Finishing can begin immediately following polymerization. The occlusal surface is grossly contoured with round, high speed carbide finishing burs or fine finishing diamond burs. Gross contouring of proximal surfaces is accomplished with flame-shaped, high speed carbide finishing burs and with garnet disks, where accessible. A No. 12 scapel blade may be used to remove gingival or proximal excess. Final finishing can be completed with a white stone or with rubber abrasive points to eliminate surface irregularities. Fine abrasive disks are used for final polishing of accessible proximal margins. A thin layer of bonding agent, following a brief etching (30 seconds) of the finished restoration, may be applied to ensure good marginal integrity.

USE OF STAINLESS STEEL CROWNS

Pre-formed or stainless steel crowns were introduced to pediatric dentistry by Humphrey in 1950. Since that time, they have become an invaluable restorative material in the treatment of

badly broken down primary teeth. They are generally considered superior to large multisurface amalgam restorations and have a longer clinical life-span than two surface amalgam restorations (Dawson et al, 1981). The crowns are manufactured in different sizes as a metal shell with some pre-formed anatomy and are trimmed and contoured as necessary to fit individual teeth.

There are three types of stainless steel crowns available.

1. Straight side crowns (Rocky Mountain Corp, Denver, CO): These crowns are neither trimmed nor contoured, requiring much adaptation. They are rarely used and are not recommended.

2. Pre-trimmed crowns (Unitek Corp, Monrovia, CA): These crowns have straight sides but are festooned to follow a line parallel to the gingival crest. They still require contouring and some trimming.

3. Pre-contoured crowns (Ion Crowns, 3M Co, St. Paul, MN; Unitek Corp, Monrovia, CA): These crowns are festooned and are also pre-contoured. Some trimming and contouring may be necessary but usually are minimal.

Indications for Use of Stainless Steel Crowns

1. Restoration of primary or young permanent teeth with extensive carious lesions. These include primary teeth that demonstrate caries on three or more surfaces or where the caries extends beyond the anatomic line angles. First primary molars with mesial interproximal lesions are included in the category because the morphologic appearance that the tooth exhibits results in inadequate support for mesial interproximal restorations.

2. Restoration of hypoplastic primary or permanent teeth.

3. Restoration of primary teeth following pulpotomy or pulpectomy procedures.

4. Restoration of teeth with hereditary anomalies such as dentinogenesis imperfecta or amelogenesis imperfecta.

5. Restorations in disabled individuals or others in whom oral hygiene is extremely poor and failure of other materials is likely.

6. As an abutment for space maintainers or prosthetic appliances.

7. Temporary restoration of a fractured tooth.

Steps of Preparation and Placement of Stainless Steel Crowns

(Note: Several different preparation designs have been advocated over the years. Only one such preparation, requiring minimal tooth reduction, is discussed here. Either Unitek or 3M crowns may be used following these steps.)

1. Evaluate the preoperative occlusion. Note the dental midline and the cusp-fossa relationship bilaterally.

2. Administer appropriate local anesthesia, ensuring that all soft tissues surrounding the tooth to be crowned are well anesthetized, and place a rubber dam.

3. Establish access with a No. 330 bur in the high speed handpiece, then remove decay with a large, round bur in the slow speed handpiece or with a spoon excavator.

4. Reduction of the occlusal surface is carried out with a No. 169L taper fissure bur or a thin, tapered diamond in the high speed handpiece. Make depth cuts by cutting the occlusal grooves to a depth of 1.0–1.5 mm, and extend through the buccal, lingual, and proximal surfaces. Next, place the bur on its side and uniformly reduce the remaining occlusal surface by 1.5 mm, maintaining the cuspal inclines of the crown (Fig. 19–9).

5. Proximal reduction is also accomplished with the taper fissure bur or thin, tapered diamond. Contact with the adjacent tooth must be broken gingivally and bucco-lingually, maintaining vertical walls with only a slight convergence in an occlusal direction. The gingival proximal margin should have a feather edge finish line. Care must be taken not to damage adjacent tooth structure. Ledges formed by deep caries should not be removed.

6. Round all line angles, using the side of the bur or diamond. The occluso-buccal and occluso-lingual line angles are rounded by holding the bur at a 30–45 degree angle to the occlusal surface and sweeping it in a mesio-distal direction. Bucco-lingual reduction for the stainless steel crown preparation is generally limited to this bevelling and is confined to the occlusal one third of the crown. If problems are later encountered in selecting an appropriate crown size or in fitting a crown over a large mesio-buccal bulge, more reduction of the buccal and lingual tooth structure may become necessary. The buccal and lingual proximal line angles are rounded by holding the bur parallel to the tooth's long axis and blending the surfaces together. All of the angles of the prepara-

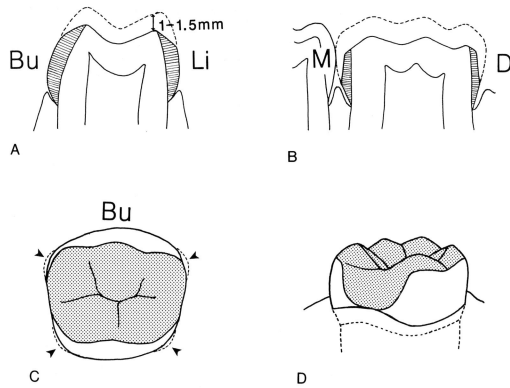

Figure 19-9 ■ Stainless steel crown preparation. Mandibular second primary molar. *A*, Proximal view (Bu = buccal; Li = lingual). *B*, Buccal view. Note feather edge gingival margins. *C*, Occlusal view. Note rounded line angles. *D*, Mesio-lingual view. Note that lingual and buccal reduction is limited to the bevelling of the occlusal one third. (From Stainless Steel Crown Preparation and Restoration, Project TAPP, Quercus Corporation, © 1977.)

tion should be rounded to remove corners but not so much as to create a round preparation.

7. Selection of a crown begins as a trial-and-error procedure. The goal is to place the smallest crown that can be seated on the tooth and to establish pre-existing proximal contacts. The selected crown is tried onto the preparation by seating the lingual first and applying pressure in a buccal direction so that the crown slides over the buccal surface into the gingival sulcus. Friction should be felt as the crown slips over the buccal bulge. Some teeth are an "in-between size," so that one crown size is too small to seat and the next larger size fits very loosely, even after contouring. Further tooth reduction may be necessary in these cases to seat the smaller crown size.

After seating a crown, establish a preliminary occlusal relationship by comparing adjacent marginal ridge heights. If the crown does not seat to the same level as the adjacent teeth, the occlusal reduction may be inadequate; the crown may be too long; a gingival proximal ledge may exist; or contact may not have been broken with the adjacent tooth, preventing a complete seating of the crown. If an extensive area of gingival blanching occurs around the crown, this indicates the crown is too long or is grossly overcontoured. Crowns are manufactured longer than necessary for the average tooth, and hence many will require some trimming. A properly trimmed crown will extend approximately 1 mm into the gingival sulcus. The Ion (3M Co) pre-contoured crowns usually require the least trimming. Before trimming, place the crown onto the preparation and lightly mark the level of the gingival crest on the crown with a sharp instrument, such as a scaler. The crowns are removed and are trimmed 1 mm below the mark with crown and bridge scissors or with a heatless wheel on the straight handpiece. The crown margins should be trimmed to parallel the contour of the gingival tissue around the tooth and should consist of a series of curves without the presence of straight lines or sharp angles.

8. Contour and crimp the crown to form a tightly fitting crown. Contouring involves bending the gingival one third of the crown's margins inward to restore anatomic features of

the natural crown and to reduce the marginal circumference of the crown, ensuring a good fit. Contouring is accomplished circumferentially with a No. 114 ball and socket pliers (Fig. 19–10A) or with a No. 137 Gordon pliers. Final close adaptation of the crown is achieved by crimping the cervical margin 1 mm circumferentially. The No. 137 pliers may be used for this; a special crimping pliers, No. 800-417 (Unitek) (Fig. 19–10B), is also available. A tight marginal fit aids in (1) mechanical retention of the crown, (2) protection of the cement from exposure to oral fluids, and (3) maintaining gingival health. After contouring and crimping, firm resistance should be encountered when the crown is seated. After seating the crown, examine the gingival margins with an explorer for areas of poor fit. Observe the gingival tissue for blanching, and examine the proximal contacts. If proximal contact needs to be established, it can be done with a ball and socket pliers after removal of the crown.

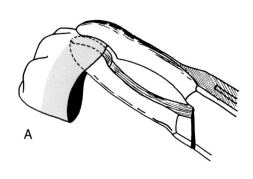

A

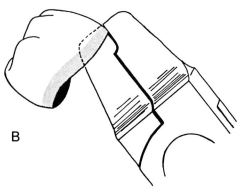

B

Figure 19–10 ■ A, Contouring is accomplished with a pair of No. 114 pliers. B, Final crimping is accomplished with a pair of No. 800-417 pliers. (From Stainless Steel Crown Preparation and Restoration, Project TAPP, Quercus Corporation, © 1977.)

When removing the crown, a scaler or amalgam carver can be used to engage the gingival margin and dislodge the crown. A thumb or finger should be kept over the crown during removal so that the movement of the crown is controlled.

9. Appropriate pulp protection must be placed, the rubber dam removed, and the crown replaced so that the occlusion may be checked. Examine the occlusion bilaterally with the patient in centric occlusion. Look for movement of the crown occluso-gingivally with biting pressure, and check for excessive gingival blanching.

After the rubber dam is removed, special care must be taken when handling the crown in the mouth. A 2 × 2 inch gauze pad should be placed posterior to the tooth being crowned to act as a safety net to prevent the crown from dropping into the oropharynx.

10. Final smoothing and polishing of the crown margin should be performed before final cementation. Smoothing is begun with the heatless stone to create smooth, flowing curves and to thin the margin of the crown slightly. Rotation of the stone should be toward and at a 45 degree angle to the edge of the crown. A rubber wheel is used to remove surface scratches, using light, brushing strokes. A wire brush can be used to polish the margins to a high shine.

11. Rinse and dry the crown inside and out, and prepare to cement it. A zinc phosphate, polycarboxylate, or glass ionomer cement is preferred. If zinc phosphate is used, two coats of cavity varnish should be placed on vital teeth before cementation and the cement should be of a consistency whereby it strings about 1½ inches from the mixing pad with the spatula. The crown is filled approximately two thirds with cement, with all inner surfaces covered.

12. Dry the tooth with compressed air, and seat the crown completely. Cement should be expressed from all margins. The handle of a mirror or a band pusher may be used to ensure complete seating, or the patient may be instructed to bite on a tongue blade. Before the cement sets, have the patient close into centric occlusion and confirm that the occlusion has not been altered.

13. Cement must be removed from the gingival sulcus. Zinc phosphate cement can be easily removed with an explorer or scaler. Polycarboxylate cement, after it has partially set, will reach a rubbery consistency. Excess cement should be removed at this stage with an explorer tip. The interproximal areas can be

cleaned by tying a knot in a piece of dental floss and drawing the floss through the interproximal region.

14. Rinse the oral cavity well, and re-examine the occlusion and the soft tissues before dismissing the patient.

Special Considerations for Stainless Steel Crowns (Nash, 1981)

Placement of adjacent crowns ■ When quadrant dentistry is practiced, it will often be necessary to place stainless steel crowns on adjacent teeth. The tooth preparation and crown selection for placing multiple crowns are similar to that previously described for single crowns, but a few areas of consideration need to be discussed.

1. Prepare the occlusal reduction of one tooth completely before beginning the occlusal reduction of the other tooth. When reduction of two teeth is performed simultaneously, the tendency is to under-reduce both.

2. Insufficient proximal reduction is a common problem when adjacent crowns are placed. Contact between adjacent proximal surfaces should be broken, producing approximately a 1.5 mm space at the gingival level.

3. Both crowns should be trimmed, contoured, and prepared for cementation simultaneously. It is generally best to begin placement and cementation of the more distal tooth first. However, most importantly, the sequence of placement of crowns for cementation should follow the same sequence as that when the crowns were placed for final fitting. Sometimes crowns will seat quite easily in one placement sequence and will seat with great difficulty if the sequence is altered.

Preparing crowns in areas of space loss ■ Frequently, when the tooth structure is lost as a result of caries, a loss of contact and drifting of adjacent teeth into space normally occupied by the tooth to be restored occur. When this happens, the crown required to fit over the buccolingual dimension will be too wide mesio-distally to be placed and a crown selected to fit the mesio-distal space will be too small in circumference. The larger crown, which will fit over the tooth's greatest convexity, is selected and an adjustment is made to reduce mesio-distal width. This adjustment is accomplished by grasping the marginal ridges of the crown with Howe utility pliers and squeezing the crown, thereby reducing the mesio-distal dimension. Considerable recontouring of proximal, buccal,

and lingual walls of the crown with the No. 137 or No. 114 pliers will be necessary. If difficulty is still encountered in crown placement, this may necessitate additional tooth reduction of the buccal and lingual surfaces and selection of another, smaller crown.

Restoration of Primary Incisors and Canines

The indications for restoration of primary incisors and canines are generally based upon (1) caries, (2) trauma, or (3) developmental defects of the tooth's hard tissue. Class III and Class V composite resins are frequently placed in primary anterior teeth. Class IV resins may be used also; however, if a great deal of tooth structure has been lost, full coverage with a crown will provide a superior restoration.

CLASS III RESIN RESTORATIONS (Fig. 19–11)

Conservative restorations with composite resin are indicated for small interproximal carious lesions of incisors and for the mesial surface of canines. Because of the large size of the pulps of these teeth, the preparations must be kept very small. Retention is gained with retentive locks on the facial or lingual surface and by bevelling the cavosurface margin to increase the surface area of the enamel etched.

Restoring the distal surface of primary canines (Fig. 19–12) requires a preparation slightly different from the preparation for incisors. The proximal box is directed at a different angle toward the gingiva. Either amalgam or resin may be used as the restorative material in this location. The preparation, with the exception of a short cavosurface bevel for the resin, is identical regardless of the restorative material chosen. The dovetail is placed on the facial surface, except when amalgam is chosen as the material of choice for a maxillary canine; in that situation, the dovetail is placed on the palatal surface.

Steps in Preparation and Placement of a Class III Composite Restoration

1. Administer appropriate anesthesia, and place the rubber dam. Ligation of individual teeth with dental floss provides the best stability.

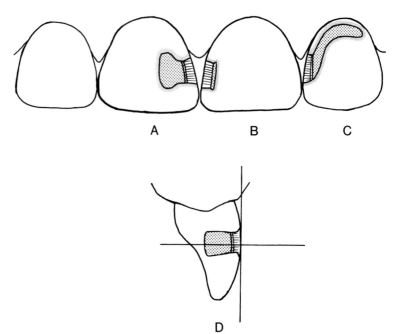

Figure 19–11 ■ Class III cavity preparations (A, B, C—labial view). Note that a short bevel is placed on the cavo-surface margin of all three preparations. A, Slot preparation with a dovetail — the most frequently utilized Class III preparation. The dovetail provides additional retention. B, Slot preparation—used for very small Class III carious lesions. C, Modified slot preparation—used when extensive gingival decalcification is evident adjacent to interproximal caries. D, The interproximal box is placed perpendicular to a line tangent to the labial surface.

2. Create access, and remove caries with a No. 330 bur or a No. 2 round bur in the high speed handpiece, utilizing a facial access. The axial wall is ideally placed 0.5 mm into dentin. A round bur in the slow speed handpiece can be used to remove deep decay. The gingival and lingual walls should just break contact with the adjacent tooth. The incisal wall of the preparation need not have contact broken to ensure adequate tooth structure remaining.

3. A dovetail or lock is placed on the labial surface, just into dentin. The lock should not extend more than halfway across the labial surface and is kept in the middle horizontal third of the tooth.

4. Place a short bevel (0.5 mm) at the cavo-surface margin. This may be accomplished with a fine, tapered diamond or with a flame-shaped composite finishing bur.

5. Clean and dry the preparation with water and compressed air, and cover the deepest portion of the preparation with a thin layer of a calcium hydroxide base.

6. Etch the enamel cavosurface margin for 60 seconds. An acid gel is preferable. Avoid allowing acid to contact dentinal surfaces. In primary teeth, with their prismless layer of enamel, acid-etch retention is not as effective as in permanent teeth, but it does aid in retention and ensures improved marginal integrity and reduced marginal leakage. After etching, rinse and dry the preparation well.

Figure 19–12 ■ Class III preparation for primary canines. A, The dovetail is usually placed on the lingual surface of maxillary canines and on the labial surface of mandibular canines. A short bevel (not shown) is placed on the cavo-surface margin of preparations to be restored with composite resin. B, The proximal box is placed perpendicular to a line tangent to the surface on which the dovetail is placed.

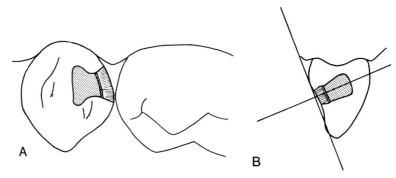

7. Place a plastic matrix. Most matrices will first need to be cut in half horizontally because they are manufactured for permanent teeth and are too wide for primary teeth. The matrix is placed interproximally, and a wedge is inserted.

8. Place a dentin bonding agent into the preparation with a small brush. Gently blow compressed air into the preparation to disperse a thin layer of bonding agent evenly over both dentin and enamel.

9. With a plastic instrument or a pressure syringe, place the composite into the preparation and pull the matrix tight around the cavity preparation with finger pressure and hold until cured. Visible light–cured composites provide a controlled polymerization time and are recommended over autopolymerizing materials. Hold the visible light as closely as possible to the composite, and polymerize according to the manufacturer's instructions. The light should be directed from both the facial and the lingual to ensure complete polymerization.

10. Finishing and polishing can be performed immediately following polymerization. The smoothest and most desirable surface of a composite is that which remains after a properly adapted matrix is removed; however, it is difficult to adapt a matrix so accurately that additional adjustment to the margins is unnecessary. Gross finishing or contouring can be performed with fine grit diamonds or with carbide finishing burs. A flame carbide finishing bur (12–20 flutes) is excellent for finishing the facial and interproximal surfaces. A scapel with a curved blade may be used to remove gingival flash. The lingual surface is best finished with a round or pear-shaped carbide finishing bur. A lubricated, pointed white stone may also be used for smoothing.

Final interproximal polishing of the restoration is completed with sandpaper strips. These strips will be best used if they are cut into thin strips 2–3 mm in width. Mounted abrasive disks can be used to finish the facial and lingual surfaces.

After polishing is completed, an unfilled resin glaze may be added to the polished restoration. The glaze helps provide a better marginal seal and a smooth, finished surface. Before adding the glaze, the restoration and surrounding enamel should first be etched for 15–20 seconds to remove surface debris. After rinsing and drying, the resin is painted onto the restoration and is polymerized. Care should be taken not to bond adjacent teeth together with the resin glaze.

11. When finishing is completed, remove the rubber dam and floss the interproximal areas to check for overhangs and to remove excess glaze material.

CLASS V RESTORATIONS FOR INCISORS AND CANINES

Class V restorations may be resins (most frequently) or amalgams. They most frequently are needed on the facial surface of canines. To prepare these restorations, penetrate the tooth in the area of caries with a No. 330 bur until dentin is reached (approximately 1 mm from the outer enamel surface). Move the bur laterally into sound dentin and enamel, thus establishing the walls of the cavity. The pulpal wall should be convex, parallel to the outer enamel surface. The lateral walls are slightly flared near the proximal surfaces to prevent undermining of enamel. The final external outline is determined by the extent of caries. Mechanical retention in the preparation can be placed with a No. 35 inverted cone bur or a No. ½ round bur, creating small undercuts in the gingivo-axial and inciso-axial line angles. For resins, a short bevel is placed around the entire cavosurface margin. Pulpal protection, etching and resin placement, and finishing is similar to that described for Class III composite placement, except that no matrix is utilized.

FULL CORONAL COVERAGE OF INCISORS (Fig. 19–13)

Indications

1. Incisors with large interproximal lesions
2. Incisors that have received pulp therapy
3. Incisors that have been fractured and have lost an appreciable amount of tooth structure
4. Incisors with multiple hypoplastic defects or developmental disturbances (e.g., ectodermal dysplasia)
5. Discolored incisors that are esthetically unpleasing
6. Incisors with small interproximal lesions that also demonstrate large areas of cervical decalcification

It is a challenging task to repair extensively destroyed anterior teeth with restorations that are durable, retentive, and esthetic. There are several methods of providing full coronal coverage to primary incisors—acid-etched resin crowns (Fig. 19–13B), stainless steel crowns,

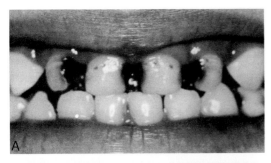

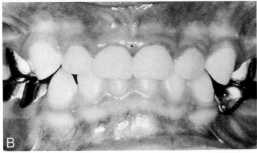

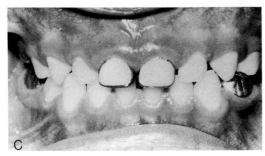

Figure 19–13 ■ Full coronal coverage of primary incisors. *A*, Extensive caries in primary incisors. *B*, Same incisors after restoration with acid-etched composite crowns. *C*, Open-face stainless steel crowns on maxillary central incisors (see Fig. 19–1 for lingual view).

and veneered or open-face stainless steel crowns (Fig. 19–13C). Each has shortcomings (Table 19–4), but each may be utilized at some time. The most esthetic and most frequently placed crown is the acid-etched resin crown. Open-face crowns enjoy popularity with many operators because of retention superior to resin crowns; however, esthetic results are compromised. Plain stainless steel crowns provide a very durable restoration but are esthetically unpleasing to most parents.

Preparation and Placement of Resin Crowns

1. Administer appropriate anesthesia.
2. Select the shade of composite resin to be used, then place and ligate the rubber dam.

3. A primary incisor celluloid crown form (Strip Crown, Unitek Corp, Monrovia, CA) is selected with a mesio-distal width approximately equal to the tooth to be restored.

4. Remove decay with a large round bur in the slow speed handpiece. If pulp therapy is required, do it at this time.

5. Reduce the incisal edge 1.5 mm, using a fine, tapered diamond or a No. 169L bur.

6. Reduce the interproximal surfaces 0.5–1.0 mm (Fig. 19–14). This reduction should allow a crown form to slip over the tooth. The interproximal walls should be parallel, and the gingival margin should have a feather edge.

7. Reduce the facial surface 0.5–1.0 mm and the lingual surface 0.5 mm. Create a feather edge gingival margin. Round all line angles.

8. Place a small undercut on the facial surface in the gingival one third of the tooth with a No. 330 bur or a No. 35 inverted cone. When the resin material polymerizes, engaging the undercut, this will serve as a mechanical lock.

9. Trim the selected crown form by cutting away excess material gingivally with crown and bridge scissors, and trial fit the crown form. A properly trimmed crown form should fit 1 mm below the gingival crest and should be of comparable height to adjacent teeth. Remember that maxillary lateral incisor crowns are usually 0.5–1.0 mm shorter than those of central incisors.

10. After the celluloid crown is adequately trimmed, punch a small hole in the incisal corner with an explorer to act as a vent for the escape of trapped air as the crown is placed with resin onto the preparation.

11. Place calcium hydroxide over the deepest areas of the preparation, and carefully etch all of the remaining enamel for 60 seconds, utilizing an acid gel. Rinse and dry the tooth thoroughly, then apply a dentin bonding agent to the entire tooth.

12. Fill the crown form approximately two thirds full with a resin material, and seat onto the tooth. Excess material should flow from the gingival margin and the vent hole. While holding the crown in place, remove the gingival excess with an explorer.

13. Allow the material to polymerize. If using a light-cured material, be certain to direct the light from both the facial and lingual directions.

14. Remove the celluloid form by using a curved scapel blade to cut the material on the facial, and then peel the form from the tooth.

15. Remove the rubber dam, and evaluate the occlusion.

Table 19–4 ■ Comparison of full coverage techniques for primary incisors

Technique	Esthetics	Durability	Time for Placement	Selection Criteria
Resin (Strip) crowns*	Very good initially; will discolor over time	Retention dependent upon amount of tooth structure present and quality of acid etch Can be dislodged fairly easily if traumatized	Time required for Optimum isolation Etching Placement Finishing	When esthetics are a great concern Adequate tooth structure remains for etching/bonding Child is not highly trauma-prone Gingival hemorrhage is controllable
Steel crowns	Poor	Very good; a well-crimped, cemented crown is very retentive and wears well	Fastest crown to place	Severely decayed teeth Esthetics of little concern Unable to adequately control gingival hemorrhage Need to place a restoration quickly because of inadequate cooperation or time
Open-face steel crowns	Good; however, there is usually some metal showing	Good—like steel crowns, are very retentive; however, facings may be dislodged	Takes longest to place because of two-step procedure Crown placement Composite placement	Severely decayed teeth Durability needed —active, accident-prone child or severe bruxism evident Esthetics are a concern

* Restoration of choice esthetically.

16. Little finishing should be required on the facial surface. A flame carbide finishing bur can be used to finish the gingival margin, should any irregularities be noted with a tactile examination with an explorer. A round or pear-shaped finishing bur may be used for final contouring of the lingual surface. Abrasive disks are used for final polishing of the areas of the crown that require contouring.

Preparation and Placement of an Open-Face (Veneered) Steel Crown

Non-veneered stainless steel crowns are not frequently used on maxillary primary incisors because of the poor esthetic result. However, they are often used on severely decayed canines and mandibular incisors, where esthetics are less noticeable. Steps for preparation and placement of both veneered (Helpin, 1983) and non-veneered crowns are discussed in this section.

The preparation for a steel crown is identical to that of a resin crown, except no facial undercut is made for the steel crown. After the preparation is completed, select a crown and try it on the tooth. Anterior steel crowns often need to have their cervical shapes changed before placement. When manufactured, the crowns have an ovoid shape with a small facio-lingual dimension. This must often be changed to allow the crown to slip onto the tooth. It is done by simply squeezing the crown slightly mesio-distally with a pair of Howe No. 110 utility pliers, thereby increasing the facio-lingual dimension. The fit of the crown should be snug, and difficulty may be encountered seating the crown with finger pressure only. An orthodontic band pusher or tongue blade may be used to aid in seating.

Anterior steel crowns do not generally require much, if any, trimming. If trimming is necessary, it is best done with a heatless wheel.

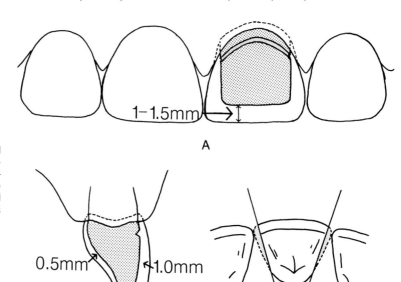

A

Figure 19–14 ■ Acid-etched (strip) composite crown preparation. *A,* Labial view. *B,* Proximal view. *C,* Incisal view. The proximal slice should be parallel to the natural external contours of the tooth.

B

C

Contouring and crimping are necessary to ensure a good marginal fit. The No. 137 Gordon pliers are best suited for this task. Check the final marginal adaptation with an explorer. Polishing and cementation procedures are identical to those for posterior steel crowns. These procedures complete the non-veneered stainless steel crown placement.

To place the open-face or veneered steel crown, the cement must be allowed to set completely, then a labial window is cut in the crown, using a No. 330 or No. 35 bur. The window extends just short of the incisal edge; gingivally, to the height of the gingival crest; and mesio-distally, to the line angles. It is desired that very little metal will be seen from the facial. With a No. 35 inverted cone bur (Fig. 19–15),

remove the cement to a depth of 1 mm. Undercuts must be placed at each margin. This can be performed with the No. 35 bur or with a No. ½ round bur. Mechanical retention is necessary because there is usually little enamel to etch. Smooth the cut margins of the crown with a fine green or white finishing stone.

A thin layer of dentin bonding agent and then composite is placed into the cut window, engaging the undercuts. Resin is added with a plastic instrument. The instrument may be wiped with alcohol to prevent resin from sticking to it. Polymerize the resin, and finish with abrasive disks. Always run the disks from resin to metal at the margins. Disks running from metal to resin will discolor the resin with metal particles.

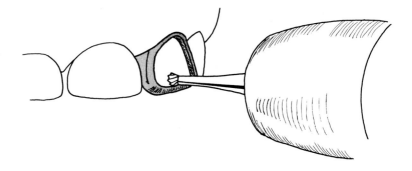

Figure 19–15 ■ Cut the window for the facing in the cemented stainless steel crown and create mechanical undercuts laterally and incisally with an inverted cone bur.

Prosthetic Replacement of Primary Anterior Teeth

Premature loss of maxillary primary incisors as a result of extensive caries, trauma, or congenital absence requires consideration for providing a prosthetic tooth replacement for the child (Steffen et al, 1971). In most instances, prosthetic replacement of primary incisors is considered an elective procedure. Space maintenance in this region is not generally necessary. The most frequent reason for placement of a prosthetic appliance is parental concern about esthetics.

Lack of compliance in appliance wear and care by the young child is the greatest limitation of and contraindication for these appliances. If a young child decides that he or she does not like the appliance, he will find a way to remove it from his mouth and will usually discard it. Education of the parents of this fact is essential before the decision to construct an appliance is made. Another contraindication for prosthetic replacement is the presence of an anterior deep bite.

Prosthetic appliances may be either fixed or removable (Fig. 19–16). When constructing either type, it is best to allow at least 6–8 weeks following the tooth loss before fabrication. This will allow for good healing and gingival shrinkage to occur and will result in a better fitting, more esthetic appliance.

The fixed appliance is a Nance-like device, constructed with two bands or steel crowns on primary molars that are connected by a palatal wire to which the replacement teeth are attached. This appliance is cemented onto the molars and is not easily removed by the child. It will require minimal adjustment. The teeth can be made to sit directly on the ridge of the edentulous space, or acrylic gingiva can be added. Disadvantages of this appliance include (1) possible decalcification around the bands; (2) more difficulty in home cleaning; and (3) bending of the wires with fingers or sticky foods, which may create occlusal interferences and the need for adjustments.

The removable appliance is a Hawley-like device that replaces the teeth and utilizes circumferential and ball clasps on the molars. These appliances require the most compliance of any of the prosthetic replacements. They are not indicated in children under 3 years old. Clasps will need adjustment, the frequency of which depends on the child's handling of the appliances. The greatest advantages of these

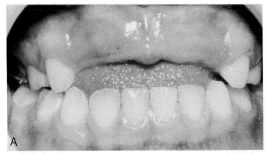

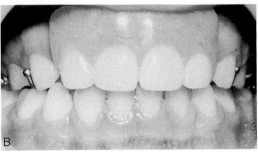

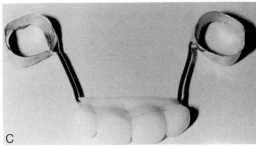

Figure 19–16 ■ Prosthetic replacement of primary anterior teeth. *A,* Edentulous space following extraction of four primary incisors. *B,* Removable prosthetic appliance in place. *C,* Example of a fixed prosthetic appliance replacing four incisors. (Courtesy of Dr. Gary Nelson, Redlands, CA.)

appliances are the ability to remove the appliance for daily cleaning and that adjustments are easily made by the dentist without having to remove and re-cement bands.

REFERENCES

Bhaskar SN, Lilly GE: Intrapulpal temperature during cavity preparation. J Dent Res 44(4):644–647, 1965.

Black GV: A Work on Operative Dentistry, Vol II, 5th ed. Chicago, Medico-Dental Publishing Co., 1924.

Bouschor CF, Matthews JL: A four-year clinical study of teeth restored after preparation with an air turbine handpiece with air coolant. J Pros Dent 16(2):306–309, 1966.

Craig RG: Restorative Dental Materials, 6th ed. St. Louis, CV Mosby Co, 1980.

Farah, JW, Powers JM: Rating permanent cements. Dent Advisor 2(1):3, 1985.

Helpin ML: The open-face steel crown restoration in children. J Dent Child 50(1):34–38, 1983.

Humphrey WP: Use of chronic steel in children's dentistry. Dent Surv 26:945–947, 1950.

Leinfelder KF, Sluder TB, Santos JF, Wall JT: Five-year clinical evaluation of anterior and posterior restorations of composite resin. Oper Dent 5:57–65, 1980.

Leinfelder KF, Vann WF: The use of composite resins on primary molars. Ped Dent 4(1):27–31, 1982.

Myers DR: Factors producing failure of class II silver amalgam restorations in primary molars. J Dent Child 44(3):226–229, 1977.

Nash DA: The nickel-chromium crown for restoring posterior primary teeth. JADA 102(1):44–49, 1981.

Phillips RW: Skinner's Science of Dental Materials, 8th ed. Philadelphia, WB Saunders Co, 1982.

Steffen JM, Miller JB, Johnson R: An esthetic method of anterior space maintenance. J Dent Child 38(3):154–157, 1971.

Waggoner WF: Composite restorations of posterior teeth—current status. J Okla Dent Assoc 74(2):39–43, 1984.

chapter *20*

Pulp therapy for the primary dentition

Gary K. Belanger

CHAPTER OUTLINE

■ **PULPAL DIAGNOSIS**
  History
  Clinical Examination
  Clinical Diagnostic Procedures
  Radiographic Examination
  Direct Pulpal Evaluation

■ **PULPAL TREATMENT PROCEDURES**
  Indirect Pulp Cap
  Direct Pulp Cap
  Pulpotomy
  Pulpectomy

The pulps of deciduous teeth vary from the pulps of permanent teeth in numerous ways, including developmental, morphologic, and histologic differences. More important clinically, they differ in their reactions to adverse stimuli and to various pulpal medications. The dentist must be aware that some medications and techniques that produce beneficial effects in permanent teeth might have a deleterious effect in primary teeth (or vice versa). An important example of this is calcium hydroxide, which can be used in different forms advantageously in several techniques in permanent teeth (e.g., direct or indirect pulp caps, apexogenesis, and apexification). In primary teeth, however, the effect of calcium hydroxide may be adverse because it frequently stimulates internal resorption (Via, 1955). Thus, the dentist must be careful not to presume a successful result in a primary pulp when using a technique that is acceptable and common for permanent pulp therapy unless he or she is certain that a beneficial response is also likely in primary teeth.

The health of the pulp in a deciduous tooth may be threatened in several ways. Dental caries that progresses through enamel and then into dentin (either partly or completely) can produce pulpal reactions, including acute and chronic inflammation and degenerative changes. A traumatic injury or excessive operative trauma (iatrogenic overpreparation) may also produce pulpal reactions. In these situations, the dentist must correctly diagnose the extent of pulpal damage and determine a treatment that will eliminate pain and promote healing to the pulp in order to maintain its health until the tooth is exfoliated.

Proper diagnosis of pulpal status will require careful evaluation of the patient's and parent's historical information, clinical examination and diagnostic checks, and accurate radiographic interpretation. In addition, the dentist must consider many other important factors, such as the following: (1) the child's overall health status, (2) the child's overall dental health picture and whether there are prematurely (or potentially) lost teeth that require planning for

257

space maintenance, (3) the reliability of the family for follow-up assessment and care, (4) the restorability of pulpally involved teeth, (5) the child's cooperative ability, and (6) the parents' motivation to save the tooth and the financial resources to do so.

Many primary teeth can be saved with appropriate pulpal intervention. Extraction may be correct and necessary in some situations but it should not be performed merely as the simplest solution, especially if loss of the tooth may lead to compromised dental arch circumference (space loss). An intact tooth successfully treated pulpally and with a restored clinical crown is a superior space maintainer.

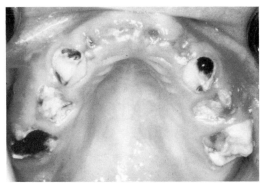

Figure 20–1 ■ Gross carious destruction of primary teeth in a child without any complaints of pain.

Pulpal Diagnosis

No single finding will predict absolutely either an affected primary pulp's histopathologic picture or a 100% successful treatment for it. Relevant information must be obtained from multiple sources.

HISTORY

Whether or not a tooth has been painful to a child (i.e., a chief complaint of a toothache) must be determined. However, pain may be very subjective and is usually interpreted by the parent. Some "emergency" visits are actually made for non-toothache conditions, such as eruption or exfoliation problems. At other times, the dentist may see children at a non-emergency appointment and detect gross carious destruction and extensive pulpal involvement, yet the child is in no apparent distress and the parent denies that the child is having any oral pain. Young children may not be able to communicate (verbalize) about pain. Furthermore, if dental problems (such as nursing bottle decay) developed early, the child may have no experience of teeth feeling any different way. Abscessed primary teeth that have adequate drainage can surprisingly manifest little or no swelling, pressure, or pain (Fig. 20–1).

The dentist should distinguish between the two main types of dental pain that children may experience. The first is *provoked* pain, which is stimulated by heat, cold, sweets, air, chewing, or other stimuli that, when removed, reduce or eliminate the pain. These signs often indicate dentin sensitivity within a deep carious lesion or around a leaking restoration. The pulpal damage is frequently minimal and reversible.

The second type of dental pain is *spontaneous* pain, which is constant, may keep the child awake at night, and is not relieved by common pain medications or remedies. This kind of pain indicates advanced (usually irreversible) pulpal damage. Furthermore, a history of redness or swelling (especially extraoral swelling, such as an eye swollen shut) must be regarded very seriously, particularly when it is accompanied by fever or other signs of systemic involvement.

Children with a history of recent orofacial trauma having affected primary teeth require immediate attention to evaluate potential dental fractures, displacements, or extrusions. Other children may be seen much later after an injury, often with a darkened incisor but without pain or other discomfort. Assessment of pulpal damage and the need for treatment must be made.

The history relating to the chief complaint must not obscure asking about the past dental history or the medical history. A youngster with serious systemic disease may require an alternative treatment approach to that for the healthy child.

CLINICAL EXAMINATION

The obvious and subtle signs of pulpal damage require a careful extraoral and intraoral inspection. Intraoral soft tissue redness, swelling and drainage, grossly decayed teeth, and traumatized teeth are all indicators of injury, inflammation, and infection, and are usually readily apparent (Fig. 20–2). However, the clinical examination should also be used to inspect for other less obvious clues suggesting problems. These include marginal ridge carious breakdown, teeth with missing or broken resto-

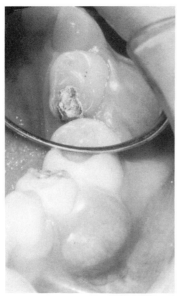

Figure 20-2 ■ Clinical view showing parulis on the buccal of tooth L.

rations, or simply any previous restorations (particularly full coverage restorations that might be indicative of extensive clinical crown loss and likely previous pulpal therapy).

CLINICAL DIAGNOSTIC PROCEDURES

Diagnostic procedures that can prove useful for primary teeth are mobility evaluation and percussion sensitivity. The dentist must be knowledgeable of normal exfoliation times so that a hypermobile tooth nearing exfoliation is not misinterpreted. Also, comparison of the mobility of a suspicious tooth with its antimere is beneficial. Significant differences would suggest abnormalities of the more mobile tooth. Percussion testing (done very gently — with the tip of finger, not with the end of a dental mirror) may be helpful in localizing a painful tooth in which inflammation has progressed to involve the periodontal ligament.

Classic pulp vitality testing in children is of dubious value, and the dentist should forego it (Kennedy and Kapala, 1985). The child in pain will be very leery and will not likely permit numerous tests, each of which require identifying an uncomfortable stimulus. Consequently, heat, cold, and electric pulse tests rarely provide accurate data for primary teeth. A child may also be so apprehensive as to react to any stimulus or react before it is even given. False results may be obtained from stimuli transmitted to

gingiva, periodontal ligament, bone, or to multi-canal pulp systems, only a part of which is vital. Teeth near exfoliation usually give unreliable results. For these reasons, information other than heat, cold, and electric pulp testing should be evaluated, especially if thermal and electrical tests might be inconclusive and cause alienation of the child's confidence.

RADIOGRAPHIC EXAMINATION

A well-taken radiograph of an area of suspicion is critical to the eventual pulpal diagnosis and treatment, since many factors can be evaluated and pathosis detected. It is very useful to take the same radiographic view of the contralateral side to allow a comparison. Factors for evaluation include the following:

1. The extent of caries and its proximity to the pulp
2. Previously placed restorations and pulpal therapy: proximity to a pulp horn or any evidence of a pulpotomy or pulpectomy procedure, whether successful or failing
3. Evidence of pulpal degenerative changes, such as calcific formations or internal resorption
4. Width of the periodontal ligament space (whether normal and uniform or not) and the lamina dura (intact or interrupted)
5. Root resorption consistent with a physiologic rather than pathologic response (left-right antimere comparisons are especially useful)
6. Radiolucencies of bone, including periapical changes (Note: for primary molars, an inter-radicular or furcation involvement is more commonly seen because accessory canals in the coronal floor make drainage more easy than through the apical foramina.) (Fig. 20-3)

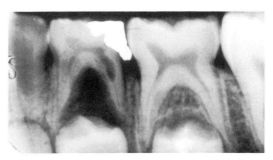

Figure 20-3 ■ Radiograph from case shown in Figure 20-2 shows poor restoration near pulp horn, internal resorption, loss of lamina dura, and bifurcation radiolucency; the tooth had previously been treated with a direct pulp cap.

7. Recognizing correctly those normal factors that complicate pediatric dental radiographic interpretation, such as larger marrow spaces, superimposition of developing secondary follicles, and the normal resorption patterns of primary teeth.

DIRECT PULPAL EVALUATION

After a diagnosis has been made, the dentist will initiate some form of treatment. The visual, tactile, and occasionally olfactory senses of the dentist then become important evaluators of actual pulpal status. The proximity of soft carious dentin to the pulp must be judged if the dentist wishes to avoid a pulp exposure. If coronal pulp amputation and a formocresol pulpotomy are planned, the nature of the bleeding from the pulp amputation site must be evaluated as normal (red color and hemostasis gained with cotton pellet pressure) or abnormal (deeper crimson color and continued bleeding after several minutes of pressure). A degenerating or necrotic pulp (dry canal) that produces a putrescent odor may be encountered. Even though the dentist may have decided upon an appropriate therapy for a damaged primary pulp, any evidence encountered during treatment that is inconsistent with the initial diagnosis must not be ignored. A change in the therapeutic approach is appropriate and preferable to continuing the initial therapy in the face of conflicting direct pulpal findings.

Pulpal Treatment Procedures

The primary pulp is affected every time an operative procedure results in exposed dentin. The dentist should always strive to protect the pulp during preparation and to avoid desiccation of exposed dentin. For amalgam preparations of normal depth, a cavity varnish prior to amalgam placement will decrease postoperative sensitivity and microleakage. For composite restorations prior to acid-etching, all exposed dentin should be covered with a calcium hydroxide liner to prevent dentinal etching and pulpal damage. The dentist must be careful not to focus just on the demands of cavity preparation but must also be alert to the goal of avoiding harm to the pulp. Neither the primary tooth's vitality (ability to respond to a stimulus) nor its viability (ability to withstand noxious stimuli and remain healthy) should be compromised during operative procedures.

The dentist's evaluation of all relevant factors of primary pulp status, as discussed previously, will provide an initial assessment of the pulp's actual histologic status. In addition, the dentist's previous experiences with various pulpal treatment options (including success rates, difficulty, and number of appointments needed) will unquestionably influence his or her judgments about appropriate treatment.

Several different types of pulp treatment have been recommended for primary pulp therapy. Ones currently considered appropriate are described.

INDIRECT PULP CAP

The indirect pulp cap procedure is described more fully for use in young permanent teeth (see Section III, Chapter 33). It is somewhat controversial for use in deciduous teeth, although some investigators advocate it as a more physiologic healing procedure for primary teeth and one preferable to the more aggressive and controversial formocresol pulpotomy (Starkey, 1980). Other professionals prefer the formocresol pulpotomy procedure, claiming it to be more predictable, have a superior success rate, and be a definitive (one appointment) rather than extended procedure. Because of these disagreements, the dentist must decide the appropriateness of either procedure after careful study and consultation.

DIRECT PULP CAP

Direct exposure of a primary pulp can occur from dental caries, from a traumatic injury with coronal fracture, or during mechanical preparation. In the direct pulp cap procedure, a calcium hydroxide preparation is placed right over the pulp exposure in an attempt to promote both pulp healing and reparative dentin formation. The only acceptable primary tooth candidate for a direct pulp cap, however, is a tooth with a small mechanical exposure (less than 1 mm in diameter) in which the following three optimal conditions exist: (1) a tooth previously asymptomatic; (2) no deep caries; and (3) rubber dam isolation, which prevents any salivary contamination.

Direct pulp capping of carious or traumatic primary pulp exposures is not indicated. Capping in these cases rarely succeeds owing to

pulpal inflammation and infection, which usually lead to internal resorption or total pulpal necrosis (Figs. 20–2 and 20–3). A formocresol pulpotomy is indicated instead. The dentist attempting an indirect pulp cap procedure in a primary tooth that unintentionally results in a carious exposure is cautioned against placing calcium hydroxide over the direct exposure. Although this treatment might be appropriate in some permanent teeth, its low success rate in primary teeth does not make it an attractive treatment option (Kennedy, 1979).

PULPOTOMY

Pulpotomy is indicated for vital primary teeth whose pulps have been exposed. It is the treatment of choice when there is *no* sign of the following: (1) spontaneous pain, (2) swelling, (3) tenderness to percussion, (4) abnormal mobility, (5) fistulas, (6) sulcular drainage, (7) internal resorption, (8) pulpal calcifications, (9) pathologic external root resorption, (10) periapical radiolucency, (11) inter-radicular radiolucency, or (12) excessive pulpal bleeding or a putrescent odor.

Formocresol has been a recommended treatment medicament for damaged primary pulps for over 50 years and actually evolved from a pulpal devitalization procedure developed prior to routine use of local anesthesia. Formocresol is widely used for pulpotomies in primary teeth, and a high rate of clinical success has been extensively documented (Berger, 1965; Redig, 1968; Morawa et al, 1975). However, concern persists over its safety and most efficacious use; the chronic inflammatory response that it produces; the effects on primary root resorption and possible hypoplasia to succedaneous teeth; as well as its immunogenic, mutagenic, and carcinogenic potential (Ranly, 1984; Myers et al, 1983). Unfortunately, long-term success with other techniques that are superior to the formocresol pulpotomy for primary teeth have not yet been shown. The use of calcium hydroxide as a primary pulpotomy medication is specifically contraindicated because of the development of internal resorption and poor clinical success. Nevertheless, research on an alternative technique includes the use of electrosurgery (Ruempling et al, 1983), glutaraldehyde (Kopel et al, 1980), and enriched collagen solution (Fuks et al, 1984).

The formocresol pulpotomy technique should be performed in the following sequence:

Access and caries removal ■ Using local anesthesia and with a rubber dam in place, remove all dental caries except that over the exposure site. Prepare an access opening that is sufficiently large by connecting the pulp horns, and then remove the entire roof of the pulp.

Coronal pulp amputation ■ Using a sterile, large spoon excavator, incise and remove all pulp tissue within the coronal chamber, being careful not to pull out the radicular pulp tissue (Fig. 20–4). A large, round bur in a slow speed handpiece is preferred by some dentists, but for the inexperienced, extreme care must be taken to avoid a pulpal floor perforation (Fig. 20–5).

Hemorrhage control and evaluation ■ One or more sterile cotton pellets should be placed over each pulp amputation site (canal orifice), and pressure should be applied for several minutes. When the pellet is removed, hemostasis should have been gained and be apparent, even though a minor amount of wound bleeding may be evident. A deep purple hemorrhage or an excessive amount of bleeding that persists in spite of cotton pellet pressure is indicative of inflammatory pulp changes that

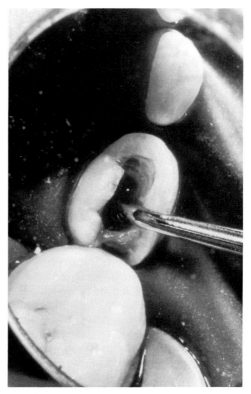

Figure 20–4 ■ Through an access opening, a spoon excavator is used to remove the coronal pulp tissue.

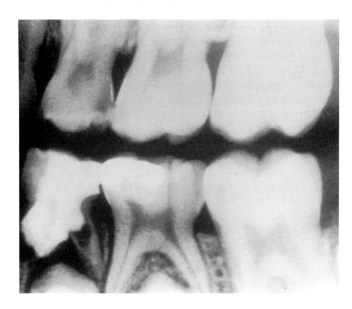

Figure 20–5 ■ Severe zinc oxide–eugenol overfill of tooth L resulting from undetected perforation of pulpal floor.

have extended into the radicular pulp. Such changes preclude the tooth from remaining a good candidate for the formocresol pulpotomy, and pulpectomy or extraction is indicated. It should be noted that no intrapulpal local anesthesia or other hemostatic agent should be used in attempting to minimize the hemorrhage, since bleeding behavior is a clinical evaluation that is critical to judging the radicular pulp status.

Formocresol application ■ A drop of one-fifth dilution of formocresol should be placed on each of several sterile cotton pellets and then blotted *very well* between the ends of a cotton roll. A pellet is placed with pressure over each radicular pulp stump for 5 minutes. While waiting, the dentist may begin the stainless steel crown preparation and its adaptation (if it is to be placed at the same visit). When the pellet is removed, the amputation site(s) should appear dark brown or black, with very little if any hemorrhage.

Zinc oxide and eugenol base and final restoration ■ A regular mix of zinc oxide and eugenol (or a reinforced product such as IRM*) should be placed at the base of the coronal pulp chamber directly on the amputation sites and should be lightly condensed so as to fill the access opening completely. The final restoration should be a stainless steel crown and, if possible, should be placed at the same appointment that the formocresol pulpotomy is completed. If that is not possible, however, the zinc oxide and eugenol will serve as an acceptable interim restoration until the stainless steel crown can be placed. An amalgam final restoration is *not* indicated because of the possibility of desiccation and fracture of the remaining tooth structure.

Many variations on the procedure as described have been used. Some dentists continue to use full strength Buckley's formocresol* rather than the one-fifth dilution, even though they have been found to be equally effective but with less concern of toxicity with the diluted solution (Morawa et al, 1975). Some dentists leave a pellet of formocresol in the coronal pulp chamber for 1 week (or more) and complete the pulpotomy as a two step procedure. Another variation is to mix a drop of formocresol with the eugenol when mixing the base material. Some dentists claim improved empirical results for these modifications, but there is little evidence that they result in superior success to the basic procedure as described previously.

PULPECTOMY

The term *pulpectomy* means the complete removal of the pulp from a tooth. When used to describe a procedure for deciduous teeth, the term also implies a root canal filling with a physiologically tolerable and resorbable material. Pulpectomy is indicated if degenerative pulpal changes have involved radicular tissues. However, as the amount and length of pulpal degeneration increases and as increasing num-

---

* L. D. Caulk Co., Milford, DE.

* Crosby Laboratories, Burbank, CA.

bers of signs and symptoms associated with a necrotic pulp are seen, the likelihood of the technique being successful decreases. A pulpectomy is the most extensive treatment available for saving a primary tooth with severe pulp involvement.

In certain critical situations, the dentist may attempt the pulpectomy even when knowing that the situation and prognosis may not be ideal. An example is when carious pulpal destruction of a primary second molar occurs before the eruption of the permanent first molar (at about age 6). Extraction of the primary second molar without provision for space maintenance would likely result in the mesial eruption of the permanent first molar with subsequent loss of space for the eruption of the permanent second premolar (Fig. 20–6). Although a distal shoe space maintainer has been suggested for this situation, maintaining the natural primary tooth is the best space maintainer. Therefore, a pulpectomy in the primary second molar is a reasonable clinical choice even if that tooth is maintained only until the permanent first molar has adequately erupted, to be followed by extraction of the primary second molar and placement of a space maintainer (Fig. 20–7).

There are a number of differences between the deciduous pulpectomy and conventional endodontic procedures in permanent teeth. They are necessitated because of several important physiologic differences between primary and permanent teeth.

1. The morphologic appearance of deciduous canals (often more dumbbell-shaped in primary molars) and the very fine, filamentous connection of the pulp system (Hibbard and Ireland, 1957) make complete débridement of the canal extremely difficult, if not impossible.

2. Deciduous roots undergo physiologic resorption prior to the exfoliation of the tooth. This necessitates using a resorbable filling material, usually a zinc oxide and eugenol paste, rather than gutta percha or silver points, which are used in permanent endodontic procedures.

3. Normal resorption of primary roots causes the actual root canal opening to be several millimeters coronal to the radiographic one, with near or actual perforation occurring along the furcation sides of the roots. Thus, compared with those of permanent teeth, the filing and shaping of primary root canals must be performed short of the radiographic apex and must be done much less aggressively to minimize the chance of mechanical perforation.

The best candidate for pulpectomy is an exposed and infected primary pulp that still has vital radicular tissue. If left untreated, the pulpal degeneration will lead to pulpal necrosis and can lead to many of the signs and symptoms as described previously. In more advanced situations, a pulpectomy can still be performed, but the dentist should be aware that success will be reduced as the severity of the pulpal degeneration increases.

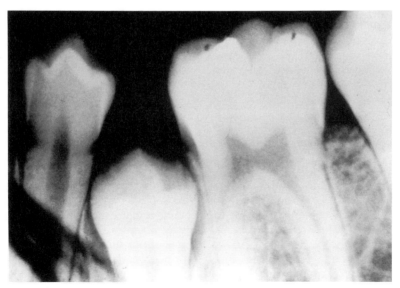

Figure 20–6 ■ Previous extraction of tooth K without placement of a space maintainer resulted in mesial drift of #19 and insufficient space for #20.

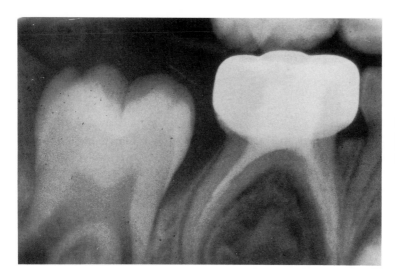

Figure 20–7 ■ Successful pulpectomy and stainless steel crown restoration of tooth T prior to eruption of #30.

The pulpectomy procedure should be performed in the following sequence:

Access Opening

If the treatment began as a pulpotomy, an access opening has already been prepared, but the walls may need to be flared more to facilitate access of the canal openings for broaches and files (Goering and Camp, 1983). Abscessed teeth are likely to have either a large carious exposure or a restoration that, when removed, very nearly exposes the roof of the coronal pulp chamber. The pulp chamber roof should be totally removed. For primary anterior teeth that have been traumatically injured with the development of facial discoloration, dentists who recommend the pulpectomy may choose to use a labial access opening so that the final restoration may also serve to improve the appearance of the discolored tooth (Mack and Halterman, 1980).

Debridement

The coronal pulp chamber may be cleaned out with rotary or hand instruments (e.g., a large, round bur or a large spoon excavator). As with a pulpotomy, the very thin pulpal chamber floor should not be compromised. Each canal orifice of the root(s) should be located. A size of barbed broach should be selected appropriate for the size of the canal. Primary anteriors have one large canal, whereas primary molars have three or four canals, one or several of which may be moderately large and the remainder of which are usually very narrow. The broach is gently used to remove as much organic material as possible from each canal. It should not be extended any closer than 2 mm from the apex (as determined by radiographs). Larger broaches may be used but not if they begin to bind in the canal, which increases the chance of instrument breakage.

Filing

Endodontic files are selected and are adjusted to stop 2 mm short of the radiographic apex of each canal after a check film is examined (Fig. 20–8). This is an arbitrary length but is intended to minimize the chance of overinstrumenting apically and causing periapical damage. In permanent teeth, files are used to remove any organic material remaining in a canal and also to remove and shape dentin, thereby creating a canal that is tapered and has an apical diameter to which the filling material — such as a gutta percha point — can be tightly fit. However, because the filling technique will be different for primary canals, the removal of organic debris is the main purpose for filing.

The very narrow canals found in primary molars require some enlargement to permit adequate access to fill them satisfactorily. A No. 25–30 file may be as large as is possible to file some molar canals (whereas primary anteriors may accept up to a No. 80–100 file). A large amount of filing should be avoided, since the primary canal wall thickness is very much reduced compared with permanent teeth and the chance of a lateral perforation increases with increased filing.

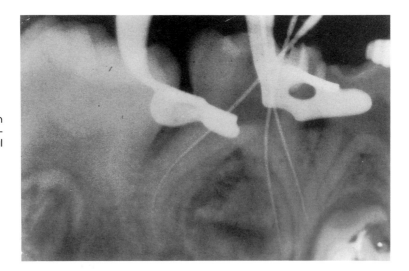

Figure 20–8 ■ Individual files in 3 canals of tooth T; the radiograph was taken at a mesial angle to separate each canal.

The canal should be periodically irrigated during filing in order to aid in debris removal. A sodium hypochlorite solution is used, since it helps dissolve organic material. However, because of concern about it being forced into the periapical tissues or through auxiliary canals into the furcation areas, the solution should be used very carefully and without excessive irrigation pressure. Sterile saline or local anesthesia may be used as an alternative solution.

Drying of the canal is accomplished with appropriately sized paper points. At this point, it must be decided whether the filling can be completed. If the tooth is abscessed or the canals are necrotic, the dentist may decide to complete the filling later and perform the pulpectomy as a two step procedure. A formocresol-impregnated pellet or paper points can be sealed in the tooth, although this is not uniformly practiced because of the controversy regarding formocresol. Many dentists feel that thorough removal of all the necrotic material and careful canal cleaning will best promote healing and allow for resolution of the infection.

Filling

A zinc oxide and eugenol mixture is used to fill primary root canals because of its ability to resorb (although this resorption occurs at a slightly slower rate than deciduous root resorption). Because zinc oxide and eugenol is a liquid and powder combination, the dentist has control over the physical quality of the mixture (i.e., its thickness), which provides an opportunity to use several different filling techniques. For the large canals in primary anteriors, a thin mixture of the zinc oxide and eugenol can be used to coat the walls of the canal. A paper point or the last file used can be coated with the thin mixture, carried to the canal, and rotated to cover the walls to the same apical level as the filing was done. A thick zinc oxide and eugenol mixture can then be made and manually condensed into the remainder of the lumen. An endodontic plugger or even a small amalgam condenser are useful to compact the paste physically to the level of the canal orifice (Fig. 20–9). Care should be taken not to overfill the canal.

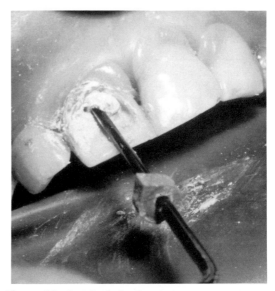

Figure 20–9 ■ Endodontic plugger being used to condense zinc oxide–eugenol into root canal of tooth E (note rubber stop).

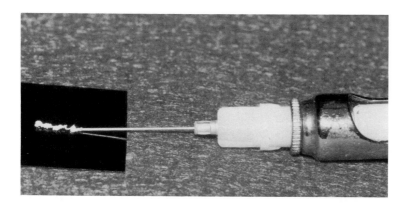

Figure 20–10 ■ Local anesthesia armamentarium, with zinc oxide–eugenol loaded into carpule and being extruded through 27 gauge needle.

In primary molars, some of the canals may be quite small even after filing. Because of the small size and difficult accessibility of these canals, an alternative delivery and filling technique is useful. This involves the use of a pressure system that carries a moderately thin zinc oxide and eugenol mixture to the correct apical level and, as it is withdrawn, fills the canal lumen. The P. C. A. Pressure Syringe* has been especially developed for this purpose, but several other filling techniques can be used in primary molars. Examples include a disposable tuberculin syringe or even a local anesthetic syringe. In the latter case, the anesthetic carpule is emptied, dried, filled with zinc oxide and eugenol, and replaced into the syringe, and the plunger is engaged to force the zinc oxide and eugenol mixture out the needle's lumen (Fig. 20–10). Each canal should be filled to the canal orifice. If it will fit, a very small endodontic plugger can be used to condense the coronal aspect of a canal. *Caution:* It is more dangerous to overfill than to underfill! A radiograph

* Pulpdent Corporation of America, Brookline, MA.

should be taken to assess the level and density of the final fill (Fig. 20–11).

Base

The pulp chamber and the access opening should be completely filled with a thick mixture of zinc oxide and eugenol or reinforced zinc oxide and eugenol. This may serve as an interim restoration if the final restoration is not completed at the same visit. However, if an anterior tooth is to be restored using a composite restoration, a zinc phosphate base should be used instead. This prevents direct contact of composite with zinc oxide and eugenol in the canal, which would cause yellowing of the restoration.

Final Restoration

A stainless steel crown is used as the final restoration for primary molars. Although it can be used also in the anteriors, esthetics is a greater concern. An open face stainless steel crown markedly improves the esthetics. A pedi-

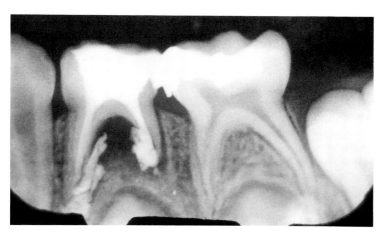

Figure 20–11 ■ Radiograph taken several days after pulpectomy fill, with the child complaining of pain, shows severe overfill of both roots.

atric strip crown former can be used to provide full composite coverage for primary incisors. If the primary incisor was intact and the facial approach was used, the large window can simply be restored, using a composite material.

REFERENCES

Berger JE: Pulp tissue reaction to formocresol and zinc-oxide–eugenol. J Dent Child 32:13–28, 1965.

Fuks AB, Michaeli Y, Sofer-Saks B, Shoshan S: Enriched collagen solution as a pulp dressing in pulpotomized teeth in monkeys. Pediatr Dent 6:243–247, 1984.

Goering AC, Camp JH: Root canal treatment in primary teeth: A review. Pediatr Dent 5:33–37, 1983.

Hibbard ED, Ireland RL: Morphology of the root canals of the primary molar teeth. J Dent Child 24:250–257, 1957.

Kennedy DB: Paediatric Operative Dentistry, 2nd ed. Chicago, Year Book Medical Publishers, 1979.

Kennedy DB, Kapala JT: The dental pulp: Biologic principles of protection and treatment. In Braham RL: Textbook of Pediatric Dentistry. Baltimore, Williams and Wilkins, 1985.

Kopel HM, Bernick S, Zachrisson E, De Romero SA: The effects of glutaraldehyde on primary pulp tissue following coronal amputation: In vivo histologic study. J Dent Child 47:425–430, 1980.

Mack RB, Halterman CW: Labial pulpectomy access followed by esthetic composite resin restoration for nonvital maxillary deciduous incisors. JADA 100:374–377, 1980.

Morawa AP, Straffon LH, Han SS, Corpron RE: Clinical evaluation of pulpotomies using dilute formocresol. J Dent Child 42:360–363, 1975.

Myers DR, Pashley DH, Whitford GM, McKinney RV: Tissue changes induced by the absorption of formocresol sites in dogs. Pediatr Dent 5:6–13, 1983.

Ranly DM: Formocresol toxicity. Current knowledge. Acta Odontol Pediatr 5:93–98, 1984.

Redig DF: A comparison and evaluation of two formocresol pulpotomy technics utilizing "Buckley's" formocresol. J Dent Child 35:22–30, 1968.

Ruempling DR, Morton TH, Anderson MW: Electrosurgical pulpotomy in primates—a comparison with formocresol pulpotomy. Pediatr Dent 5:14–18, 1983.

Starkey, PE: Treatment of pulpally involved primary molars. In Hurt WC: Current Therapy in Dentistry, Vol. 7. St. Louis, CV Mosby, 1980.

Via WF: Evaluation of deciduous molars treated by pulpotomy and calcium hydroxide. JADA 50:34–43, 1955.

chapter *21*

Patient management

J. R. Pinkham

As has been mentioned several times in this book so far, the usual and customary entrance age of children into a dentist's office has been sometime around the third birthday. The authors and editors believe that this is no longer a reasonable entry time. Strategies for effective prevention of dental disease simply must be implemented much, much earlier in life.

Before dentistry became prevention oriented, the entry at age 3 years made sense from a patient management standpoint. As reviewed in the first dynamics of change section (Section I, Chapter 11), it is not until around the third birthday that the majority of children have the communication skills and have been sufficiently socialized to be able to comply with the demands and rigors of a dental appointment.

Also, it is not until age 3 that most children have the language and communication skills to learn from the dentist those essential things about what he or she is doing that allow these youngsters to dismiss their fears about a new, unknown, and potentially threatening person and environment.

Obviously, some children as young as 2 years can go to their dentist and learn to be good patients. Conversely, some youngsters as old as 4 years will reliably have a difficult time because of their slow development. However, it is relatively safe to assert that the vast bulk of behavior management practiced, discussed in the literature, and taught in dental schools today is geared primarily toward the preschool child, ages 3–6 years. Most dentists agree that

269

the preschool child clearly requires the most energy and talent for effective management.

Putting the Challenge into Perspective

For years, this author has begun his lectures on patient management by asking the audience to consider the following challenge:

If I told you that there was a crocodile in your reception room, and that I would pay you one million dollars to fill one of its teeth (and you knew that I was telling you the truth), YOU WOULD FIND A WAY!

This challenge sets the tone for a very fundamental conclusion about dentistry for children —it is in any analysis, doable. Kids are little, and dentists are big. *Big* is superior to *little* any time there is a confrontation. Therefore, the dentist who is determined to get the dentistry done should, by his own ability, be able to develop a strategy to manage any child to the extent that he can perform dentistry for that child. However, improvising behavior management methods is not needed. There are a variety of already documented techniques that reliably help a dentist manage young children (Chambers, 1977).

The Importance of Conviction, Experience, and Good Intentions

Although dentistry for children is doable, not all dentists enjoy working with children. Any dentist who regularly sees preschool children experiences some crying, wiggling and kicking, tantrums, and a variety of other avoidance behaviors. Coping with these kinds of behaviors and devoting energy toward the interception of these behaviors exasperate some dentists. Other dentists feel guilty or anxious. Still others feel uncomfortable around the involved parents, and some may dread the next child scheduled on the appointment book.

The only reliable way to avoid inappropriate behaviors of children completely is profound pharmacologic management of their behavior. Such management, however, is beyond the educational objectives of this basic text. Drug management of children's behavior requires an extensive educational endeavor. It is important to understand that even when it is used by clinicians with special training, the pharmacologic management of children can be very risky. The utilization of drugs is discussed again later in this chapter.

One aspect of the dental treatment of children (barring burn-out) seems to be predictive of those who can manage children and those who cannot. That aspect is experience. Dental students and young practitioners may be very discouraged by the anxiety that they feel and the insecurity that they experience when certain children start to misbehave. However, with time and dedication to the techniques taught in dental school and outlined in this book, a practitioner's skills in child patient management become refined, and with this refinement comes self-confidence in this area of dentistry. Self-confidence of the dentist in his or her management skills is essential to successful interchanges with potentially unruly children.

An Embarrassment of Riches

In 1977, Dr. David Chambers, a psychologist with extensive interest in dentistry for children and considerable input into the literature on how dentists should manage children, labeled the available ways dentists can manage children as an "embarrassment of riches." Anyone knowledgeable about dentistry for children should concur with Dr. Chambers. There are so many ways of managing kids that have been described in journals and textbooks that few if any dentists can master them all.

There is, however, a basic inventory of skills that remain critical. Some of these management techniques are nice and polite, some have reasonable elegance in psychological terms, and some upon first inspection by a lay person (and perhaps by sophomore dental students, too) may appear very rigorous and authoritative.

Basics in Managing Children in the Dental Experience

PREAPPOINTMENT EXPERIENCE

The preappointment entails bringing the child to the dental office for a tour and orientation. The child is made aware of the fact before hand that *absolutely nothing* will be done that day. The child gets to meet the receptionist,

dental assistant(s), and dentist. If things go well, certain dental equipment can be shown and explained in "childese," such as Mr. Wind and Mr. Water for the triplex or Mr. Buzzer for the handpiece.

Comments

Preappointment experiences are not used much anymore because of time constraints of both the dentist and the parents. This technique is somewhat different than an observation appointment, in which a child watches his parent or brother or someone else get treated by the dentist. Observation appointments can be useful, but common sense also leads one to believe that they may backfire if the child sees something that frightens him.

Common sense also dictates that a young child's first appointment should be kept as pleasant and simple as possible. For most children 3 years old and older, an examination and prophylaxis and fluoride treatment can be made a pleasant, even enjoyable experience.

TELL, SHOW, DO

The tell, show, do method is the backbone of the educational phase of grooming an accepting, relaxed child dental patient. The technique is simple and usually works. The technique dictates that before anything is started (except the injection of local anesthetic and other procedures that defy explanation (e.g., pulp extirpation), the child be told what will be done and then shown by some sort of simulation what will happen before the procedure is started. For example,

Matt, I'm going to clean your teeth with this special dental toothbrush (prophy angle and rubber cup). You see this soft rubber cup? Well, when I step on this gas peddle this cup turns, and when it is full of toothpaste it really can make your teeth shine. Now, Matt, pinch the cup and you will see how soft it is. Now let me run it on your fingernail so you can feel how it works. Okay, Matt, please open your mouth for me. Thank you.

Comments

The choice of words is important in the tell, show, do technique. Proper accomplishment requires that the dentist has a substitute vocabulary for his or her tools and procedures that the child can understand.

At least four out of five children who are over 3 years old and have a normal social history and emotional status can be guided through a new technique successfully by the use of tell, show, do.

VOICE CONTROL

Voice control requires that the dentist interject into his or her communication with the child more authority. The tone of the voice is very important. It must have a "I'm in charge here" ring to it. The facial expression of the dentist must also mirror this attitude of confidence. In fact, a dentist can "voice control" with facial expression alone.

Comment

Voice control is a very essential technique for managing preschool children. It is extremely effective at intercepting inappropriate behaviors as they start to happen and is moderately successful once inappropriate behaviors are full-blown.

HAND-OVER-THE-MOUTH

The hand-over-the-mouth technique calls for the dentist to place his or her hand over the mouth of a hysterically crying child. It is used to intercept tantrums or other fits of rage. It has to be paired with voice control. This technique works reliably with a variety of child personality types (Levitas, 1974).

The technique is not intended to scare the child. It is intended to get the child's attention and to quiet him so that he can hear the dentist.

Comments

The hand-over-the-mouth technique has remained somewhat controversial, for obvious reasons. Critics have offered that it may be psychologically aggravating to the child. The technique remains in most dentists' repertoire of management techniques quite simply because it works. It works fast and therefore is very cost-effective. Patients who qualify for this technique usually would need management with medications, hospitalization, or significant further social and psychological maturation in order to be easily treated if the technique were not used.

PHYSICAL RESTRAINT

This literally means physically restraining inappropriate movements of the child during dental treatment. This can be done with hands, belts, tape, sheets, and some manufactured armamentaria (Fig. 21–1). Obviously, this technique, when used for the duration of an appointment, is reserved for basically unmanageable children. An alternative to physical restraint usually involves management by drugs or general anesthesia. These techniques can be expensive and sometimes dangerous.

One aspect of physical restaint is the management of jaws and keeping the child's mouth open. Figure 21–2 shows some equipment available for this job.

Comments

No matter what society's opinion becomes on physical restraint, it will survive as a technique. Leading candidates for physical restraint are the very young child (under 30 months) who needs emergency treatment of trauma and various types of disabled children, including the mentally retarded.

PRAISE AND COMMUNICATION

Praise and communication are self-explanatory. All people, including kids, react favorably to praise. Furthermore, effective dentistry for children means effective communication of the dentist to the child, and vice versa.

Comments

Praise and effective communication combined with tell, show, do is an unbeatable combination in managing children in the dental experience for the majority of children after age 3.

OTHER METHODS

There are other management techniques readily available to the dentist that are taught in at least some of the dental schools in North

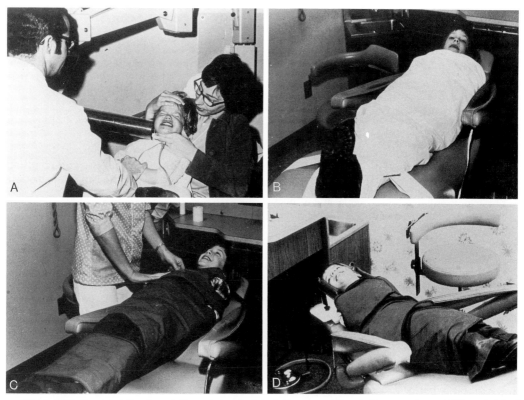

Figure 21–1 ■ Patient stabilization. *A*, Parental restraint. *B*, Sheet and ties. *C*, Papoose board (Olympic Medical Corporation, Seattle, WA). *D*, Papoose board with head stability attachment.

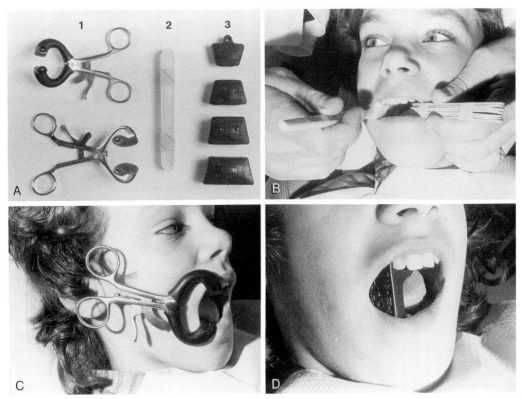

Figure 21-2 ■ Jaw stabilization devices. *A, 1,* Molt mouth gags; *2,* taped tongue blades (sizes can be varied according to size of patient); *3,* McKesson mouth props. *B, C,* and *D,* Clinical uses of devices.

America. Among these are maternal anxiety reduction techniques. (Paternal anxiety reduction has not been studied but probably would upon examination land similar conclusions.) It has been shown that as a mother's anxiety about her child's dental appointment lessens, so does her child's anxiety. Pairing a frightened child with a "brave" child in the clinic has had some success. Hypnosis and relaxation techniques have some devotees. Play therapy, listening to music or white sound, desensitization sessions, gift giving, and observation appointments have all been advocated to some degree at one time or another.

Children's behavior can also be managed with chemicals. Nitrous oxide with accompanying oxygen is very popular in parts of the United States for managing children's behavior in the dental office. This technique is very helpful for some children. It is not, however, the answer for every misbehaving child, and there are some children whom it seems to excite more

than it relaxes, albeit those are few and far between. If a dentist uses nitrous oxide and oxygen, he or she must develop ways of introducing children to the machinery, nosepiece, and feelings that they will experience.

A variety of drugs can be used to relax or sedate a child. These can be swallowed, injected intramuscularly or submucosally, given in a vein, or given rectally. There are published indications for these drugs. It is important to remember, however, that the stronger and therefore potentially more useful the drug is in dampening misbehavior, the greater the danger of drug-related side effects. Also, the younger and therefore smaller patient is at a greater risk of overdose than the older and larger one. The monitoring of the vital signs of sedated children is absolutely essential.

Lastly, there is general anesthesia. This works reliably but is expensive and time consuming. There is a slight morbidity risk with this technique also (see Chapter 22).

Profile of the Good Child Dental Patient

When new acquaintances find out that a dentist treats children, they often offer the conclusion that he or she must be a remarkably patient person. Actually, anything but that conclusion is necessarily true. The reason that these people make this false assumption stems in part from a misconception about what it takes to successfully treat a child dentally. These people probably perceive that the dentist must sit in his clinic, lovingly holding the hand of every child he treats and searching for words and phrases that will get the child to cooperate.

Such a perception is generally wrong. The fact remains that the great majority of children over 36–40 months of age are astonishingly well-behaved, complying dental patients when handled correctly. In fact, they may be the easiest of all patient types to treat. They don't demand exceptional patience from the dentist. They don't need it.

Performing dentistry for these kids is a very pleasant, rewarding professional experience. In many cases, the dentist will feel a personal attachment to the child ("He's mine"). It's fun to talk to these children, to ask them questions, to find out what they will wear at Halloween or get for Christmas, to know their favorite television show or food, or to find out how they feel about their new baby brother. Conversing with children is fun and should be overall a relaxing part of a general practitioner's day.

The good child dental patient reacts to "crisis moments" of the dental appointment appropriately. This means he reacts *as well as he can*. The most frequent "crises" in dentistry for children and how the good child dental patient manages them are as follows.

Crises in the Dental Appointment and the Good Child Dental Patient

SEPARATION FROM THE PARENT

Separation from the parent is not always done. Under 36–40 months of age, the child often behaves better if the parent accompanies him or her to the dental operatory. Often the parent of a child younger than age 3 has an opinion as to whether the youngster will be better or worse if he or she is present. Over this age, most children do not need their parents to accompany them, but the dentist may wish that the parents be present during the appointments. The dentist's preference should be known by the parent and child *at least* before the first treatment (fillings, extractions, etc.) appointment.

If the parent of a child older than 2 ½ – 3 years does accompany the child to the operatory, he or she should be prepared to leave if the youngster does not behave. This agreement between parent and dentist about leaving needs to be made before the child is seated in the dental chair. It is important that the child know about the agreement.

The good child dental patient separates from the parent easily. This is not to say that the separation is easy for the child emotionally, but it does mean that the child has the wherewithal to do it. At his best, the child looks eager to get started, shows no observable fear, and talks freely with the dental assistant who escorts him from the reception room.

GETTING INTO THE CHAIR

As simple as it sounds, some kids have difficulty in getting into the dental chair. This may stem from natural fears and the perceived vulnerability that goes along with getting off one's feet. Some kids need assistance and will have to be guided by the hand or even picked up and put into the chair.

However, the good child dental patient gets right into the chair. It is really nice when this happens, since it provides the first real opportunity to praise the child for his good behavior and ability to do things asked of him. ("Wow, John, look at you. I bet your daddy couldn't have gotten into this chair any faster.").

DENTIST SEATED AT CHAIR

The dentist coming to the chair represents to the child that treatment is imminent. The well-adjusted child can handle this. She will respond to her name (most dentists have learned the value of nicknames), answer questions, and accept and react to praise. ("What a pretty dress." "Thank you, Mommy got it for me.")

The dentist also represents the most authoritative figure in the dental office, and the good child patient realizes that his or her directives need to be followed. Directives such as "Hands

on your tummy and open wide-tall" are obeyed by the child and obeyed quickly.

THE INJECTION

Without question, the injection is the most universally feared procedure in dentistry for children and maybe dentistry in general. It is, however, not a major obstacle for most children. A large percentage of children will not react at all to the injection. The technique is now so painless that many little kids never know that they even got a "shot" when the dentist gave them "sleepy water." A good-tasting topical anesthetic is usually indicated. It is not indicated in the obviously agitated child who appears to be getting worse.

A percentage of young children know from siblings, parents, and peers that they will get an injection. Unfortunately, many youngsters have been given a very frightening description of the needle. They expect pain. Fortunately, many of these kids will still accept the procedure with only a few tears and with virtually no avoidance behaviors. These kids then learn that the "shot" isn't bad at all, and at later appointments the "pinch" is just that, a little pinching feeling in their mouth. The dentist must not lie about the needle. If asked if the injection will hurt, he or she should say, "You will feel a little pinch."

If the child starts avoidance behaviors, firm voice control needs to be established. Seldom will delaying the injection bring better behavior. Few dentists have found any utility in showing the syringe to the child who "wants to see what it looks like." Therefore, clinicians are encouraged not to be hesitant with this procedure. In fact, not using a topical anesthetic may, in certain situations, be wise because of the additional waiting time involved.

A child can cry during the injection and perhaps even need some momentary restraint of arms and body by a dental assistant and still qualify as a very good dental patient. The test is that the crying and squirming go away when the needle goes away.

Figure 21–3 shows a recommended method for the dental assistant to pass the needle from

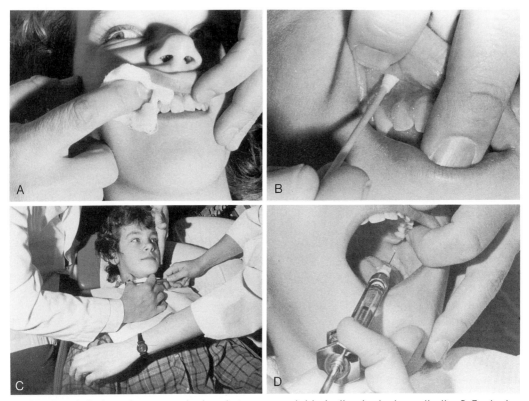

Figure 21–3 ■ *A,* Drying of mucosa prior to using an acceptable-tasting topical anesthetic. *B,* Topical anesthetic application. This step can be eliminated for very apprehensive children. *C,* Under the chin transfer of syringe. Note that the dental assistant is prepared to restrain the child's arms. *D,* Introduction of syringe to oral cavity. Note how the syringe is stabilized by a finger touching the patient's chin.

the tray to the dentist. Obviously, the use of needles around wiggling, thrashing children must be done very cautiously.

THE DENTAL PROCEDURE

Nine times out of ten, the dental procedure is restorative treatment if an injection for anesthesia has been given. Fortunately, dentists do not need to extract many teeth in children anymore. For the good child patient, the procedure itself (i.e., the drilling) is easy, compared with the injection. Many youngsters will fall asleep during the procedure. This may come as a surprise, but most children, even 3-year-olds, can tolerate a fairly long dental appointment without becoming restless. As said before, most kids are great dental patients.

There still is some need for extractions. Here again, most kids do well, but clinical experience still leads many dentists to believe that this can be a very scary procedure for little ones. Some investigators have assigned Freudian castration implications to this fear. The author believes that it is the force and torquing of the tooth that arouses anxiety. Luckily, most extractions in children are quick and simple.

END OF THE APPOINTMENT

It may seem silly to label the end of the appointment as a crisis, but sometimes people spend all their emotional reserves for the heat of battle and then afterwards become unglued. A good child dental patient ends his appointment on a high note. He is eager to leave yet is patient enough and human enough to stay around to be congratulated and praised for his behavior in the chair.

RETURN TO THE PARENT

The return of the child to the parent also may not seem like a crisis event. However, when one understands how some misbehaving child dental patients handle this aspect of their dental appointment, this time and its importance become more clear. Some children will want their parents to feel guilty about making them go to the dentist and will portray themselves as victims. This dramatization is often intercepted if the dentist or auxiliary is present.

Good child dental patients return to their parent beaming with pride. They know they have done well and that they have pleased their parents. They are pleased themselves. The dentist's compliments to their parent about them are returned by way of smiles and bright eyes. For the dentist, this is a really nice occasion.

In summary, somebody is doing something right with most children because most kids turn out to be good, accepting dental patients. However, there are exceptions, and these exceptions need to be understood.

Misbehaving Child Dental Patients

It is now appropriate to explore the types of children who reliably misbehave at the dental office. These are children who just can't cope or, importantly, just *won't* cope with the stimuli and behavioral demands of the dental experience.

The first group are special children who are emotionally compromised. This is not a large group of children, but they do exist. Dentistry as well as many other challenges of life are difficult for these children because of their psycho-emotional problems. It is important to realize that the problem may be undiagnosed.

The next largest group are the "shy birds." These are the introverted, poorly socialized children who are afraid of the social challenges associated with going to the dentist. The best management technique with these children is to break the barrier of shyness with friendship.

The third group are those children who have a hard time with dentistry because they are frightened. (Fear of dentistry is discussed later.) It is the author's opinion that fear of needles is 90% of the fear of dentistry.

Another group of misbehaving children are those who do not like authority. These children don't like dental appointments, and their dislike is based on an aversion to compliance to adult directives.

CATEGORY I: THE EMOTIONALLY COMPROMISED CHILD

A reliable finding with emotional illness is anxiety. When the anxiety of an emotional illness is compounded with the anxiety attendant to a dental appointment, a behavioral explosion often occurs. Emotionally compromised children are generally very bad dental patients. At best, they are no fun. It is as if there is no child left in a child's body.

The problem with these patients is that often there is no confirmed diagnosis. Parents, even very intelligent, well-informed ones, have no idea that anything is wrong. Having grown accustomed to the behaviors of their child, they often overlook the abnormalities of their child's behavior or they have rationalized an explanation for why their child behaves in certain ways. This should be regarded as extremely unfortunate, since most emotional diseases are diagnosable and treatable and as is so often the case, the earlier the upset is addressed, the faster and more effective is the therapy.

Emotional illness can also be a problem for children from broken homes and other less than desirable parenting circumstances. The children of poverty probably suffer from more emotional compromises than do children from more privileged classes. As a group, abused and neglected children (see Introduction, Chapter 1) certainly have a high percentage who are emotionally aggravated.

The author has had very little success in convincing parents that their child's misbehavior during a dental appointment might be due to an unknown emotional problem. However, it is professional to share any convictions a dentist has that are for the child's best welfare. Of course, if abuse and neglect are suspected, the dentist is legally obligated to report the children to the appropriate authorities.

CATEGORY II: THE SHY, INTROVERTED CHILD

Introversion or shyness is a problem for many people, including children, especially very young children. Because the dental experience for children is a fairly intense human encounter that demands rapport and communication between the adult dentist and the child patient, it is obvious that a very shy child will be stressed by the experience. This stress can lead the child to an avoidance behavior, such as crying. Usually, the crying takes on the form of compensatory whimpering. Rarely does the introverted child display aggressive avoidance behavior, such as a tantrum. These children can be likened to puppies in some respects. When threatened, they go limp and tremble.

The dental profession has long recognized that shy children will have a hard time adjusting to the expectations of a dental appointment. As with all children, the dentist's first objective is to establish rapport, trust, and communication. With shy children, this requires patience

because they are unskilled at "feeling people out" and they are categorically mesmerized by the challenge of communicating.

Yet, as formidable as the challenge may seem, the techniques of talking to these children on their level; praise; and tell, show, do reliably penetrate the oyster shell that these youngsters have secreted around their personality and in time, sometimes startlingly fast, they open up. When they open up, they usually become fantastic patients because the dental appointment means for them socially that somebody knows their name, is interested in them, and is willing and ready to talk to them. This opening up does not always happen, but it often does occur.

CATEGORY III: THE FRIGHTENED CHILD

A child who is frightened represents a formidable challenge to the dentist as well as to teachers, physicians, parents, and everyone else who encounters him. In treating such a child, the dentist has a particular problem in that even though the dental encounter is not very long, it is intense and requires, ideally, enormous cooperation by the child. The dentist also contends with the problem of fear to probably a greater degree than do most other adults who react with the child. These fears range from fear of needles to fear of bodily harm to general fears of the unknown. If someone really wanted to make a complete and specific list of all the possible sights, sounds, smells, and expectations that are reasonably unique to the dental experience, it could probably fill up a legal pad. The hand-held instruments alone would be an extensive list of possibilities.

The answer to the question of whether a child can misbehave in dentistry because of fear is definitely in the affirmative. The answer as to how one knows whether a misbehaving child's behavior is fear-motivated misbehavior or otherwise is, as one would expect, a more challenging proposition. Yet, information paired with experience and common sense reliably allows the dentist to determine what is motivating the child.

Some of the established reasons that a parent and clinician can use to help identify a child who is very fearful of dentistry are the following:

● The child is unable to arrest intellectually, even when educated by parent or dentist, his fears about the dental appointment either

because of his chronological age (roughly, for normal children, 36–40 months is when most children are intellectually able to arrest their fears when given information about what will happen) or because of slow development (perhaps mental retardation).

● The child is overreacting to fears because of other emotional upsets in his life. This category includes children who are coming from homes that are in acute chaos because of impending divorce or separation, children who are abused, and children grieving because of the loss of a grandparent or friend. Children who have been coping with other health problems are included in this category. These circumstances often yield self-limiting emotional disturbances. The problems resolve themselves in time, but when present they make dentistry, particularly some of the more rigorous appointments such as tooth extraction, very difficult for these children to endure.

● The child has been "sold" a set of fears by peers, siblings, or parents. Such fears have been called *acquired fears*.

● The child has had a previous bad and painful experience at a physician's or dentist's office or at a hospital. These are *learned* fears.

● The child is emotionally ill.

All the above children, with perhaps the exception of the emotionally ill, are easy to define and identify. Emotional illness, as has been discussed, is something parents often do not address at home, and the real clues that some kids are not well emotionally do not often emerge until these youngsters are enrolled in a formal educational process and are observed by a teacher(s) daily.

One major point is in order here. If the misbehavior is because of an intense dread or fear of dentistry, it is important that the parent and the dentist establish this fact in no uncertain terms. If a child is so frightened that good behavior is impossible, it is the obligation of both of these adults to make sure that everything is done not to further the child's anxieties attendant to dentistry. This may mean postponing dentistry, it may mean the utilization of drugs, and it may even mean performing the dentistry under general anesthesia. Whatever it requires, it is important that the most appropriate measures be taken regardless of cost, convenience, and efficiency. That is the only humane course to take.

As said before, dreadfully fearful children usually can be screened and identified before

dentistry begins. The only gray zone is the child who would seem to have an emotional illness. In cases of a high suspicion of emotional illness (no one has an explanation as to why the youngster would be *so* frightened), it remains the most professional and humane recommendation that the dentist refer the child for examination to a psychiatrist, psychologist, or other counselor. The parent should accept this referral in the spirit in which it is given, that is, the best thing at this time that can be done for this child is to establish whether in fact he or she is emotionally healthy enough to go through a dental appointment without maladaptive behavior and sequelae.

CATEGORY IV: THE CHILD ADVERSE TO AUTHORITY

The Duke of Windsor, during one of his visits to the United States, noted tongue-in-cheek that one of the things that he liked about America was how well American parents minded their children. Much has been written in the dental literature over the years about children who are difficult because they cannot follow adult directives well (Pinkham, 1983). Some labels for these youngsters have been spoiled children, incorrigible and overindulged children, and defiant children.

Certainly, even the most casual observer can verify that there are a variety of misbehaviors of children. One trip to a grocery store, a fast food restaurant, or even a public swimming pool where parents and children congregate will reliably show misbehaving children. If children will misbehave in a shopping mall, in the automobiles of their parents, and even in their own homes, why should they not misbehave at the dentist's office? Well, obviously they do.

What is the nature of this misbehavior? Why does it happen? There is a child for whom emotional illness, introversion, or fear simply is not the reason for his or her inappropriate behavior at the dental office. The reason is instead that the child has an aversion to authority. Upon analysis, it is easy to see that a dentist is a very strong authoritative figure in his own office and therefore is a prime candidate to stimulate this kind of child's worst behavior.

Where did the aversion to authority come from? The thoughts and literature of Dr. Alfred Adler, who was a contemporary of Freud and Jung, and Dr. Rudolph Dreikurs, a student and devotee of Adler, point out that there are four potential misdirected goals in the life of a child

(Adler, 1958; Dreikurs, 1964). These goals seep into the personality repertoire of a child, where they satisfy subtly the strong human craving of a quest for superiority, which Adler felt was the main force that drives all human behavior. Noting that one potential way of feeling superiority comes about by the manipulation of people, both authors project a warning to parents that their child may adopt a style of behavior with them that will carry over to other authority figures that the child encounters in life, such as the dentist. These misdirected goals and what they mean to the involved children are as follows:

1. *Undue attention*: "In order to satisfy my intense appetite for feeling superior, I will through manipulative behavior make sure that my parents pay attention to me any time that I want them to. Since this paying attention to me quickly relieves my insecurities about my being superior, I am likely to want much more attention than is reasonable."
Behavioral characteristics: Annoying, irritating, teasing, disruptive.

2. *Struggle for power*: "In order to satisfy my intense appetite for feeling superior, I am prepared to have a power struggle with my parents about getting attention. This is a challenge and I do intend to win. They will pay attention to me or else."
Behavioral characteristics: Argues and contradicts, does the opposite of instruction, causes people anger, throws temper tantrums.

3. *Retaliation and revenge*: "In order to satisfy my intense appetite for feeling superior, if I do not get what I want, which in a nutshell is attention, I will get even with my parents and I will punish them. I will not let them do this to me without hurting them back."
Behavioral characteristics: Has violent temper, says things that hurt people, seeks revenge, gets even.

4. *Inadequacy*: "In order to satisfy my intense appetite for feeling superior, I have convinced myself that I am special in the worst sort of way. I am totally unable to grow up, unable to achieve, and in fact I plan to do nothing at all for either myself, my parents or anyone else on the face of this earth."
Behavioral characteristics: Gives up easily, rarely participates, acts as if he is incapable, displays inadequacy.

Space does not permit a detailed discussion of misdirected children. It seems obvious to conclude that each of the four misdirected goals gets more serious from one level to the next. The child who simply wants some attention may very likely find dentistry a nice experience in that it is such a personal one on one occasion. The child who engages in power struggling has a bully's attitude and may not have any compulsions at all about arguing with a dentist or challenging a dentist's authority. The retaliation and revenge child can quite frankly be dangerous. This is the type of child who may bite. This child is not warm and fun and probably will not respond to praise. The child who thinks about himself in a defeated, inadequate way is very likely to show a variety of misbehaviors if the dentist asks him to cooperate. Overcoming the challenges of the dental appointment is beyond the grasp of this child. When challenges arise, this child tells himself that he is inferior and can't possibly measure up.

It should also be noted that severely misdirected children present problems in a variety of social circumstances and certainly have troubles in school. Fortunately, most of these children will in time outgrow their misdirection. One will find only behavioral remnants or subtleties of their misdirections in adolescence and young adulthood.

SUMMARY: MISBEHAVING CHILDREN

The discussion of the four categories of misbehaving children are outlined in what is believed to be the relative incidence in which a practitioner in dentistry will encounter them. In other words, there are fewer emotionally disturbed children than there are introverted children, fewer introverted children than frightened children, and fewer frightened children than children who just do not like to comply with authoritative adults. Blends of the four problem groups are obvious. In fact, a blend is probably the norm.

It is the author's feeling that dental students and clinicians with very little experience in dentistry for children and certainly the parents of misbehaving children often assign the majority of the reason for why children misbehave in the dental office to their fear of dentistry. Conversely, older and more experienced clinicians do not endorse the fear theory as much but instead assert that the inappropriate behavior really does not have very much to do with the dental appointment. They note that these children do not cope well with any sort of stress and that they really often simply do not like to work

with any adults who make demands on them. Authority, not dentistry, is what these children dread.

The child who has a genuine dreadful fear of dentistry has to be handled very specially, and the handling of this child has got to be, whenever possible, a cooperative effort of the dentist and the parents. Mild to modest fear of dentistry, particularly to the needle, is normal. Importantly for normal children over 3 years of age who have a competent dentist and one who will take the time to educate them with tell, show, and do as the primary technique, these fears can be arrested or put into a manageable status.

REFERENCES

Adler A: What Life Should Mean to You. New York, Capricorn Books, 1958.

Chambers DW: Behavior management techniques for pediatric dentists: An embarrassment of riches. 44(1):30–34, 1977.

Dreikurs R, Soltz RN: Children, The Challenge. New York, Hawthorn Books, 1964.

Levitas TC: HOME—Hand over mouth exercise. J Dent Child 41(3):23–25, 1974.

Pinkham JR: Classifying and managing child dental patients' misbehaviors: A three-step adlerian approach. J Dent Child 5(4):437–441, 1983.

chapter 22

Hospital dentistry

Stephen Wilson

This chapter on hospital dentistry and general anesthesia is designed to convey a basic understanding of dentistry in the hospital. The hospital can be a valuable asset for the dentist in the treatment of individuals regardless of their age, provided that there is a sound and reasonable basis for its use.

The dentist has a continuum of management techniques that may be used to intercept maladaptive behaviors of child dental patients (see Chapter 21). At one end of this continuum are the sound psychological principles of behavior management associated with "tell, show, do," and on the other end is general anesthesia in the hospital. In between these two extremes are other sophisticated and skillful management techniques, such as desensitization, flooding (voice control or hand-over-the-mouth), "time out," hypnosis, or psychopharmacology.

General anesthesia should be considered a last resort in this continuum of managing patients. Moreover, the basis for its use should be dependent not only on the patient's behavior but also on the patient's overall needs. For instance, the hemophiliac has special medical needs that will usually require more elaborate care and treatment, which is found in the hospital setting. Because of the special needs of these kinds of patients, other medical personnel (physicians, laboratory technicians, and nurses) will need to be involved in the appropriate management of the patient. A list of indications for the use of general anesthesia may include the following:

1. A patient with a significant medical diagnosis or problem. This may include blood dyscrasias, congenital heart disease, a known allergy to local anesthesia, severe kidney and liver dysfunction, and some seizure disorders.

2. A patient with a severe sensory, physical, or mental dysfunction or condition that prevents routine dental treatment in the office.

3. A patient who despite all other management techniques remains recalcitrant, uncooperative, or extremely fearful and who is in need of extensive dental care. This may include the very young child with rampant nursing bottle caries.

4. A patient with a significant craniofacial anomaly (e.g., cleft palate) with extensive dental needs.

5. A patient with extensive dental needs and who lives in a remote area where dental care is unavailable or where transportation is compromised.

6. A patient who has suffered significant orofacial or dental trauma.

General anesthesia in the hospital has certain risks and potential side effects. These include but are not limited to sore throat or croup from intubation, avulsion of teeth with the laryngoscope, psychological trauma from patient mismanagement, emphysema, brain death, malignant hyperthermia, and death. The patient benefit-risk ratio must be maximized through careful patient selection, appropriate medical consultations, patient history and physical examination, psychological preparation of the patient, and a competent anesthesiology staff.

Another point of practicality that the dentist must consider is the cost of general anesthesia and hospitalization. The cost can be substantial and, in many cases, prohibitive for the patient or the family. The dentist who uses hospital facilities should be aware of the hospital and anesthesia fees and any financial management programs that may be available to the parents. The parents or patient must be informed of these costs during the treatment planning session. Although many insurance companies will not cover dental treatment under general anesthesia, it is wise to contact the patient's insurance company prior to treatment under general anesthesia in a hospital.

Hospital Staff Privileges

For hospital privileges to be obtained, most hospitals in the United States require that the dentist have the following minimal background: (1) be a graduate of an accredited American or Canadian dental school, and (2) have a dental license in the same state as the hospital. Many hospitals also require some advanced training in which hospital experience was included.

Dentists obtain hospital staff privileges through the same process as physicians. Application is made through the medical staff office. The completed application and the credentials of the applicant are thoroughly reviewed by a member of the medical staff or by the credentials committee of the hospital. Recommendations for staff privileges and appointment are made and then acted upon by the medical staff of the hospital. Final approval is made by the board of directors of the hospital.

Various categories of staff membership with associated privileges are available. In general, they are reflective of the member's degree of

activity in the hospital and of his or her responsibility to participate in medical staff governance. For example, the active staff category is usually for those individuals who utilize a hospital on a daily or regular routine basis, whereas the courtesy staff category refers to those individuals who employ the services of a hospital on a less frequent basis. It is the duty and responsibility of each member of the hospital staff, including the dentist, to become routinely familiar with and abide by specific policies and governing bylaws of the hospital.

The dentist should carefully select a hospital to which he or she wishes to become a member. Considerations in selecting a hospital should include the following:

1. Strong medical support and consultation for dentistry
2. Convenience to the dentist's office
3. Other dental members and specialists on the hospital staff
4. Administrative attitude toward dentistry
5. The experience of the anesthesiology staff
6. Availability of dental equipment
7. Positive support of hospital policies for patient orientation to the hospital environment
8. Support staff trained for managing disabled patients
9. Availability of outpatient surgery that is particularly useful to dental admission

Inpatient vs. Outpatient Care

Patients may be admitted to a hospital and spend a minimum of one night (inpatients) or they may be admitted and discharged on the same day (outpatients), depending on their specific needs, requirements, or complications associated with surgery. Obviously, patients who have a medically compromising or traumatized condition that will require special medical management are candidates for inpatient status when elective dental procedures are to be considered.

With the increasing cost of inpatient hospital care and the recognition of new anesthetic and surgical management of patients in recent years, third party carriers are attempting to minimize health care costs by encouraging outpatient surgery. However, it is worth reiterating that consultation with the patient's physician or other medical specialists is absolutely essential for appropriate management of the patient

under general anesthesia, regardless of inpatient or outpatient status, expense, or insurance coverage.

Preoperative Preparation and Informed Consent

The parents and patient must be adequately informed of the treatment that is to be rendered in the hospital. This includes psychological preparation of the parents and patient for the hospital experience. Many hospitals will provide hospital orientation sessions, which familiarize the patient and family with the environment, procedures, and services of the hospital. These sessions are very important, as it has been shown that mismanagement and insufficient psychological preparation can be detrimental to the continual well-being of the patient. If the patient is to be admitted to the hospital overnight, a parent should be encouraged to spend the night with the child (Table 22–1).

In addition to orally describing to the parents why the child should be treated under general anesthesia and all the steps involved in the hospital experience, a preoperative letter should be sent to them a minimum of 2 weeks prior to admission. In the letter, detailed steps, including times, dates, documentation, places, and the possibility of postponement if either the patient's health changes or instructions were not followed, should be enumerated. The dentist should never assume that the parents understand all details. It is wise to contact the parents and patient and satisfactorily determine that they understand all their responsibilities. Finally, it is absolutely essential that the dentist obtain informed consent for treatment of the patient under general anesthesia from the parent or legal guardian prior to admission.

Physical Examination

The patient's physician or a physician on the active medical staff should be contacted and arrangements made for a history and physical examination within 72 hours prior to general anesthesia. The physician should clear the patient for general anesthesia, based upon his or her findings, and document the clearance for general anesthesia in the patient's hospital chart or in a letter that is incorporated in the chart at the time of admission. Normally, only

Table 22–1 ■ Key steps for dental care in the hospital

Step	Explanation
1. Patient and parent evaluation	Physical, emotional, dental findings; reliability of parents
2. Preoperative letter	To confirm time and date of operating room case, parent's responsibilities
3. Arrangements/appointments	Patient history and physical, hospital orientation, treatment planning, financial considerations, reservations (operating room and ward), medical consultations, laboratory requirements, informed consent
4. History and physical examination	Past and present medical history reviewed, social and family history, review of systems and oral findings
5. Laboratory tests	Blood, electrolyte, urinary, radiographic, and others as needed
6. Admission	Inpatient or outpatient status
7. Orders	Preoperative orders
8. Operating room	Anesthesia, patient preparation, dental procedures
9. Recovery room	Postoperative orders
10. Family visitation	Convey patient's status and summary of procedures accomplished
11. Operative note	Formal narrative of operating room procedures
12. Discharge summary	Narrative of patient's stay in the hospital
13. Postoperative instructions	Given to parents/guardian; special instructions
14. Follow-up appointment	Set time and date of follow-up evaluation

Table 22–2 ■ Guidelines for general evaluation and classification of patient status according to the American Society of Anesthesiologists (ASA)

I. No organic, physiologic, biochemical, or psychiatric disorders; healthy patient

II. Mild to moderate systemic disturbances without significant physical limitations

III. Severe systemic disturbances and physical limitations

IV. Life-threatening systemic disorder

V. Moribund patient and emergency situations

Class I or II: Usually reserved for elective dentistry only.
Class III or IV: Routine elective dentistry is not performed on patients in these categories.

individuals who are ASA (American Society of Anesthesiologists) Class I or II (Table 22–2) are considered for elective dental treatment under general anesthesia.

The patient should have a work-up that is as careful and complete as possible prior to admission. The preoperative work-up will aid in the decision to admit the patient in an inpatient or outpatient status. This work-up should include (1) dental records as complete as possible; (2) obtaining a history and physical examination from a physician, with clearance of the patient for general anesthesia; (3) requesting consultations with other specialists as indicated; (4) ensuring that special needs of the patient are or will be met in a timely manner (psychological preparation, antibiotic prophylaxis, factor replacement in hemophiliacs, etc.); and (5) scheduling the procedure with the operating room coordinator and reserving an overnight room when necessary.

Hospital Documentation and Procedures

Complete, legible, and accurate record-keeping is imperative. All entries in a hospital chart should include the date, time, and signature of the person making the entry. The dentist who is a staff member of a hospital should become familiar with the divisions of a hospital chart (Fig. 22–1). Hospitals routinely audit records for thoroughness and can suspend or withdraw privileges of staff members whose records are incomplete. When the patient is admitted, the dentist should write an admittance note. This note will give a brief medical history of the patient and a preoperative diagnosis, with emphasis on oral findings. It also describes the procedure to be accomplished during the admission.

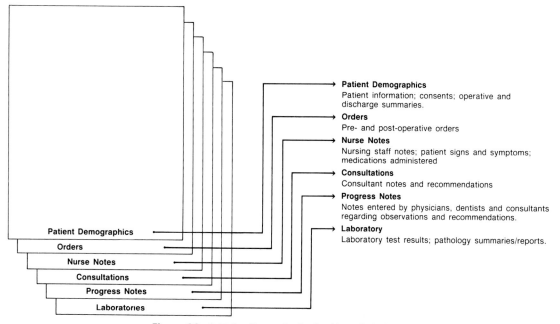

Figure 22–1 ■ Sections of a typical hospital chart.

Patient Demographics
Patient information; consents; operative and discharge summaries.

Orders
Pre- and post-operative orders

Nurse Notes
Nursing staff notes; patient signs and symptoms; medications administered

Consultations
Consultant notes and recommendations

Progress Notes
Notes entered by physicians, dentists and consultants regarding observations and recommendations.

Laboratory
Laboratory test results; pathology summaries/reports.

Laboratory and diagnostic tests can be ordered either immediately prior to or during the admission process. The specific requirements for general anesthesia in the hospital or by the anesthesiology staff often dictate which tests should be ordered by the dentist, but these may include a complete blood count with differential (white blood cell discrimination), prothrombin time (PT), partial thromboplastin time (PTT), platelet count, electrolyte screening (Sequential Multiple Analyzer 6/60 or 12/60), posteroanterior (PA) and lateral chest radiographs, and a routine urinalysis (UA). These tests will provide valuable information on oxygen transport capacity, infectious processes, coagulation adequacy, kidney and liver function, and airway and lung adequacy. If the patient is to be treated as an outpatient, these tests can be performed 24 hours prior to admission. If the patient has an unusual medical problem, specialized tests may be ordered. Consultation with the dentist's medical colleagues is a must to make this determination. The results of all of these diagnostic tests will be entered in the laboratory section of the hospital chart.

The attending dentist should visit the patient at the hospital on the eve of the scheduled surgery (inpatient) and/or early in the morning to review laboratory results, answer any questions of the parents or patient, attempt to allay any anxiety that may arise in the patient or family, and, if necessary, write any last preoperative orders. Also, the dentist should evaluate the physical status of the patient and review the patient's systems. Any changes in the physical status of the patient should be brought to the attention of the anesthesiology staff members, who may alter or postpone the administration of general anesthesia. These findings are entered in the progress notes. Immediately following the surgery, the dentist should write postoperative orders for the proper management of the patient in his or her recovery from general anesthesia.

Routinely, these orders include (1) monitoring of the vital signs every 15 minutes until they are stable and then every half hour, (2) monitoring potential hemorrhage sites and providing for hemostasis, (3) maintaining fluid and electrolyte balance through intravenous replacement, (4) providing moist air at bedside, (5) ordering medications (analgesics, antibiotics, vitamins, etc.), (6) managing minor tissue trauma from the surgery (ice packs), and (7) prescribing an appropriate diet. It is also wise to include a telephone or beeper number for the nursing personnel to contact the dentist, if necessary.

An operative report is dictated immediately after visiting with the family. This report is highly standardized, and an example of its summarized contents can be seen in Table 22–3.

If the patient is staying in the hospital overnight, the dentist should visit the patient later in the day and note his or her progress. The patient's postoperative status will determine when he or she can be released from the hospital. It is also important to consider and determine the parent's ability to manage the patient at home properly. The parents should be told when to return to the dental office for a follow-up evaluation (usually in 1 week).

Finally, a discharge summary report should be dictated. This report includes the patient's name, admission and discharge dates, history of present illness, physical findings, hospital course and laboratory analysis, operation performed, postoperative diagnosis, condition of

Table 22–3 ■ Items that should be included in a typical operative report

1. Dentist's name
2. Other surgeons, assistants
3. Date
4. Patient's name and hospital number
5. Preoperative diagnosis with oral findings
6. Postoperative diagnosis
7. Time patient transported to operating room
8. Time of induction
9. Induction agents and methods
10. Anesthetic maintenance agents
11. Intubation technique
12. Throat pack placement
13. Patient preparation and draping
14. Complete and detailed description of operation
15. Time of completion of case
16. Condition of and time patient taken to recovery area
17. Extubation time and place
18. Postoperative condition
19. Estimation of blood loss
20. Fluid replacement

patient at discharge, and follow-up instructions, which are also conveyed to the parents.

Operating Room Protocol

Many hospitals have nursing personnel who will provide instruction in proper scrubbing, gowning techniques, and operating room protocol. Dentistry in the operating room is considered a clean, but not sterile, technique because of the inability to sterilize the operating field (viz., the mouth). Despite the objections of many dentists that sterile gloves interfere with tactile sensitivity and therefore may not be utilized, it is strongly recommended that sterile gloves be worn. Adaptability to the supposedly decreased tactile sensitivity occurs rapidly, and the reduction in the possibility of cross-contamination is minimized. Masks and protective eye apparel are also highly recommended.

Besides the anesthesiologist, a circulating and/or scrub nurse is usually present in the operating room (Fig. 22 – 2). He or she has multiple duties, including the setup of the operating room, retrieval of requested instruments and supplies, gowning and gloving of the surgeons, and assisting in the patient preparation prior to and following the surgery. Many hospitals will permit the dentist to bring a dental assistant to assist in the procedure. The assistant should be minimally aware of proper operating room protocol. It should be emphasized that assistants must either carry malpractice insurance or be covered through the dentist's umbrella policy; otherwise, most hospitals forbid their presence. The dentist should also understand that he or she is the individual who is primarily legally responsible for the patient and for the activities that occur in the operating room.

A patient under general anesthesia typically has the following systems monitored: the heart's electrical activity by electrocardiogram (ECG), blood pressure, heart rate, respiratory rate and sounds (via a precordial stethoscopic bell), and body temperature. An intravenous line (IV) is started in a hand, forearm, or leg vein to maintain proper fluid and electrolyte balance and to administer drugs prior to, during, and following the dental procedures. The IV line may have been started prior to the patient being transported to the operating room.

Once the patient has been connected to appropriate monitors, the anesthesiologist will begin the process of inducing anesthesia. The anesthesiologist usually starts this process with the administration of oxygen and nitrous oxide via a mask. Other drugs or inhalation agents are introduced either through the IV line (e.g., barbiturates, atropine, curare, and/or succinylcholine) or by the mask (e.g., halothane or fluorane), and the patient rapidly progresses to a surgical plane of anesthesia. Next, endotracheal intubation via the nasal orifices (this should be

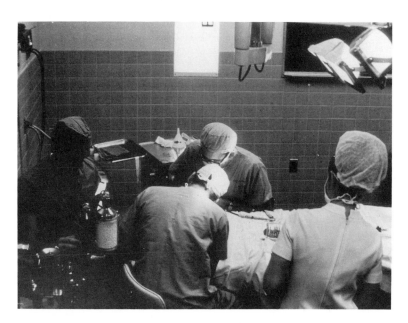

Figure **22 – 2** ■ Photograph showing typical operating room and personnel.

requested by the dentist for maximal freedom in the oral operating field) is accomplished by the anesthesiologist. The anesthesiologist maintains the patient at the proper level of anesthesia by regulating the concentration and combination of the inhalation gases with possible drug supplementation through the IV line.

The patient's eyes should be lubricated and taped shut or protected by goggles. The patient's body should be draped. At this time, any radiographs that are clinically indicated may be obtained. The radiology department usually will assist by developing the films, but previous arrangements and notification of the department should be made. The patient and anesthesiologist must be protected by lead aprons. A pharyngeal throat pack (usually a vaginal pack, which must be moistened with sterile saline to protect the mucosal lining) is placed. The pack is gently but firmly placed from side to side to occlude the posterior pharyngeal area. This keeps the throat free of debris. The end of the pack should extend out of the corner of the mouth as a reminder to remove it following the operation. Care and caution must be taken not to dislodge the endotracheal tube.

A thorough dental prophylaxis is now performed, and re-evaluation of the dental lesions is indicated to confirm or alter the previously established treatment plan. A rubber dam should be applied and the teeth restored. Topical fluoride should be applied before the rubber dam is removed. Exodontia and soft tissue surgery should be performed last, as it is very important to maintain a clear field during restorative procedures and to obtain hemorrhage control prior to awakening the patient. The anesthesiologist should be notified approximately 5–10 minutes prior to the completion of all procedures so that he or she may be prepared to reverse anesthesia and awaken the patient. The throat pack should be removed slowly and the throat and mouth carefully examined and thoroughly suctioned. The patient may be extubated either in the operating room or in the recovery room, depending on the discretion of the anesthesiologist.

The dentist should accompany the patient to the recovery room, write postoperative orders, and inform the recovery room personnel of any special instructions. It is especially important for the recovery room personnel to monitor oral hemorrhage and be instructed to apply a 4 × 4 inch gauze compress in the event of hemorrhage. The personnel members in the recovery room are most adept at managing the patient and his or her needs.

Logistical Problems

The dentist must be aware that treating a patient in the hospital requires him or her to be out of the office for a variable period of time. Problems to consider are: (1) time to and from the hospital, (2) visiting with the patient and family, (3) waiting in line for operating room access, (4) turn-around time associated with the preparation of the operating room from one surgical procedure to the next, and (5) ensuring that all paperwork and dictations are completed. Consequently, hospital cases may significantly impact on the economics of a routine dental practice. Nonetheless, hospital dentistry can be very self-satisfying and certainly provides a conducive atmosphere for establishing and maintaining strong ties with other medical professionals. These colleagues can be sources both for referrals and for consultation. This type of interaction can only benefit dental patients as well as dentists themselves.

BIBLIOGRAPHY

Davis MJ, Bierenbaum HJ: Hospital care in pedodontics: A survey of current practices. Pediatr Dent 4:245, 1982.

Enger DJ, Mourino AP: A survey of 200 pediatric dental general anesthesia cases. J Dent Child 52:36, 1985.

Ferretti GA: Guidelines for outpatient general anesthesia to provide comprehensive dental treatment. Dental Clin North Am 28:107, 1984.

Gonty AA, Racey GL: Nasal endotracheal intubation for outpatient anesthesia. J Oral Surg 38:191, 1980.

Hooley JR, Daun LG (eds): Hospital Dental Practice. St. Louis, CV Mosby Co, 1980.

chapter *23*

Periodontal considerations

Paul Casamassimo

The periodontium of the preschooler traditionally has been characterized as generally healthy, with disease confined mainly to marginal gingivitis. A very few children develop systemic illness involving bone loss and premature exfoliation of primary teeth. A practitioner can count on seeing only a handful of these children in a practice lifetime. The generalizations that children neither have gingivitis of any consequence nor accumulate calculus are inaccurate, since many children do.

What *does* appear to be a truism is that the role of gingivitis in progressing to periodontitis is altered in children. Gingivitis in children, especially preschoolers, does not lead to any appreciable or irreversible tissue damage. The goal of good periodontal health in the preschooler is not to prevent tissue destruction, but rather to maintain healthy oral supporting tissues, establish a low plaque environment with normal microflora, and give the child a pleasant appearance and good personal hygiene.

Epidemiology of Periodontal Disease in Preschoolers

Numerous studies have addressed the periodontal status of preschoolers, with differing results. One study of 3-year-olds found gingivitis in virtually all of the children examined (Poulsen and Møller, 1972), while another noted it in about half of those in that age group (Kruger, 1955). The extent or seriousness of gingivitis in relation to plaque formation was studied by Cox and colleagues in 1974, who found children to have more plaque than adults but less inflammation proportionately than adults in relation to the amount of plaque. In 1973, Mackler and Crawford had similar results with preschoolers suffering from minimal gingivitis despite not having brushed for several weeks. Knowledge about gingivitis in preschoolers can be summarized as follows:

1. Children do experience gingivitis in varying amounts.

2. Gingivitis, though common, does not appear to have irreversible effects on the primary periodontium.

3. Gingivitis in children is largely reversible.

4. Gingivitis does not seem to occur with the same severity as it does in the adult in response to similar levels of plaque.

Histologic evidence supports a difference between childhood and adult gingivitis. Several researchers have noted a lymphocytic infiltrate in gingivitis in children as compared with the plasma cell–dominated infiltrate seen in gingivitis in adults (Ranney et al, 1981).

The clinical significance of the epidemiologic data is that the majority of periodontal problems in children are reversible, with little or no tissue damage. Children appear to have some resistance factor, probably immune, that prevents progression of the gingival lesion to periodontitis.

Normal Periodontium in the Primary Dentition

The periodontium of the primary dentition differs from that of the adult in several ways. The gingivae are more red, flabbier, and lack the stippling of adult gingivae. The tissue is less fibrous and is more vascular. The periodontal membrane is wider, with less density of fibers. Alveolar bone is also different, with fewer trabeculae, larger marrow spaces, and less calcification. The blood supply and lymphatic drainage is also more extensive in bone (Ruben, 1979). Figure 23–1 depicts the periodontium of a healthy primary dentition.

The size, shape, and spacing of primary teeth also may contribute to the periodontal health of children. The interdental papillae are flatter and, with spacing, more accessible to cleaning. The underlying bone is flatter at the alveolar crest. The short crowns of anterior teeth may minimize occlusal forces on the alveolus. The widely spaced flat roots of the posterior teeth may help distribute forces and account for the lack of occlusal trauma seen in the primary dentition.

Periodontal Conditions in the Three- to Six-Year-Old

GINGIVITIS

Gingivitis appears first as an inflammation of the gingival margin that progresses to include the free gingivae and occasionally the attached gingivae. In many cases, the inflammation will confine itself to the free gingivae, despite large accumulations of plaque. The gingival tissue becomes reddened and swollen and will bleed upon probing or brushing as the condition worsens. The individual response to plaque as an etiologic agent is variable, with some children showing a minimum of response to local factors.

Gingivitis can also be associated with gross caries and poor quality restorations. Traumatic injuries and pulpal conditions can also involve gingival inflammation (Figure 23–2). Removal of the offending agent or appropriate therapy will correct the problem, and tissues should re-

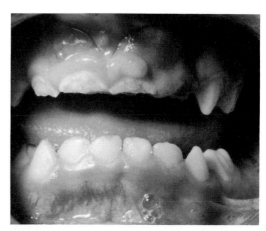

Figure 23–2 ■ Gingival inflammation secondary to a large accumulation of plaque, dental caries, and pulpal pathosis in an incomplete primary dentition.

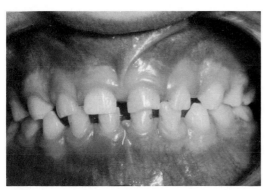

Figure 23–1 ■ A healthy primary dentition with well-formed and disease-free gingivae.

turn to health. It is noteworthy that the long-term consequence of such local inflammation is not clear. Because with the turnover of dentitions the gingival tissues change dramatically, it is unlikely that inflammatory injury is of any future consequence.

OTHER GINGIVAL CONDITIONS

Children in this age group are subject to a variety of gingival problems related to systemic illness, its treatment, or infections by organisms such as the herpes simplex virus. These are discussed elsewhere in the text in greater detail.

BONE LOSS CONDITIONS IN THE THREE- TO SIX-YEAR-OLD

Because gingivitis rarely progresses to periodontitis in the preschooler, bone loss is extremely rare. Loss of attachment with breakdown of alveolar bone, exposure of root surfaces, tooth mobility, and tooth loss are seldom seen except in cases of systemic disease or its treatment. Table 23–1 lists those conditions known to result in bone loss in the primary

Table 23–1 ■ Conditions associated with bone loss in the primary dentition

Dental Abnormalities
Dentin dysplasia
Juvenile periodontitis
Papillon-Lèfevre syndrome
Malignancies
Histiocytosis X conditions
Leukemia
Hematologic/Immune Disorders
Neutrophil function disorders
Neutropenia
Metabolic Disorders
Scurvy
Hypophosphatasia
Diabetes
Gaucher's disease
Toxicities
Mercury
Radiation

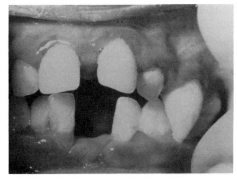

Figure 23–3 ■ Bone loss associated with hypophosphatasia in a 3-year-old. Note exposed roots and malposition secondary to loss of bone support.

dentition. In most cases, damage is irreversible and results in the loss of teeth prematurely. Treatment in these cases is usually palliative unless the systemic problem can be solved. Even when general health is stabilized, some teeth may be lost early. Figures 23–3 and 23–4 depict examples of bone loss conditions in the preschooler.

PERIODONTAL THERAPY

The nature of periodontal disease in this age group has shaped the procedures commonly utilized to treat conditions. By far, simply cleaning and polishing is the most common procedure performed. Gingivectomy may be used for treatment of phenytoin-induced gingival overgrowth.

The frequency or need for semi-annual prophylaxis has been a topic of recent controversy.

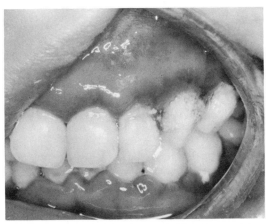

Figure 23–4 ■ Severe periodontal involvement in a child with chronic neutropenia. Note severe inflammation and root exposure on anterior teeth.

Evidence suggests that frequent prophylaxis is beneficial to tissues, but for reasons suggested throughout this chapter, the cost-benefit ratio does not justify the service for many children. Stain and calculus removal and removal of plaque prior to a thorough examination are some justifications for a pediatric prophylaxis. Preparation of teeth for a fluoride treatment is not, since evidence now suggests that fluoride uptake is not altered by overlying plaque (Tinanoff et al, 1974).

Occlusal Wear and Temporomandibular Joint Disorders

The preschooler is relatively free of both occlusal traumatism and temporomandibular joint (TMJ) disorders. Many clinicians have noted the extreme yet asymptomatic attrition of the primary dentition in the late preschool years as well as the preschooler's ability to tolerate large occlusal interferences in restorations. Parents commonly ask what to do about bruxism in the young child. One study of 5- to 6-year-olds found 15% of children to be reported to brux by parents, while another 15% demonstrated wear facets suggestive of bruxism yet were unknown to grind their teeth (Kuch et al, 1979).

Although some children may experience real TMJ pain, it is rare and most commonly the result of trauma. The following can be said to be true about TMJ disorders and bruxing in children:

1. Bruxism is common in children.
2. Primary teeth can show significant wear without symptoms of oral or extraoral pain.
3. Objective signs of TMJ malfunction such as clicking or deviation upon opening may be present without any symptomatic pain.
4. Actual TMJ pain is rare in children.

REFERENCES

Cox MO, et al: Oral leukocytes and gingivitis in the primary dentition. J Periodontol Res 9:23, 1974.

Kruger BJ: Incidence of gingivitis among samples of Brisbane school and preschool children. Aust J Dent 59:237, 1955.

Kuch EV, et al: Bruxing and non-bruxing children: A comparison of their personality traits. Pediatric Dent 1:182, 1979.

Mackler SB, Crawford JC: Plaque development and gingivitis in the primary dentition. J Periodontol 44:18, 1973.

Poulsen S, Møller IJ: The prevalence of dental caries, plaque, and gingivitis in 3-year-old Danish children. Scand J Dent Res 80:94, 1972.

Ranney R, et al: Pathogenesis of gingivitis and periodontal disease in children and young adults. Pediatric Dent 3 (Special Issue):89, 1981.

Ruben MP: Nature of periodontal disease in children and adolescents. In Richardson ER (ed): Periodontal Diseases in Children and Adolescents: State of the Art. Proceedings of a Symposium, May 21–23, 1978, Meharry Medical College, Nashville, Tennessee, 1979, p 7.

Tinanoff N, et al: Effect of a pumice prophylaxis on fluoride uptake in tooth enamel. JADA 88:384, 1974.

Space maintenance in the primary dentition

John Christensen □ Henry Fields

General Considerations

Management of premature tooth loss in the primary dentition requires careful thought by the clinician, because the consequences of proper or improper space management may influence dental development well into adolescence. Early loss of primary teeth may compromise the eruption of succedaneous teeth if there is a reduction of space in the arch length. On the other hand, timely intervention may save space for the eruption of the permanent dentition. The key to space maintenance in the primary dentition is to know which problems to treat.

Premature tooth loss in this age group is best thought of in terms of anterior (incisors and canines) and posterior (molars) teeth. The causes for and treatment of missing teeth differ in these two regions. Anterior tooth loss is due primarily to trauma and secondarily to tooth decay. Injuries to the primary incisors are common, because a child of this age is learning to crawl, walk, and run. Although the prevalence of dental decay appears to be declining, a small number of children still suffer from nursing bottle and rampant decay. These decay patterns result in tooth loss in both the anterior and posterior regions. The majority of posterior tooth loss is due to dental caries; rarely are primary molars lost to trauma. If no space loss has occurred following tooth loss, space maintenance is appropriate. If space loss has occurred, a comprehensive evaluation is required to determine whether space maintenance, space regaining, or no treatment is indicated. This type of evaluation and decision-making is described in the mixed dentition section, Chapters 29 and 34, because most space regaining is attempted at that time.

Missing primary incisors are usually replaced for four reasons: space maintenance, function, speech, and esthetics. Some dentists feel that early removal of a primary incisor will result in space loss as adjacent teeth drift into the space formerly occupied by the lost incisor. However, this does not seem to be true in most clinical situations. There may be some rearrangement of space between the remaining incisors, but there is not a net loss of space. Intuitively, this makes sense because there is no apparent movement or drifting of teeth when developmental spacing is present in the primary dentition.

Poor masticatory function has also been proposed as a reason for replacing missing primary incisors. Concerns have been expressed about a child's ability to eat after four maxillary incisors have been removed as a result of nursing bottle decay. Feeding is not a problem, and when given a proper diet, the child will continue to grow normally.

Slowed or altered speech development has been cited by some investigators as a justification to replace missing maxillary incisors. This may be valid if the child has lost a number of teeth very early and is just beginning to develop speech. Many sounds are made with the tongue touching the lingual side of the maxillary incisors, and inappropriate speech compensations may develop if these teeth are missing. However, if the child has already acquired speech skills, the loss of an incisor is not particularly important (Rieckman and ElBadrawy, 1985).

Probably the most valid reason for replacing missing incisors is esthetics. Esthetic concerns are voiced by some parents and not by others. If parents do not indicate a desire to replace missing teeth, certainly no treatment is appropriate. If the parents do wish to replace the missing teeth, either a fixed lingual arch or a removable partial denture with attached primary teeth can serve as a prosthetic replacement (Fig. 24–1). The dentist should present both alternatives and let the parents make an educated decision.

Loss of a primary canine as a result of either trauma or decay is rare. Because it is so rare, there is some debate whether space loss will occur if the tooth is not replaced. From a conservative point of view, a band and loop space maintainer (see later discussion) or a removable partial denture may be placed if the patient is very cooperative. Either of these appliances will need to be remade when the permanent lateral incisor erupts because it will require more space than the primary lateral incisor and will interfere with the space maintenance. If a space maintainer is not placed in the maxilla, a midline shift to the affected side should be anticipated when the permanent incisors erupt. In the mandible, lingual movement of the incisors and movement of the midline to the affected side will occur. A lingual arch may be appropriate after the permanent incisors erupt to prevent the midline shift.

Therefore, space maintenance is mostly concerned with the replacement of primary molars. Loss of interproximal contact as a result of decay, extraction, or ankylosis of an adjacent tooth will result in space loss owing to mesial and occlusal drift of the tooth distal to the newly created space. There is also evidence that the tooth mesial to the affected molar will drift distally into the space (Owen, 1971). Therefore, loss of space or arch length can occur from both directions (Fig. 24–2).

Space maintenance begins with good restorative dentistry. The dentist should strive for ideal restoration of all interproximal contours. Early restoration of interproximal caries will ensure that no space loss occurs. In some instances, however, large carious lesions may make ideal restoration of the tooth impossible and space loss inevitable. Even if the pulpal tissues have

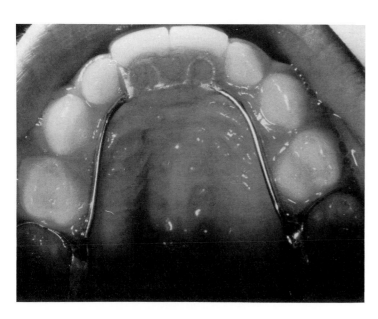

Figure 24–1 ■ A fixed (as shown here) or removable partial denture can be used to replace missing anterior teeth in the primary dentition. In most cases, the partial denture is placed for esthetic reasons and not to prevent space loss in the anterior dental arch.

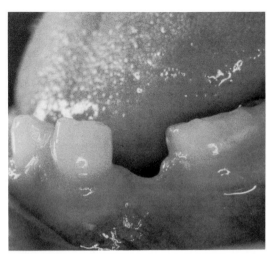

Figure 24–2 ■ Premature loss of the primary first molar results in loss of space from both directions. The primary second molar drifts mesially, while the primary canine drifts distally.

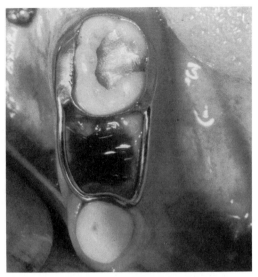

Figure 24–3 ■ The band and loop appliance is used to maintain the space after the premature loss of a single tooth. The band and loop is indicated when there is unilateral loss of a primary first molar before or after the eruption of the permanent first molar. The loop is constructed of .036 inch round wire and is soldered to the band.

been compromised, pulp therapy should be initiated and the tooth maintained, if at all possible, because the natural tooth is still superior to the best space maintainer available. In cases of ankylosis, the tooth should be maintained until space loss is imminent, then extracted and the space maintained. Ankylosed teeth usually show limited vertical change in the primary dentition years.

Appliance Therapy

BAND AND LOOP

Four appliances are used to maintain space in the primary dentition. The first appliance, the band and loop, is used to maintain the space of a single tooth. This appliance is inexpensive and is easy to fabricate. However, it requires continuous supervision and care and does not restore the occlusal function of the missing tooth. The majority of space maintenance cases in the primary and mixed dentitions will use the band and loop appliance. The appliance is indicated in the following situations:

1. Unilateral loss of the primary first molar before or after eruption of the permanent first molar (Fig. 24–3)
2. Bilateral loss of a primary molar before the eruption of the permanent incisors (Fig. 24–4)

The initial step in constructing a band and loop appliance is to select and fit a band on the abutment tooth. Band selection is a trial-and-error affair, and bands are fit until one can be nearly seated on the tooth with finger pressure (Fig. 24–5A). A band pusher and band biter are used to achieve the final occluso-gingival position (Fig. 24–5 B and C). A properly placed band will be seated approximately 1 mm below the mesial and distal marginal ridges (Fig. 24–5D). If a band cannot be easily fitted, orthodontic separators should be placed to create space for the band material (Fig. 24–5E). This same technique is used to place orthodontic bands on posterior teeth when fixed orthodontic therapy is indicated. The next step is to make a quarter arch impression of the band and edentulous area with either compound or alginate impression material. If alginate impression material is used, the tray should be perforated so that the material can flow through the perforations and prevent the impression from distorting when it is removed. Following the impression, the band is gently removed with a band remover and is placed in the correct position and orientation in the impression.

The impression is poured in stone with the band in place. The cast is separated, and an .036 inch wire is formed into a loop and contoured to fit the band and alveolar ridge. The loop should parallel the edentulous ridge 1 mm off the gingival tissue and should rest against the adjacent

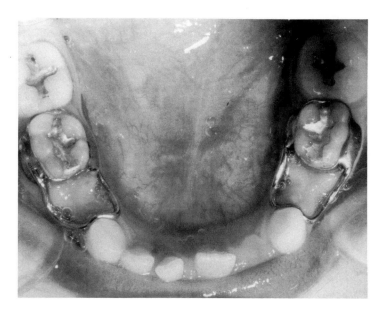

Figure 24–4 ■ If both primary first molars are lost prematurely in the mandibular arch and the permanent incisors have not erupted, bilateral band and loop appliances are used to maintain space. A lingual arch is not indicated in this situation because it may interfere with the subsequent eruption of the permanent mandibular incisors.

tooth at the contact point. The facio-lingual dimension of the loop should be approximately 8 mm. This dimension should allow the permanent tooth to erupt freely yet not impinge on the buccal mucosa or tongue. The loop should not restrict any physiologic tooth movement, such as the increase in intercanine width that occurs during eruption of the permanent lateral incisors.

When the band and loop appliance returns from the laboratory, it should be tried in and adjusted if necessary. Following the try-in, the band should be cemented on a clean, dry abutment tooth with zinc phosphate cement. The patient is then recalled every 3–4 months to check that the appliance still fits properly and that the cement has not washed out. The eruption of the permanent tooth is an easily recognized indication for removal.

Two modifications of the band and loop appliance are not recommended for use in space maintenance therapy. The bonded band and loop is a contoured wire similar to the loop portion of the band and loop that is bonded to the abutment tooth with composite resin. There are two reasons that the bonded band and loop is not recommended. First, it is difficult to keep the wire bonded to the tooth because of the shearing force of occlusion. If the bond breaks, there is a potential for space loss and the added danger of aspiration of the wire. Second, the bonded band and loop is nearly impossible to adjust. The other band and loop variation not recommended is the crown and loop appliance. The crown and loop technique advocates pre-

paring the abutment tooth for a stainless steel crown and then soldering a space-maintaining wire directly to the crown. If the solder joint fails and the wire breaks loose, there is no way to repair the appliance intraorally. The crown must be cut off, a new crown fit, and the wire resoldered. It is much easier to restore the abutment tooth with a stainless steel crown and then make a band and loop that fits the crown. Care and maintenance of the band and loop appliance is also easier than the crown and loop if the appliance is damaged or needs to be modified.

LINGUAL ARCH

The second appliance used to maintain posterior space in the primary dentition is the lingual arch. The lingual arch is often suggested in cases in which teeth are lost in both quadrants of the same arch. Bands are fit on the posterior abutment teeth, and an impression of the arch is made. In the primary dentition, the primary second molars are banded, whereas the permanent first molars are usually banded in the mixed and permanent dentitions. An .036 inch wire is soldered to the molar bands, although the arch can be made removable by welding attachments to the band if the arch needs to be removed periodically for adjustments or for other reasons. The lingual arch should have an ideal anterior arch form that is positioned to rest on the cingula of the incisors 1–1.5 mm above the soft tissue. The arch should be stepped to the lingual in the canine region to avoid im-

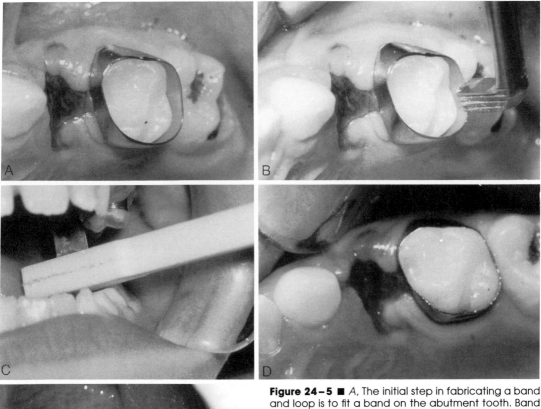

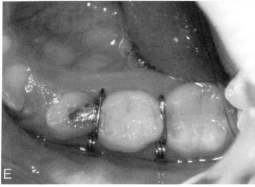

Figure 24–5 ■ *A*, The initial step in fabricating a band and loop is to fit a band on the abutment tooth. Band selection is a trial-and-error procedure and continues until a band is nearly seated on the tooth with finger pressure. *B*, A band pusher is used to seat the band to near ideal position. The dentist should maintain a good finger rest because soft and hard tissue injury can occur if the pusher slips without proper support. *C*, Final occlusogingival position is achieved with a band biter. In the maxillary arch, the band biter should be placed on the distolingual portion of the band for final positioning. In the mandibular arch, the band biter should be placed on the distofacial portion of the band. *D*, A properly fitted band is seated approximately 1 mm below the mesial and distal marginal ridges. *E*, If a tight interproximal contact prevents the band from seating properly, orthodontic separators are placed to create space for the band material. The separators are removed within 7–10 days, and the band is fitted.

pinging on the primary molars and the unerupted premolars. Small adjustment loops mesial to the abutment teeth are incorporated into this keyhole configuration so that the appliance can be either modified to fit properly or activated to move teeth.

Because the permanent incisor tooth buds develop and erupt somewhat lingual to their primary precursors, a mandibular lingual arch is not recommended in the primary dentition because the wire resting adjacent to the primary incisors may interfere with the eruption of the permanent dentition. Instead, bilateral band

and loop appliances are recommended in this situation. The maxillary lingual arch is feasible because it can be constructed to rest away from the incisors. Two types of lingual arch designs are used to maintain maxillary space, the Nance and transpalatal arches. These appliances use a large wire to connect banded teeth on both sides of the arch that are distal to the extraction site. The difference between the two appliances amounts to where the wire is placed in the palate. The Nance arch incorporates an acrylic button that rests directly on the palatal rugae (Fig. 24–6). The transpalatal arch (TPA) is

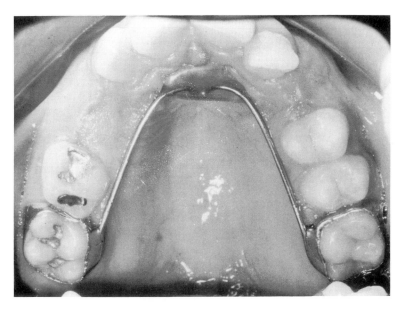

Figure 24-6 ■ The Nance arch is a fixed lingual arch appliance used to maintain space in the maxilla when there has been bilateral loss of teeth. An acrylic button rests directly on the palatal rugae and prevents the abutment teeth from drifting mesially. This button is attached to the .036 inch palatal arch wire that is soldered to the bands. Food and debris may lodge under the button, creating a hygiene problem if the appliance is not thoroughly cleaned.

made up of a wire that traverses directly across the palate without touching it (Fig. 24–7). Although the TPA is a cleaner appliance and is easier to construct, many clinicians feel that it allows the teeth to move and tip mesially, resulting in space loss.

DISTAL SHOE

The distal shoe appliance is used to maintain the space of a primary second molar that has been lost before the eruption of the permanent first molar (Fig. 24–8). An unerupted perma-

nent first molar will drift mesially within the alveolar bone if the primary second molar is lost prematurely. The result of the mesial drift will be loss of arch length and the possible impaction of the second premolar. The appliance is constructed very much like the band and loop. The primary first molar is banded and the loop extended to the former distal contact of the primary second molar. A piece of stainless steel is soldered to the distal end of the loop and is placed into the extraction site. The stainless steel extension acts as a guide plane for the permanent first molar to erupt into proper position and should be positioned 1 mm below the me-

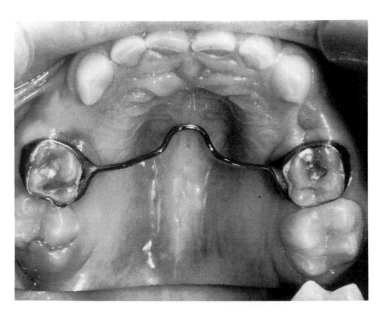

Figure 24-7 ■ The transpalatal arch (TPA) is another fixed lingual arch appliance used to maintain space following bilateral loss of maxillary teeth. The TPA is more hygienic than the Nance appliance because it only consists of the .036 inch palatal wire, but it allows the abutment teeth to tip mesially in some cases, resulting in space loss.

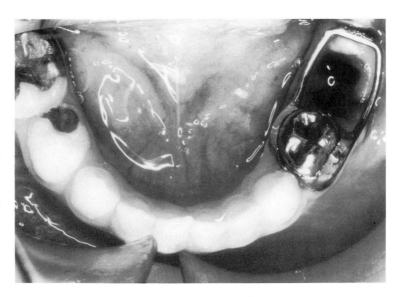

Figure 24–8 ■ The distal shoe appliance is used to maintain the space of a primary second molar that has been lost prematurely before the eruption of the permanent first molar. A stainless steel extension is soldered to the distal end of the band and .036 inch loop; this extension is positioned 1 mm below the mesial marginal ridge of the unerupted permanent first molar. The extension serves to guide the eruption of the permanent first molar.

sial marginal ridge of the unerupted molar in the alveolar bone. After the permanent molar has erupted, the extension can be cut off or a new band and loop appliance can be constructed. To ensure that the stainless steel extension is in proper position and in close proximity to the permanent first molar, a periapical radiograph is taken before the appliance is cemented (Fig. 24–9).

There are many problems associated with the distal shoe appliance. Because of its cantilever design, the appliance can only replace a single tooth and is somewhat fragile. No occlusal function is restored owing to this lack of

strength. In addition, histologic examination shows that complete epithelialization does not occur after placement of the appliance (Mayhew et al, 1984). Because the epithelium is not intact, the distal shoe appliance is contraindicated in medically compromised patients and in patients who require subacute bacterial endocarditis (SBE) coverage.

REMOVABLE APPLIANCE

A final type of appliance used to maintain space in the primary dentition is the removable

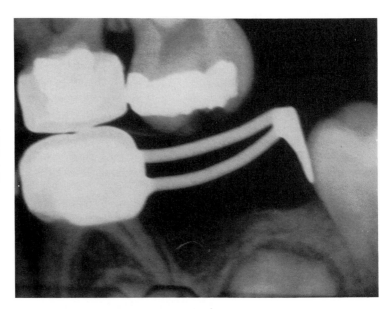

Figure 24–9 ■ A periapical radiograph is taken prior to cementing the distal shoe appliance to ensure that it is properly positioned in relation to the unerupted permanent first molar.

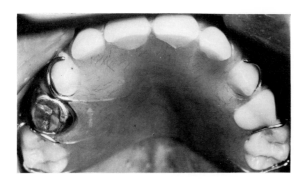

appliance (Fig. 24–10). The appliance is typically used in situations in which more than one tooth has been lost in a quadrant. The removable appliance is often the only alternative because there are no suitable abutment teeth and because the cantilever design of the distal shoe or the band and loop is too weak to withstand occlusal forces over a two-tooth span. Not only can the partial denture replace more than one tooth, it can also replace occlusal function.

Two real drawbacks of the appliance are retention and compliance. Retention is a problem because primary canines do not have large undercuts for clasp engagement. If tooth loss is unilateral, retention problems can be overcome by placing sturdy retention clasps on the opposite side of the arch. However, if loss of teeth is bilateral, retention problems are almost inevitable. Compliance is a problem closely related to retention. Three- to six-year-old children will not tolerate an ill-fitting appliance and will not use it. In fact, some children will not tolerate a retentive appliance. The dentist is then resigned to waiting until permanent teeth (molars) erupt so that they can be used as abutments for lingual arch appliances. Partial dentures need clasp adjustment and acrylic modification occasionally to maintain good retention and allow eruption of the permanent teeth.

Summary

Space maintenance in the primary dentition should be thought of in terms of anterior and posterior space loss. Space maintenance is not required for missing primary incisors. Primary incisors should only be replaced if there are esthetic concerns. Posterior space maintenance is a necessity in this age group and should be undertaken in cases in which primary molars are lost prematurely and the space is adequate. The band and loop appliance is used most often; other appliances can be used as different situations dictate. Judicious space maintenance is very beneficial to the child patient and may prevent future alignment and crowding problems.

REFERENCES

Mayhew MJ, Dilley GJ, Dilley DCH, Jacoway J, Johnson PT: Tissue response to appliances in monkeys. Pediatr Dent 6: 148–152, 1984.

Owen DG: The incidence and nature of space closure following the premature extraction of deciduous teeth: A literature survey. Am J Orthod 59:37–48, 1971.

Rieckman GA, ElBadrawy HE: Effect of premature loss of primary maxillary incisors on speech. Pediatr Dent 7:119–122, 1985.

chapter 25

Oral habits

John Christensen □ Henry Fields

The presence of an oral habit in the 3- to 6-year-old child is an important finding in the clinical examination. An oral habit is no longer considered to be normal for children near the end of this age group. If the habit has resulted in movement of the primary incisors, some form of intervention is indicated prior to the eruption of the permanent incisors. If no dental changes have occurred, no treatment can be advocated based on dental health, but some patients and parents may want to seek treatment based on the fact that digit or pacifier habits become less socially acceptable as the child becomes older. Efforts to discourage the habit may involve as little as a conversation between dentist and child or involve more complex appliance therapy. The most important thing to remember about any intervention is that the child must want to discontinue the habit for treatment to be successful.

Thumb and Finger Habits

Thumb and finger habits make up the majority of oral habits. Dentists are often questioned about the kinds of problems these habits may cause. The types of dentitional changes that a digit habit may cause vary, depending on the intensity, duration, and frequency of the habit. Intensity is the amount of force that is applied to the teeth during sucking. Duration is defined as the amount of time spent sucking a digit. Frequency is the number of times the habit is practiced throughout the day. Duration plays the most critical role in tooth movement caused by a digit habit. Clinical and experimental evidence suggest that 4–6 hours of force per day are necessary to cause tooth movement. Therefore, a child who sucks intermittently with high intensity may not produce much tooth movement at all, whereas a child who sucks continuously (for greater than 6 hours) can cause a significant dental change. The classic symptoms of an active habit are reported to be the following:

1. Anterior open bite
2. Facial movement of the upper incisors and lingual movement of the lower incisors
3. Maxillary constriction

Anterior open bite, the lack of vertical overlap of the upper and lower incisors when the teeth are in occlusion, develops because the digit rests directly on the incisors (Fig. 25–1). This creates a slightly increased vertical opening. The digit impedes eruption of the anterior teeth, while the posterior teeth are free to erupt.

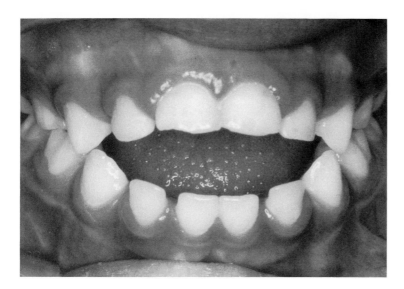

Figure 25–1 ■ This patient exhibits an anterior open bite that is a direct result of an active thumb habit. An open bite results when the thumb impedes the eruption of the anteror teeth, moves them facially, and allows the posterior teeth to erupt passively. Actual intrusion of the anterior teeth is possible but unlikely.

Passive eruption of the molars will result in an anterior open bite. Anterior open bite may also be caused by intrusion of incisors. However, inhibition of eruption is easier to accomplish than true intrusion.

Facio-lingual movement of the incisors depends on how the thumb or finger is placed in the mouth. Usually, the thumb is placed so that it exerts pressure on the lingual surface of the maxillary incisors and on the labial surface of the mandibular incisors (Fig. 25–2). A child who actively sucks can create enough force to tip the upper incisors facially and the lower incisors lingually. The result is an increased overjet.

Maxillary arch constriction is due to the change in equilibrium balance between the oral musculature and the tongue. When the thumb is placed in the mouth, the tongue is forced down and away from the palate. The obicularis oris and buccinator muscles continue to exert a force on the buccal surfaces of the maxillary dentition, especially when these muscles are contracted during sucking. Because the tongue no longer exerts a counterbalancing force from the lingual, the posterior maxillary arch collapses into crossbite.

Timing of treatment is critical in this age group. The child should be given an opportunity to stop the habit spontaneously before eruption of the permanent teeth. Hence, treatment is usually undertaken between ages 4 and 6 years. Three different approaches to treatment have been advocated, depending on the willingness of the child to stop the habit. The first approach, reminder therapy, is appropriate for those who desire to stop the habit but need some help to stop completely. An adhesive bandage taped to the offending finger can serve as a constant reminder not to place the finger in the mouth. The bandage remains in place until the habit is extinguished. Unpleasant stimuli, such as an ill-tasting solution painted onto the finger, also remind the child to refrain from sucking. This type of therapy is perceived as punishment, however, and may not be as effective as a neutral reminder.

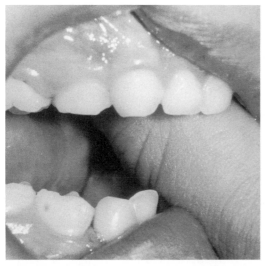

Figure 25–2 ■ With most thumb habits, the thumb exerts pressure on the lingual surface of the maxillary incisors and on the facial surface of the mandibular incisors. This causes the maxillary incisors to tip facially and the mandibular incisors to tip lingually, resulting in increased overjet.

A second means of influencing oral habits is through a reward system. A contract is drawn between the child and parent or between the child and dentist. The contract simply states that the child will discontinue the habit for a specified period of time and in return receive a reward if the requirements of the contract are met. The reward does not need to be extravagant but should be special enough to motivate the child. The more involvement the child can take in the project, the more likely the project will succeed. This may include placing stick-on stars on a homemade calendar when the child has successfully avoided the habit for an entire day. At the end of the time period, the reward is presented with verbal praise for meeting the conditions of the contract (Fig. 25–3).

If the habit continues to persist following reminder and reward therapy and the child truly wants to eliminate the habit, appliance therapy is necessary. This type of treatment involves placing an appliance in the mouth that will physically discourage the habit by making it difficult to suck a thumb or finger. The dentist should explain to the patient and parent that the appliance is not a punishment but rather a permanent reminder not to place the finger in the mouth. The two appliances used most often to discourage the sucking habit are the quad helix and the palatal crib. The quad helix is a fixed appliance used to expand a constricted maxillary arch (Fig. 25–4). The helices of the appliance serve to remind the child not to place the finger in the mouth. The quad helix is a versatile appliance because it can correct a posterior crossbite and discourage a finger habit at the same time.

The palatal crib is designed to interrupt a digit habit by interfering with finger placement and sucking satisfaction. The palatal crib is generally used in cases in which no posterior crossbite exists. However, it may also be used as a retainer following maxillary expansion with a quad helix. Bands are fitted on the permanent first molars or primary second molars. A heavy lingual arch wire (.038 inch) is bent to fit passively in the palate and is soldered to the molar bands. Additional wire is soldered onto this base wire to form a crib or mechanical obstruction for the digit. It is advised that a lower cast be made at the same time so that the appliance can be constructed so as not to interfere with normal occlusion (Fig. 25–5). The parent and child should be informed that certain side effects temporarily appear after the palatal crib is cemented. Eating, speaking, and sleeping patterns may be altered during the first few days following appliance delivery. These difficulties usually subside within 3 days to 2 weeks (Haryett et al, 1970). The major problem with the palatal crib and, to a lesser degree, the quad helix is oral hygiene. The appliance traps food and is difficult to clean thoroughly. Halitosis and tissue inflammation can result.

Habit discouragement appliances should be left in the mouth for 6 months. The palatal crib stops the child from sucking immediately but requires another 6 months of wear to extinguish

Figure 25–3 ■ A personalized calendar can be used to motivate a child to stop a sucking habit. Stick-on stars are applied to the calendar on days the child has successfully avoided the habit. At the end of the month or the specified period of time, a reward and verbal praise can be provided for discontinuing the habit.

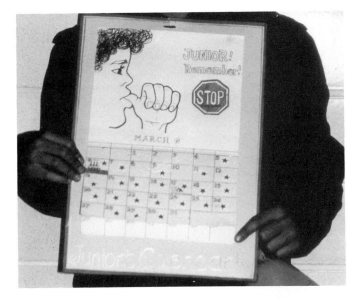

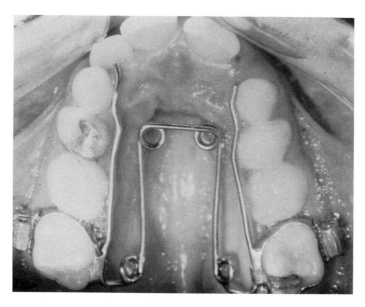

Figure 25–4 ■ The quad helix is a fixed appliance used to expand a constricted maxillary arch. The anterior helices also serve to discourage a sucking habit by reminding the child not to place a finger in the mouth. Therefore, this appliance is often used in cases in which there is an active sucking habit and a posterior crossbite.

the habit completely (Haryett et al, 1970). The quad helix also requires 6 months of treatment. Three months are needed to correct the crossbite, and 3 months are required to stabilize the movement.

Pacifier Habits

Dental changes created by pacifier habits are similar to changes created by thumb habits (Fig. 25–6). Anterior open bite and maxillary constriction are seen consistently in pacifier suckers. Labio-lingual movement of incisors may not be as pronounced as with a digit habit but is usually present nonetheless. Manufacturers have developed pacifiers that claim to be more like a mother's nipple and not as deleterious to the dentition as a thumb or conventional pacifier. Research has not substantiated these statements. Pacifier habits are theoretically easier to stop than digit habits because the pacifier can be discontinued gradually or at one point in time under the control of the parent. This type of control is obviously not possible with digit habits, which makes a notable difference in the degree of patient compliance required to eliminate the two types of habits. In a few cases, the

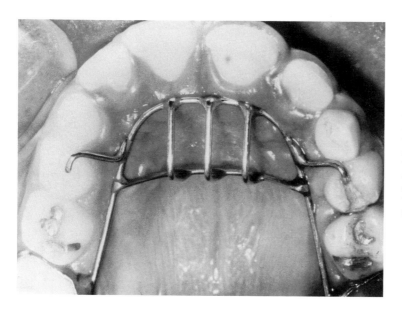

Figure 25–5 ■ A palatal crib is a fixed appliance designed to stop a digit habit by mechanically interfering with digit placement and sucking satisfaction. The patient should expect temporary disturbances in eating, speaking, and sleeping patterns during the first few days following appliance delivery.

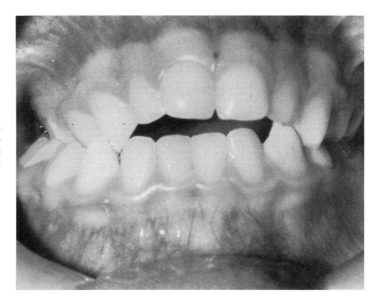

Figure 25–6 ■ A pacifier can create dental changes nearly identical to that of a digit habit. The labiolingual movement of the incisors is usually not as pronounced as with a digit habit.

child may subsequently start sucking a finger and elimination of the finger habit may become necessary.

Lip Habits

Habits that involve manipulation of the lips and perioral structures are termed lip habits. A number of lip habits exist, and their influence on the dentition is varied. Lip licking and lip pulling habits are relatively benign as far as dentitional effects are concerned. Red, inflammed, and chapped lips and perioral tissues during cool weather are the most apparent changes associated with these habits. Little can be done to stop these habits effectively, and treatment is usually palliative and limited to moisturizing the lips.

Although most lip habits do not cause dental problems, lip sucking and lip biting certainly can maintain an existing malocclusion. Whether these habits can create a malocclusion is questionable and not easily answered. The most common presentation of lip sucking is the lower lip tucked behind the maxillary incisors (Fig. 25–7). This places a lingually directed force on the mandibular teeth and a facial force on the maxillary teeth. The result is a proclination of the maxillary incisors, a retroclination of the mandibular incisors, and an increased amount of overjet. This problem is most common in the mixed and permanent dentitions. Treatment depends on the skeletal relationship

of the child and on the presence or absence of space in the arch. If the child has a Class I skeletal relationship and increased overjet that is solely the result of tipped teeth, the clinician can tip the teeth to their original or a more normal position with either a fixed or a removable appliance. However, if a Class II skeletal relationship exists, a more involved growth modifi-

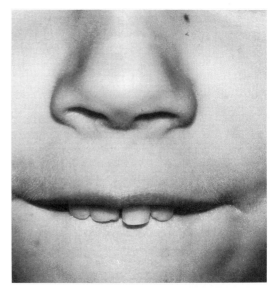

Figure 25–7 ■ The most common habit involving the lips is tucking the lower lip behind the maxillary incisors. The lower lip forces the maxillary teeth facially and the mandibular teeth lingually, resulting in an increased overjet. In addition, the lower lip and other perioral tissues can become chapped and inflamed as a result of constant wetting of the tissue.

cation procedure will be needed to treat the malocclusion.

Tongue Thrust and Mouthbreathing Habits

Recently, a great deal of attention has been given to tongue thrust and mouthbreathing habits as sources of malocclusion. As discussed in Chapter 13, tongue thrust is characteristic of the infantile and transitional swallows, both considered normal for the neonate. Epidemiologic data indicate that the percentage of individuals with infantile and transitional swallowing patterns is greater than the percentage of individuals with open bite (Kelly et al, 1973). This indicates there is not a simple cause-and-effect relationship between tongue thrusting and open bite. Furthermore, data measuring the duration, intensity, and frequency of force associated with tongue thrust suggest that the habit may be able to sustain an open bite but not create one (Proffit and Mason, 1975). Therefore, tongue thrusting should be considered a finding and not a problem to be treated.

Mouthbreathing and its association with malocclusion is a complex issue. Research designed to answer questions about their association has been flawed and not well controlled. The major problem of this research has been the reliable identification of mouthbreathers. Some individuals may appear to be mouthbreathers because of their mandibular posture or incompetent lips. It is normal for a 3- to 6-year-old to be slightly lip incompetent (see Chapter 17, Fig. 17–2). Other children have been labeled mouthbreathers because of suspected nasal airway obstruction. Two locations consistently have been suggested to be sites of obstruction, the nasal turbinates and the nasopharyngeal adenoidal tissues. Clinical judgment is not accurate enough to make a diagnosis of nasal airway impairment. The only reliable method of determining the mode of respiratory function is to use a plethysmograph and air flow transducer to determine total nasal and oral air flow. Despite the difficulties in identifying mouthbreathing individuals, there is an indication that a weak relationship may exist between mouthbreathing and malocclusions characterized by a long lower face and maxillary constriction. However, it should be noted that this relationship is very weak and does not imply that turbinectomies and adenoidectomies are advocated to clear the nasal airway (Bresolin et al, 1984; Wenzel et al, 1985).

Nail Biting

Nail biting is a habit rarely seen before 3–6 years of age. The number of individuals who bite their nails is reported to increase until adolescence, but there are very little data on this subject. It has been suggested that the habit is a manifestation of increased stress in the individual. There is no evidence that nail biting can cause malocclusion or dental change; therefore, there is no recommended treatment. However, nail biting may damage the fingernail beds themselves, so it may be necessary to use appropriate nail care products to protect the nails.

Bruxism

Bruxism is a grinding or gnashing of the teeth and is usually reported to be nocturnal. However, some children grind their teeth during the day. Most children engage in some bruxism that results in moderate wear of the primary canines and molars. Rarely, with the exception of handicapped individuals, does the wear endanger the pulp by proceeding faster than secondary dentin is produced. Masticatory muscle soreness and temporomandibular joint pain have also been attributed to bruxism. The exact cause of significant bruxism is unknown, although most explanations center around local, systemic, and psychological reasons (Kuch et al, 1979). The local theory suggests that bruxism is a reaction to an occlusal interference, high restoration, or some irritating dental condition. Systemic factors implicated in bruxism include intestinal parasites, subclinical nutritional deficiencies, allergies, and endocrine disorders. The psychological theory submits that bruxism is the manifestation of a personality disorder or increased stress. Children with musculoskeletal disorders (cerebral palsy) and children who suffer from mental retardation commonly grind their teeth. This last type of bruxism is the result of the underlying physical and mental condition of the patient and is difficult to manage dentally.

Treatment should begin with simple measures. Occlusal interferences should be identified and equilibrated if necessary. If occlusal interferences are not located or equilibration is not successful, referral to appropriate medical personnel should be considered, to rule out any systemic problems. If neither of these two steps is successful, a mouthguard-like appliance can be constructed of soft plastic to protect the teeth

and try to eliminate the grinding habit. If the habit is deemed to be due to psychological factors, which is unlikely, referral to a child development expert is warranted. Rarely will occlusal wear be so great that stainless steel crowns are necessary to prevent pulpal exposure or eliminate tooth sensitivity.

Self-Mutilation

Self-mutilation, repetitive acts that result in physical damage to the individual, is extremely rare in the normal child. However, the incidence of self-mutilation in the mentally retarded population is between 10 and 20% (DenBesten and McIver, 1984). It has been suggested that self-mutilation is a learned behavior. This may be the case, because it is one of the few behaviors that is reliably reinforced, that is, attention is always gained. A frequent manifestation of self-mutilation is biting of the lips, tongue, and oral mucosa. Any child who willfully inflicts pain or damage to himself should be considered psychologically abnormal. Such children should be referred for psychological evaluation and treatment. Self-mutilation has also been associated with biochemical disorders, such as Lesch-Nyhan and de Lange's syndromes. Besides behavior modification, treatment for self-mutilation includes use of restraints, protective padding, and sedation. If restraints and protective padding are unsuccessful, extraction of selected teeth may be necessary.

REFERENCES

Bresolin D, Shapiro GG, Shapiro PA, Dassel SW, Furukawa CT, Pierson WE, Chapko M, Bierman CW: Facial characteristics of children who breathe through the mouth. Pediatrics 73:622–625, 1984.

DenBesten PK, McIver FT: Oral self-mutilation in a child with congenital toxoplasmosis: A clinical report. Pediatr Dent 6:98–101, 1984.

Haryett RD, Hansen FC, Davidson PO: Chronic thumbsucking: A second report on treatment and its psychological effects. Am J Orthod 57:164–178, 1970.

Kelly JE, Sanchez M, Van Kirk LE: An assessment of the occlusion of teeth of children. National Center for Health Statistics, US Public Health Service, 1973, DHEW Publ No. HRA 74-1612.

Kuch EV, Till MJ, Messer LB: Bruxing and non-bruxing children: A comparison of their personality traits. Pediatr Dent 1:182–187, 1979.

Proffit WR, Mason RM: Myofunctional therapy for tongue-thrusting: Background and recommendations. J Am Dent Assoc 90:403–411, 1975.

Wenzel A, Hojensgaard E, Henriksen JM: Craniofacial morphology and head posture in children with asthma and perennial rhinitis. Eur J Orthod 7:83–92, 1985.

chapter 26

Orthodontic treatment in the primary dentition

John Christensen □ Henry Fields

The goals of orthodontic treatment in the primary dentition are to maintain good interdental relationships and to intercept developing problems that may influence those relationships. The clinician needs to differentiate skeletal problems from dental problems in order to fulfill these goals. Treatment of skeletal malocclusions in this age group is ordinarily deferred until a later age. Three general reasons are offered for delaying treatment. First, the diagnosis of skeletal malocclusion is difficult in this age group. Subtle gradations of skeletal problems and immature soft tissue development make diagnosis of all but the most obvious cases difficult. Second, although the child is growing at this stage, the amount of facial growth remaining when the child enters the mixed dentition years is sufficient to aid in the correction of most skeletal malocclusions. Third, any treatment at this age would require prolonged retention because the initial growth pattern tends to re-establish itself when treatment is discontinued.

Skeletal Problems

Skeletal problems are addressed only if there is a progressive asymmetry as a result of a functional disturbance. The reason for treating these cases early is that treatment at a later time may be more difficult and complex if the child continues to grow asymmetrically and if dental compensation increases. The goal of early treatment is to prevent the asymmetry from becoming worse or to alter growth so that the asymmetry actually improves. The majority of progressive asymmetry cases are treated with functional, removable appliances that are designed to alter growth by manipulating skeletal and soft tissue relationships and allowing differential eruption of teeth. Orthognathic surgery is a second treatment for progressive asymmetry but is reserved for only the most severe cases. It is usually necessary to operate a second time when the child is older because growth tends to remain asymmetric even after surgical correction. Because the diagnosis and treatment of progressive asymmetry are difficult, it is recommended that these cases be referred to a specialist.

Early treatment of patients with dentofacial anomalies is also advocated. Dentofacial anomalies include a number of environmentally and genetically induced conditions that have altered the relationship of the facial structures. Examples of such anomalies include cleft lip and palate, hemi-facial microsomia, and man-

dibulofacial dysostosis (Treacher-Collins syndrome). A specialist or specialty team works to minimize the facial disfigurement through early surgical and orthodontic intervention.

Dental Problems

Dental malocclusion in the primary dentition is readily treated by the general practitioner with a knowledge of fixed and removable appliances. The key to successful orthodontic treatment is careful diagnosis and treatment planning, which are dependent on the data base obtained at the initial examination. In this age group, tooth movement should be restricted to tipping teeth into proper positions. Orthodontic appliances designed to move teeth bodily are not indicated.

Before specific treatment problems are discussed, the biology of tooth movement should be reviewed briefly. A force that is applied to a tooth will cause alterations in the periodontal ligament and surrounding alveolar bone. Whether the alterations cause biochemical or electrical changes in these cells is not completely known. However, a remodeling process begins to allow the tooth to move. This remodeling process may take as little as 3 days or as much as 2 weeks, depending on the amount of force applied to the tooth. After the tooth has moved a certain distance, the force exerted by the orthodontic appliance diminishes to an amount that is below that necessary for tooth movement. During this time, remodeling is completed and the periodontal ligament and alveolar bone cells begin to return to their normal state. This reorganization period is necessary to prevent injury to the tooth and supporting structures. The clinical implication of cellular change, tooth movement, and cellular reorganization is that orthodontic appliances should only be reactivated at 4–6 week intervals to avoid injury to the periodontium. Therefore, there is some biologic reasoning behind monthly dental visits during orthodontic treatment (Proffit et al, 1986).

After tooth movement is complete, the patient enters the retention phase of treatment. Retention is the period of time that the teeth are held in their new position. Retention is necessary because teeth that have been moved orthodontically tend to move back or relapse into their original position after appliances have been removed. Relapse may be due to many factors; however, gingival fibers are reported to play a major role. During treatment, gingival fibers tend to be stretched or compressed. They will return to their original size unless some reorganization of the fiber network occurs, which generally takes 3–4 months (Reitan, 1959). Hence, most clinicians recommend a 3 month retention period after minor tooth movement to allow for reorganization.

Incisor Protrusion and Retrusion

In addressing the anteroposterior plane of space, the clinician is mainly concerned with the position of the incisors, particularly the maxillary incisors. The majority of anteroposterior problems involve anterior crossbite, a condition in which the maxillary incisors occlude lingual to the mandibular incisors. A lingual arch or a removable appliance can be used to correct the crossbite. The lingual arch can be designed in one of two ways. The arch may be activated to tip maxillary teeth into proper position, or it may have soldered auxiliary wires to exert the tipping forces. The lingual arch is activated approximately 1 mm per visit. The auxiliary wires can be activated 2 mm. Generally, a tooth moves 1 mm per month during treatment. Therefore, if a tooth requires 3 mm of movement to be properly aligned, 3 months of treatment will be necessary. In a removable appliance, wire finger springs are incorporated into the palatal acrylic to move the teeth facially. The appliance is stabilized by placing retentive clasps on the posterior teeth (Fig. 26–1). The finger springs are activated 1.5–2.0 mm per month. If the patient exhibits a positive overbite and overjet after treatment, retention is probably not necessary because the occlusion will generally hold the tipped incisor in its new position. If there is no overbite, the appliance should be maintained until overbite is established to ensure that relapse will not occur.

One further point should be made about anterior crossbite. In some cases of posterior crossbite or occlusal interference, a child will posture the jaw forward to achieve maximum intercuspation and an anterior crossbite will result. This type of anterior crossbite is due to jaw posturing rather than tooth or jaw malposition. In these cases, treatment is directed toward the posterior crossbite or the occlusal interference and not toward the anterior crossbite.

Excessive overjet in the primary dentition is usually due to a non-nutritive sucking habit or to a skeletal mismatch between the upper and

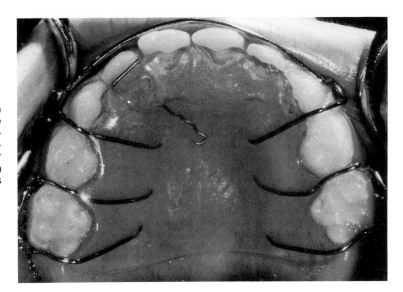

Figure 26-1 ■ In this case, an anterior crossbite involving the primary maxillary right lateral incisor is being treated with a removable appliance. The finger spring is activated 11/2-2 mm per month until the incisor is tipped out of crossbite.

lower jaws. As mentioned previously, owing to the tendency for abnormal growth patterns to recur, most skeletal problems should not be treated at this time. Incisor protrusion as a result of a sucking habit can be addressed, however. Treatment is usually directed at eliminating the habit and not at correcting the incisor protrusion. Incisor protrusion will usually correct itself if the habit is discontinued and if the equilibrium between the tongue, lips, and perioral musculature is re-established. The quad helix and palatal crib have already been discussed and are the appliances of choice (see Chapter 25, Figs. 25-4 and 25-5). Studies designed to determine how long the appliance must remain in place to terminate the habit effectively suggest that 6 months is a minimum time period (Haryett et al, 1970).

Posterior Crossbite

Posterior crossbite in the primary dentition is primarily a result of constriction of the maxillary arch. Constriction is often the result of an active thumb habit, although there are many cases in which the origin of the crossbite is undetermined. The first step in treating a posterior crossbite is to establish whether there is an associated mandibular shift. If a mandibular shift is present, treatment should be implemented to correct the crossbite. A mandibular shift has been implicated by some as the cause of asymmetrical growth of the mandible and dental compensation. The asymmetry is believed to occur because the condyles are positioned dif-

ferently within each fossa. Muscle and soft tissue stretch exert forces on the underlying skeletal and dental structures that may alter normal growth and arch development. If no shift is detected, the mandible should grow symmetrically. When there is no shift, treatment is usually delayed until the permanent first molars erupt, unless gross crowding is present. In this situation, expansion of the arch should result in more room for the primary and permanent teeth. If the permanent molars erupt into crossbite, treatment can be initiated if no other malocclusion exists. When the permanent molars erupt normally and there is no mandibular shift, treatment may not be indicated for the crossbite of the primary molars until the premolars erupt. Correction of the crossbite in the primary molar region during the mixed dentition does improve the chances that the premolars will not erupt in crossbite (Thilander et al, 1984).

There are three basic approaches to the treatment of posterior crossbite in children: (1) equilibration to eliminate mandibular shift, (2) expansion of the constricted maxillary arch, and (3) repositioning of specific teeth to correct intra-arch alignment. In a small number of cases, the mandibular shift is due to an interference caused by the primary canines. These cases can be diagnosed by repositioning the mandible and noting the interference. Selective removal of enamel with a diamond bur in both arches will eliminate the interference and the lateral shift into crossbite.

In cases of bilateral maxillary constriction, expansion is needed to correct the crossbite and

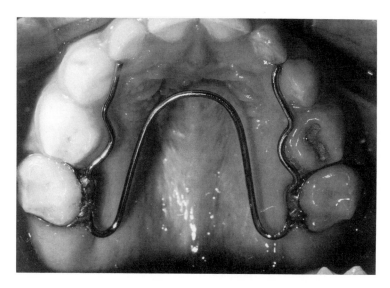

Figure 26–2 ■ The W-arch is a fixed appliance used to correct posterior crossbites in the primary dentition. The appliance is activated 3–4 mm beyond its passive width or so that one arm of the W rests over the central grooves of the teeth when the other arm is in proper position.

lateral shift. This type of case should be treated as soon as it is diagnosed unless it is anticipated that the permanent first molar will erupt within 6 months. In this situation, it is better to allow the permanent molars to erupt and to incorporate these teeth into treatment if necessary.

Both fixed and removable appliances can be designed to correct maxillary constriction, although fixed appliances are reliable and require little patient cooperation. Fixed appliances are variations of a lingual arch bent into the shape of a W. In fact, one of the most popular appliances used to treat crossbites is named the W-arch (Fig. 26–2). Another popular appliance is the quad helix (see Chapter 25, Fig. 25–4). The W-arch is constructed of .036 inch wire that rests 1.0–1.5 mm off the palate to avoid soft tissue irritation. The W-arch is activated 3–4 mm wider than its passive width or so that one arm of the W is resting over the central grooves of the teeth when the other arm is in proper position. To move teeth preferentially in the anterior region of the mouth, the appliance is activated by bending the palatal portion of the arm near the solder joint, as demonstrated in Figure 26–3. If more correction is needed in the molar region, the appliance is activated by bending the anterior palatal portion. The appli-

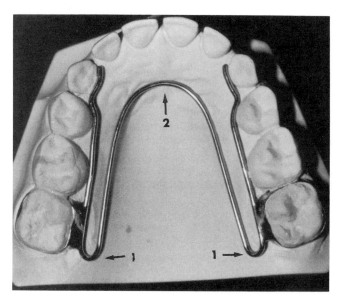

Figure 26–3 ■ To preferentially move teeth in the anterior region of the mouth, the W-arch is activated by bending the arm of the W in the area marked location 1. If more movement is desired in the molar region, the appliance is activated by bending the anterior portion of the W in the area marked location 2.

ance expands the arch approximately 1 mm per side per month. Expansion should continue until the crossbite is slightly overcorrected and until the lingual cusps of the maxillary teeth occlude on the lingual inclines of the buccal cusps of the mandibular teeth. Most crossbites are corrected in 3 months, and the teeth are retained for an additional 3 months. The patient should return monthly for the dentist to check the treatment progress and to reactivate the W-arch if needed. The appliance may be activated intraorally, although the force and direction of activation may be difficult to approximate and unwanted tooth movement can result. Usually it is easier and more accurate to remove, activate, and recement the appliance.

The quad helix is designed much like the W-arch but incorporates more wire into the appliance, making it more flexible. It is constructed of .038 inch wire with two helices in the anterior palate and two helices near the solder joint in the posterior palate. The helices are wound away from the palate and can serve to remind the digit-sucking patient to refrain from the habit. Therefore, this is the preferred appliance in a patient with a finger habit and posterior crossbite. Because the quad helix has more wire than the W-arch, it has a greater range of action and can be activated nearly twice as far as the W-arch and deliver an equivalent amount of force. Overcorrection and retention are required for the quad helix as well. Despite activating the W-arch or quad helix on one side only, teeth on both sides of the arch feel an equivalent amount of force. In other words, the teeth should all move an equal amount. This is desirable in a situation in which there is bilateral maxillary constriction. If, however, the crossbite is due to a true unilateral maxillary constriction, it would be more appropriate to move only the teeth at fault. One way to accomplish this with a fixed appliance is to construct an unequal W-arch or quad helix that has a long and short arm (Fig. 26–4). The short arm touches only the teeth that need to be moved, and the long arm touches as many contralateral teeth as possible. The theory behind the unequal W-arch is to pit movement of a large number of teeth against a small number of teeth. The side with the smaller number of teeth will tend to move more than the side with the larger number, although there will be expansion on both sides of the arch. An alternative method of unilateral treatment is to place a mandibular lingual arch to stabilize the lower arch and attach cross-elastics to the constricted maxillary

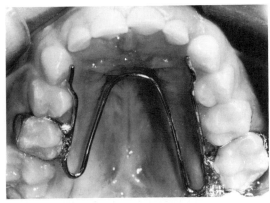

Figure 26–4 ■ An unequal W-arch is used to treat a true unilateral crossbite in the primary dentition. The short arm is placed on the constricted side of the arch against the teeth to be moved out of crossbite. The long arm of the arch is placed on the opposite side of the arch and rests against as many teeth as possible to resist tooth movement on that side. In theory, the constricted side of the arch will move more than the opposite side. (From Fields HW, Proffit WR: Orthodontics in general practice. *In* Morris AL, Bohannan, HM, Casullo DP: The Dental Specialties in General Practice, Philadelphia, WB Saunders Co, 1983, p 315.)

teeth. This results in true unilateral movement of the maxillary teeth. This alternative requires more cooperation from the patient and is technically more difficult.

Removable appliances can also be used to correct posterior crossbites but are more difficult to use unless the appliances have good retention. The forces used to expand the dental arch are large enough that they tend to dislodge removable appliances. Most removable appliances are Hawley split plate designs that use a variety of clasps to provide retention (Fig. 26–5). If the crossbite is due to a bilateral maxillary constriction, the appliance is split down the middle of the palate. A wire spring or a jackscrew embedded in the acrylic is activated to provide force necessary for movement. The wire spring is activated approximately 2 mm per month. The jackscrew is turned one time per day; each turn provides .025 mm of activation. The wire spring appliance is probably easier for the patient to place and remove than a jackscrew appliance, and compliance may be better as a result. If the crossbite is unilateral or if only one or two teeth are in crossbite, the palatal acrylic can be cut so that the spring exerts force in a manner similar to the unequal W-arch (Fig. 26–6).

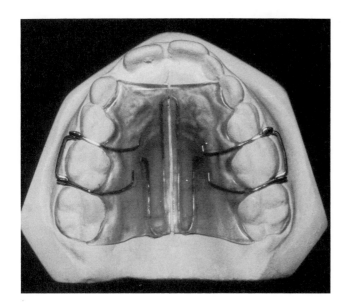

Figure 26–5 ■ Removable appliances can be used to correct posterior crossbites in the primary dentition. The split plate appliance is activated by opening the wire spring 2 mm per month. The appliance is more hygienic than the W-arch or quad helix because it can be removed to clean the teeth. However, the appliance requires multiple retention clasps because it tends to dislodge when activated.

Figure 26–6 ■ The unequal split plate appliance is used to treat true unilateral crossbites. Like the unequal W-arch, the appliance is designed to move the constricted teeth preferentially out of crossbite and minimize movement elsewhere. The extent of the crossbite and the number of teeth in crossbite determine where the unequal split is made in the appliance. In this case, the left side is in crossbite.

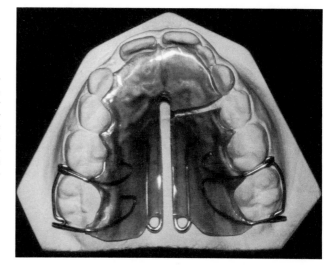

Open Bites

Vertical problems in the primary dentition are principally the result of a finger or pacifier habit. Treatment of an anterior open bite that is due to a sucking habit has been discussed previously, and the reader is referred back to the appropriate section. Deep bite in the primary dentition is generally not treated at this time. The depth of bite usually improves with the eruption of the permanent first molars if the problem is due to dental malocclusion. Skeletal problems, whether anterior open bite or deep bite, are extremely difficult to treat and are appropriately referred to a specialist.

REFERENCES

Haryett RD, Hansen FC, Davidson PO: Chronic thumb-sucking: A second report on treatment and its psychological effects. Am J Orthod 57:164–178, 1970.

Proffit WR, et al: Contemporary Orthodontics. St. Louis, CV Mosby Co, 1986, pp 228–245.

Reitan K: Tissue rearrangement during retention of orthodontically rotated teeth. Am J Orthod 29:105–113, 1959.

Thilander B, Wahlund S, Lennartsson B: The effect of early interceptive treatment in children with posterior cross-bite. Eur J Orthod 6:25–34, 1984.

Local anesthesia and oral surgery in children

Stephen Wilson □ R. Denny Montgomery

Successful management of patients, especially pediatric patients, in terms of allaying their anxiety and discomfort during restorative and surgical procedures, is facilitated by the attainment of profound local anesthesia.

Good operator technique in obtaining local anesthesia in pediatric patients is essential and requires mastery of the following areas: (1) child growth and development (physical and mental), (2) behavior management, (3) physiologic pain modulation, and (4) pharmacology of local anesthetics.

Oral surgery procedures in children are similar to and possibly easier than those in adults. There are some important differences as well. In this chapter, an overview of the principles of local anesthesia and oral surgery in children is presented.

Local Anesthesia in Children

TOPICAL ANESTHESIA

Topical anesthesia is used to obtund the discomfort associated with the insertion of the needle into the mucosal membrane. The usefulness of topical anesthesia has been debated. For instance, the taste of the anesthetic, the period of time for the patient to anticipate the needle, and the establishment of a conditioned patient response from the needle immediately following the application of topical anesthetic have been considered to be detrimental factors. However, the operator's effectiveness in interacting with children to distract and increase

317

their suggestibility toward managing their own anxieties may supercede the disadvantages of topical anesthesia. Therefore, the authors recommend the use of a benzocaine topical anesthetic that is good tasting and that is available in an easy to control gel.

A small amount of the topical anesthetic should be applied with a cotton-tipped applicator to the mucosa, which has been adequately dried and isolated with a 2 × 2 inch cotton gauze pad (Fig. 27–1). The time required for the topical anesthetic to reach its full effectiveness may vary from 30 seconds to 5 minutes. Although toxic responses to topical anesthesia are rare, excessive amounts should be avoided.

GENERAL CONSIDERATIONS FOR LOCAL ANESTHESIA

The exact mechanism of action of local anesthetics has not been determined. It is known that a local anesthetic alters the reactivity of neural membranes to propagated action potentials that may be generated in tissues distal to the anesthetic block. Action potentials that enter an area of adequately anesthetized nervous tissue are blocked and fail to transmit information to the central nervous system (Bennett, 1984).

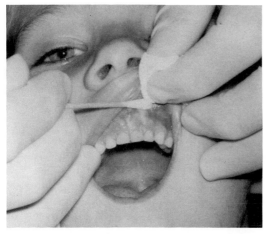

Figure 27–1 ■ Application of topical anesthetic to vestibular tissues for buccal infiltration of incisors. Note a minimal amount of anesthetic on the cotton tip applicator.
Technique: 1. Reflect tissue to expose injection site. 2. Dry soft tissue with 2 × 2 gauze pad. 3. Apply topical gel with cotton-tipped applicator. 4. Maintain applicator on tissue site for minimum of 30 seconds (see manufacturer's recommendations). 5. Remove applicator and proceed with injection.

The efficacy of local anesthesia depends upon the concentration of the anesthetic on a segment of the nerve. Beyond a fixed amount of local anesthetic necessary for blockage of neuronal impulses, any excess is wasteful and potentially dangerous. Failure to obtain anesthesia is most likely due either to operator error in depositing the solution sufficiently close to the nerve or to anatomic aberrations (e.g., accessory innervation).

Local infection and inflammation can modify the normal local physiology of tissue by causing the release of neuroactive substances (e.g., histamine, kinins, and prostaglandins) and by lowering the pH. These changes reduce the lipid solubility of the anesthetic and interfere with its ability to penetrate the nervous tissue. Blocking the nerve at a more proximal site distant from the infected area may be a viable alternative. Antibiotic administration may reduce the extent of infection and permit definitive treatment under local anesthesia that would otherwise be impossible.

Local anesthesia may be obtained anatomically by one of three means:

1. *The nerve block,* which is the placement of anesthetic on or near a main nerve trunk. This results in a wide area of tissue anesthesia.

2. *The field block,* which is the placement of anesthetic on secondary branches of a main nerve.

3. *Local infiltration,* which is the deposition of the anesthetic on terminal branches of a nerve. Adequate diffusion of local anesthetic from local infiltration readily occurs in children because their bones are less dense than those of adults.

Local anesthetics used in dentistry are classified as esters or amides. Amides are more frequently used because of their reduced allergenic characteristics and greater potency at lower concentrations. The concentration of the different agents varies, and care must be taken to prevent overdose (Table 27–1). As an example, two full cartridges (Carpules) of 2% lidocaine (Xylocaine) without vasoconstrictor may be easily tolerated by an adult, but the same amount exceeds the maximal allowable dosage (2 mg/lb body weight) for a 20 pound child.

Local anesthetic Carpules (1.8 ml) also contain preservatives, organic salts, and, in some, vasoconstrictors. The preservatives (e.g., methylparaben) may be a source of allergic reactions. The vasoconstrictors (e.g., epinephrine) are used to constrict blood vessels, counteract the

Table 27-1 ■ Dosages of two amide local anesthetics used in dentistry

Lidocaine 2% (Xylocaine) with epinephrine 1:100,000
Maximum dosage: 2 mg/pound
Mg/cartridge: 36
Absolute maximum dosage: 300 mg

Mepivacaine 2% (Carbocaine) with neo-cobefrin 1:20,000
Maximum dosage: 2 mg/pound
Mg/cartridge: 36
Absolute maximum dosage: 300 mg

Patient Weight (pounds)	Maximum Dosage	
	mg	*No. of Cartridges*
20	40	1
40	80	2
60	120	3
80	160	4
100	200	5.5
120	240	6.5
140	280	7.5
160	300	8
180	300	8

vasodilatory effects of the local anesthetic, and prolong the duration of the anesthetic.

OPERATOR TECHNIQUE

Communication in a language that the child is capable of understanding is important and necessary. The dentist may have to modify his or her wording to accommodate the level of the child's understanding when discussing the injection. For instance, the child may be told that the tooth will be "going to sleep" after a "little pinch" is felt near his tooth. The dentist should not deny that the injection may hurt, as this denial may cause the child to lose trust and lack confidence. The dentist should minimize but not reinforce the child's anxieties and fears about the "pinch."

The discomfort of the injection may be lessened by counter-irritation, distraction, and a slow rate of administration. Counter-irritation refers to the application of vibratory stimuli (e.g., rapid displacement of loose alveolar tissue) or of moderate pressure (e.g., with a cotton-tipped applicator) to the area adjacent to the site of injection. These stimuli have a physical and psychological basis for modifying noxious input. Distraction can be accomplished by

continuing a constant monologue with the child and by maintaining his or her attention away from the syringe. The operator should always aspirate and alter the depth of the needle if necessary prior to slowly injecting the anesthetic. The time of deposition of a single Carpule should take at least 1 minute. Rapid injections tend to be more painful because of rapid tissue expansion. They also potentiate the possibility of a toxic reaction if the solution is inadvertently deposited in a blood vessel.

The role of the dental assistant is very important during transfer of the syringe and in anticipation of patient movement. During the transfer of the syringe from the assistant to the dentist, the child's eyes tend to follow the dentist's. The eyes of the dentist should be focused on the face of the patient (Fig. 27-2). The hand of the dentist that is to receive the syringe is extended close to the head or body of the child. The body of the syringe is placed between the index and middle finger, with the ring of the plunger being slipped over the dentist's thumb by the assistant. The plastic sheath protecting the needle is then removed by the assistant. The dentist's peripheral vision will guide the syringe to the mouth in a slow, smooth movement.

Reflexive movements of the child's head and body should be anticipated (Sanders, 1979, p 106). The head can be stabilized by holding firmly but gently between the body and arm or hand of the dentist. The assistant passively extends his or her arm across the chest of the child so that potential arm and body movements can be intercepted. The area of soft tissue that is to receive the injection is reflected by the free hand of the dentist. The hand can also be used to block the vision of the child as the syringe approaches the mouth. Once tissue penetration by the needle has occurred, the needle should not be retracted in response to the child's reactions. Otherwise, the child's behavior may deteriorate significantly if he or she anticipates reinjection. Finger rests are strongly advocated.

MAXILLARY PRIMARY AND PERMANENT MOLAR ANESTHESIA

The innervation of maxillary primary and permanent molars arises from the posterior superior alveolar nerve (permanent molars) and middle superior alveolar nerve (mesio-buccal root of the first permanent molar, primary molars, and premolars).

In anesthetizing the maxillary primary molars or permanent premolars, the needle

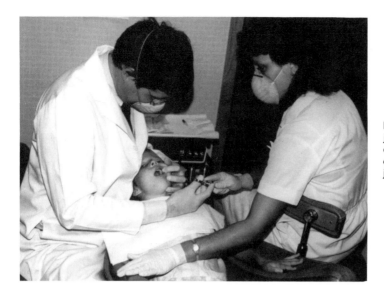

Figure 27–2 ■ Preparing for the injection. Note the hand positions of the dentist and assistant to stabilize the child's head and body during the injection.

should penetrate the muco-buccal fold and be inserted to a depth that approximates that of the apices of the buccal roots of the teeth (Fig. 27–3). The solution should be deposited adjacent to the bone. The maxillary permanent molars may be anesthetized with a posterior superior alveolar nerve block or by local infiltration.

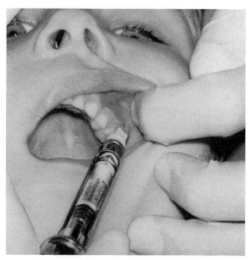

Figure 27–3 ■ Buccal infiltration for anesthetizing maxillary primary molars.
Technique: 1. Reflect tissue to expose injection site. 2. Orient bevel of needle to be parallel to the bone. 3. Insert needle in mucobuccal fold. 4. Proceed to depth that approximates the apices of the buccal roots of the molar(s). 5. The bevel of the needle should be adjacent to the periosteum of the bone. Aspirate. 6. Deposit the bolus of anesthetic slowly. 7. Remove needle and apply pressure with a 2 × 2 gauze for 1 minute to obtain hemostasis.

MAXILLARY PRIMARY AND PERMANENT INCISOR AND CANINE ANESTHESIA

The innervation of maxillary primary and permanent incisors and canines is by the anterosuperior alveolar branch of the maxillary nerve. Labial infiltration commonly is used to anesthetize the primary anterior teeth. The needle is inserted in the muco-buccal fold to a depth that approximates that of the apices of the teeth (Fig. 27–4). Rapid deposition of the solution in this area is contraindicated because it produces discomfort during rapid expansion of the tissue. The innervation of the anterior teeth may arise from the opposite side of the midline. Thus, it may be necessary to deposit some solution adjacent to the apex of the contralateral central incisor.

The infraorbital block injection is an excellent technique that may be used in place of local infiltration of the anterior teeth. All ipsilateral anterior maxillary teeth are anesthetized by this block. The needle is inserted anywhere in the muco-buccal fold from the lateral incisor to the first primary molar and is advanced next to bone to a depth that approximates the infraorbital foramen. The foramen is readily palpated as a notch on the infraorbital rim of the bony orbit. The solution is deposited slowly.

PALATAL TISSUE ANESTHESIA

The tissues of the hard palate are innervated by the anterior palatine and nasal palatine

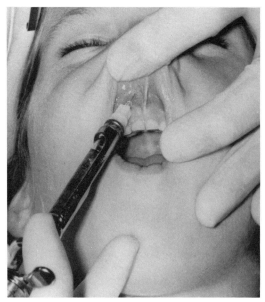

Figure 27–4 ■ Labial infiltration of maxillary incisor area.

Technique for maxillary primary and permanent incisors and canines: 1. Reflect tissue to expose injection site. 2. Orient bevel of needle to be parallel to the bone. 3. Insert needle in mucobuccal fold. 4. Proceed to depth that approximates the apices of the roots. This depth is less in the primary dentition than that of the permanent dentition. 5. The bevel of the needle should be adjacent to the periosteum of the bone. Aspirate. 6. Inject the bolus of anesthetic very slowly. 7. Remove needle and apply pressure to area with 2 × 2 gauze for hemostasis.

nerves. Surgical procedures involving palatal tissues usually require a nasal palatine nerve block (Fig. 27–5) or anterior palatine anesthesia (Fig. 27–6). These nerve blocks are painful, and care should be taken to prepare the child adequately. These injections are not usually required for normal restorative procedures. However, if it is anticipated that the rubber dam clamp will impinge on the palatal tissue, a drop of anesthetic solution should be deposited into the marginal tissue adjacent to the lingual aspect of the tooth. A blanching of the tissue will be observed.

MANDIBULAR TOOTH ANESTHESIA

The inferior alveolar nerve innervates the mandibular primary and permanent teeth. This nerve enters the mandibular foramen on the lingual aspect of the mandible. The position of the foramen changes by remodeling more superiorly from the occlusal plane as the child matures into adulthood. The foramen is at or

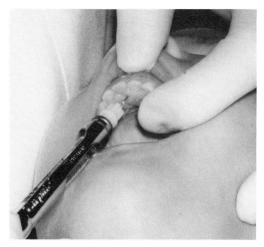

Figure 27–5 ■ Nasal palatine block. The needle is inserted to the left or right side of the papilla. Note the blanching of tissue at the injection site.

slightly above the occlusal plane during the period of the primary dentition (Benham, 1976). In adults, it averages 7 mm above the occlusal plane. The foramen is approximately midway between the anterior and posterior borders of the ramus of the mandible.

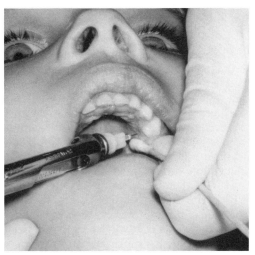

Figure 27–6 ■ Palatal infiltration of primary molars anesthetizing the anterior palatine nerve. The cotton-tipped applicator is being held firmly against the palatal tissue. The needle is inserted in the area between the applicator and tooth. The applicator may provide a masking or distracting effect.

Technique: 1. Apply pressure with cotton-tipped applicator to site that is to receive the needle. 2. Insert needle with bevel oriented parallel to the bone immediately adjacent to the applicator. 3. Proceed to a depth at which the bevel of the needle is adjacent to the periosteum and aspirate. 4. Inject the bolus of anesthetic very slowly. 5. Remove needle and apply pressure to area with a 2 × 2 gauze for hemostasis.

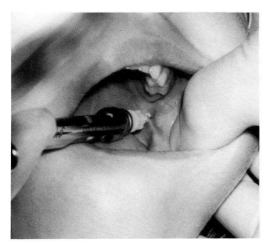

Figure 27 – 7 ■ Inferior alveolar block.
Technique: 1. With patient's mouth opened as wide as possible, place the ball of the thumb on the coronoid notch on the anterior border of the mandible. 2. Position the index and middle fingers on the external posterior border of the mandible. 3. Insert the needle with bevel oriented parallel to the bone and at the level of the occlusal plane between the internal oblique ridge and the pterygomandibular raphe. The barrel of the syringe will be exiting the mouth adjacent to the lip commissure contralateral to the side that is to be anesthetized. 4. Insert the needle to a depth that is adjacent to the bone. Aspirate. 5. Slowly inject the bolus of anesthetic. 6. Remove the needle and apply pressure to area with 2 × 2 gauze for hemostasis.

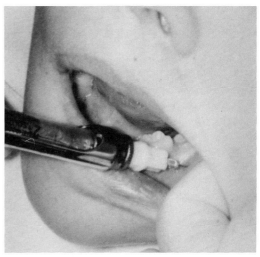

Figure 27 – 8 ■ Long buccal nerve block.
Technique: 1. Reflect tissue to expose site of injection. 2. Insert needle in the mucobuccal fold at a point distal and buccal to the most posterior molar. The bevel of the needle should be oriented parallel to the bone. 3. Insert needle to a depth that is adjacent to the bone. Aspirate. 4. Slowly inject the bolus of anesthetic. 5. Remove the needle and apply pressure to area with 2 × 2 gauze for hemostasis.

For the inferior alveolar nerve block, the child is requested to open his or her mouth as far as possible. Mouth props may aid in maintaining this position for the child. The ball of the thumb is positioned on the coronoid notch of the anterior border of the ramus, and the fingers are placed on the posterior border of the ramus. The needle is inserted between the internal oblique ridge and the pterygomandibular raphe (Fig. 27 – 7). The barrel of the syringe overlies the two primary mandibular molars on the opposite side of the arch and parallels the occlusal plane. The needle is advanced until it contacts bone, aspiration is completed, and the solution is deposited slowly.

Occasionally, the inferior alveolar nerve block is not successful. A second attempt may be attempted; however, the needle should be inserted at a level higher than that of the first injection. Care must be taken to prevent an overdose of anesthetic (see Table 27 – 1).

The long buccal nerve supplies the molar buccal gingivae and may provide accessory innervation to the teeth. It should be anesthetized along with the inferior alveolar block. A small quantity of solution is deposited in the muco-

buccal fold at a point distal and buccal to the most posterior molar (Fig. 27 – 8).

Some operators advocate the use of a periodontal ligament injection for anesthetizing singular teeth (Malamed, 1982). An advantage of this method is that soft tissue is not anesthetized, which may prevent inadvertent tissue damage from chewing following dental procedures. However, there is some evidence that this type of injection may produce areas of hypoplasia or decalcification on succedaneous teeth (Brannstrom et al, 1984).

COMPLICATIONS OF LOCAL ANESTHESIA

The complications of local anesthesia may include local and systemic effects (Malamed, 1986). Local complications may include masticatory trauma (Fig. 27 – 9), hematomas, infections, nerve damage by the needle, trismus, and, rarely, needle breakage in the soft tissue. These types of complications may be minimized by aspirating, decreasing needle deflection, and warning the parent and child that the soft tissue will be anesthetized for a period of up to 1 – 2 hours following the restorative procedure.

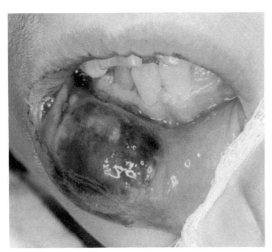

Figure 27-9 ■ Masticatory trauma to lower lip that has been anesthetized with an inferior alveolar block.

Systemic complications include allergic reactions and cardiovascular and central nervous system (CNS) dysfunctions. The CNS responses to local anesthetics are complex and depend on plasma concentrations. These responses range from dizziness, blurred vision, and anxiety to tremors, convulsions, CNS depression, and death. The primary effect of local anesthetics on the heart is that of myocardial depression.

The management of overdoses will vary, depending on the presenting symptoms and/or signs. Mild reactions require little more than patient reassurance and, if necessary, termination of the planned treatment. Severe reactions require oxygen supplementation and ventilatory support.

Oral Surgery in Children

In many ways, oral surgical procedures for children are similar to and possibly easier than those performed for adults. There are some very important differences as well. The purpose of this section is to present basic techniques and surgical principles necessary to perform oral surgical procedures safely and competently for the child and adolescent patient. This section discusses the extraction of teeth, minor soft tissue procedures (i.e., biopsies and frenectomies), odontogenic infections, and the recognition and initial care for facial injuries and fractures.

PREOPERATIVE EVALUATION

The dentist treating the child patient must be careful to evaluate the entire patient and not focus only on the oral cavity. Important considerations in caring for the child patient include the following:

1. Obtaining a good medical history
2. Obtaining appropriate medical and dental consultations
3. Anticipating and preventing emergency situations
4. Being fully prepared to treat emergency situations properly when they occur

In addition to the medical preoperative evaluation, it is important to perform a thorough dental preoperative evaluation, which includes taking appropriate preoperative radiographs. These often include two or more periapical radiographs of the same area in order to determine buccal, lingual, facial, or palatal relationships of impacted teeth. Another preoperative consideration is the future need for space maintenance as a result of the premature loss of primary teeth. Failure to provide immediate space maintenance may allow for the mesial migration of permanent first molars after premature primary molar loss.

TOOTH EXTRACTIONS

Armamentarium

Many dentists choose to use the same surgical instruments for their child patients as they routinely use for their adult patients. However, most pediatric dentists and oral and maxillofacial surgeons prefer the smaller pediatric extraction forceps, like the No. 150S and 151S (Fig. 27-10), for the following reasons:

1. Their reduced size more easily allows placement in the smaller oral cavity of the child patient.
2. The smaller pediatric forceps are more easily concealed by the operator's hand.
3. The smaller working ends (beaks) more closely adapt to the anatomy of the primary teeth.

The choice of the proper instrumentation can also depend on special considerations unique to the child and the adolescent. The use of cow horn mandibular forceps is contraindicated for primary teeth, owing to the potential injury to the developing premolars. Great care must also

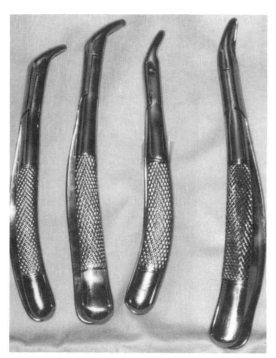

Figure 27–10 ■ Extraction forceps; left to right, No. 151S, No. 151, No. 150S, No. 150.

be given to the routine use of elevators and forceps adjacent to large restorations such as chrome crowns and especially restorations adjacent to erupting single rooted teeth that may easily become dislodged with the slightest force.

General Considerations

The manual technique used to perform extractions in the child patient is similar to the manual extraction technique utilized in the adult. The greatest difference is in patient management. It is essential that the dentist take the time to describe the ensuing procedure completely and accurately to the child. The extraction appointment should always begin with proper topical and local anesthesia, with consideration given to oral, intravenous, or nitrous oxide psychosedation on an individual basis (see Chapter 21). A few children may require general anesthesia for the surgical procedure to be accomplished. The choice of proper local anesthesia-sedation-general anesthesia technique depends upon the psychological constitution of the child and upon the extent and nature of the surgical procedure. The appropriate local anesthetic technique for each type of tooth is described earlier in this chapter.

There are a number of aspects of the extraction procedure that should be performed with every extraction. The dentist should consult with the child and the parents prior to surgery in order to prepare them for the upcoming procedure. The dentist should provide any preoperative needs such as prescriptions or any dietary restrictions that might be necessary as a result of the planned sedative techniques. The entire surgical procedure and the expected postoperative recovery course should also be described. This will allow the parents to prepare for any special postoperative arrangements, such as the need for a soft diet or child care support. As noted before, the dentist should perform a thorough review of the patient's medical history, looking especially for medical conditions that might complicate treatment.

There is no other type of dental treatment in which the principles of tell, show, and do are more important than during extractions. The dentist should be sure to obtain profound anesthesia because once the patient has felt pain, it may be difficult to regain the child's confidence to a level in which he or she will behave in a manner that will allow completion of the procedure. Just prior to the actual extraction, the dentist should place the balls of the index finger and thumb in the area of the extraction and demonstrate to the child the types of pressures and movements that he or she will encounter during the extraction. This digital pressure should be firm enough to rock the child's head from side to side in the headrest.

There are several factors that make it possible for the child patient to aspirate or swallow foreign objects during dental treatment. These factors include (1) the common practice of treating the child patient in a reclining position; (2) poor visibility as a result of the smaller opening into the oral cavity and the proportionately larger tongue of the child, and (3) the increased likelihood of unexpected movements by the child patient. To prevent this from happening, the patient should be positioned in the chair so that the upper jaw is at a no more than 45 degree angle with the floor (Fig. 27–11). If a greater than 45 degree angle is preferred by the operator, consideration should be given to either placing a light gauze pack in the posterior oral cavity (Fig. 27–12) or performing the extraction with the use of a rubber dam.

The dentist should be placed in the position in which he or she can easily control the instrumentation, have good visual access to the surgical site, and control the child's head. The nondominant hand of the dentist is then placed in

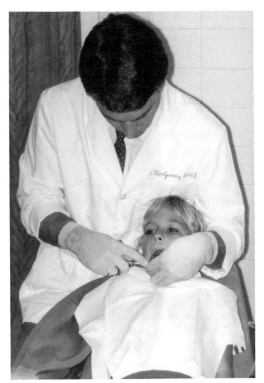

Figure 27–11 ■ To help prevent aspiration of extracted teeth, the child is positioned so that the upper jaw is at a 45 degree angle with the floor.

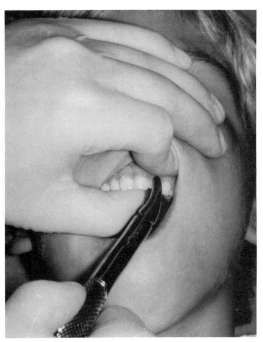

Figure 27–13 ■ The dentist's non-dominant hand helps control the child's head, supports the jaw being treated, retracts adjacent soft tissues, and palpates the alveolar process and adjacent teeth during extraction.

the patient's mouth. The role of the non-dominant hand is to help control the patient's head; to support the jaw being treated; to help retract the cheek, lips, and tongue from the surgical field; and to palpate the alveolar process and adjacent teeth during the extraction (Fig. 27–13).

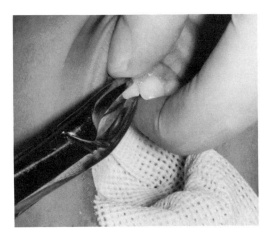

Figure 27–12 ■ A gauze screen in the oral cavity helps prevent aspiration of extracted teeth.

Once the proper operator and non-dominant hand positions are established, the actual extraction technique may begin. Variations in technique for individual teeth are discussed later in this chapter, but the following general principles apply to all extractions (Kruger, 1984). An instrument such as a dental curette or periosteal elevator is used to separate the epithelial attachment of the tooth to be extracted (Fig. 27–14). Then appropriate elevators may be used to luxate the tooth to be extracted, but great care must be utilized in order not to damage adjacent or underlying teeth. The appropriate forceps are then placed on the tooth to be extracted, usually seating the lingual or palatal beak first and then rotating the facial beak into proper position. During the entire extraction technique, firm apical pressure should be placed on the forceps. The extraction is then performed, using the proper forceps technique.

After the tooth is removed from its socket, the surgical site is evaluated visually and with the use of a curette. The curette should be used as an extension of the dentist's finger to palpate and evaluate the extraction site. No attempt should be made to scrape the extraction site. If a pathologic lesion such as a cyst or periapical granuloma is present at the apex of a permanent

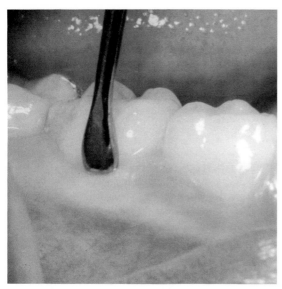

Figure 27–14 ■ A periosteal elevator is used to separate the epithelial attachment of the tooth prior to extraction.

tooth socket, it should be gently enucleated. Aggressive manipulation of a curette in a primary tooth socket is contraindicated, owing to the potential for damage to the succeeding tooth bud. The operator should palpate both the facial and palatal or buccal and lingual aspects of the surgical site to feel for any bone irregularities or alveolar expansion. Any bone sharpness should be very conservatively removed with the use of either a rongeur or a bone file. Digital pressure should be able to return the alveolus to its pre-surgical configuration if gross expansion has occurred.

The extraction site should now be evaluated for the need for sutures, although they are rarely indicated following extraction of primary teeth. The first postoperative concern is that of obtaining initial hemostasis by way of an intraoral gauze pack. In the anesthetized, deeply sedated, or very young child, a pack that extends out of the oral cavity should be used in order to prevent swallowing of the gauze. Before the patient is dismissed, a written list of postoperative instructions should be given and explained to both the patient and the parents (Table 27–2). The postoperative instruction list should explain how to contact the dentist after hours in case of an emergency.

Maxillary Molar Extractions

Primary maxillary molars differ from their permanent counterparts in that the height of

Table 27–2 ■ Postoperative instruction list for patients

POSTOPERATIVE INSTRUCTIONS:

1. Bite on gauze for 30 minutes. Don't chew on the gauze.

2. Do not use a straw to drink for 24 hours.

3. Brush remaining teeth daily, but don't rinse or use a mouthwash the day of the surgery.

4. Take pain pills and any other medication as directed.

5. If pain increases after 48 hours or if abnormal bleeding continues, call our office.

6. To prevent bleeding and swelling, keep your head elevated on 2 or 3 pillows while you rest and/or sleep.

7. Do not spit. Spitting will cause more bleeding. Excess saliva and a little blood appears as a lot of bleeding.

8. If bleeding starts again, put gauze, a clean white cloth, or a damp tea bag over the bleeding area and bite on it with firm steady pressure for 1 hour. Do not chew on it.

9. Ice packs can be used immediately after surgery and for the next 24 hours to reduce swelling. Keep ice packs on 10 minutes and off 10 minutes.

10. Black and blue marks are bruises and often occur after surgery. Usually you don't notice them. Sometimes the skin is discolored. Do not worry about this.

11. Drink lots of liquids and eat anything you can swallow.

Call our office about any complications or if you need to change your appointment.

Dr. E. X. Traction
Office No: 555-0123
After hours call 555-3210

contour is closer to the cemento-enamel junction and their roots tend to be more divergent and smaller in diameter. Because of the root structure and potential weakening of the roots by the eruption of the permanent tooth, it is not uncommon for root fracture to occur in primary maxillary molars.

Another important consideration is the relationship of the primary molar roots to the succeeding premolar crown. If the roots encircle the crown, the premolar can be inadvertently extracted with the primary molar (Fig. 27–15). After the epithelial attachment is separated, a No. 301 straight elevator is used to luxate the tooth (Fig. 27–16). The extraction is completed, using a maxillary universal forceps (No. 150S).

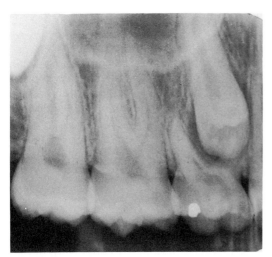

Figure 27–15 ■ Primary molars with roots encircling the developing premolar may need to be sectioned to prevent accidental extraction of the premolar.

Palatal movement is initiated first, followed by alternating buccal and palatal motions with slow continuous force applied to the forceps. This will allow expansion of the alveolar bone so that the primary molar with its divergent roots can be extracted without fracture.

Extraction of Maxillary Anterior Teeth

The maxillary primary and permanent central incisors, lateral incisors, and canines all have single roots that are usually conical in shape. This makes them much less likely to fracture and allows for more rotational movement during extraction than is possible with multirooted teeth. A No. 1 forceps is useful in the extraction of maxillary anterior teeth (Fig. 27–17).

Mandibular Molar Extractions

When extracting mandibular molars, the dentist must give special care to the support of the mandible with the non-extraction hand so that no injury to the temporomandibular joints is inflicted (Fig. 27–18). Following luxation with a No. 301 straight elevator, No. 151S forceps are used to extract the tooth with the same alternating buccal and palatal motions used to extract maxillary primary molars.

Extraction of Mandibular Anterior Teeth

The mandibular incisors, canines, and premolars are all single rooted. Because of this fact, one must take great care that the elevator and

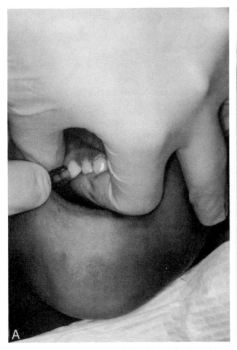

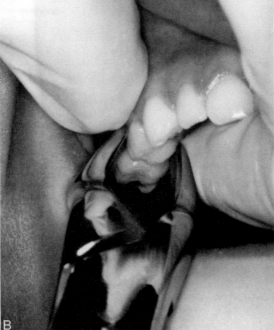

Figure 27–16 ■ A, A No. 301 straight elevator is used to luxate the tooth. Extreme care is taken to prevent accidental luxation of adjacent teeth. B, The molar is extracted using slow continuous force in alternating buccal and palatal directions.

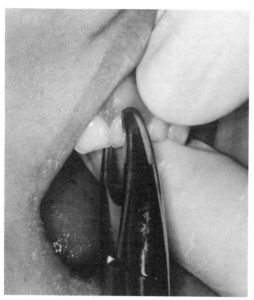

Figure 27–17 ■ Rotational movements and buccal-lingual motions are used to extract primary incisors.

forceps do not place any force on adjacent teeth, as they can become easily dislodged. This also enables the dentist to use rotational movements in the extraction process. Then slow, continuous force applied in alternating labial and lingual movements will enable these teeth to be removed easily.

Management of Fractured Primary Tooth Roots

Any dentist who extracts deciduous molars will have the opportunity on occasion to treat

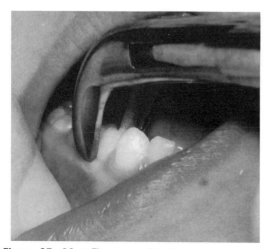

Figure 27–18 ■ The non-extraction hand supports the mandible during extraction of mandibular molars.

root fractures. Once the root has fractured, the dentist must consider the following factors. Aggressive surgical removal of all root tips may cause damage to the succedaneous teeth. On the other hand, leaving the root *may* increase the chance for postoperative infection and *may* increase the theoretical potential of delaying permanent tooth eruption, although most primary root tips will resorb. A common sense approach is best. If the tooth root is clearly visible and can be removed easily with an elevator or root tip pick, the root should be removed. If several attempts fail or if the root tip is very small or is situated very deep within the alveolus, the root is best left to be resorbed most probably by the erupting permanent tooth. In some cases, the root tips do not resorb but are situated mesially and distally to the succeeding premolar and do not impede its eruption (Fig. 27–19). The patient and parents should be notified that a root fragment has been retained, and they should be assured that the chance of unfavorable sequelae is remote.

If the preoperative evaluation indicates that a root fracture is likely or that the developing succedaneous tooth may be dislodged during the extraction, an alternative extraction technique should be utilized. In these cases, the crown should be sectioned with a fissure bur in a buccolingual direction so that the detached portions of the crown and roots can be elevated separately (Sanders, 1979, p 148).

SOFT TISSUE SURGICAL PROCEDURES

A number of soft tissue procedures occasionally must be performed for the child patient. Careful pre-surgical consideration should be given to the following:

1. The expected change in the condition with maturation
2. The optimal time (or age) for the procedure
3. The type of anesthetic or sedation required
4. Postoperative complications or sequelae
5. Expected results

Biopsies

Biopsy techniques in children are similar to those in adults. A very small lesion is probably best treated with an excisional biopsy, whereas lesions 0.5 cm or larger should probably have an incisional biopsy, especially if there is any

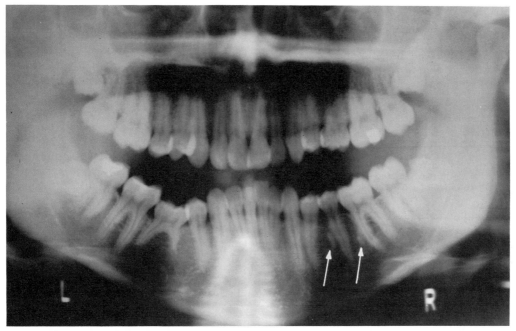

Figure 27–19 ■ In this patient, unresorbed primary root tips *(arrows)* did not impede the eruption of the succeeding premolar. Also note the congenitally missing lower left second premolar. The left mandibular second primary molar roots are not resorbing, and the occlusal surface of this tooth is well below the occlusal plane.

doubt regarding the diagnosis of the lesion. Before performing a biopsy on any lesion, the dentist should consider the possibility of a vascular lesion. Any such area should be palpated for intravascular turbulence (thrill), auscultated with a stethoscope for the presence of a bruit, and checked by needle aspiration for the presence of blood within the lesion. Biopsies should not be performed on vascular lesions until a thorough work-up has been completed (Gibilisco, 1985).

Some areas of the oral cavity, such as the mucosa and lips, are easily accessible, whereas other areas, such as the tongue, can be difficult and may require sedation or general anesthesia in order to accomplish the biopsy. The biopsy area should be carefully evaluated for proximity to important anatomic structures, such as the mental nerve or salivary ducts or their orifices. Resorbable sutures are preferred, to prevent the necessity of removing sutures in the child patient. The disadvantage of some resorbable sutures is that the knot can be very hard and stiff and irritating to the child. Soaking gut sutures in glycerin prior to their use softens them considerably.

Frenectomies

Maxillary labial frenectomies ■ Recent trends justify significantly fewer maxillary labial frenectomies. These procedures should only be performed after it has been shown that the frenum is a causative factor in maintaining a diastema between the maxillary central incisors. This cannot be determined until after the permanent canines have erupted. Therefore, a maxillary labial frenectomy prior to the age of 11 or 12 is probably not indicated.

Lingual frenectomies ■ Evidence from speech pathologists indicates that only the most severe ankyloglossia (tongue-tied) conditions significantly affect speech. Therefore, lingual frenectomies should not be performed until after an evaluation and therapy by a qualified speech therapist.

DENTOALVEOLAR SURGERY

More difficult dentoalveolar procedures may involve the use of mucoperiosteal flaps and bone openings of the maxilla or mandible. These are indicated for procedures such as retained roots, bone cysts, impacted teeth (canines, supernumerary teeth, etc.), or intrabone pathologic lesions. Basic technique involves the preparation of an adequate mucoperiosteal flap as well as an adequate bone opening. At the same time, the operator must be cautious to avoid injury to such structures as the mental or

inferior alveolar nerves, developing or erupting teeth, and the maxillary sinus.

Procedures to uncover impacted maxillary canines are highly successful (Fifield, 1986). Preoperative radiographs are taken to locate the canine within the alveolus accurately. It is often necessary to take two or more periapical radiographs, using the buccal object rule to predict the labio-palatal position of an impacted tooth. The appropriate soft tissue approach (either labial or palatal) is used in a conservative bone uncovering of the crown. Great care is taken not to disturb the root of the impacted canine because it is believed that there is an increased chance of ankylosis if the cementum is disturbed. If root development has not been complete, the exposed canine may be allowed to erupt passively. If the impacted canine has complete root development or is poorly positioned, an orthodontic bracket may be bonded to the exposed portion of the crown with autopolymerized resin. The exposed canine can now be orthodontically positioned within the maxillary arch.

FACIAL INJURIES

The dentist may be the first health care professional consulted for injuries to the teeth, lips, jaws, or soft tissues of the face. The dentist should be aware of potential problems with each type of injury and treat the patient appropriately or refer him or her to a qualified specialist.

Initial care should be directed toward pain control, hemorrhage control, patient reassurance, wound toiletry if possible, and tetanus prophylaxis. Care should be taken to account for all teeth. Chest or abdominal radiographs may be necessary to find swallowed or aspirated teeth. Traumatic injuries to the teeth are discussed in Chapters 14 and 33.

Facial trauma is rarely life threatening. A significant number of patients who present with facial trauma may also have acute life-threatening injuries such as chest or abdominal trauma, or more commonly, serious head or neck injury. The dentist must be sure that there are no other serious injuries before treating the facial injuries.

Soft tissue injuries of the face or oral cavity can usually be treated with primary closure. Great care must be taken to be certain that no foreign objects are left hidden within the wound. Gravel or dirt left embedded in soft tissue may leave a permanent tattoo on the face.

Puncture type wounds often carry glass or debris deep within the wound. When a doubt exists about the presence or absence of a foreign body within the soft tissue, a soft tissue radiograph may be helpful in identifying the presence of embedded material (see Fig. 14–5).

Small lacerations of the wet portion of the lips, gingivae, alveolar mucosa, or tongue usually heal very well even if left unsutured. Large lacerations should be closed, regardless of their location. A resorbable suture is most commonly used intraorally, although some practitioners prefer using silk suture material because it has a softer texture. The disadvantage of silk suture is that it requires removal in 5–7 days and the patient is still generally tender to manipulation of that area. Lacerations that extend from the face into the oral cavity (through-and-through lacerations) require a layered closure. Principles of a layered closure include a watertight mucosal closure, followed by closure of the muscular, facial, subcutaneous, and skin layers as necessary. Facial lacerations are always reapproximated first at significant anatomic structures, such as the vermilion border, columella of the nose, or eyebrows. Malalignment of these structures produces a very noticeable cosmetic defect.

Facial Fractures

The definitive treatment of facial fractures is best handled by an experienced dental practitioner, such as an oral and maxillofacial surgeon. Often the patient will present to the dentist with an unsuspected fracture.

Patients with maxillary or midface fractures may present with any or all of the following signs or symptoms:

   1. Altered occlusion
   2. Numbness in the infraorbital nerve distribution
   3. Double vision
   4. Periorbital ecchymosis (bruising)
   5. Facial asymmetry or edema
   6. Limited mandibular opening
   7. Subcutaneous emphysema (skin cracking upon palpation)
   8. Nasal hemorrhage
   9. Ecchymosis of the palatal or buccal mucosa
  10. Mobility or crepitus upon manipulation of the maxilla

Patients with mandibular fractures may present with any or all of the following signs or symptoms:

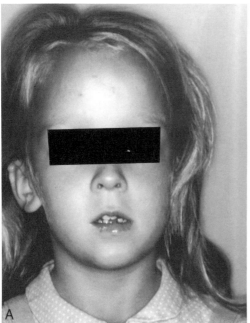
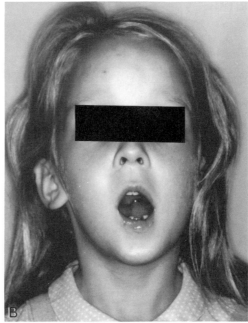

Figure 27–20 ■ *A*, This child suffered a fracture of her left condyle. Note the deviation of the mandible to the left. *B*, The deviation of the mandible toward the side of the condylar fracture is more evident upon opening.

1. Mandibular hemorrhage
2. Numbness in the mental or inferior alveolar nerve distribution
3. Altered occlusion
4. Ecchymosis or abrasion of the chin
5. Ecchymosis of the floor of the mouth or buccal mucosa
6. Periauricular pain
7. Mandibular deviation on opening (Fig. 27–20)
8. Mobility or crepitus upon manipulation of the mandible.

Initial treatment of facial fractures should be directed toward the immobilization of fractured segments, early antibiotic therapy for open fractures, and pain control (Rowe and Williams, 1985). Definitive treatment should then be performed by a qualified specialist.

ODONTOGENIC INFECTIONS

Infections of odontogenic origin are common in the child and adolescent patient. Classic signs and symptoms of infection include redness, pain, swelling, and local and systemic temperature increases. Because of wider marrow spaces in the child, an odontogenic infection can rapidly spread through the bone, possibly resulting in damage to the erupting teeth. Most odontogenic infections in the child are not serious and can be easily treated by pulp therapy or removal of the involved tooth. There are serious complications that uncommonly arise from an odontogenic infection, including cavernous sinus thrombosis, brain abscess, airway obstruction, and mediastinal spread of infection. Signs and symptoms of a more serious infection include an elevated systemic temperature (102–104°F), difficulty in swallowing, difficulty in breathing, nausea, fatigue, and sweating. The child with an odontogenic infection may become dehydrated as a result of his or her refusal to take fluids because of oral pain.

Treatment of odontogenic infections is directed toward providing adequate drainage of the infection. This can be accomplished in minor infections by way of a pulpectomy or extraction. The treatment of more serious odontogenic infections is best accomplished by way of surgical incision and drainage (Sanders, 1979, p 186). It is often necessary to identify the causative organism or organisms in order to prescribe the most appropriate antibiotic. Because most oral infections are mixed infections (aerobic and anaerobic), penicillin remains the antibiotic of choice for initial therapy.

REFERENCES

Benham NR: The cephalometric position of the mandibular foramen with age. J Dent Child 43:233, 1976.

Bennett CR: Monheim's Local Anesthesia and Pain Control in Dental Practice, 7th ed. St. Louis, CV Mosby, 1984, p 68.

Brannstrom M, Lindskog S, Nordenvall KJ: Enamel hypoplasia in permanent teeth induced by periodontal ligament anesthesia of primary teeth. JADA 109:735, 1984.

Fifield CA: Surgery and orthodontic treatment for unerupted teeth. JADA 113:590, 1986.

Gibilisco JA: Oral Radiographic Diagnosis. Philadelphia, WB Saunders Co, 1985, p 224.

Kruger G: Textbook of Oral and Maxillofacial Surgery, 6th ed. St. Louis, CV Mosby, 1984, p 52.

Malamed SF: The periodontal ligament (PDL) injection: An alternative to inferior alveolar nerve block. Oral Surg 53:117, 1982.

Malamed SF: Handbook of Local Anesthesia, 2nd ed. St. Louis, CV Mosby, 1986, p 230.

Rowe N, Williams J: Maxillofacial Injuries. Edinburgh, Churchill Livingstone, 1985, p 538.

Sanders B: Pediatric Oral and Maxillofacial Surgery. St. Louis, CV Mosby, 1979.

SUMMARY FOR SECTION II

Practically speaking, children between 3 and 6 years of age probably present the potential of being the greatest challenge to today's practicing dentist. Children who do not require any restorative, pulpal, or surgical therapy would be the exceptions. These children need only to phase into a progressively more sophisticated regimen of prevention and experience examinations that are somewhat more rigorous than those before age 3.

However, for the child who suffers various destructions of the primary dentition, not only is the dentist confronted with needing to master the techniques of restoring, treating, or extracting these teeth after acquiring anesthesia of the teeth; importantly, the dentist must also be able to manage the behavior of the child such that the child complies with him or her to the extent that the dentistry can be performed safely, efficiently, and effectively. A variety of psychological techniques have been developed to allow dentists to treat the vast majority of children of this age group who may seek to avoid dental treatment. When a child does seek avoidance of treatment and the dentist is unable to manage him, the dentist needs to understand the severity of the reasons behind this child's avoidance and take appropriate steps (e.g., refer the youngster to the pediatric dentist).

With regard to the behavioral management of children, all dentists inevitably will encounter some children who need pharmacologic management, including hospitalization and treatment with general anesthesia, or who should be referred to a specialist. Children with certain special needs, such as a disability, must also be addressed by the dentist who treats this age group.

The dental development of a child during this age readies him or her for the next pivotal stage of the dentition, and that is the advent of the permanent dentition. This is a gradual process, lasting from age 6 to age 12. However, generally by the time a child reaches age 6, the eye of the well-trained dentist can catch many predictors of future occlusal, space, and other alignment problems.

In summary, the dentist has four ultimate responsibilities to a child during these years. First, prevention of hard and soft tissue diseases remains paramount. Management of insults, both those of disease and of trauma, to the primary teeth is second. Third is the management of the integrity of the primary arches. Fourth, and very important, is the grooming of an accepting, unafraid dental patient.

section III

The transitional years: six to twelve years

If one examines a group of children younger than 6 years, there tends to be homogeneity in these children regarding such characteristics as height, weight, dental appearance, and facial esthetics. If one could re-examine this group later, when they are over 12 years old, there would be much less overall similarity provided to the observer of these characteristics. Indeed, there would be noticeably tall individuals and short individuals, heavy and slight individuals, dentally ideal and dentally unesthetic individuals, and facially appealing and facially plain or perhaps even disadvantaged individuals.

The dentist during these years must be concerned with the development of the permanent occlusion, the harmonious relationships of the two jaws, facial posture, and dental appearance. During these years, the child will increasingly become more conscious of his or her appearance. This consciousness will continue to heighten until it is at its most profound point in the adolescent years.

Additionally, parents will begin to notice increasingly the appearance of their children from a dental standpoint. In fact, age 6 itself, with the eruption of the two lower permanent central incisors, usually is accompanied by questions by the parents directed to the dentist. A usual question about the two lower permanent central incisors is why they come in rotated and what will happen to these teeth in the future. The maxillary permanent central incisors often appear to parents to be extraordinarily large and very yellow. In the vast majority of cases, these are of normal size and the yellowness is natural when compared with the very white enamel of the primary teeth. However, the permanent incisors do look strange to the parent uninformed about the difference in color of the enamel of the permanent dentition and the primary dentition.

From age 6–12, the prevention program of the child will continue at home and the parents will still need to continue supervision. It is hoped that as the child progresses toward adolescence, the need of the parent to supervise the youngster in oral hygiene will begin to diminish.

In the dental office, prevention procedures will often become more intense during these years. The advent of the first permanent molars in the 6- and 7-year-old, with the possibilities of these teeth having buccal pit fissures, lingual pit fissures, and deep grooves on the occlusal surface, may signal a need for preventive sealants to stop the possibility of pit and fissure caries. Calculus accumulations also loom as more of a problem than in younger years.

With children starting to participate in team sports, ball throwing sports, and riding bicycles, the chances for facial trauma and trauma to the early permanent dentition increase. This is particularly true for children who for whatever reason present maxillary incisors that are flared forward in their arch and that are likely to absorb the blow from any insult to the face between the nose and the chin.

In summary, everything that the dentist knows how to do for children between 3 and 6 years of age remains important for children between ages 6 and 12, because these youngsters will still have primary teeth, particularly the posterior ones, during these years. Some children will continue to need space maintenance. Others will need interceptive orthodontic treatment. There will be children who misbehave and who will need to be managed, although the incidence of misbehavior will be much less than in younger age groups. Obviously, prevention needs remain and sealants may be indicated. Fluoride supplementation should be encouraged throughout this transitional time. Because of the advent of the permanent dentition, different pulpal therapies and restorative techniques must be mastered to treat the problems presented by this age group effectively. Lastly, the fact that the child in this age range can give the dentist more information for deciding on his or her orthodontic needs is very important, particularly if early treatment is to be attempted.

chapter 28

The dynamics of change

PHYSICAL CHANGES

BODY

J. R. Pinkham

The average 6-year-old in the United States is approximately 3 feet, 10 inches tall and weighs about 48 pounds. By the time the child reaches age 12, he will be about 5 feet tall and will weigh about 85 pounds. This represents from age 6–12 an approximately 5–6% weight increase per year and a weight adjustment of about 10% per year (Watson and Lowrey, 1967).

By age 6, the child's overall bodily proportions are fairly close to what he or she will be as an adult. The most remarkable proportional change in the body during these years will result from the lengthening of the child's limbs.

During the years between ages 6 and 12, boys as a group are generally slightly taller than girls as a group until around age 10. From age 10 to around age 15, girls will be slightly taller than boys. From a weight standpoint, boys are slightly heavier than girls until around age 11, when girls overtake boys weight-wise for a brief time. Why boys eventually become taller than girls is dealt with in the discussion of the body's physical changes in the adolescence section of this book (Section IV, Chapter 35).

Other growth and developmental changes that are noteworthy during these years are the further increases in blood pressure, the continuing decrease in the pulse rate, the increased mineralization of the skeleton, and the increase in muscular tissue. In addition, the lymphatic tissues reach a peak in their development during these years to the point that they exceed the amount that the adult will have.

REFERENCE

Watson EH, Lowrey GH: Growth and Development of Children, 5th ed. Chicago, Year Book Publishers, 1967.

HEAD AND NECK

Jerry Walker

The years from ages 6 through 12 represent a continuous progression of the head and neck growth noted in the 3- to 6-year old. The periodic variations in growth rate for various aspects of the male head and face are depicted in Figure 28–1. It can be observed that, with the exception of maxillary antral height, by age twelve 90% or almost 90% of all other facial measurements are complete.

In a comparison of differential growth center rates of craniofacial components from age 5– 10, the remainder of neural growth is almost entirely complete (Fig. 28–2). During this same age span, the jaws (A-2 and B-3 of Fig. 28–2) will grow at a rate faster than the neural growth rate. Despite this faster rate, considerable general growth will be experienced after age 10. The final structuring of the face and head will take place during puberty (Behrents, 1985).

Any discussion of facial growth would not be complete without a description of the different types of bone growth. In 1980, Ranly reported that the deposition and calcification of bone tissue can occur in one of two ways, directly (intramembranous) or indirectly (cartilage replacement). In intramembranous formation, osteoblasts secrete a matrix composed of collagen and proteoglycans and additionally pro-

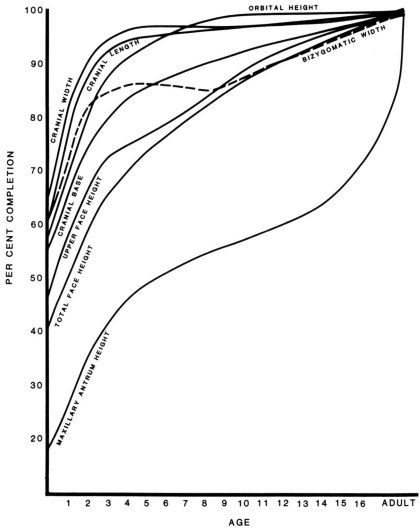

Figure 28–1 ■ Male craniofacial dimensional change. (From Behrents RG: Growth in the Aging Craniofacial Skeleton. Center for Human Growth and Development. The University of Michigan, Ann Arbor, Michigan, 1985.)

GROWTH INCREMENTS

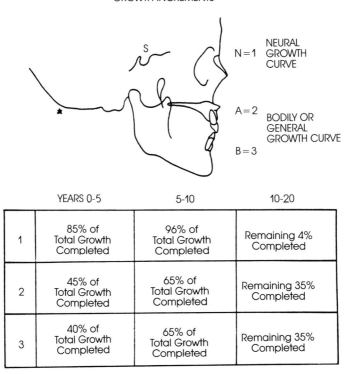

YEARS 0-5	5-10	10-20
1	85% of Total Growth Completed	96% of Total Growth Completed	Remaining 4% Completed
2	45% of Total Growth Completed	65% of Total Growth Completed	Remaining 35% Completed
3	40% of Total Growth Completed	65% of Total Growth Completed	Remaining 35% Completed

Figure 28–2 ■ Differential growth center rates of craniofacial components. (From Behrents RG: Growth in the Aging Craniofacial Skeleton. Center for Human Growth and Development. The University of Michigan, Ann Arbor, Michigan, 1985.)

mote the deposition of calcium hydroxyapatite into this matrix.

Intramembranous bone formation occurs in the outer surface of bone (periosteum), in the inner surface of bone (endosteum), and, in the case of a few bones in the skull, at the edges in specialized structures called sutures. Sutures consist of soft tissue interposed between two bones. The division of labor in the sutures allows for differential growth, whereby one bone of the skull might grow at a greater rate than its neighbor.

The indirect method is more circuitous, using a scaffold or precursor of cartilage on which to deposit bone. In this situation, cartilage is first formed by chondroblasts; it then undergoes a degenerative process associated with mineralization and finally is invaded by bone-resorbing cells that reduce the cartilage to a framework. The osteoblasts in turn deposit bone matrix around this cartilage model. In time, the remnants of the cartilage matrix are completely lost in the process of growth and remodeling.

There are three cartilage replacement mechanisms in the head, each of them unique from the rest of the body. They are as follows:

1. *Spheno-occipital synchondrosis*: The structure on the skull most resembling the growth plates of long bones is the cartilage remnant, located between the sphenoid and the occipital bone along the midline of the cranial base. Its cellular organization can be visualized by putting together the reserve cartilage layers of two growth plates. Owing to this architecture, interstitial expansion is bidirectional, increasing the size of bones simultaneously.

2. *Nasal cartilage*: The nasal septum seen in the adult skull divides the nasal cavity into two parts. At birth this septum is formed entirely of cartilage, but in the adult all of it is converted into bone except the anterior segment, which unites the tissues of the nostrils. The advancing bone tissue sweeps diagonally across the cartilage, downward and forward.

3. *Condyles*: In the long bone, the load-bearing surface and the articular cartilage are separated from the cartilage growth zone by epiphyseal bone. In the condyle, however, the articular surface and cartilage replacement tissue are juxtaposed. The most peripheral zone of the condylar articulation is not composed of cartilage, as it is in long bones, but rather of connective tissue.

In the condyle, the replacement mechanism during growth differs from other areas both in the source of new cartilage cells and in the orientation they assume. In the condyle, new cartilage cells are derived from non-cartilage precursors (in the long bones, new cartilage cells are derived from other cartilage cells through division). The cells of the condylar cartilage remain random or embryonic and are thus unable to form the specialized columnar arrangement of the growth plate (Ranly, 1980).

REFERENCES

Behrents RG: Growth in the Aging Craniofacial Skeleton. Monograph 17, Craniofacial Growth Series, Ann Arbor, Michigan, Center for Human Growth and Development, 1985.

Ranly DM: A Synopsis of Craniofacial Growth. New York, Appleton-Century-Crofts, 1980.

DENTAL CHANGES

C. A. Full

Early during this period of time, many children will experience the eruption of all four first permanent molars and the exfoliation of the mandibular and maxillary primary central and lateral incisors with a subsequent eruption of permanent incisors between the ages of 6 and 7 years (see Table 11–6). The maxillary permanent lateral incisors may be seen later than age 7 for some children.

With the exception of the third molars, all of the permanent teeth will usually have erupted by the end of the twelfth year. Except for the third molars, the enamel of all of the permanent teeth will have been completed by age 8. In the mandibular arch and following the first permanent molars and central incisors, the teeth erupt in immediate succession — that is, centrals, laterals, cuspids, first and second premolars, and second permanent molar from 6–7 years through 11–13 years of age. The same sequence takes place in the maxillary arch except for the maxillary cuspid, which usually erupts after the bicuspids or premolars and at about the time or before the eruption of the second permanent molars (Fig. 28–3).

The mandibular central incisor roots are complete by age 9. The roots of the four first permanent molars, the maxillary central incisors, and the mandibular lateral incisors are usually complete by age 10. The roots of the maxillary lateral incisors are complete by age 11.

Because the position of the dental lamina of the permanent teeth was located to the lingual of all of the primary teeth (except for the dental lamina coming off of the second primary for the three permanent molars), the anterior teeth develop in their vault or crypt lingual to and near the apex of the primary incisors. When the roots begin to form on the permanent teeth, they start to migrate toward the oral cavity. Generally, they follow a pattern such that they come across the primary root, resorbing it and erupting slightly labial to the location sustained by the primary tooth (Fig. 28–4). Therefore, the permanent teeth are usually always found angulated more buccally when compared with their primary predecessors (Fig. 28–5). The developing bicuspids develop between the roots of the primary molars and continue to erupt in a slight mesial position. The permanent molars develop from one dental lamina and like the bicuspids or premolars erupt in or at a mesial inclination or angle.

Compared with the primary incisors, the permanent incisors are larger and develop in a more restricted area (Finn, 1973). Their growth, although perpetual, is at a much slower rate during their eruption as compared with the pri-

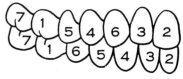

Figure 28–3 ■ Desirable eruption sequence for the permanent teeth. (Reproduced by permission from McDonald RE, Avery DR: Dentistry for the Child and Adolescent, 4th ed. St. Louis, 1983, The C. V. Mosby Co.)

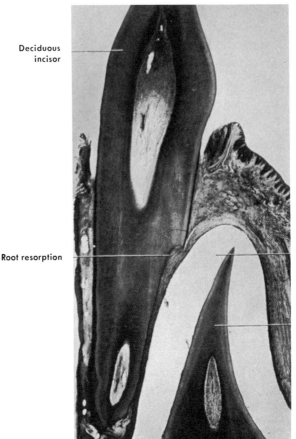

Deciduous incisor

Root resorption

Enamel of permanent incisor

Dentin

Figure 28–4 ■ Resorption of root of primary incisor owing to pressure of erupting successor. (Reproduced by permission from Bhaskar, S. N., editor: Orban's Oral Histology and Embryology, ed. 10, St. Louis, 1986, The C. V. Mosby Co.)

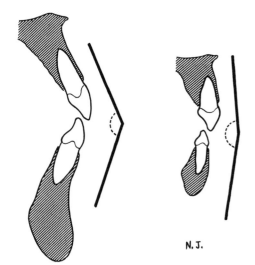

N. J.

Figure 28–5 ■ Angulation of permanent and primary incisors. (Reproduced with permission from Moyers, R. E.: HANDBOOK OF ORTHODONTICS, 3rd edition. Copyright © 1973 by Year Book Medical Publishers, Inc., Chicago.)

mary incisors. The inclinations of the eruptive paths of the permanent incisors account for their flared appearance. Also, it is natural to find diastemata between the incisors, particularly in the maxilla. The permanent canine in the maxillary arch is usually the last permanent tooth to erupt mesial to the first permanent molar. As the permanent canine begins to erupt, its mesial component of force is often adequate to straighten the incisors and close the diastemata. This period of development has been called the "ugly duckling stage" (Fig. 28–6) (Finn, 1973).

REFERENCE

Finn SB: Clinical Pedodontics, 4th ed. Philadelphia, WB Saunders Co, 1973.

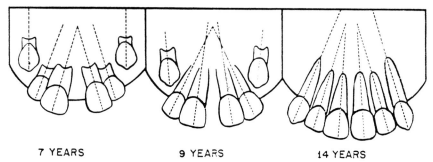

7 YEARS   9 YEARS   14 YEARS

Figure 28–6 ■ The "ugly duckling" stage. (From Finn SB: Clinical Pedodontics, 4th ed. Philadelphia, WB Saunders Co, 1973; after Broadbent BH: Angle Orthodont 1:183–208, 1937.)

COGNITIVE CHANGES

J. R. Pinkham

A book could easily be written describing the incredible cognitive acquisitions, adjustments, and sophistications made by a child from age 6 to age 12. Mental capacity alone grows exorbitantly. For example, by age 12 a child can outline on paper or mentally recall the travels of Marco Polo. At age 6 the concept of an ancient man from Italy going to China would not be remarkable and probably would be mentally unretainable.

In 1970, White concluded that between ages 5 and 7 years there may be a reorganization of the central nervous system that accounts for a dramatically increased ability to remain diligent at a task or attentive to a problem. Unquestionably, the attention span of the child after age 7 is substantially more than the child under 5 years of age.

The school age years of 6–12 are the years when a child becomes literate. Before age 6, few children can do much more than print their names. After age 12 most children will have accomplished an appropriate approach to grammar and syntax and will have the ability to increasingly sophisticate both oral and written communications. In some parts of the world, it is not uncommon for a child to be fluent in a second language by age 12.

According to Piaget, the ages between 6 and 12 roughly approximate his third major developmental stage of cognition, the phase of con-

crete operations. Piaget theorized the following four major periods of intellectual development:

1. *Sensorimotor*: birth to 18 months
2. *Preoperational*: 18 months to 7 years
3. *Concrete operations*: 7 to 12 years
4. *Formal operations*: 12 years and onward

So far this book has presented a study of the child through his sensorimotor and preoperational stages. In the concrete operations stage, Piaget has described numerous sophistications in the child's mental abilities. For instance, the 5-year-old may be able to walk "two blocks down, one block right to the second white house" to get to his aunt's residence, but this same 5-year-old could not draw this route out on a piece of paper. However, by age 7 or 8, the same child could portray the route by a self-drawn map. In other words, mental representations of actions become a part of the cognitive abilities of the child during these years. For the dentist who instructs children on the process of tooth decay, it may be helpful in designing his or her preventive presentation to understand the difference in mental representation ability of preschoolers and school age children. Obviously, two different presentations are needed.

During the years of 6–12 (7–12, according to Piaget) children will acquire abilities to understand the constancies between length, mass,

number, and weight despite external differences. Relativity will also emerge in the child's evaluation system. To the 4-year-old, the word "dark" means black. The 10-year-old can talk about a "dark" green car.

In summary, the child from age 6–12 cognitively grows up. By age 12 years, his mind and mental prowess have matured and he is capable of the assimilation of real as well as theoretical abstract information.

REFERENCE

White SH: Changes in Learning Processes in The Late Preschool Years. Presented at a meeting of The American Education Association, Chicago, Illinois, 1968.

EMOTIONAL CHANGES

J. R. Pinkham

The years of 6–12 are years of matriculation toward the acceptance of societal norms for behavior by the child. Crying, tantrums, and other rages will, for normal children, be relinquished as possible modes of expression of frustration. Whereas the preschooler needs, perhaps demands, immediate rewards and satisfaction, the child in the transitional years masters the emotional ability to delay gratification. This awareness of delay is reinforced by the child's schooling, and increasingly the child is guided toward the appropriate investment of his or her time into worthwhile activities. Homework, chores at home, caring for pets, newspaper delivery, scouting, team sports, and piano lessons are some of the behaviors expected of this age group, which were almost impossible during the preschool years.

Another emotional refinement that happens from age 6–12 is the ability to utilize life's tasks in ways effective enough to stave off boredom. Previously, the preschooler immersed his mental preoccupation into something until all his energy and attention was spent. Then, at the point of burn-out, he looked for his parents or other attendants to find something else for him to do. However, between ages 6 and 12 the need of adults to direct the child's attention rapidly recedes, and by age 12 a child usually has a ledger of wants and desires, a sense of the time that should be spent in their pursuit, and an ability to prioritize which wants and desires should come first or last.

In this age range, body image starts to become an emotional feature of the child's life. Unquestionably, for the majority of children the importance of body image will be most dramatic during adolescence, but its emergence is certainly during these years. Whereas the 6-year-old usually couldn't care less about ketchup on his face or mud on his pants, the 12-year-old may agonize over a blemish or over not having clothes that are stylish. In summary, bodily appearance becomes an emotional awareness and emphasis during these years. Unquestionably, this has dental ramifications. The mottled enamel of the 6-year-old may have disturbed only the child's parents. The child was indifferent. By age 12, this condition may account for a lack of smiling, social withdrawal, and forlornness by the child. Teasing could make these findings worse.

Although there certainly are exceptions, the majority of children from age 6–12 will find overall emotional satisfaction only when they are accepted by peers socially. Lack of acceptance, outright ostracism, and teasing can certainly be very emotionally damaging. During these years, with the help of parents, teachers, role models, and other significant people, it is important for the child to become emotionally resilient. The abilities to handle and recover from humiliation, frustration, loss, and disappointment need at least to start to emerge during these years. If they don't, adolescence presents a real danger.

SOCIAL CHANGES
J. R. Pinkham

The years between ages 6 and 12 are often referred to as middle childhood. These years are clearly more complicated socially than earlier years because of school, increasing importance of peers, and the enormous expansion of the child's social environment. These years will see the child intensify his focus on and pursuit of some already existing motives, while others are minimized or diminished completely.

School is certainly extremely important for this age group and represents an extrafamilial world that may reinforce social responses learned at home, portray new ones, and even retrain or deny others. Whether he or she is encountered earlier in preschool or now at school, the teacher is likely to be the first significant, day-by-day, authoritative adult outside the child's immediate family. Also, as opposed to baby sitters and relatives, the teacher is encountered by the child in an environment that the teacher has control over. In 1964, Franco concluded that a child's feelings about his first teacher correlate closely with the child's feelings about his mother.

Perhaps suprisingly, most children anticipate school positively and remain enthusiastic about their experiences there. It has also been noted that children's self-importance, self-control, and ability to be independent (e.g., getting one's own cereal for breakfast) heighten quickly during the first few months of school (Stendler and Young, 1951). These findings are less true for children from disadvantaged homes. Also, unfortunately, enthusiasm for school and teachers tends to decline in later years and this decline appears to be more significant in children from disadvantaged homes than in those from higher, more fortunate social classes. It has been speculated by some investigators that middle- and upper-middle-class parents may be better role models regarding school, since their children see them reading, studying, and pursuing other intellectual activities.

Unquestionably, teachers have an important impact on the socialization of a child. Space is far too limited in this text to discuss how different teacher attributes affect pupils, but unquestionably the characteristics of being fair and consistent, the capacity to maintain order without being overly authoritative, and the ability to praise effectively are appreciated by children and have very positive social effects.

The peer group that a child joins also can have powerful socializing forces. Sometimes the values of the peer group will be antithetical to those of the teacher and parents. This presents a conflict for the child in that he may risk reprimand from authoritative adults or ridicule or rejection from his peers if he conforms to one or the other's expectations. It is important for parents to understand these conflicts and how socially strong peer pressure can be in this age group. It is also important to note that the child who eagerly accepts a peer value that disappoints his parents may in fact be doing so for the feelings of acceptance and nurturing that were not sufficiently instilled in him at home.

One last factor marks the middle childhood years. This is the advent of increasingly stronger, more stable, and more meaningful friendships. Generally, friendships will be with the same sex. Friends at this age level also share as a rule similar socioeconomic status, intelligence, maturity, and interests.

REFERENCES

Franco D: The child's perception of "the teacher" as compared to his perception of "the mother." Dissert Abstr 24:3414–3415, 1964.

Stendler CB, Young N: Impact of first grade entrance upon the socialization of the child: Changes after eight months of school. Child Develop 22.:113–122, 1951.

Examination, diagnosis, and treatment planning

Paul Casamassimo □ John Christensen □ Henry Fields

The examination of the child in the transitional years presents the diagnostic dilemma of managing oral health at a dynamic stage of development. Although the preschooler's dentition is relatively stable, the child in the transitional years will go from a full complement of primary teeth, through a mixed dentition, to a full adult set of teeth, excluding the third molars. The ease and success of this transition constitute the main challenge for the dentist treating this age group. A large part of this chapter is devoted to orthodontic considerations, but the other elements of significance in dental management of this group should not be ignored. They are as follows:

1. *Preventive considerations related to tooth sealants, nutrition, and fluoride intake:* The eruption of permanent teeth may require a decision about sealant application. The entry into the more heterogeneous, less controlled environment of school places the child at risk for increased carbohydrate exposure. Finally, the child's access to fluoride in school, diet, and other sources makes re-evaluation of fluoride exposure necessary.

2. *Prevention and management of trauma:* The child in school may be active in sports; at the very least, he or she has expanded social interaction. For a period in the school years, the maxillary incisors are at greater risk for traumatic injury, especially if they protrude.

3. *Development of skills in personal oral hygiene:* The child emerging from the school years should have the skills and knowledge to provide effective personal oral hygiene.

4. *Participation in health care decisions:* Classic thought in dentistry sees the school age child as a passive recipient of care. Unfortunately, the result may be poor compliance and a tendency to consider the dentist rather than oneself as responsible for health.

The History

Elements of history taking and recording are discussed in Chapter 17. The parent remains the historian of choice, yet the older school age child can provide valid and corroborative information. An important aspect of history taking

in this group should be involvement of the child, whose role initially should be that of listener but whose role can evolve into that of participant. By adolescence, the child can provide accurate, valuable information. Some instances in which this involvement may have a profound benefit for provider and patient are when (1) antibiotic premedication for heart disease is required, (2) there is a history of illness that accompanies a complicated medical history, or (3) there is a history of a positive reaction to the hepatitis antigen. The payoff for imparting this knowledge to the young patient through a good physician-patient relationship many not be evident until the child seeks care alone as an adolescent.

A health history form should address issues similar to those for the younger child but with different expectations. The differences in patient history for this age child in general are the following:

1. Medical intervention has usually occurred. Most children will have a physician and may have had an emergency visit or an operation. School enrollment will have required a physical examination and other treatment for the majority of children.

2. A health history will have evolved. The child will have, by virtue of years, tested his or her coagulation and immunologic systems and possess a developmental profile. Most childhood-onset disorders will manifest themselves at some time during this period, if not already noted; therefore, symptomatology remains an important aspect of history taking.

3. A dental history should be evolving, with caries experiences, caries prevention, care delivery, and dental development as established parameters. Children usually will have had a dental visit as part of school enrollment.

The Examination

As in younger children, the examination includes a behavioral assessment; general appraisal; and head and neck, facial, intraoral, and radiographic examinations.

BEHAVIORAL ASSESSMENT

Another advantage for the dentist is the child's emergence into a period when few chil-

dren experience behavioral problems that cannot be resolved with simple tell, show, and do. Even early in this period, the child can be reasoned with to accept dental treatment. The child who resists attempts at careful and compassionate explanation of care may be suffering from a more significant emotional or psychological problem. The diagnostic process for behavioral problems is clearer in this age group because so few children will resist care. The dentist's diagnostic approach should include ruling out major behavioral problems by history and general appraisal. The next step is to "chair-test" the child, using the dentist's proven techniques of managing children. The technique used may be tell, show, do, positive reinforcement, voice control, or some other method that has worked consistently in the past. If this fails, the dentist should consider further evaluation or referral. Some causes of extreme behavior problems in this age group include substance abuse, physical or sexual abuse, family problems, or a minor learning disability.

GENERAL APPRAISAL

The school age population provides a wide range of physical and emotional profiles, yet the general appraisal should be easier from several standpoints. First, the school age child should have developed gross motor skills, and any variations from normal findings should be obvious. For example, the toddler may be active yet still clumsy. The school age child, even at the early end of this age group, can play with skill. Speech development should also well exceed that of the preschooler, as should emotional and intellectual status. This adaptation is really a manifestation of development of the brain and is one reason why schooling begins at this age.

An advantage available to the dentist examining children in this age group is the host of health professionals with whom to work if problems are noted. School placement has usually identified problem areas, and the appropriate therapy has usually been initiated. These professionals can assist in clarifying findings made at the dental visit. Table 29–1 lists some characteristics of the school age child that are important in the diagnostic process.

Table 29–1 ■ Selected developmental characteristics of the seven- to twelve-year-old child

Intellectual Development

Demonstrates school readiness early in this period

Should be able to read and write in this period

Becomes capable of logical thought

Psychological Development

Acquires sense of accomplishment for tasks

Learns responsibility for actions

Develops a sense of right and wrong

Looks outside the home for standards or values

Physical Development

Refinement of motor skills occurs as central nervous system develops

Spine straightens to improve posture

Sinuses enlarge

Lymphoid system reaches high point of development

Physiologic Development

6-Year-Old	9-Year-Old	12-Year-Old
Height		
Boys = 121 cm	Boys = 140 cm	Boys = 154 cm
Girls = 119 cm	Girls = 137 cm	Girls = 157 cm
(Growth rate is approximately 6 cm per year in this period.)		
Weight (75th percentile)		
Boys = 24 kg	Boys = 33 kg	Boys = 44 kg
Girls = 23 kg	Girls = 32 kg	Girls = 45 kg
(Growth rate is approximately 3–3.5 kg per year.)		
Pulse (average for age)		
100/min	90/min	85–90/min
Respiration (50th percentile)		
23/min	20/min	18/min
Blood pressure (average for age)		
105/60 mm Hg	110/65 mm Hg	115/65 mm Hg

HEAD AND NECK EXAMINATION

The head and neck examination should be completed in a manner similar to that outlined in Chapter 17.

FACIAL EXAMINATION

Facial examination of the 6- to 12-year-old child is a systematic description of the face in three planes of space. It is essentially the same as the facial examination described in Chapter 17, and the reader should review the substance

of this examination if needed. This section elaborates on findings that are particularly important to the 6- to 12-year-old.

The profile examination notes the anteroposterior and vertical dimensions of the face and the position of the lips and incisors relative to the face. The ideal soft tissue profile is slightly convex to straight (Fig. 29–1). Most clinicians find that detection of anteroposterior skeletal problems is somewhat easier in this age group, possibly owing to reduced soft tissue thickness. A mild mandibular deficiency in a 4-year-old child may have been difficult to diagnose initially, but it is more apparent at age 8 and even more obvious at age 12. If a skeletal problem exists, the source of the discrepancy is identified by comparing the position of the maxilla and mandible with a vertical reference line (see Chapter 17).

In this age group, vertical profile assessment continues to concentrate on the proportionality of the upper, middle, and lower facial thirds. At this point, growth has increased the vertical lin-

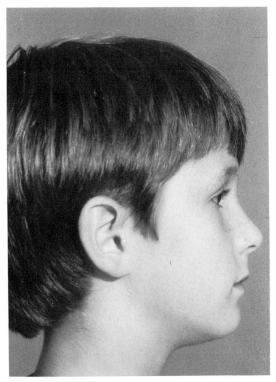

Figure 29–1 ■ The ideal soft tissue profile is slightly convex to straight when considering the bridge of the nose, the base of the upper lip, and the depth of the labio-mental fold in the anteroposterior dimension for the 6- to 12-year-old child.

ear facial dimensions; however, the proportionality of the well-balanced face remains basically the same. Research has indicated that vertical dysplasia is confined to the lower facial third in this age group (Fields et al, 1984). If this is true, the middle and upper thirds can be used as standards to compare with the lower facial third.

Incisor and lip position should be examined carefully in this age group. The child is entering the mixed dentition period, and the position of the erupting permanent incisors will be reflected in the position of the lips. The upper lip is of fairly uniform size and thickness and gives a good indication of the underlying position of the maxillary incisor. The position of the lower lip is also dependent on the position of the maxillary incisor. This is because the lower lip normally covers 1–2 mm of the maxillary inci-

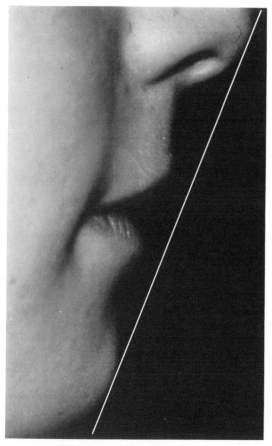

Figure 29–2 ■ In this age group, the lips are positioned on or slightly behind a line connecting the tip of the nose with the soft tissue chin. Lip position must be considered in the context of the nose and chin. A large nose and chin will be more able to accommodate protrusive lips than will a small nose and chin.

sal edge at rest. Therefore, lip posture is a strong indicator of maxillary dental protrusion. Lip and incisor position should always be considered in the context of the nose and chin. The lips should be positioned on or slightly behind a line connecting the tip of the nose with the chin (Fig. 29–2). A large nose and chin will be more able to accommodate protrusive incisors and lips than will a small nose and chin.

INTRAORAL EXAMINATION

The procedures for oral examination are similar to those in the preschool group and include the charting of teeth and dental caries. Less emphasis needs to be placed on developing behavior with the examination process, since these children will be more cooperative. The areas of evaluation that require more emphasis are the periodontal, preventive, and orthodontic aspects.

Periodontal Evaluation

A thorough examination of this age group involves both periodontal probing and use of a gingival index if inflammation is a problem. The periodontal examination should address the following:

1. *Selective probing of anterior teeth and first permanent molars:* The likelihood of bone loss and migration of the attachment is slight, but some children in this age group will experience juvenile periodontitis. Erupting teeth will usually have a deep sulcus until the crown is fully erupted. Gingival inflammation in early puberty may also confound pocket depth measurements.

2. *Evaluation of tissue attachments, especially those of the lower anterior teeth:* Facial clefts as a result of malposition and abnormal muscle attachments, if identified early, can be successfully managed with grafting, tooth movement, or a combination of both (Fig. 29–3).

3. *Identification of problem areas, such as mandibular and maxillary anterior teeth:* Calculus accumulation, inflammation secondary to anterior crowding, mouth breathing and poor cleaning, and eruptive gingivitis are examples of localized problems.

Numerous gingival indices exist to assess inflammation. The gingival index (GI) (Loe and Silness, 1963) can be adapted for pediatric use. The GI uses the following scoring system:

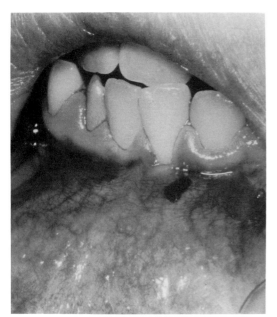

Figure 29 – 3 ■ The labial gingival cleft is caused by a lack of attached gingival tissue, abnormally high (coronal) muscle attachment, anterior crossbite, or a combination of any or all of these factors.

0   Normal gingiva
1   Mild inflammation: slight change in color, slight edema, no bleeding on probing
2   Moderate inflammation: redness, edema, and glazing; bleeding on probing
3   Severe inflammation: marked redness and edema; tendency for spontaneous bleeding; ulceration

In the private practice setting, it may be easier to modify an existing index, using key teeth to provide baseline readings and progress. These readings can be recorded on the examination form adjacent to the data for the teeth being examined. Full mouth probing performed routinely is not warranted.

Oral Hygiene Evaluation

The assessment of clinical needs and patient skills in oral hygiene is a part of the examination process. The history should reveal a pattern of personal care, while the clinical examination should address problem areas in the oral cavity. A patient's brushing skills and dexterity for flossing can be judged at chairside with direct correlation to clinically identified deficiencies, such as plaque accumulation opposite the side on which the brush is held, buccally placed canine teeth, difficult to reach lingual surfaces, and sensitive areas. The information should be used to formulate a hygiene strategy for that child.

Occlusal Evaluation

The occlusal evaluation is organized around a systematic approach of alignment and around the anteroposterior, transverse, and vertical planes of space.

Alignment

The intraoral occlusal examination in the mixed dentition begins with assessment of arch form and alignment characteristics. An ideal arch should be symmetrical in the anteroposterior and transverse dimensions. Minor asymmetry may exist but is usually confined to the anterior region if there is inadequate space for the eruption of the permanent incisors. Significant asymmetry is rare and is usually indicative of skeletal asymmetry or some type of oral habit that has displaced the teeth and alveolus. Arch form is described as being either U- or V-shaped.

After the form and symmetry of each arch have been characterized, it is imperative to count the number of permanent and primary teeth. A clinical examination and a panoramic radiograph will allow the practitioner to determine which teeth are present, developing, or missing. Disturbances in the initiation and proliferation stage of tooth development may lead to an abnormal number of teeth. Teeth that do not form are termed congenitally missing teeth (Fig. 29 – 4). The most common missing teeth in the permanent dentition, with the exception of the maxillary and mandibular third molars, are the maxillary lateral incisor and the mandibular second premolar (Shafer et al, 1974). In general, the most distal tooth in a class of teeth is congenitally missing most often.

Supernumerary teeth are extra or in addition to the normal complement of teeth. These teeth are most often found in the maxillary midline region and are called mesiodens (Fig. 29 – 5). Supernumerary teeth also are found frequently distal to the maxillary molars and in the mandibular premolar regions (Shafer et al, 1974).

Although not a tooth in the strictest sense, the odontoma is discussed in this section on tooth number. The odontoma is a benign, mixed tumor of enamel and dentin that is diagnosed radiographically. Two types of odontomas are identified. Odontomas that resemble teeth are

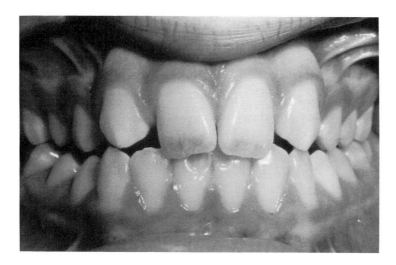

Figure 29-4 ■ This patient is congenitally missing both maxillary lateral incisors. The most common missing teeth in the permanent dentition, besides the third molars, are the maxillary lateral incisor and the mandibular second premolar.

called compound odontomas; those that are irregular in shape are labeled as complex. Both types may interfere with normal tooth eruption and are usually treated by surgical removal before eruption problems arise but late enough to avoid surgical trauma to adjacent developing teeth (Fig. 29-6).

Disturbances in the morphodifferentiation and histodifferentiation stages of tooth development will result in alterations of tooth size and shape. Each arch should be examined for generalized large (macrodontia) or small (microdontia) teeth and for localized tooth size discrepancies. Generalized large or small teeth

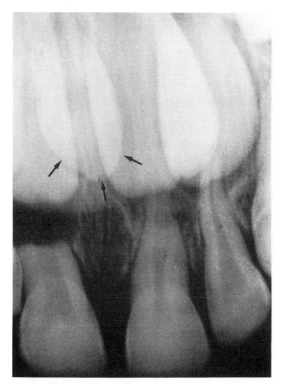

Figure 29-5 ■ A midline supernumerary tooth, or mesiodens, is situated between the unerupted maxillary central incisors. Arrows indicate the position of the mesiodens, which can cause eruption and tooth formation disturbances.

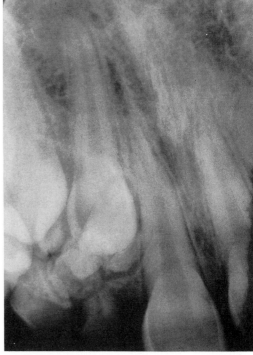

Figure 29-6 ■ In this radiograph, a complex odontoma is impeding the eruption of the maxillary right lateral incisor and canine. The odontoma should be surgically removed before eruption problems arise but late enough to avoid surgical trauma to the adjacent developing teeth. (Courtesy of Dr. Phillip R. Parker.)

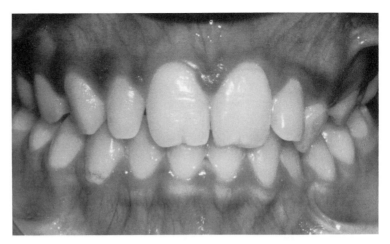

Figure 29-7 ■ This maxillary right lateral incisor is smaller than normal in size; such a tooth is often called a peg lateral, owing to its mesio-distal tapered form. Localized tooth size problems of this type make it difficult to establish good dental relationships.

usually can be aligned so that there is a compatible occlusal relationship. However, localized tooth size problems make it difficult to establish good dental relationships. Undersized maxillary lateral incisors and mandibular second premolars are the most common isolated tooth size problems (Fig. 29-7). Again, the most distal tooth in the dental class is most often affected. Sometimes, complex orthodontic and restorative treatment is necessary to achieve a harmonious occlusal relationship and meet esthetic requirements when local tooth size problems exist.

Teeth with abnormal crown and root structures may create occlusal problems. Careful clinical and radiographic examination is necessary to diagnose these problems. If the abnormality involves the crown (maxillary peg lateral or talon cusp), the crown will need to be recontoured by adding restorative material to increase the crown size or reduced in size by selective equilibration to eliminate occlusal interferences. Either condition usually requires tooth movement prior to definitive restorative care to obtain an esthetic and functional result. Root structure abnormalities such as dilaceration may make orthodontic movement of teeth very difficult (Fig. 29-8). Often the portion of the root apical to the irregularity is resorbed during tooth movement. Additionally, if a tooth with root abnormalities is scheduled for extraction, it may be prudent to refer the patient to a specialist because the abnormality will certainly complicate the extraction.

The position of erupted and unerupted permanent teeth in this age group should be noted and compared with the normal sequence and time of eruption. Minor asymmetry in dental eruption is normal, and there is little concern if

less than 6 months difference in eruption exists between contralateral sides of the mouth.

Three tooth positioning problems are associated with the mixed dentition: ectopic erup-

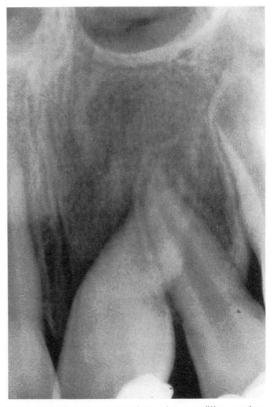

Figure 29-8 ■ Root structure abnormalities, such as this dilacerated maxillary left central incisor, make orthodontic movement of teeth very difficult. A dilaceration of this magnitude makes the root more susceptible to apical resorption and complicates final crown and root positioning.

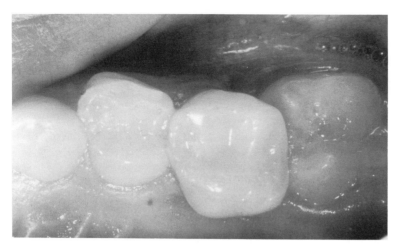

Figure 29–9 ■ In ectopic eruption, the permanent first molar resorbs a portion of the distal root of the primary second molar. In this case, the permanent first molar has lodged under the primary second molar crown. In other cases, the permanent molar will spontaneously "jump" or move distally and erupt into normal position.

tion, impaction, and the midline diastema. Ectopic eruption is a term used to describe a path of eruption that causes root resorption of a portion or all of the adjacent primary tooth. Ectopic eruption is most often associated with the permanent maxillary first molar and mandibular lateral incisor (Pulver, 1968; Gellin and Haley, 1982). In ectopic eruption, the permanent first molar resorbs a portion of the distal root of the primary second molar (Fig. 29–9). In many cases, the permanent molar will spontaneously "jump" or move distally and erupt into correct position. In other cases, the permanent molar will lodge under the primary molar crown and no longer erupt. There is no pain or discomfort associated with ectopic eruption unless a communication develops between the oral cavity and the pulpal tissue of the primary molar, causing an abscess.

The prevalence of permanent first molar ectopic eruption is reported to be 3–4% (Kimmel et al, 1982). Several reasons have been proposed to explain ectopic molar eruption: (1) the maxillary teeth are larger in size than normal, (2) the maxilla is smaller than normal, (3) the maxilla is positioned further posteriorly than normal in relation to the cranial base, and (4) the angulation of the erupting maxillary permanent first molar is abnormal (Pulver, 1968). Although ectopic molar eruption may occur in the mandibular arch, it is more common in the maxilla.

Ectopic eruption of the permanent lateral incisor is most often seen in the mandibular arch. The erupting incisor resorbs all or a portion of the primary canine root because the path of eruption is abnormal or arch length is deficient (Fig. 29–10). The primary canine will either exfoliate prematurely or impede further eruption of the lateral incisor.

A related phenomenon is lingual eruption of the permanent incisors, predominately the mandibular incisors. The prevalence of lingually erupting mandibular incisors is about

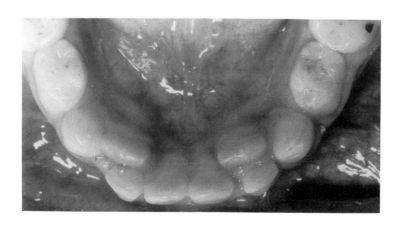

Figure 29–10 ■ Ectopic eruption of the permanent lateral incisors is most often seen in the mandibular arch. In this example, the mandibular lateral incisors erupted lingual to their ideal position and the primary laterals are still present. In some cases, the lateral incisors will erupt into more normal position but will cause the premature exfoliation of the primary canine.

10% (Gellin and Haley, 1982). The cause of ectopic and lingually erupting incisors is not well established. One explanation suggests that ectopic and lingual eruption of the incisors is due to an abnormal pattern of resorption. Alternatively, it has been suggested that lingual eruption is a variation of the normal eruption pattern because the lower incisor tooth buds form lingual to the primary incisors and may not migrate facially.

Tooth impaction is diagnosed during the clinical examination or from appropriate radiographs. Impaction of anterior teeth is caused by overretained primary teeth, supernumerary teeth, severe crowding, or failure in the eruption mechanism (Fig. 29–11). The permanent tooth usually erupts if the overretained primary tooth or supernumerary is removed. If the tooth is impacted as a result of crowding, it is necessary to provide space either orthodontically or by extraction to allow eruption. Treatment is discussed in the next section.

Posterior tooth impaction is normally the result of inadequate arch length. Inadequate arch length is caused by a tooth-jaw size discrepancy or space loss as a result of premature primary tooth loss. If the arch length problem is generalized, either permanent teeth need to be removed or the arch needs to be expanded to allow eruption of all the permanent teeth. Limited, localized crowding from space loss can be treated by regaining the lost space orthodontically.

Primary failure of eruption is an unusual eruption problem affecting posterior teeth. It is diagnosed when a tooth fails to erupt despite the fact there is adequate space and no overlying hard tissue to prevent eruption. Furthermore, all teeth distal to the affected tooth also fail to erupt. The cause of primary failure of eruption is unknown (Proffit and Vig, 1981).

A small, maxillary midline diastema in the early mixed dentition is normal. Typically, it is caused by the position of the unerupted lateral incisors and/or canines (Fig. 29–12). The unerupted teeth are positioned superior and distal to the roots of the central incisors and direct the central incisor roots toward the midline and the crowns to the distal. As the lateral incisors or canines erupt, the incisors upright slowly and

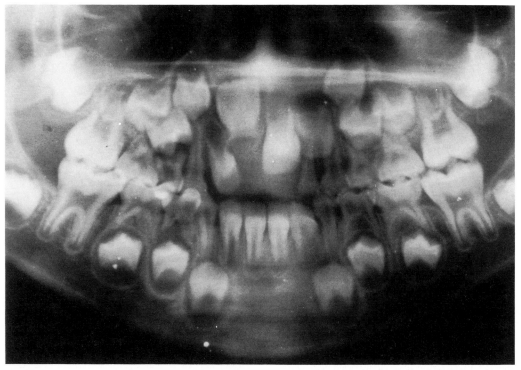

Figure 29–11 ■ In this age group, tooth impaction in the anterior region is usually caused by overretained primary teeth, supernumerary teeth, or severe crowding. In a small number of cases, a failure in the eruption mechanism is responsible for the delayed eruption. In this case, the maxillary right central incisor is completely inverted and is directed toward the nasal cavity.

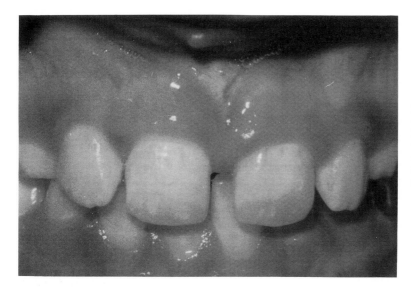

Figure 29-12 ■ A small maxillary midline diastema is normal in the mixed dentition. The diastema will tend to close with the eruption of the permanent maxillary lateral incisors and canines.

the midline space begins to close. Treatment to close a diastema is usually delayed until the permanent canines are fully erupted.

If the diastema is larger than 3 mm, the cause may be a mesiodens, a localized tooth size problem, or abnormal incisor positioning. A mesiodens is usually discovered in the radiographic examination, and its removal will normally allow the diastema to close. A size mismatch between the upper and lower teeth may result in a diastema. Normally, the maxillary incisor crowns are small or excessively tapered, although the mandibular teeth may be too large in relation to the maxillary teeth. If large spaces are present, a combination of tooth movement and anterior restorations will be required to correct a size discrepancy. Abnormal incisor positioning and protrusion also may result in a midline diastema. The positioning may be due to past or present finger habits or to abnormal eruption and is best treated by retracting the incisors orthodontically and consolidating space.

During the examination of each arch, a detailed inspection of the periodontium should be completed. Orthodontic treatment may be delayed or the treatment plan altered if the periodontal tissues are not healthy. Orthodontic treatment initiated during periods of active gingival or periodontal disease may further compromise periodontal health because fixed appliances are difficult to keep clean and existing inflammatory conditions will be exacerbated and result in further loss of supporting structures. A periodontal probe is necessary to evaluate the health of the tissues properly (Fig. 29–13). The probe measures the depth of the sulcus and the amount of free marginal and attached gingiva. Sulcular depths greater than 3 mm and attached gingiva of less than 1 mm indicate possible periodontal disease, and further evaluation is warranted. The amount of attached gingiva should also be considered in the context of the type of tooth movement being planned. Facial movement of a lower incisor with minimal attached gingiva may cause further loss of attachment, and a gingival grafting procedure should be considered. Lingual movement of the same incisor does not involve the same risk of loss of attachment and may even contribute to an increase in attached tissue.

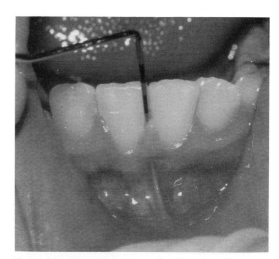

Figure 29–13 ■ During examination of each arch, a periodontal probe is used to evaluate gingival health. Orthodontic treatment initiated during periods of active gingival or periodontal disease may further compromise periodontal health.

Oral hygiene and gingival health should be evaluated by using plaque, gingival, and bleeding indices. Oral hygiene instructions should be given before orthodontic treatment is started and should be consistently reinforced during the treatment. Lastly, the position of frena and their height of attachment on the alveolar ridge should be determined by gently manipulating the lips and cheeks. Occasionally, frenal attachments near the crest of the ridge need to be repositioned prior to or following orthodontic treatment because they pull on attached mar-

ginal tissue and compromise gingival health or prevent space closure.

Anteroposterior Dimension

Permanent molar and canine relationships should be noted and compared with the anteroposterior skeletal relationships that were determined during the extraoral examination. Permanent molar and canine relationships are illustrated in Figure 29–14. Dental relationships normally reflect the underlying skeletal

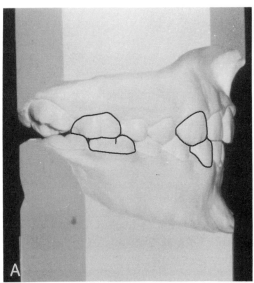

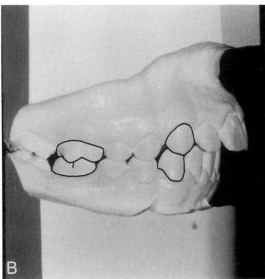

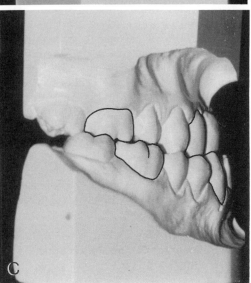

Figure 29–14 ■ A, In the permanent dentition, permanent molar and canine relationships are determined and compared with the anteroposterior skeletal relationships. To determine molar relationships, the position of the mesio-buccal cusp of the permanent maxillary first molar is related to the position of the facial groove of the permanent mandibular first molar. If the mesio-buccal cusp occludes in the facial groove, the molar relationship is termed Class I. The canine relationship is determined by the relationship of the maxillary canine to the embrasure between the mandibular canine and first premolar (or primary first molar). If the maxillary canine occludes in the embrasure, the canine relationship is also called Class I. B, If the mesio-buccal cusp of the permanent maxillary first molar occludes mesial to the mandibular facial groove, the molar relationship is termed Class II. The canine relationship is Class II if the maxillary canine occludes mesial to the mandibular canine–first premolar embrasure. C, If the mesio-buccal cusp of the permanent maxillary first molar occludes distal to the mandibular facial groove, the molar relationship is termed Class III. The canine relationship is Class III if the maxillary canine occludes distal to the mandibular canine–first premolar embrasure.

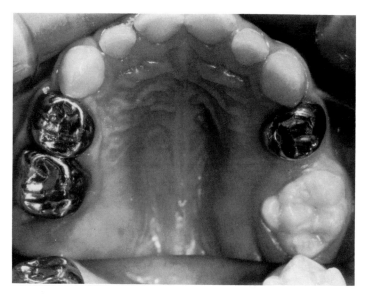

Figure 29–15 ■ Dental relationships usually reflect the underlying skeletal relationships, although it is possible to have different dental and skeletal relationships. In this case, the molar relationship on the left side is different from the molar relationship on the right side, as well as different from the skeletal relationship. This is because the primary maxillary left second molar was lost prematurely and the permanent maxillary left first molar drifted mesially during eruption.

relationships, although it is feasible to have different dental and skeletal relationships if teeth are missing or have drifted. For example, an individual with a Class I skeletal relationship may have a Class II molar relationship on one side if a primary maxillary second molar was lost prematurely and if the permanent maxillary first molar was allowed to drift forward into the space (Fig. 29–15).

If the permanent teeth are properly aligned in the alveolar bone at a normal angulation, overjet is a direct measurement of the relationship between the dental arches. Normal overjet is approximately 2 mm; therefore, the discrepancy between the arches can be calculated by subtracting 2 mm from the measured overjet. Incisor position is not always ideal, however, and estimates of dental arch discrepancies must be adjusted if both upper and lower anterior teeth are not protrusive or retrusive.

Transverse Relationship

Dental midline and posterior crossbite evaluation is conducted in the same manner as described in Chapter 17. Functional deviations of the mandible are identified by noting discrepancies between centric relation and centric occlusion. Posterior crossbites are determined to be either unilateral or bilateral. As the child becomes older, it becomes more critical to identify whether a crossbite is due to skeletal or dental causes. In the early mixed dentition years, treatments for both skeletal and dental crossbites are essentially the same. However, treatment of posterior crossbite in the complete permanent dentition differs, depending on whether the crossbite is skeletal or dental in origin.

Vertical Dimension

The vertical dental examination is concerned with overbite–open bite measurements and ankylosis. Normal overbite in this age group is approximately 2 mm. If there is a deviation from normal, the clinician should try to determine if the deviation is due to a dental or a skeletal problem. Treatment of the malocclusion varies, depending on the source of the problem.

Ankylosis of primary teeth can present several problems because of the magnitude of vertical dentoalveolar growth. Dental eruption and vertical growth of the alveolus may be as much as 10 mm from age 6–12. Thus, ankylosis of a primary tooth at an early age may result in large marginal ridge discrepancies, tipping of adjacent teeth, and vertical bone loss. Most of these problems, with the exception of space loss, will resolve when the succedaneous tooth erupts. Ankylosis and associated problems are discussed in Chapter 17, and the reader is referred there for more detail.

Supplemental Orthodontic Diagnostic Techniques

Orthodontic treatment in the mixed dentition is more complex than treatment in the primary dentition. The clinician must consider the difference in size between the primary and perma-

nent dentitions, the amount of space available for the permanent dentition, and the dental and skeletal relationships of the patient. This formidable job requires supplemental information to make accurate orthodontic diagnoses and to develop coherent treatment plans.

Diagnostic study casts are an essential part of a thorough evaluation. Findings recorded during the intraoral examination are reviewed and are confirmed on the study models. Alignment and tooth position characteristics should receive special attention because appliance design must be appropriate for each rotation and displacement.

After the diagnostic casts are studied, analyses are performed to determine tooth size relationships and arch length adequacy. The tooth size analysis attempts to compare the size of teeth in one arch with the size of teeth in the other. Tooth size must be compatible to ensure that teeth fit together correctly after treatment. The arch length analysis attempts to predict whether there is sufficient space available in the dental arch for the unerupted permanent teeth.

Tooth Size Analysis

The tooth size analysis is calculated, using a method development by Bolton (1958). Bolton selected 55 cases of excellent occlusion and measured the mesio-distal diameter of all teeth on the casts except for the permanent second and third molars. From the measurements, Bolton determined that a certain ratio existed between the size of the upper and lower teeth. A ratio could be determined for either the 6 anterior teeth or all 12 of the measured teeth. Little constructed a table based on the Bolton ratios to simplify tooth size determinations (Proffit et al, 1986). To use the table, the mesio-distal width of each individual tooth is measured with a needle-pointed divider or Boley gauge (Fig. 29–16). The widths of the teeth are summed, and the intersection of the mandibular and maxillary totals is located on the table. The intersection gives the tooth size discrepancy in mm (Fig. 29–17). Because there is some error in measuring the casts and some error in the analysis itself, tooth size discrepancies of 1.5 mm or less are not considered significant.

Several clinical situations contribute to tooth size discrepancy. The maxillary lateral incisor is commonly smaller than normal, resulting in a mandibular anterior tooth size excess. The second premolar often exhibits size variability in the posterior segment. When significant tooth size discrepancies are discovered, the child is best referred to a specialist because simple tooth movement will not produce good esthetics or occlusion. Treatment of tooth size discrepancies often requires a combination of tooth movement and restorative dentistry.

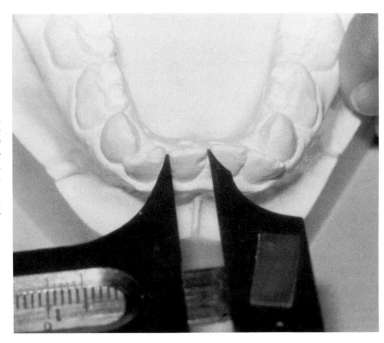

Figure 29–16 ■ To complete the tooth size analysis developed by Bolton, the mesio-distal width of each permanent tooth (except for second and third molars) is measured with a Boley gauge or a needle-pointed divider. The measurements are added together to provide totals for the six anterior teeth and for the overall arch.

BOLTON ANALYSIS

Maxillary Anterior Excess

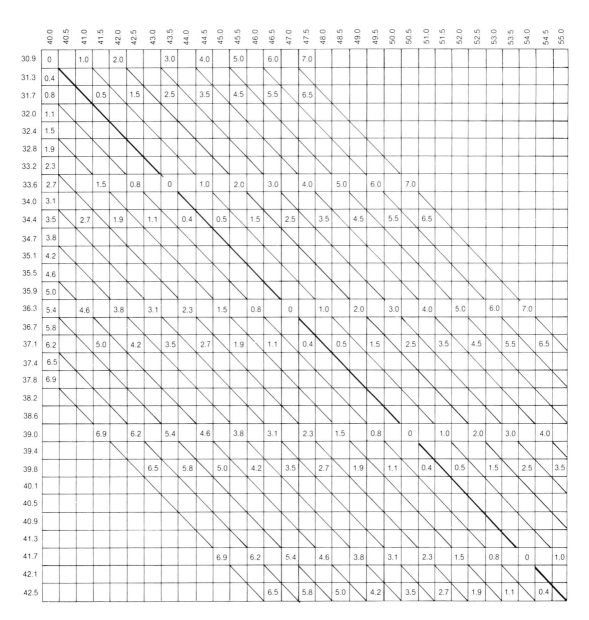

A

Mandibular Anterior Excess

Figure 29–17 ■ To determine if there is an anterior or overall tooth size discrepancy, the intersection of the maxillary and mandibular totals is located on the appropriate table. *A*, The width of the mandibular anterior teeth is indicated on the vertical axis, and the width of the maxillary anterior teeth is found on the horizontal axis. The intersection indicates if a tooth size discrepancy exists, whether it is a maxillary or mandibular excess, and the size of the discrepancy in mm. *B*, This table provides the same information for overall tooth size relationships. (Courtesy of Dr. Robert Little. Reproduced by permission from Proffit WR, Ackerman JL: Orthodontic diagnosis: The development of a problem list. *In* Proffit WR, et al: Contemporary Orthodontics. St. Louis, 1986, The C. V. Mosby Co.)

BOLTON ANALYSIS

Maxillary Overall Excess

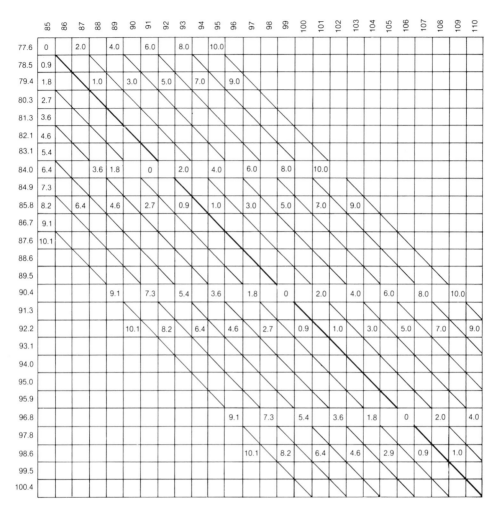

Mandibular Overall Excess

B

Figure 29–17 ■ *(Continued)*

Space Analysis

The space analysis is normally completed in the mixed dentition and is used to predict the amount of space available for the unerupted permanent teeth. A number of different space analyses exist; however, all space analyses have two features in common. First, the permanent first molars and the mandibular incisors must be erupted to perform the analysis. Second, the mandibular incisors (sometimes in addition to other measurements) are used to predict the size of the unerupted canines and premolars.

The following four assumptions are made in calculating a space analysis:

1. All permanent teeth are developing normally. Although this seems obvious, the analysis is meaningless if teeth are congenitally missing.

2. There is a correlation between the size of the erupted mandibular incisors and the remaining succedaneous teeth. The stronger the correlation, the more accurate will be the prediction of unerupted tooth size.

3. The prediction tables are valid for a broad population. The ethnic background of the patients used in most space analysis studies is Northwest European. If the patient is not of Northwest European descent, the analysis should be interpreted with some caution.

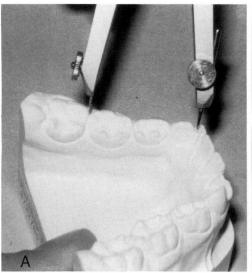
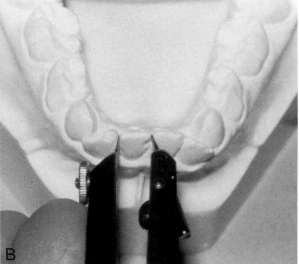

$$\frac{\text{sum of incisors}}{2} + 10.5 \text{ mm} = \begin{array}{c}\text{predicted width of canine}\\ \text{and 2 premolars in one}\\ \text{mandibular quadrant}\end{array}$$

C

$$\begin{array}{c}\text{total arch}\\\text{length}\end{array} - \begin{array}{c}\text{sum of}\\\text{incisors}\end{array} - \begin{array}{c}\text{2 (predicted}\\\text{width)}\end{array} = \begin{array}{c}\text{available}\\\text{arch length}\end{array}$$

D

Figure 29 – 18 ■ *A*, The first step in the Tanaka-Johnston space analysis is to determine available arch length. This is accomplished by dividing the arch into several segments and measuring each segment over the contact points and incisal edges of the teeth. *B*, The second step is to measure the width of the four mandibular incisors and add them together. *C*, The mesio-distal width of the unerupted canine and premolars in one quadrant is calculated by the above formula. In the mandibular arch, 10.5 mm is used to determine the canine-premolar widths. In the maxillary arch, half the sum of the mandibular incisors is still used but 11.0 mm is substituted for 10.5 mm because the unerupted permanent maxillary teeth are slightly larger. *D*, The final step in the analysis is to subtract the width of the four incisors and the predicted canine-premolar widths from the total arch length. The remainder is the available arch length. If the remainder is positive, there is adequate space in the arch. If the remainder is negative, the permanent teeth require more room to erupt than is available in the arch.

4. Arch dimensions remain stable throughout growth. This assumption is made to simplify the procedure, even though it is recognized that the intercanine width, intermolar width, and arch length dimensions do change slightly with age and eruption of teeth. Skeletal growth patterns may also affect arch dimension stability. Class II mandibular deficient individuals tend to have proclined mandibular incisors to compensate for the deficiency, whereas Class III individuals tend to have more upright or retroclined mandibular incisors.

The most accurate space analysis currently available is a modification of the Hixon-Oldfather analysis (Staley et al, 1984). This analysis uses lower incisor widths and the width of the unerupted premolars measured from radiographs to predict permanent tooth size. The Tanaka-Johnston analysis is most clinically useful because it requires no additional radio-

graphs or tables to predict tooth size (Tanaka and Johnston, 1974). The first step in the Tanaka-Johnston analysis is to determine available arch length. The distance from the mesial of the permanent first molar to the mesial of the contralateral permanent first molar is measured by dividing the arch into several segments (Fig. 29 – 18*A*). Each segment is measured over the contact points and incisal edges of teeth. The segments are added together to provide an approximation of total arch length. The second step in the analysis is to measure the width of the four mandibular incisors (Fig. 29 – 18*B*). The widths of the four incisors are added together to provide the amount of room necessary for ideal alignment. The mesio-distal width of the unerupted canine and premolars in one quadrant is predicted by adding 10.5 mm to one half the width of the four lower incisors (Fig. 29 – 18*C*). The final step in the space analysis is to subtract the width of the lower incisors and two times

the calculated premolar and canine width (both sides) from the total arch length approximation (Fig. 29–18D). If the result is positive, there is more space available in the arch than is needed for the unerupted teeth. If the result is negative, the unerupted teeth require more space than is available to erupt in ideal alignment.

The maxillary space analysis is conducted in the same way. Maxillary arch length is measured, the width of the maxillary incisors is determined, and 11.0 mm is added to half the width of the four lower incisors to predict the size of the unerupted maxillary canine and premolars in one quadrant. The incisor width and the predicted canine-premolar width is subtracted from the total arch length to determine the amount of space available in the maxillary arch.

After the arch length predictions are made, the clinician should return to the cast and decide if the results make sense. For example, if the arch appears to be crowded and the analysis predicts 5 mm of excess space, the analysis should be repeated or examined for mistakes. Furthermore, the results should be thought of in the context of the patient's soft tissue profile. The space analysis may indicate that the patient is moderately short of space, yet because the patient has very retrusive lips and incisors the treatment of choice would be to expand the arch by moving the incisors facially to provide better lip support (Fig. 29–19). Conversely, an analysis may predict that there is no crowding, yet extractions are considered necessary because the patient has very protrusive teeth and

lips (Fig. 29–20). Dental protrusion and dental crowding are actually manifestations of the same problem. Whether the arch is crowded or the incisors protrusive is dependent on the interaction between the pressure of the resting tongue and circumoral musculature.

Two factors must be considered when using the Tanaka-Johnston analysis. It tends to overpredict the width of the unerupted teeth slightly in the study sample. This makes the amount of crowding appear more severe than it actually is. In addition, if the patient is not of Northwest European background, it is difficult to know if the prediction will be over- or understated. An alternative method to determine available space is to measure arch length and incisor width as noted previously and then obtain periapical radiographs of the canines and premolars. The mesio-distal widths of the unerupted teeth are measured on the periapical films and then corrected for magnification by comparing the width of erupted teeth on the films with the actual width of these teeth on the cast. By using this technique, an individual space analysis can be performed for every patient. The disadvantage of this technique is that the patient is exposed to more radiation.

Analysis of Cephalometric Head Films

Analysis of lateral cephalometric head films is an additional diagnostic aid used to determine the relationship of the skeletal and dental structures. The cephalometric head film is normally ordered when significant skeletal dis-

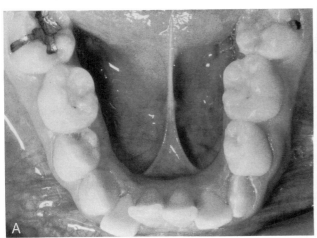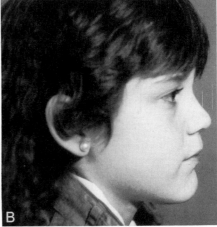

Figure 29–19 ■ The results of the space analysis (A) are thought of in the context of the patient's soft tissue profile. In this example, the space analysis indicates that the patient is short of arch length. However, the profile analysis (B) indicates that the patient cannot tolerate further loss of lip support. It is more prudent to expand the arch in this case to provide additional space than to extract teeth.

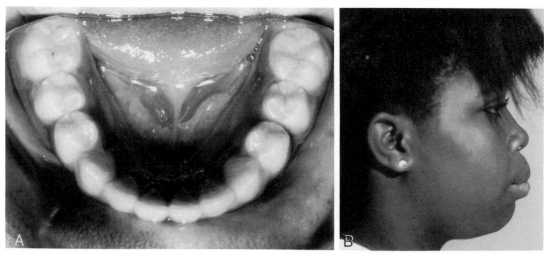

Figure 29–20 ■ In this example, the space analysis (A) indicates that there is no shortage of arch length. However, the profile analysis (B) indicates that the patient has extremely protrusive lips and incisors. It is more prudent to extract teeth and retract the incisors and lips in this case. This illustrates the fact that dental crowding and dental protrusion are actually manifestations of the same problem.

crepancies exist and comprehensive orthodontic treatment is being considered. The cephalometric analysis does not replace the facial profile analysis; it provides more specific information about the contribution of each skeletal and dental component to the malocclusion. The facial profile analysis should be used by the clinician to gather basic information about the spatial relationships of the teeth and jaws. If the clinician identifies significant anteroposterior or vertical discrepancies, the patient should be evaluated by a specialist. At that time, a lateral cephalometric radiograph may be used to obtain a precise assessment of the problem.

A large number of cephalometric analyses exist; however, the common goal of all analyses is to determine the size and position of the skeletal structures and the position of the teeth. The first step in the cephalometric analysis is to obtain a diagnostic head film. For the radiograph to be diagnostic, the head must be positioned within a cephalostat in a natural, relaxed posture (Fig. 29–21). In other words, the patient's head should not be tipped up or down, because this will alter the perceived relationship of the skeletal structures. A mandibular deficiency may not be apparent if the patient's head is tipped upward. Natural head position is produced by having the patient look at the distant horizon. The teeth should be together and the lips relaxed when the film is exposed.

After the head film is made, the radiograph should be screened for pathologic findings. If

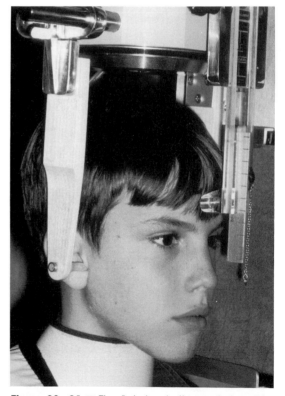

Figure 29–21 ■ The first step in the cephalometric analysis is to obtain a diagnostic head film. After the patient has been appropriately draped with lead aprons, the head is placed in the cephalostat in a natural, relaxed position. Natural head position is produced by having the patient look at the distant horizon.

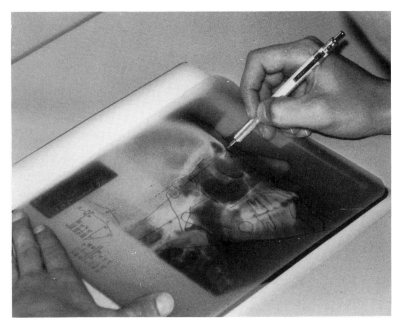

Figure 29–22 ■ After the head film has been screened for pathologic findings, a piece of matte acetate paper is placed over the film, and the anatomic structures are traced and landmarks are identified. Linear and angular measurements made from this tracing provide the basis for the cephalometric analysis.

none exists, a piece of matte acetate paper is placed over the film and the anatomic structures are traced and landmarks identified (Fig. 29–22). Linear and angular measurements made from this tracing provide the basis for the analysis. The analysis should evaluate the position of the maxilla and mandible with that of the cranial base and the relationship of the maxilla and mandible to one another. It should evaluate the position of the teeth in each jaw and the relationship of the upper denture to the lower. Vertical relationships between total, upper, and lower facial heights of the anterior face should be determined. Finally, the analysis should evaluate the soft tissue profile and the position of the lips in relation to the nose and chin.

A cephalometric analysis requires two reference lines to orient the position of the teeth and jaws. Historically, the Frankfort horizontal plane has been used as the horizontal reference line because it was felt to be parallel to the true horizontal when the patient was looking at a distant point. The Frankfort horizontal plane connects the upper rim of the external auditory meatus (porion) with the inferior border of the orbital rim (orbitale) (Fig. 29–23). Although the Frankfort horizontal plane is not always parallel to the true horizontal, it is still the most widely used horizontal reference line. The vertical reference line can be either a true perpendicular (to the horizon) through nasion, the

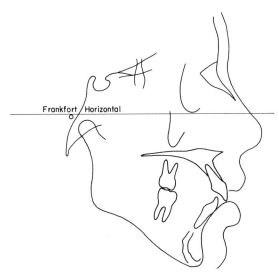

Figure 29–23 ■ Cephalometric analysis requires two reference lines to orient the position of the head and teeth. Historically, the Frankfort horizontal plane has been used as the reference line because it was felt to be parallel to the true horizontal when the patient is looking at the horizon. The Frankfort horizontal plane is constructed by connecting the upper rim of the external auditory meatus (porion) with the inferior border of the orbital rim (orbitale). The vertical reference line is either a true perpendicular to nasion, the bony bridge of the nose, or a perpendicular to the Frankfort plane through nasion.

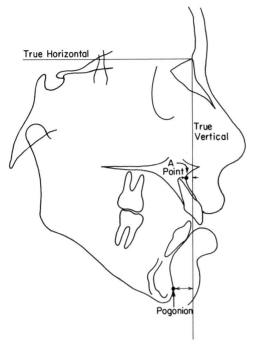

Figure 29–24 ■ The position and size of the maxilla and mandible are evaluated by comparing A point (maxilla) and pogonion (mandible) with a vertical reference line. In a well-positioned maxilla, A point is located 1–2 mm behind the vertical reference line. Pogonion is normally 5 mm behind the vertical line in a properly positioned mandible.

bony bridge of the nose, or a perpendicular to the Frankfort plane through nasion.

The position and size of the maxilla and mandible are evaluated by comparing A point (maxilla) and pogonion (mandible) to the vertical reference line. Normal maxillary position and size should place A point 1–2 mm behind the vertical line (Fig. 29–24). Pogonion is normally 5 mm behind the vertical in a well-positioned mandible (McNamara, 1983).

Angular and linear measurements can be used to compare the position of the maxilla with that of the mandible. The angle formed by connecting A and B points with nasion has traditionally been used to describe the position of the two jaws (Fig. 29–25). In normally related jaws, the angle is between 2 and 5 degrees. Larger positive values suggest a Class II relationship, whereas negative values indicate Class III tendencies. The difference between the size of the lower and upper jaw as determined from the Harvold measures can also be used to relate the jaws (Harvold, 1974).

Vertical facial proportions can be measured in two ways. The most direct method of determining vertical proportions is to measure total,

upper, and lower facial heights and construct facial height ratios or compare linear measurements to age appropriate norms (Isaacson et al, 1971; Harvold, 1974). Total facial height is normally measured from nasion to menton. The division between upper and lower facial height is made at the anterior nasal spine (Fig. 29–26). The upper facial height should compose approximately 45% of the total facial height in a well-proportioned individual (Wylie and Johnson, 1952). Vertical facial height can be indirectly determined from the mandibular plane angle (the angle between the mandibular plane and the Frankfort horizontal plane). A long face individual will tend to have a large mandibular plane angle, whereas a short face individual will exhibit a small mandibular plane angle (Fig. 29–27).

Maxillary and mandibular dental position is evaluated by measuring overjet, overbite, and the axial and bodily position of the incisors. Overjet and overbite are simple measurements from the facial surfaces and incisal edges of the incisors, respectively (Fig. 29–28). The axial and bodily position of the maxillary incisor is

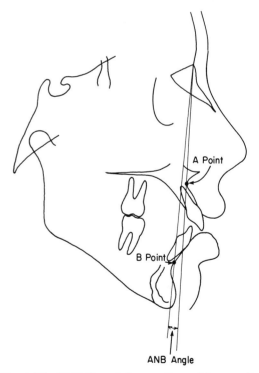

Figure 29–25 ■ The relative positions of the maxilla and mandible also are compared by using an angular measurement. In normally related jaws, the angle formed by connecting A and B points with nasion is between 2 and 5 degrees. Larger positive values suggest a Class II relationship, whereas negative values indicate a Class III tendency.

It is important to realize that the numbers derived as norms serve as diagnostic tools and not as the diagnosis itself. Certain measurements may suggest that a discrepancy exists, and this should be verified by the clinical examination. The clinician should also remember that hard and soft tissue analyses vary according to the ethnic background of the patient, and an appropriate analysis should be used. A cephalometric analysis or superimposition should

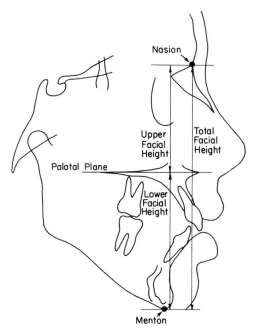

Figure 29–26 ■ Vertical facial proportions are determined by measuring total, upper, and lower facial heights. Total facial height is normally measured from nasion to menton. The division between upper and lower facial height is made at the palatal plane (a line connecting the anterior and posterior nasal spines). The measurements are used to construct facial height ratios or are compared with age appropriate norms.

determined relative to the nasion–A point line; the mandibular incisor position is related to the nasion–B point line. Axial inclination is determined from the angle formed by the intersection of the long axis of the incisor with the appropriate nasion–A point or nasion–B point line. Bodily position is a measure of linear distance from the facial surface to the reference line (Steiner, 1960) (Fig. 29–29).

A number of soft tissue analyses exist to describe the facial profile. The major problem with soft tissue analysis is that the head film is a static representation of a dynamic object. Lip position may be quite different on the head film, depending on whether the patient was in a relaxed pose or was straining to put the lips together when the film was made. This makes clinical assessment of the profile all the more important. Nevertheless, lip position is usually compared with the nose and chin. The Ricketts "E" line is convenient to use and is a line connecting the tip of the nose to the anterior contour of the chin (Fig. 29–30). In the permanent dentition, the upper lip is normally 1 mm behind the line and the lower lip is on the line or slightly behind it. (Ricketts, 1981).

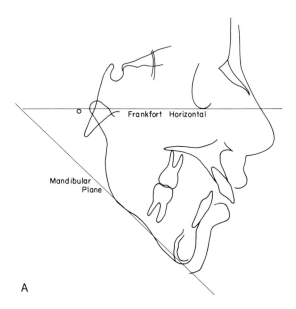

A

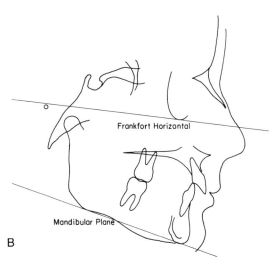

B

Figure 29–27 ■ A, Vertical facial height is determined indirectly from the mandibular plane angle (the angle between the mandibular plane and the Frankfort horizontal plane). This angle is usually approximately 24 degrees. A large mandibular plane angle is normally indicative of a long lower facial height. B, Conversely, a small mandibular plane angle is indicative of a short lower facial height.

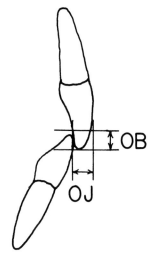

Figure 29–28 ■ The position of the maxillary and mandibular incisors and indirectly the entire dentition is evaluated by measuring the overjet and overbite. Overjet (OJ) is a horizontal measure of the distance between the most anterior points on the facial surfaces of the maxillary and mandibular central incisors. Overbite (OB) is a vertical measure of the overlap between the incisal edges of the maxillary and mandibular incisors.

also be performed at the end of orthodontic treatment to compare the results of treatment with the original treatment goals.

Serial cephalometric head films taken before, during, and after treatment can be superimposed to illustrate changes in jaw and tooth positions. The observed change is a combination of tooth movement and growth, and it is very difficult to differentiate one from another. To superimpose head films, one must locate an area within the head that is not changing, that is, an area not affected by growth or treatment from which change can be determined. Traditionally, three superimpositions are made when growth and treatment change are being evaluated.

The first superimposition illustrates overall changes in the face. The comparison is made by superimposing structures of the anterior cranial base or along the sella–nasion line registering at sella. The amount and direction of change in the soft tissue profile and position of the jaws

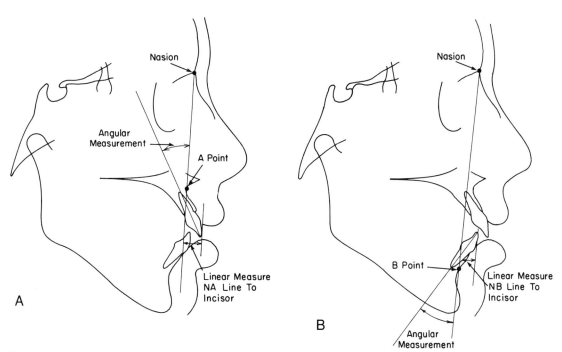

Figure 29–29 ■ A, The axial and bodily positions of the maxillary incisor are determined by an angular and a linear measurement. Axial position is determined by an angle formed by the intersection of the long axis of the incisor with the nasion–A point line. A large angle (greater than approximately 22 degrees) suggests that the incisor is axially protrusive; a small angle suggests that the incisor is upright. The bodily position of the incisor is determined by measuring the linear distance between the facial surface of the incisor and the nasion–A point line. On the average, this distance is 4 mm. A large measurement suggests that the incisor is positioned too far anteriorly, whereas a small or negative measurement indicates that the incisor is positioned too far posteriorly in relation to the maxilla. B, The position of the mandibular incisor is similarly evaluated, although the nasion–B point line is used as a reference line. For these measurements, the average inclination is 25 degrees and the average linear distance is 4 mm.

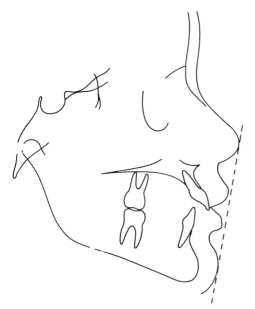

Figure 29–30 ■ The Ricketts "E" line is a convenient reference line to assess the position of the lips in relation to the nose and chin. In the permanent dentition, the upper lip is normally 1 mm behind a line connecting the tip of the nose to the anterior contour of the chin. The lower lip is usually on or slightly behind this line.

are readily apparent (Fig. 29–31A). To demonstrate the amount and direction of dental change, structures of the maxilla and mandible are superimposed (Fig. 29–31 B and C). In the maxilla, the superimposition is a best fit of the maxilla, pterygomaxillary fissure, and zygomatic process. The mandibular superimposition is made on the inner surface of the mandibular symphysis, the outline of the mandibular canal, and the unerupted third molar crypts.

RADIOGRAPHIC EVALUATION

The transition into the mixed dentition requires modification of the basic pediatric survey. Some considerations for radiographs of children in this period are the following:

1. Identification of missing teeth, supernumerary teeth, and the developmental status of permanent anteriors and premolars requires greater periapical coverage on films. The permanent second premolars are usually evident on radiographs at age 4, but they may not be apparent until age 8.

2. Potential eruption problems may be diagnosed from the radiographs by studying the unerupted teeth. Ectopic eruption of permanent first molars has been discussed and is diagnosed from routine bitewing radiographs. Ectopic eruption of incisors and canine impaction, another maxillary eruption problem, are often diagnosed from a panoramic radiograph. Labial or palatal positioning of the canine is determined by using a split image panoramic film or two periapical radiographs. The image of the canine on the two films will shift as the angulation of the central x-ray beam changes. If the image of the canine moves in the same direction (relative to the other teeth) as the central x-ray beam from the first film to the second, the canine is positioned lingual or palatal to the other teeth. If the image moves in the opposite direction of the beam from the first film to the second, the canine is located buccal to the teeth. This technique may also be used to locate supernumerary teeth or other abnormal structures.

3. Small palate size, especially early in the school age period, prevents or complicates maxillary periapical radiography using a long cone film stabilizing apparatus.

4. Greater anteroposterior length to the posterior occlusion requires more bitewing coverage.

In the early mixed dentition, a radiograph should be taken to detect supernumerary or missing teeth in the anterior maxilla. It is also recommended that all tooth-bearing areas be surveyed during the early mixed dentition years. This survey could consist of a panoramic radiograph and posterior bitewings. The panoramic radiograph offers the advantage of showing the temporomandibular joint (TMJ). Definitive temporomandibular joint films are indicated when there are clinical signs of dysfunction or a history of TMJ abnormalities. A traditional intraoral film survey in this age group would use appropriate anterior occlusal views and at least one periapical film in each posterior quadrant and posterior bitewings (Fig. 29–32). The number of films should be dictated by the size of the tooth-bearing areas, the adequacy of tissue coverage by the size of films tolerated, and the needs of the child. A 12 film survey (4 posterior periapicals, 6 anterior periapicals, and 2 posterior bitewings) should suffice even for the older school age child if performed well.

The techniques for the child, especially for those early in this age group, may include modifications. The anterior area requires placement of the film positioner deeper in the palate to obtain proper orientation. Two alternatives are

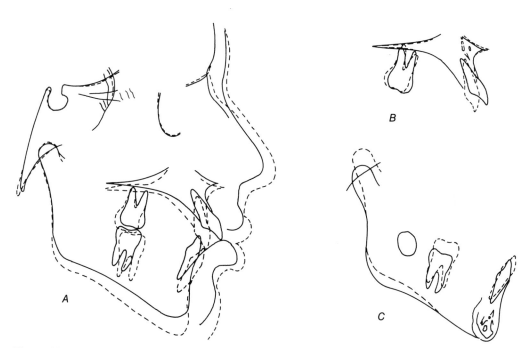

Figure 29–31 ■ *A,* Serial cephalometric head films are superimposed to illustrate changes in jaw and tooth positions during growth and orthodontic treatment. To assess overall change, a stable area within the head that is not influenced by growth or treatment is located. These overall changes in the face are illustrated by superimposing them on structures of the anterior cranial base. In this case, the solid line represents the individual before orthodontic treatment was initiated. The second or dashed line represents the individual after treatment was completed. During treatment, the maxilla moved slightly forward and downward. The horizontal position of the mandible remained virtually unchanged. However, the mandible did move vertically. The position of the lips improved during the treatment period as well. *B,* To illustrate the amount and direction of dental change, structures within the maxilla and mandible are superimposed. In this case, the maxillary superimposition, made by a best fit of palatal morphologic appearance, shows that the incisor and molar were both tipped distally. In addition, there was a change in the vertical position of the incisor. The change in incisor and molar position contributed to the improvement in molar relationships and overjet reduction. *C,* The mandibular superimposition, made by overlaying the inner aspect of the mandibular symphysis, the canal of the inferior alveolar nerve, and the unerupted third molar crypt, shows that both the incisor and molar erupted vertically.

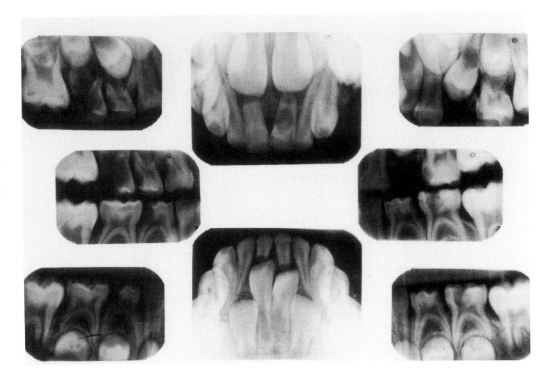

Figure 29–32 ■ An appropriate radiographic examination in this age group consists of anterior occlusal radiographs, at least one periapical film in each posterior quadrant, and posterior bitewing radiographs. The number of films should be dictated by the size of the tooth-bearing areas, the adequacy of tissue coverage by the size of the films, and the needs of the child.

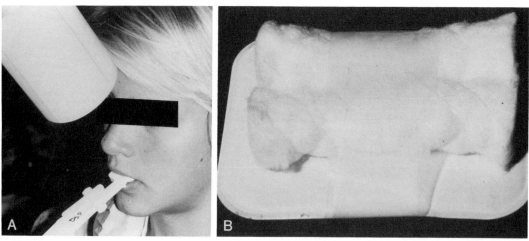

Figure 29–33 ■ *A*, The Snap-A-Ray device can be used as an anterior film stabilizer. The prong end of the Snap-A-Ray is used to hold a film in place by the child. A bisecting angle technique is used. *B*, Alternatively, cotton rolls can be used to stabilize the film. Taping two or three cotton rolls can help fill the space in the palate and stabilize an anterior film. Care must be taken not to bend the film. Bisecting angle technique is used.

to use the prong end of the Snap-A-Ray device with bisecting angle technique or to use a film with cotton rolls attached (Fig. 29–33). The long cone technique for posterior teeth is the same as for adults, with two modifications to help improve the product. Figure 29–34 demonstrates increasing vertical angulation to pick up the developing teeth. Figure 29–35 shows placement of cotton rolls on the bite block to facilitate positioning in small mouths or when teeth needed for stabilization are absent. A styrofoam bite-block may be used to obtain anterior films, using a bisecting angle technique

(Fig. 29–36). The bitewing technique for this age group is essentially the same as for the pre-schooler. It may take more skill to open contacts by very careful positioning of the beam. Larger films may be preferable, since they cover more area in each exposure.

Selection criteria also apply to this age group. Justification of a full-mouth survey of some type is based on the need to identify dental developmental problems and pathosis. The numbers of films made should reflect the composite adequacy of exposure of individual views. This translates to making as few films as

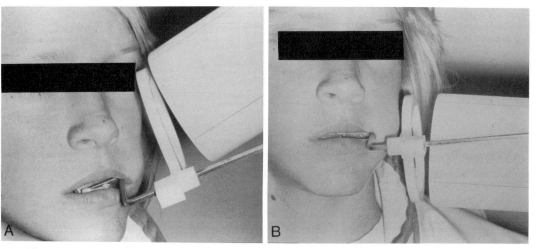

Figure 29–34 ■ *A* and *B*, Increasing vertical angulation of posterior periapical films will provide more coverage of periapical tissue. This helps the radiographs to include developing premolar roots in this age group.

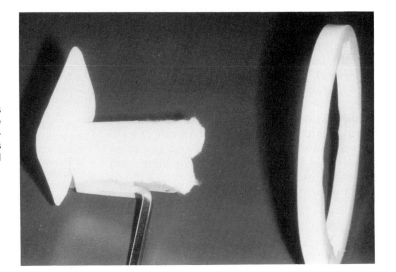

Figure 29–35 ■ Several cotton rolls will help hold the film holder in place in cases in which palate depth is insufficient or teeth are missing. Rolls can be taped to both above and below the holder's bite-block.

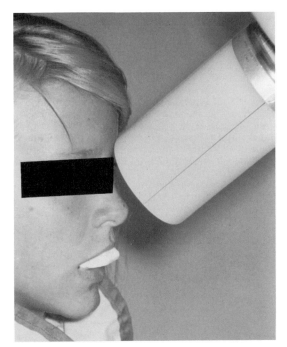

Figure 29–36 ■ A styrofoam bite-block can be used to aid in film positioning. Most plastic holders can be cut down to fit the child in the transitional dentition better.

needed to reveal tissue areas. Within the ages of 6 and 12 years, a variety of combinations of films are possible. No single set of projections is considered best.

Treatment Planning for Non-orthodontic Problems

The planning of care for this age group usually centers around orthodontic considerations, although many patients require additional management. Some elements of treatment planning that may need to be addressed but that are only peripherally related to orthodontics are the following:

1. *Management of primary caries:* Within this age period, many primary teeth are within a short time of normal exfoliation. A decision to extract a tooth or restore it must be made with its remaining lifespan in mind, as well as the length of time that the child will be without a replacement. Prosthetic replacement for a short time may not be indicated if adequate functional surfaces are available elsewhere and space maintenance is not indicated.

2. *Management of pathosis:* Some forms of oral pathosis, such as supernumerary teeth, odontomas, or missing teeth, are left to this period for definitive management, owing to the child's better ability to cooperate and impending effects of the problem.

3. *Prevention of dental disease:* The choice of sealants is also made during this period, as are decisions about how to manage incipient interproximal lesions of permanent teeth. Topical

fluoride regimens may be considered if the caries pattern changes for the worse.

4. *Health issues:* Children with disabilities or serious illnesses are in a transitional time. The child with cancer, orofacial clefting, cerebral palsy, or a host of other conditions may need special consideration of such issues as life-span, realistic functional requirements, retention of teeth for growth purposes, and the role of teeth in social acceptance. The decisions regarding these issues are often complex, with input from parents, the child, and other professionals helpful in decision-making.

The dentist's role is to provide information about the need for care, the benefit anticipated, the alternatives (including no treatment) to care, and the burden of maintenance of care. These special patients may tax the dentist's skills in planning care and may require consideration of careful and frequent observation rather than treatment.

REFERENCES

Bolton WA: Disharmony in tooth size and its relation to the analysis and treatment of malocclusion. Am J Orthod 28:113–130, 1958.

Fields HW, Proffit WR, Nixon WL, Phillips C, Stanek E: Facial pattern differences in long-faced children and adults. Am J Orthod 85:217–223, 1984.

Gellin ME, Haley JV: Managing cases of overretention of mandibular primary incisors where their permanent successors erupt lingually. ASDC J Dent Child 49:118–122, 1982.

Harvold EP: The Activator in Orthodontics. St. Louis, CV Mosby Co, 1974.

Isaacson JR, Isaacson RJ, Speidel TM, Worms FW: Extreme variation in vertical facial growth and associated variation in skeletal and dental relations. Am J Orthod 41:219–229, 1971.

Jacobson A: The "Wits" appraisal of jaw disharmony. Am J Orthod 67:125–138, 1975.

Kimmel NA, Gellin ME, Bohannan HA, Kaplan AL: Ectopic eruption of maxillary first permanent molars in different areas of the United States. ASDC J Dent Child 49:294–299, 1982.

Loe H, Silness J: Periodontal disease in pregnancy. I. Prevalence and severity. Acta Odont Scand 21:553, 1963.

McNamara JA, Jr: A method of cephalometric analysis. *In* McNamara JA, Ribbens KA, Howe, RP (eds): Clinical Alteration of the Growing Face, Monograph 12, Craniofacial Growth Series, Ann Arbor, 1983, University of Michigan, Center for Human Growth and Development. 81–105.

Proffit WR et al: Contemporary Orthodontics. St. Louis, CV Mosby Co, 1986.

Proffit WR, Vig KWL: Primary failure of eruption: A possible cause of posterior open-bite. Am J Orthod 80:173–190, 1981.

Pulver F: The etiology and prevalence of ectopic eruption of the maxillary first permanent molar. ASDC J Dent Child 35:138–146, 1968.

Ramfjord SP: The periodontal index. J Periodontol 38:610, 1967.

Ricketts RM: Perspectives in the clinical application of cephalometrics. Angle Orthod 51:115-150, 1981.

Shafer WG, Hine MK, Levy BM: A Textbook of Oral Pathology. Philadelphia, WB Saunders Co, 1974.

Staley RN, O'Gorman TW, Hoag JF, Shelly TH: Prediction of the widths of unerupted canines and premolars. J Am Dent Assoc 108:185–190, 1984.

Steiner CC: The use of cephalometrics as an aid to planning and assessing orthodontic treatment. Am J Orthod 46:721–735, 1960.

Tanaka MM, Johnston LE: The prediction of the size of unerupted canines and premolars in a contemporary orthodontic population. J Am Dent Assoc 88:798–801, 1974.

Wylie WL, Johnson EL: Rapid evaluation of facial dysplasia in the vertical plane. Angle Orthod 22:165–182, 1952.

Prevention of dental disease

Arthur Nowak □ *James Crall*

The patient between 6 and 12 years of age presents an interesting professional challenge for the dentist. At the beginning of this period, the patient who the dentist is dealing with is one who continues to be dependent upon the parents but who is now thrust into a new environment for approximately 8 hours a day—the school setting. By the end of this period, the child is a patient who has gained partial independence from the parents and who is about ready for junior high school. In the case of the female patient, womanhood will soon be encountered.

In addition, all through this period a number of orofacial changes are taking place. Most or even all of the primary teeth will have been replaced with permanent teeth. The alignment and occlusion of the teeth are developing, and the adult face is emerging. "What I look like" becomes important, not only to the patient but to all the people he or she meets each day, especially peers.

Diet and dietary practices are severely challenged by the educational environment and social pressures, both during the day and after school hours. Nutritional requirements vary from year to year in this period. As the growth of the patient changes from one of slow, pro-gressive physical growth early in the period to one of substantial physical growth during the end of the period, the diet of the child needs to stay in tune. Not only are the dietary requirements dependent on growth and development; they are also dependent on the level of physical and mental activity the child is engaged in. Snacking becomes a common practice during this period. With vending machines easily available, convenience stores on many street corners, and the influence of radio and television, children are constantly reminded of their hunger needs.

Many changes in manual dexterity take place during this period. Although continuing gross motor development prevails, this is the period when fine motor activity begins to mature. This is fortunate, because during this period the child is challenging the parents for independence, especially in areas of personal hygiene, clothes selection, and dietary choices. Conflicts emerge between the parents' desires and the child's wishes. It is a time when parents must have a strong daily influence on all types of activities, including oral care. With the eruption of the permanent teeth, the fluoride needs begin to shift from systemic administration to topical application. Periodic review of those

needs by the dentist is important so that the child receives the optimal protection available.

From 6–12 years of age, many children will become athletically involved. For those children playing contact or other trauma prone sports, the dentist should provide mouth protectors (see Section IV, Chapter 40).

Fluoride Administration

The period from 6–12 years of age is extremely important with regard to fluoride administration for three major reasons: (1) the crowns of many permanent teeth will continue to form during this period, (2) the posterior permanent teeth will erupt and will be at greater risk to develop caries until the process of posteruptive maturation has occurred, and (3) the child will be increasingly responsible for the maintenance of his or her oral health. The optimal use of all forms of fluoride should be employed to provide protection during this first phase of carious attack upon those teeth that will eventually constitute the permanent dentition.

SYSTEMIC FLUORIDES

Studies suggest that a substantial portion of the anti-caries protection provided by water fluoridation in humans occurs during the pre-eruptive period (van Eck, 1985). Additional studies in laboratory animals have reported that daily doses of fluoride administered via gastric intubation during the period of tooth formation reduced the incidence of caries in these teeth following their eruption (Hunt and Navia, 1975). Because systemically acquired fluoride may become deposited and redistributed in developing teeth during the mineralization phase as well as during the subsequent period prior to eruption, current recommendations call for systemic fluoride supplements to be provided for all children residing in areas where the water is fluoride-deficient until the age of 14. This protocol should help to ensure maximum protection for the posterior teeth, which are more vulnerable to carious attack. The dosage of supplemental fluoride does not change for children beyond the age of 3.

TOPICAL FLUORIDES

During the period from 6–12 years of age, the child should become increasingly responsi-

ble for the maintenance of his or her dentition. Many forms of topical fluoride are appropriate for children in this age group, including fluoride toothpastes, fluoride mouthrinses, and concentrated fluoride preparations for professional and home application.

Evidence continues to accumulate to support the effectiveness of frequent applications of agents with relatively low concentrations of fluoride. The two principal forms of these agents in the United States are fluoride toothpastes and fluoride mouthrinses.

Fluoride Toothpastes

The daily use of a fluoride-containing dentifrice should form the foundation of a child's preventive dental activities. Although many toothpastes have fluoride in their formulations, those products that have obtained approval by the Council on Dental Therapeutics of the American Dental Association (ADA) should be recommended. The formulations of those toothpastes that have not obtained ADA approval may impede the release of fluoride from these products, thereby compromising their effectiveness (Stookey, 1985). Currently approved fluoride toothpastes contain sodium fluoride (NaF) or sodium monofluorophosphate (MFP) as active ingredients. The maximum allowable concentration of fluoride in dentifrices at this time is 1000 ppm (Stookey, 1985).

Fluoride Mouthrinses

The use of fluoride mouthrinses has grown considerably in recent years as a result of their increased usage in the home as well as in school-based mouthrinsing programs. The most popular preparations contain neutral NaF, although stannous fluoride and acidulated phosphate fluoride rinses also are available. Several fluoride mouthrinses, including many 0.05% NaF products, are available on an over-the-counter (non-prescription) basis.

Numerous clinical trials conducted in the 1960's and 1970's reported caries reductions in the 20–40% range among children in non-fluoridated areas who rinsed with either 0.2% NaF on a weekly basis or 0.05% NaF on a daily basis (Torrell and Ericsson, 1974; Driscoll, 1974). More recent studies, conducted since the overall decline in dental caries in children became evident, have reported that (1) the expected benefits from fluoride rinsing in terms of the actual number of tooth surfaces saved from

becoming carious are generally less than previously reported, and (2) rinsing appears to have a greater effect in older children (10 years of age or older) (Bell et al, 1984; Poulsen, et al, 1984). Nevertheless, the observation that fluoride rinsing provides greater protection to teeth erupting during the time when rinses are being applied would seem to provide a rationale for their use in the 6- to 12-year-old age group.

Mouthrinses would seem to be particularly indicated for individuals deemed to be at high risk to develop caries. Included in this category would be those children who lack the motivation or manual dexterity necessary to carry out effective oral hygiene procedures; patients wearing orthodontic appliances or prostheses, which may complicate the process of plaque removal; and patients with medical conditions that place them at increased risk for caries. Examples of individuals in the last group would be patients undergoing head and neck radiation therapy, which may compromise their salivary flow, and patients who are required to take frequent doses of liquid or chewable medications having a high sugar content.

Concentrated Fluoride Agents for Professional Application or Home Use

Applications of more concentrated forms of fluoride should be considered for individuals who cannot or do not make optimum use of the high frequency–low concentration forms of fluoride therapy. Generally, this implies semiannual applications of concentrated fluoride gels in the dental office.

Several fluoride gels and solutions, including combinations of acidulated phosphate fluoride (APF) and stannous fluoride, are available for home use. Practitioners should be aware that some of these products contain concentrations of fluoride that are similar to those found in fluoride toothpastes or over-the-counter rinses and, in most cases, have not undergone clinical testing. Some of these low concentration products also have been advocated for professional application but are unlikely to be effective when used on an infrequent basis (Crall and Bjerga, 1984). Therefore, the advantage of these less concentrated products over commercially available fluoride toothpastes and mouthrinses is questionable. More concentrated fluoride gels (0.5% APF) have been shown to be effective in reducing the incidence of caries and may be useful in high risk patients or in patients with rampant caries.

Home Care

With school and school activities now emerging as a major influence in the daily schedule of the child, routine personal hygiene must be scheduled. It is hoped that the development of such a routine will have been reinforced with the routines established during the preschool period. Life between 6 and 12 years of age becomes increasingly busy. It is not only the school activities that fill the daily schedule. Music lessons, sports activities, dancing and singing lessons, homework, religious instructions, daily chores, babysitting, and the delivering of newspapers all begin to influence the daily schedule and therefore the time remaining for personal hygiene.

Although brushing after all meals is ideal, it appears that it is unrealistic. A compromise needs to be worked out. An appropriate recommendation would be for a thorough cleaning of the teeth and massaging of the gingivae before bed, with additional brushing after breakfast and the evening meal. Brushing after lunch in school is inappropriate because most children will not remember their toothbrush and because they are more interested in physical activity after completing lunch. Recommending that they swish vigorously with water after lunch will help to dislodge any large particles of remaining food as well as neutralize any acid that is present.

Parents need to remain quite active in supervising mouth care during this period. Interference from television, radio, and stereos cannot be tolerated. A firm stand with appropriate discipline, if required, is recommended to develop and maintain this important hygiene practice. Periodic inspection of the mouth by the parents is indeed appropriate. Because fine motor activity is further developing during this period, parental assistance is required to remove all plaque, especially on the buccal surfaces of the posterior maxillary molars and the lingual surfaces of the mandibular posterior molars. Appropriate sized and contoured toothbrushes should be selected to meet the child's needs. With increasing oral dimensions and the number of teeth, larger brushes should be considered. Soft, nylon-bristled brushes are recommended over other varieties.

With the increased size and independence of the child, the bathroom becomes the ideal location for cleaning. Previously recommended supine positioning to increase visibility and stability are no longer appropriate. A well lit

bathroom with a wall mirror or hand mirror will greatly assist in the cleaning process.

Use of disclosing tablets or solutions will assist the child and parent to evaluate the thoroughness of the cleaning. At least weekly, a disclosing agent should be used and with the parent's supervision the child's mouth should be inspected. Areas of disclosed plaque should be noted, and instructions on modifications of routines should be given so that the plaque will be removed daily.

With the exfoliation of primary teeth and the eruption of permanent teeth the mouth may be sore, causing the child to be hesitant to do a thorough cleaning. Generally with the loosening of a primary tooth, the gingiva will be tender and even swollen. Mild wiping of this area with the toothbrush should maintain the health of the tissues. As the permanent teeth erupt, their alignment may be irregular and the gingival tissues may lose their "knife edge" anatomy with the tooth. Instead, a ledge of gingival tissue may emerge that will allow plaque to accumulate (Fig. 30 – 1). Careful manipulation of the toothbrush will be necessary until the gingival contour transforms into a smooth margin with the tooth. In mouths with developing arch length – tooth size discrepancy, the resulting poor alignment of teeth will cause increased retention of food and plaque. Until this is corrected, additional manipulation of the brush by both child and parent may be necessary.

Toward the end of this developmental period, the child may have enough digital fine motor activity to be able to learn the process of flossing. Like any other motor activity, flossing must be patiently learned and practiced frequently to be mastered. Parents can be very helpful in assisting the child. Inappropriate use of the floss by snapping it into the interproximal surfaces can injure the gingiva. Once passed through the contact, the floss must be carefully manipulated along one surface of the tooth and then along the opposite, making sure that the floss reaches the area just under the gingival crevice. One of many floss holders available commercially may greatly assist in the process.

Children with developmental disabilities will require partial or total assistance in oral care, depending on their mental and physical capabilities. If a parent must either assist or be totally responsible for mouth care, a mouth prop may be helpful (Fig. 30 – 2). With good head stability and mouth propping, the cleaning process will be enhanced. With severely disabled children, more than one person may be necessary. Stabilization and positioning may be necessary, and if so the bathroom may be an inappropriate place for oral care. The bedroom or other living areas with available floor space, beds, or couches will allow the child to be placed in a supine position and stabilized. In these situations, the use of a dentifrice will further complicate the process because of the foaming and the need to expectorate.

Lastly, as the child grows older his or her social activities, overnight trips, weekends, or extended periods away from home will increase. As children "pack their bags," toothbrushes, dentifrices, and floss will probably be thought of last, if at all. Again, parents must be responsible to make sure that the appropriate tools are available for oral care. Whether they will be used is another question.

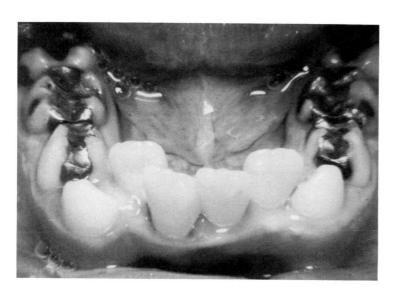

Figure 30 – 1 ■ Early mixed dentition. Note crowding of teeth and ledge of gingiva.

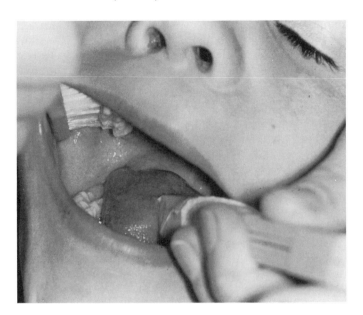

Figure 30-2 ■ A tongue blade mouth prop can be used to facilitate mouth care in a disabled child.

Diet

Although children are introduced to a variety of new foods during the preschool years, it is during the primary grades that the challenge to the well-established dietary habits begins. Again, the exposure to a full day in school with frequent treats; school lunches, either from home or purchased at school; and the multitude of after-school activities, usually associated with food; will all influence the child's eventual dietary habits. In addition, the child will be under heavy influence from the commercial media, especially television. The effect of food choices and purchases on children's oral health has been carefully studied, and although advocacy organizations have attempted to influence the number of commercials related to food, it remains common for the school age child to be exposed to many enticements during a period of television or radio entertainment. If children accompany parents to the market — a practice not encouraged — the purchases are frequently related to television and radio commercials.

Although some dramatic changes have been witnessed recently in food selections and dietary practices, it is known that a large percentage of family's meals are still eaten on the run, eaten in fast food restaurants, seldom eaten with the entire family, or eaten too often in front of the television set. Today's per capita consumption of caloric sweeteners in the United States is around 123 pounds annually, even though there has been substantial decrease in the use of ordinary refined table sugar in the home. Per capita consumption of soft drinks has almost doubled since the early 1970's, from 250 (12 ounce) cans to over 400 cans in the early 1980's. Eighty per cent of the sugar in America's diets is from soft drinks, candy, baked goods, and bread, whereas only a small percentage is from milk, milk products, and fruits.

Nevertheless, caries rates have been dramatically reduced during the last 10 years, even though dramatic changes have been taking place in dietary practices. Can dentists make any further impact on the way children eat and what they eat? In order to help some children, the answer to this question must be in the affirmative because poor diet may be the biggest predictor of the dental health dilemma of children.

For children with severe caries problems, the dentist must evaluate all causative factors, including diet and dietary practices. As reported earlier, the dietary history, whether a 24 hour recall or a 3-7 day history, is recommended. Once the history is received, the dentist or a designated staff person reviews it with the parent, paying particular attention to the number of exposures to carbohydrates per day and when these foods were eaten (mealtimes, after meals, or between meals). Every exposure of a food containing a refined carbohydrate, especially one that adheres to the teeth and dissolves slowly, will produce acid in and around the plaque. If a promiscuous pattern emerges, it

should be defined and recommendations for substitute foods or modifications of a practice should be provided. Identifying particular areas of concern and providing specific recommendations will be accepted more readily by parent and child than making sweeping changes of the entire diet. A series of small changes, successfully modified over a period of time, will eventually lead to a better diet for dental health.

As more is learned of the cariogenic potential of foods, "foods safe for teeth" will be identified and marketed. In the meantime, it is unrealistic to recommend to parents of 6- or 7-year-olds that all candy and baked goods be eliminated. It is better to advise parents of favorable compromises. For example, a dentist could encourage that a chocolate candy be eaten instead of a caramel, or that candy and baked goods be eaten only after meals and not before or between meals. Children can learn appropriate eating habits, but these recommendations must be realistic and the parents must be enthusiastic to change. The parents also should be urged to work with school authorities to provide meals that are not only wholesome and nutritious but also eye-appealing to the child. In addition, parents should work with their children's teachers to encourage appropriate snacks and party foods for special occasions.

The diets of children with developmental disabilities may be modified for a number of reasons. To meet caloric requirements, supplements are frequently added to routine foods. Unfortunately, these supplements are frequently refined carbohydrates and therefore increase the risk of acid production. Foods may be altered—minced, pureed, or mashed—to assist in swallowing and to minimize the need for chewing. Because of these modifications, retention in the mouth is enhanced and oral clearance is decreased. Because of chewing and swallowing difficulties, fresh fruits and vegetables are sometimes withheld from the diets of these children. Substitutes include pastries, canned fruits, puddings, and gelatin desserts, all with a high percentage of refined carbohydrates. The dentist and his or her staff must be aware of these modifications and must be realistic in providing dietary recommendations to parents of children with developmental disabilities.

REFERENCES

Bell RM, Klein SP, Bohannan HM, Disney JA, Graves RC, Madison R: Treatment Effects in the National Preventive Dentistry Demonstration Program. Santa Monica, CA, Rand Corporation, 1984.

Crall JJ, Bjerga JM: Fluoride uptake and retention following combined applications of APF and stannous fluoride in vitro. Pediatr Dent 6:226–229, 1984.

Driscoll WS: The use of fluoride tablets for the prevention of dental caries. In Forrester DJ, Schultz EM, Jr (eds): International Workshop on Fluorides and Dental Caries Reductions. Baltimore, University of Maryland, 1974.

Hunt CE, Navia JM: Pre-eruptive effects of Mo, B, Sr, and F on dental caries in the rat. Arch Oral Biol 20:497–501, 1975.

Poulsen S, Kirkegaard E, Bangsbo G, Bro K: Caries clinical trial of fluoride rinses in a Danish public child dental service. Community Dent Oral Epidemiol 12:283–287, 1984.

Stookey GK: Are all fluoride dentifrices the same? In Wei SHY (ed): Clinical Uses of Fluoride. Philadelphia, Lea and Febiger, 1985, pp 105–131.

Torrell P, Ericsson Y: The potential benefits to be derived from fluoride mouthrinses. In Forrester DJ, Schultz EM, Jr (eds): International Workshop on Fluorides and Dental Caries Reductions. Baltimore, University of Maryland, 1974.

van Eck AAMJ, Groenveld A, Backer Dirks O: Pre and post-eruptive caries reduction by water fluoridation. Caries Res 19:163, 1985, Abs 28.

The acid-etch technique in caries prevention: pit and fissure sealants and preventive resin restorations

M. John Hicks

Increasingly, the attention of the dental profession has been directed toward prevention of dental caries in occlusal surfaces. For a number of decades, the prime area of concern has been related to reducing the incidence and prevalence of caries occurring on smooth surfaces. The most recent reports regarding caries prevalence and incidence in pediatric and adolescent age groups have indicated a dramatic reduction in dental caries during the past decade, especially with respect to smooth surface lesions. This significant change in the dental caries status of children and adolescents has been at-tributed to a number of factors (Hicks et al, 1985). First, this generation of children may have benefited from the optimal use of both systemic and topical fluorides. Second, parents have become more aware of the importance and need for dental care with the young child, resulting in parents bringing their child to the dentist at an earlier age when perhaps only preventive measures or minimal restorative needs are indicated. Third, group dental insurance programs that include dental care for the pediatric patient have become available. The availability of such programs has removed some of

the financial burden for the children's dental care from the family. Fourth, the increase in dental manpower has allowed for easy access to dental care. Fifth, the interest of the dental profession in preventive dentistry has increased as the effects of preventive regimens on dental disease have been shown to have both scientific and clinical bases.

Epidemiology of Occlusal Caries

During the past decade, the pattern of caries experience has changed significantly in the pediatric population. Approximately 44% of children between 6 and 11 years of age were considered to be caries free when examined in 1974 for a caries prevalence study conducted by the National Center for Health Statistics. In the 1980 National Caries Prevalence Survey conducted by the National Institute of Dental Research (NIDR), 57% of children in this same age group were found to be caries free. In the 12- to 17-year-old age group, less than 10% of adolescents were clinically caries free in 1974. Just a single decade later, more than 17% of adolescents were considered to be caries free. In fact, at the present time at least 11% of 17-year-old young adults are caries free.

With the increasing proportion of children and adolescents that remain caries free, there has also been a reduction in the number of decayed, missing, and filled surfaces (DMFS) for those affected by caries. In the 6- to 11-year-old age category, this reduction in DMFS has been shown to be 35% when the caries prevalence studies of 1974 are compared with those for 1980. In the 12- to 17-year-old adolescent group, a 26% reduction was found in DMFS from 1974 to 1980. In the 1974 study, the mean DMFS for 17-year-old adolescents was 16.9 surfaces. In contrast, the mean DMFS for 17-year-olds in the 1980 study was 11.0 surfaces, a reduction of almost 35% in the total number of surfaces involved by dental caries.

The occlusal surface is particularly vulnerable to caries development. Caries involving occlusal surfaces accounts for 54% of the total caries experience in children and adolescents, according to both the National Preventive Dentistry Demonstration Program completed in 1984 (Bell et al, 1984) and the 1980 NIDR National Caries Prevalence Survey. In 1974, occlusal caries represented 49% of the total caries experience in children and adolescents. This apparent increase in the proportion of caries experience attributed to occlusal caries is due to a 45% reduction in caries prevalence in interproximal surfaces that occurred between 1974 and 1980. The fact that occlusal caries is responsible for over half the total caries experience in children and adolescents is remarkable, considering the fact that occlusal surfaces represent only 12.5% of the total number of tooth surfaces exposed to cariogenic challenges. The reason for this high degree of caries is due to the presence of pits and fissures in occlusal surfaces. When dental caries that occurs in pits and fissures on buccal and lingual surfaces are considered, pit and fissure caries has been shown to account for at least 80% of the total caries experience in children and adolescents, according to information from the National Preventive Dentistry Demonstration Program.

Occlusal caries represents a disease process that has an early onset. Approximately one third of children between the ages of 1 and 3 years have experienced dental caries in the primary dentition, with 67% of these lesions being occlusal caries. With the permanent dentition, 65% of first molars in 12-year-old children either have been restored because of occlusal caries or presently have occlusal caries. In fact, with elementary school children from a fluoridated community, 90% of all lesions in first permanent molars have been shown to be due to pit and fissure caries (Bohannan et al, 1984; Hennon et al, 1969; Graves and Burt, 1975).

Morphology of Surfaces With Pits and Fissures

The dental profession has known for some time that caries susceptibility on tooth surfaces with pits and fissures is related to the form and depth of these pits and fissures. Because of the interest in caries formation in pits and fissures, attempts have been made to provide an elaborate classification system for pits and fissures. However, for the sake of simplicity, two main types of pits and fissures are usually described: (1) a shallow, wide, V-shaped fissure (Fig. 31–1A); and (2) a deep, narrow, I-shaped fissure (Fig. 31–1B) that is quite constricted and may resemble a bottleneck in that the fissure may have an extremely narrow slit appearance with a larger base as it extends toward the dentinoenamel junction. These fissures may also have a number of different branches. The typical fissure usually contains an organic plug composed

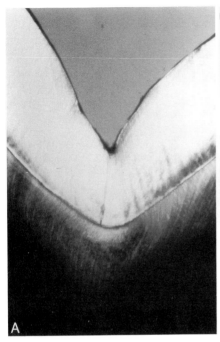
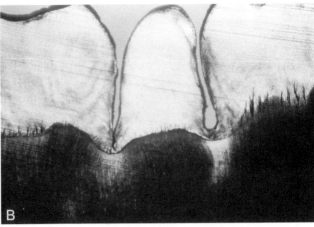

Figure 31–1 ■ Histologic appearance of the main types of pits and fissures in occlusal surfaces (polarized light microscopy; water imbibition). *A*, Shallow, wide V-shaped fissure. *B*, Deep, narrow I-shaped fissure.

of reduced enamel epithelium, microorganisms forming a dental plaque, and oral debris. Examination of fissures, even with low levels of magnification, reveals the reason for the caries susceptibility of tooth surfaces with pits and fissures. The fissure provides a niche for dental plaque accumulation that is difficult to remove. The speed with which dental caries occurs in the surface is, most likely, related to the fact that the depth of the fissure is in close proximity to the dentino-enamel junction and to the underlying dentin, which is highly caries susceptible (Hicks and Flaitz, 1986; Ngano, 1961; Galil and Gwinnett, 1975).

The morphology of occlusal surfaces varies from tooth to tooth and from individual to individual. In general, however, the "typical" premolar tooth (Fig. 31–2A) will have a primary fissure with usually three or four pits. With a "typical" molar tooth (Fig. 31–2B), as many as ten separate pits may be present in primary, secondary, and supplemental fissures. In addition, certain surface porosities that would not be noticeable clinically become apparent when the surface is examined microscopically.

Histopathology of Caries in Pits and Fissures

At one time, caries formation in fissures was thought to occur at the base of the fissure and involve the deeper aspects of the underlying tooth structure prior to the fissure walls and cuspal inclines being affected by the caries process. This would be expected, owing to the extension of the fissure into the tooth surface for a considerable depth. However, such is not the case. Rather, the inclines forming the walls of the fissure are affected first by the caries process. The first histologic evidence of lesion formation is found at the orifice of the fissure and is usually represented by two independent bilateral lesions in the enamel composing the opposing cuspal inclines (Fig. 31–3A). As the lesion progresses, the fissure walls become involved and coalescence of the two independent lesions into one lesion occurs at the base of the fissure. The enamel present at the base of the fissure is affected to a greater degree than that of the cuspal inclines, and the lesion spreads both laterally within the enamel adjacent to the fissure and readily toward the dentino-enamel junction (Fig. 31–3B). Once the caries process involves dentin, the progress of the lesion is enhanced as a result of the increased caries susceptibility of dentin when compared with enamel. Eventually, cavitation of the fissure occurs as a result of loss of mineral and structural support from the adjacent enamel and underlying enamel, resulting in a clinically detectable lesion. The unique process of caries formation in pits and fissures is due to the presence of the organic plug in the fissure.

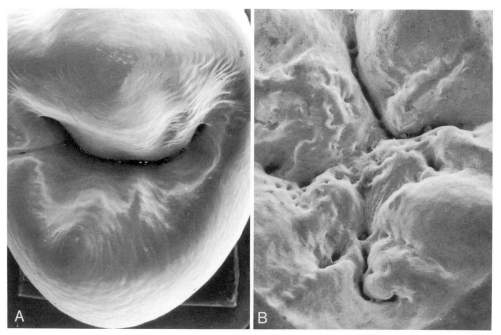

Figure 31–2 ■ Surface morphologic appearance of caries-free premolar (A) and permanent molar (B) (scanning electron microscopy).

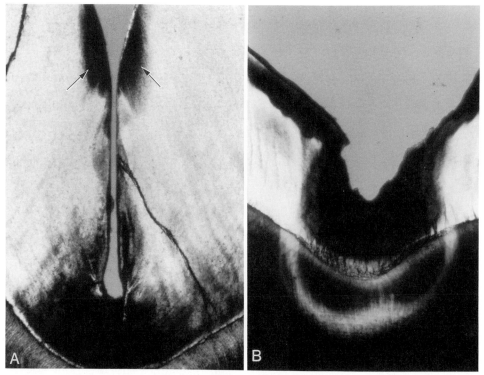

Figure 31–3 ■ Histologic appearance of pit and fissure caries (polarized light microscopy; water imbibition). A, Caries formation (arrows) begins in the cuspal inclines just above the fissure orifice. The darkened appearance at the base of the fissure is due to the organic material present. B, The lesion progresses to the point at which the base of the fissure and underlying dentin become involved. With further progression, cavitation will occur, resulting in a clinically detectable lesion.

This organic plug acts as a buffer against the acid by-products of dental plaque and provides a diffusion barrier, resulting in a lessened acid attack at the fissure base during the initial phase of caries formation (Hicks and Flaitz, 1986).

Although systemic and topical fluoride utilization has been shown to be highly effective in prevention of dental caries in smooth surfaces, enamel surfaces with pits and fissures have received minimal caries protection from either systemic or topical fluoride agents. The reason why fluoride appears to be ineffective in preventing caries in fissured surfaces may be related to the total depth of enamel on smooth surfaces in comparison with that underlying the fissure (Hicks and Flaitz, 1986; Silverstone, 1984). With smooth surfaces, approximately 1 mm of enamel is found superficial to the dentino-enamel junction, whereas the base of a fissure present in an occlusal surface may be relatively close or lie within dentin. Should caries develop in an occlusal fissure, the underlying dentin becomes involved rapidly, resulting in a frank, clinically detectable lesion. When caries formation occurs in enamel composing a smooth surface, a considerable amount of enamel must become involved in the caries process prior to dentinal involvement. It is thought that it may take as long as 3–4 years for dentinal involvement to occur. During this time period, remineralization of the smooth surface lesion may occur as a result of exposure to various fluoride agents and result in the arrest of lesion progression. When fissures are present in smooth surfaces, a pattern of caries involvement similar to that for occlusal surfaces is found and would appear to be related to the lessened thickness of enamel available (Fig. 31–4).

Prevention of Pit and Fissure Caries: Historical Perspective

During the 1920's, two different clinical techniques were introduced in an attempt to reduce the extent and severity of pit and fissure caries in occlusal surfaces. In 1924, Thaddeus Hyatt advocated the prophylactic restoration. This procedure consisted of preparing a conservative Class I cavity that included all the pits and fissures and then placing an amalgam restoration. The rationale for this procedure was that the prophylactic restoration prevented further insult to the pulp from caries and required less time for restoration than when the tooth eventually succumbed to dental caries. A more conservative approach to prevention of pit and fissure caries was presented by Bodecker. Initially, he advocated cleaning the fissures with an explorer and flowing a thin mix of oxyphosphate cement into the fissures, essentially an attempt to seal the fissure. Later, he introduced an alternative method for caries prevention, the prophylactic odontotomy, involving eradication of the fissures in order to transform deep, retentive fissures into cleanable ones. These two clinical techniques were employed until the widespread use of sealants became prevalent.

The development of pit and fissure sealants was based upon the discovery that etching of enamel with phosphoric acid would increase the retention of resin restorative materials and improve the marginal integrity considerably. The initial studies regarding the effects of acid-etching on enamel were performed by Buonocore in 1955. The first sealant material that utilized the acid-etch technique was introduced in the mid-1960's and was a cyanoacrylate mate-

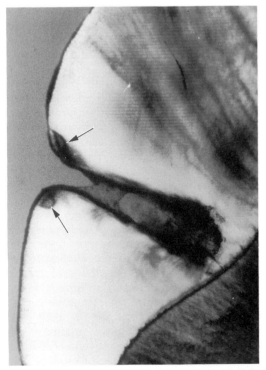

Figure 31–4 ■ Histologic appearance of a pit in the buccal surface of a permanent molar tooth. Caries formation (*arrows*) is evident at the orifice of the fissure. An organic plug is present in the fissure. The base of the pit approaches the dentino-enamel junction (polarized light microscopy; water imbibition).

rial. Cyanoacrylates were not suitable as sealant materials, owing to bacterial degradation of the material in the oral cavity over time. By the late 1960's, a number of different resin materials had been tested and a viscous resin was found to be resistant to loss and produced a tenacious bond with etched dental enamel. This resin is formed by reacting bisphenol A with glycidyl methacrylate, and this class of resins has become known as dimethacrylate (BIS-GMA) (Bowen, 1982). BIS-GMA is a relatively large epoxy, resin-like hybrid monomer in which epoxy groups are replaced by methacrylate groups. BIS-GMA incorporates the rapid polymerization characteristic of methyl methacrylate and the minimal polymerization shrinkage property of epoxy resins. The vast majority of restorative resin materials are based upon the BIS-GMA formulation and vary from sealants in that restorative materials include filler particles such as quartz, glass, and porcelain in order to improve their strength, whereas the majority of sealants either are unfilled BIS-GMA or have relatively few filler particles added.

BIS-GMA sealants differ in the way in which the material is polymerized. Two methods of polymerization have been employed. Autopolymerized (chemical-cured) systems involve mixing two liquids, a base resin and catalyst resin. The material sets by an exothermic reaction, usually within 1–2 minutes. Photoactivated (light-cured) polymerization has also been used with sealants. Initially, ultraviolet light of 365 nm was used to initiate the setting reaction. However, owing to the inconsistency of the wavelength of light and possible retinal damage with long-term use, photoactivation of sealant materials with exposure to a visible light source of 440–448 nm was introduced. Use of visible light sources also requires eye protection, owing to the intensity of the light created. The benefits of light-cured versus chemical-cured sealants are the following: (1) setting of the sealant occurs in only 10–20 seconds; (2) no mixing of resins is required, eliminating incorporation of air bubbles that may occur with chemical-cured materials; and (3) the viscosity of sealant remains constant during the infiltration of the etched enamel pores, and the sealant does not set until it is light-initiated. The disadvantage of light-cured sealants is the cost of the visible light unit. A number of units may be needed in a dental practice if sealants are placed by auxiliaries.

Tinted and clear sealant materials are also available. The tinted materials are usually either opaque white or transparent pink. Tinted sealants have been advocated because of ease of detection by both the dentist and the parents, which allows for monitoring of sealant retention. With clear sealants, detection of the sealant requires tactile exploration of the sealed surface. No apparent differences have been reported between tinted and clear sealants for retention rates and caries prevention.

Pit and Fissure Treatment Alternatives

With pits and fissures, there are four treatment alternatives that may be considered by the dental practitioner: (1) observation only, (2) sealant placement, (3) preventive resin restoration, and (4) amalgam or posterior composite restoration. The diagnostic criteria and recommended treatments are presented in Table 31–1.

The indications for sealant placement are the following: (1) deep, retentive pits and fissures, which may cause wedging or catching of an explorer; (2) patient has positive history of previous occlusal lesions in other teeth; (3) patient is receiving other preventive treatment, such as systemic and topical fluoride therapy, to inhibit interproximal caries formation; and (4) tooth considered for sealant application erupted less than 4 years ago.

Contraindications for sealant placement are the following: (1) well-coalesced, self-cleaning pits and fissures; (2) patients with many interproximal lesions and no preventive treatment to inhibit interproximal caries formation; and (3) tooth has remained caries free for 4 years or longer. These contraindications are general ones that should be taken into consideration when pits and fissures are being evaluated. However, if the clinical impression is a questionable one with respect to whether to seal an occlusal surface, it would be more appropriate to err toward sealant placement than toward observation of the surface and development of occlusal caries over a period of time.

A clinical procedure for restoration of isolated pits and fissures and simultaneous caries prevention in the remaining, unaffected pits and fissures, known as the preventive resin restoration, utilizes the acid-etch technique. This technique was introduced in 1978 by Simonsen as an alternative to either sealing over a questionable occlusal surface or restoring the entire surface with an amalgam restoration. The technique involves widening of the pits and fissures

Table 31–1 ■ Protocol for pit and fissure treatment alternatives

Diagnosis	Treatment
Caries Free Surface No explorer wedging* Well-coalesced, self-cleanable fissures or no identifiable fissures	**No Treatment** Observation only
Caries Free Surface No explorer wedging Stained fissure Tooth erupted more than 4 years ago	**No Treatment** Observation only
Caries Free Surface No explorer wedging Stained or decalcified appearance of fissures Tooth erupted less than 4 years ago	**Sealant Placement** Adequate isolation from saliva: place sealant Adequate isolation not possible: allow further eruption, and place sealant within 3 months
Caries Free Surface Explorer wedging as a result of anatomy of fissures Stained or decalcified appearance of fissures	**Sealant Placement** Adequate isolation from saliva: place sealant Adequate isolation not possible: allow further eruption, and place sealant within 3 months
Incipient Caries Explorer catch† as a result of incipient caries limited to isolated pits and fissures Decalcified appearance of pit and fissures indicative of incipient caries	**Preventive Resin Restorations** Type A Type B Type C
Carious Surface Obvious clinical caries with explorer catch Loss of enamel adjacent to fissures Demineralized appearance to occlusal surface Generalized involvement of fissures with caries	**Restoration** Amalgam restoration *or* Posterior composite restoration

* *Explorer wedging:* Defined as a catch of a sharp explorer in pits or fissures on a clean, dry surface with the following characteristics: (1) pit or fissure is probed vertically, (2) explorer engages a fissure with no clinical or radiographic evidence of caries, (3) action may or may not be reproducible, (4) explorer penetrates into enamel only, and (5) probing by the explorer may elicit slight discomfort.

† *Explorer catch:* Defined as an obvious catch of a sharp explorer in pits or fissures on a clean, dry surface with the following characteristics: (1) pit or fissure is probed vertically, (2) explorer engages a fissure with clinical evidence of incipient enamel or dentinal caries, (3) action is definitely reproducible, (4) explorer engages the fissure such that the explorer's weight is supported with minimal stabilization by the operator, (5) explorer penetrates both enamel and dentin, (6) fissure may or may not have radiographic evidence of caries, and (7) explorer possibly elicits slight discomfort or pain on probing.

and removal of enamel and/or dentin that appears to be affected by caries. Depending on the extent of caries removal, either a filled or unfilled resin is used to restore the cavity, while a sealant material is placed over the remaining, intact pits and fissures.

The indications for a preventive resin restoration are the following: (1) An explorer catch in isolated pits and fissures, indicating the presence of caries; (2) deep pits and fissures that either prohibit complete penetration of sealant material or may possibly have caries of clinical significance at their bases; (3) an opaque, chalky appearance along the pits and fissures, indicative of incipient caries of clinical significance;

and (4) absence of interproximal caries and preventive treatment to decrease the likelihood of interproximal caries formation.

The contraindications for a preventive resin restoration are the following: (1) interproximal caries requiring restoration, and (2) extent of caries involvement requiring restoration of the entire surface with either an amalgam or a posterior composite (Hicks, 1984a).

Three types of preventive resin restorations have been described (Simonsen, 1980; Hicks, 1984b). Type A preventive resin restorations require minimal preparation of pits and fissures with a No. ¼ or ½ round bur prior to sealant placement. A diluted composite consisting of a

mixture of unfilled resin and posterior composite material is preferred to fill a Type B cavity that is prepared with a No. 1 or 2 round bur. Caries removal with a Type B preventive resin usually results in more than one half of the total depth of enamel being involved; however, the cavity is still within enamel. The Type C restoration requires the use of a No. 2 or larger round bur. This cavity usually extends into dentin and may require a calcium hydroxide base. A Type C cavity should be restored with a posterior composite material, following application of either an unfilled bonding resin or a dentinal bonding agent. It must be emphasized that only pits and fissures with caries of clinical significance are prepared, and intact pits and fissures with no clinical evidence of caries are not included in the preparation.

Retention and Caries Prevention with Sealants and Preventive Resin Restorations

Numerous clinical trials have been carried out to assess the retention rates and caries reduction associated with sealant placement (Fig. 31–5A). One of the longest-running clinical trials has involved periodic evaluations of a single application of a chemical-cured sealant to over 313 sites in first permanent molars in 205 children aged 6–10 years (Houpt and Shey, 1983). The retention rate for the sealants was followed over a 6-year period. The caries incidence for the sealed teeth was compared with contralateral, paired first molar teeth that were caries free at the beginning of the study. One year following sealant application, 94% of the sealants were completely retained and caries had occurred in 3% of the sealed teeth. Over 23% of control teeth either were found to have occlusal caries or had been restored. By year 3 of the study, 83% of the sealants were completely retained. Although caries occurred in 12% of the sealed teeth, 54% of the control teeth either had been restored or had occlusal caries. By year 6 of the study, 74% of the control teeth had experienced caries, whereas only 25% of the sealed teeth either had been restored or had occlusal caries. The retention rate for the sealants was 58% after the sixth year. It is interesting to note that even though 42% of the occlusal surfaces had lost their sealants, only 25% had developed caries. This implies that even if sealant material is not detected clinically, it may be present in the depth of the fissure and provide protection against caries formation. The results from this study would be considered representative for most other studies using the current generation of sealant materials. The level of caries prevention shown within this study is

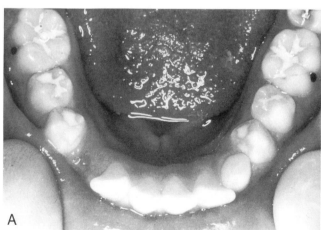

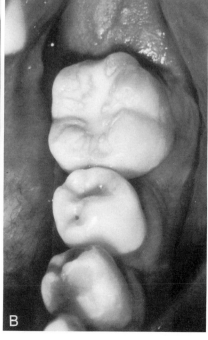

Figure 31–5 ■ Clinical appearance of fissure sealants and a preventive resin restoration. A, These sealants have been retained for 6 years with the permanent first molars and for 2 years with the premolar teeth and are protecting these teeth from occlusal caries formation. B, After 5 years, this preventive resin restoration is still present and is responsible for the occlusal surface of the first molar remaining caries-free.

quite remarkable, considering that only a single application of sealant material occurred. Should a sealant be lost in a private practice setting, reapplication of the sealant would occur, whereas in the vast majority of clinical sealant trials, the research protocol allows for only a single application of sealant.

Reapplication of sealants to occlusal surfaces that have lost their sealants may provide a much greater reduction in caries than reported by most single-application sealant studies. In fact, a study was completed that incorporated reapplication of sealant following sealant loss as part of its research protocol (Charbeneau, 1982). This study reported that over a 4-year period 54% of sealed surfaces required no reapplications, 32% required one reapplication, 10% required two reapplications, and 5% required three reapplications. The retention rate at the end of the first year was 92%. With the reapplication protocol, the lowest retention rate was 85% after the third year of the study, with 93% retention occurring at the end of the fourth year. This study indicated that an 8% reapplication rate per year may be necessary. Of great interest was the fact that this type of preventive dentistry program was found to be 100% effective in occlusal caries prevention over a 4-year period. It appears as though in a dental practice that maintains an adequate recall system for sealant evaluation and that reapplies sealant material to occlusal surfaces that have lost their sealants, a relatively high degree of caries prevention would be experienced.

Similar levels of caries reduction and retention may be expected when sealants are applied to primary molars. In a clinical study involving a single application of sealant to 436 primary molars and 583 permanent molars, 94.9% of the primary teeth had retained their sealants after 3 years, while 93.5% of the permanent molars had retained their sealants (Simonsen, 1981).

Preventive resin restorations appear to have a relatively high retention rate and a significant effect on caries formation in surfaces with pits and fissures (Fig. 31–5B). A 5-year clinical trial has evaluated retention and caries incidence associated with 332 preventive resin restorations placed in predominately first molar teeth of 110 children aged 6–14 years (Houpt et al, 1986). Complete retention of preventive resin restorations was found in 72% of cases. Partial loss occurred with 22% of the restorations, whereas only 6% of the restorations had been completely lost. Caries had occurred in only 7% of cases. It would appear that preventive resin res-

torations are retained as well as, if not to a higher degree than, sealants are on occlusal surfaces. However, preventive resin restorations appear to prevent occlusal caries to a much higher level than sealant placement. Similar results were found in a clinical trial of 3 years duration in which caries occurred in less than 1% of patients treated with preventive resin restorations (Simonsen, 1980).

Clinical Technique: Sealant Application and Preventive Resin Restoration Placement

SEALANT APPLICATION

Step 1 ■ Isolation of the tooth from salivary contamination should be carried out, preferably using rubber dam isolation (Fig. 31–6). If rubber dam isolation is not possible, cotton roll isolation with adequate suction to remove saliva from the operating field is necessary.

Step 2 ■ Prophylaxis of the tooth surface to be sealed should be carried out, using a fluoride free pumice slurry applied with a rubber cup or brush using a slow speed handpiece. An alternative prophylactic method is cleaning the fissure with a sodium bicarbonate slurry applied with an ultrasonic unit. Rinse the tooth surface thoroughly to remove the prophylactic paste and oral debris. Dry the tooth surface.

Step 3 ■ Apply the etching agent to the tooth surface with a fine brush, a cotton pledget, or a mini-sponge for 60 seconds with permanent teeth and 120 seconds with primary teeth. Gently rub the etchant applicator on the tooth surface and periodically add etching agent to the tooth surface.

Step 4 ■ Rinse the tooth surface with an air-water spray for 10 seconds. This will remove both the etching agent and reaction products from the etched enamel surface. Dry the tooth surface for approximately 5 seconds. The etched enamel will take on a frosted white appearance. If the enamel does not have this appearance, repeat the etching step. If cotton roll isolation has been used, replace the cotton rolls at this time, making certain that salivary contamination of the etched enamel does not occur. If salivary contamination does occur at this stage, rinse the tooth surface, dry thoroughly, and repeat the etching process for a full 60 seconds.

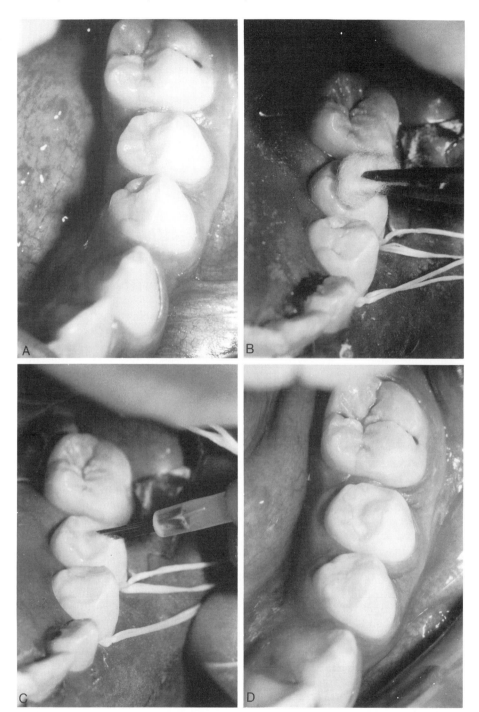

Figure 31-6 ■ Sealant application. *A*, Sealant application to the occlusal surfaces of these premolar teeth is necessary because of the presence of deep retentive fissures. *B*, Following rubber dam isolation and pumice prophylaxis, phosphoric acid is applied to the teeth for 60 seconds, using a cotton pledget. The etched surface is then rinsed thoroughly and dried. *C*, An opaque sealant is applied with a fine brush. Polymerization of the sealant is completed with a visible light unit for 20 seconds. With chemical-cured sealants, setting time varies from 1 to 2 minutes following mixing of the materials. *D*, Following removal of the rubber dam, the occlusion should be evaluated to determine if adjustment is necessary.

Step 5 ■ Apply the sealant material to the etched surface with a fine brush, a mini-sponge, or an applicator provided by the manufacturer. Place an adequate amount of sealant to cover all fissures on the occlusal surface. A thin layer of sealant should be carried up buccal and lingual inclines of the occlusal surface in order to seal supplementary fissures. With chemical-cured sealants, working time varies from 1–2 minutes. With light-cured sealants, curing is initiated by exposing the sealant to visible light and requires 10–20 seconds.

Step 6 ■ Explore the entire occlusal surface for pits and fissures that have not been sealed and for voids in the material. If deficiencies are found, apply additional sealant. Usually, a sticky layer of apparently unreacted sealant will be present on the surface. This is an air-inhibited layer of sealant that does not undergo polymerization. Remove the rubber dam.

Step 7 ■ Evaluate the occlusion of the sealed surface to determine if excessive sealant material is present and needs to be removed. A small discrepancy in occlusal interference is easily tolerated because the sealant will abrade, allowing for proper interdigitation of the teeth.

PREVENTIVE RESIN RESTORATION PLACEMENT

Placing a preventive resin restoration utilizes the same principles of the acid-etch technique as those of sealant placement, with the exception of caries removal from isolated pits and fissures.

Step 1 ■ Isolate teeth as described previously (Fig. 31–7).

Step 2 ■ Remove caries from isolated pits and fissures, using a round bur in a high speed handpiece. The size of the round bur will be dictated by the amount of caries present. Only caries should be removed, and no attempt should be made to incorporate retention into the preparation.

Step 3 ■ Perform prophylaxis of occlusal surface as described previously, followed by rinsing and drying.

Step 4 ■ If dentin is exposed, a calcium hydroxide base should be placed prior to acid-etching.

Step 5 ■ Acid-etch the occlusal surface as described previously.

Step 6 ■ Place a thin layer of resin bonding

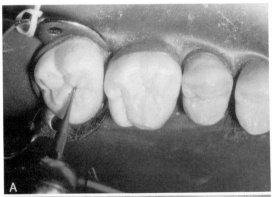
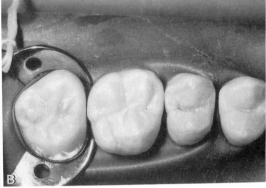
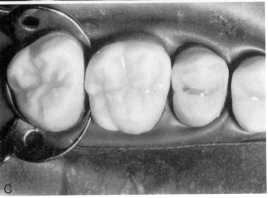

Figure 31–7 ■ Preventive resin restoration placement. *A*, Following isolation with a rubber dam, pits and fissures with caries of clinical significance are removed with a round bur in a high-speed handpiece. *B*, Following minimal cavity preparation, a pumice prophylaxis is carried out. If dentin is exposed, a cavity base should be placed prior to etching the occlusal surface. *C*, Type A preventive resin restorations have been completed. The occlusion should be evaluated to determine if adjustment is necessary.

agent or dentinal bonding agent into the cavity preparation, followed by a diluted posterior composite for a Type B cavity or a posterior composite material for a Type C cavity. If the restorative material is chemically cured, allow to set. If a light-cured material is used, expose the material to a visible light source. Once the material is set, apply sealant material over the restored area and adjacent intact, etched fissures. With a Type A preventive resin restoration, only sealant material is applied to the occlusal surface, including the prepared enamel.

Step 7 ■ Explore the surface for exposed pits and fissures and voids in the material. If necessary, apply additional sealant material. Remove the rubber dam.

Step 8 ■ Evaluate the occlusion, and adjust if necessary.

Although both techniques involved in sealant application and placement of preventive resin restorations appear to be simple, a high degree of failure may occur if the operator does not pay strict attention to the steps in the acid-etch technique. Of particular importance to the success of the acid-etch procedure is avoidance of salivary contamination of the enamel once the surface has been etched.

Scientific Basis for the Acid-Etch Technique

Initial studies involving acid-etching of surface enamel utilized 85% phosphoric acid. Since the 1950's, a considerable number of both laboratory and clinical studies have been performed to determine the appropriate acid type and concentration that would yield optimal bonding characteristics with the least loss of surface enamel. Phosphoric acid in the range of 30–40% (weight to weight) with an application time of 60 seconds for permanent teeth and 120 seconds for primary teeth has been shown to produce optimal bonding characteristics while minimizing loss of surface enamel. Primary teeth have been shown to require increased etching times as a result of the decreased mineral content and increased organic content of primary enamel. The majority of commercially available sealant materials utilize either 35 or 37% phosphoric acid as the etching agent. One sealant material utilizes 50% phosphoric acid with 7% zinc oxide added to reduce the effects of surface enamel loss (Silverstone, 1974; Silverstone et al, 1975).

Acid-etching of surface enamel has been shown to produce a certain degree of porosity (Silverstone, 1975). In fact, sound enamel etched with phosphoric acid has been shown to be affected at three levels, using imbibition studies with polarized light microscopy (Fig. 31–8). First, there is a narrow zone of enamel that is removed by etching. In this manner, plaque and surface and subsurface organic cuticles are effectively removed. Fully reacted mineral crystals in the surface enamel are also removed, resulting in exposure of a more reactive surface, an increase in surface area, and a reduced surface tension that allows for resin to wet the etched surface more readily. This zone is approximately 10 μm in depth and has been called the etched zone. The second zone is the qualitative porous zone, which is 20 μm in depth. This zone is rendered porous by the etchant and may be identified qualitatively using polarized light microscopy. The third histologic zone of etching is qualitatively indistinguishable from the adjacent enamel and may be detected only with quantitative polarized light techniques. This zone is approximately 20 μm deep and is called the quantitative porous zone.

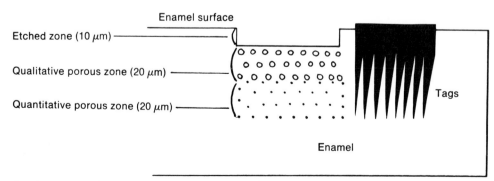

Figure 31–8 ■ Histologic zones created in sound enamel by the acid-etch technique. Resin penetrates into the porosities in etched sound enamel, forming retentive resin tags.

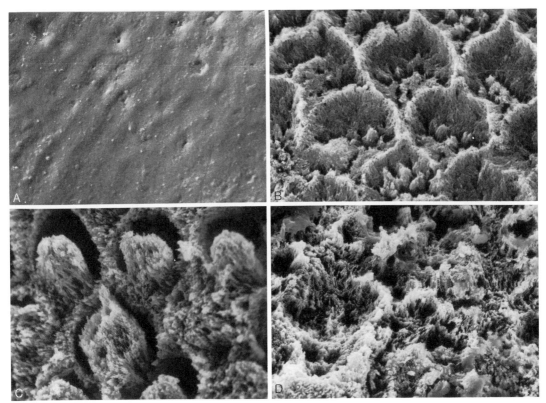

Figure 31–9 ■ Effects of the acid-etch technique on surface morphology (scanning electron microscopy). *A*, The surface of sound enamel is relatively smooth, with occasional depressions representing terminations of enamel prisms. *B*, Type 1 etching pattern, with loss of prism cores following etching. *C*, Type 2 etching pattern, with loss of prism peripheries following etching. *D*, Type 3 etching pattern, with surface porosities but without a distinct prism morphologic appearance.

When a sealant material is applied to an etched enamel surface, the resin material penetrates into the porosities created within the sound enamel by the etching procedure.

Three characteristic etching patterns occur when surface enamel is exposed to phosphoric acid (Fig. 31–9). The type 1 etching pattern demonstrates a generalized roughening of the enamel surface but with a distinct pattern (Fig. 31–9B). The enamel prism cores have been lost as a result of the etching procedure, leaving the prism peripheries relatively intact. The average diameter of the hollowed prism core measures 3 μm. With the type 2 etching pattern, the prism peripheries appear to be lost (Fig. 31–9C). The prism cores remain behind, projecting toward the original enamel surface. Some regions of enamel possess neither type 1 nor type 2 etching patterns. Within these regions, areas in which the etching patterns do not conform to prism morphology may be seen (Fig. 31–9D). These regions are referred to as having a type 3 etching pattern. No specific etching pattern is preferentially created during the etching procedure, and types 1, 2 and 3 etching patterns will oftentimes be found adjacent to one another (Silverstone et al, 1975; Silverstone, 1974).

Enamel-Resin Interface

Following application of a sealant material to an etched occlusal surface, the pits and fissures that were present in the surface are occluded with resin material (Fig. 31–10A). The surface morphology of the occlusal surface changes from a surface in which plaque and debris can accumulate easily to a surface with no readily apparent pits and fissures that may be relatively self-cleansing. When the interface between the enamel and resin are examined, it is found to be an intimate one with no detectable space present between the resin and underlying etched enamel (Fig. 31–10B).

Sealant materials do not simply bond to the enamel surface but rather penetrate into micro-

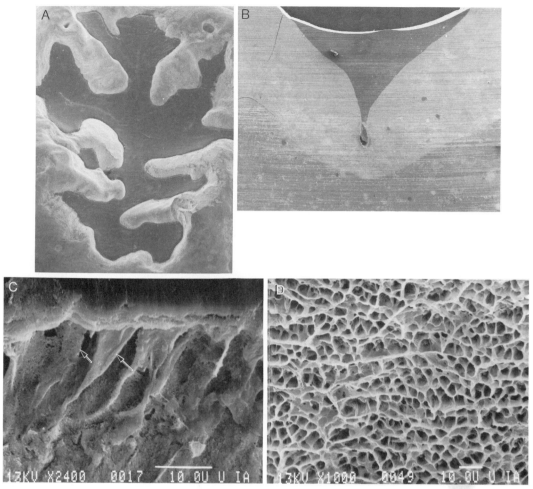

Figure 31–10 ■ The enamel-resin interface (scanning electron microscopy). *A,* Following sealant placement, the pits and fissures on this occlusal surface are protected from cariogenic challenges by the acid-resistant sealant. *B,* The interface between the enamel forming the fissure and the sealant appears to be an intimate one, with no apparent space between the etched enamel and sealant. *C,* Following partial demineralization of enamel that has been sealed, resin tags *(arrows)* may be seen in the etched enamel. *D,* Complete demineralization of enamel that has been sealed allows one to visualize the appearance of the acid-resistant resin tags.

pores created in enamel during the etching procedure. This infiltration of the enamel results in the formation of resin tags within the etched enamel, which allows the sealant to be retained (Fig. 31–10C and D). The depth of penetration by the resin may be determined by measuring the resin tag length following partial or complete demineralization of the tooth structure in dilute acid. Resin tags, on the average, penetrate etched enamel to a depth of 25–50 μm, with some tags terminating at depths of up to 100 μm from the surface (Silverstone, 1974, 1984).

Resin tags serve a number of functions. They provide a mechanical means for retention of the sealant. The resin tags surround the enamel crystals and may provide resistance to demineralization by acids. BIS-GMA sealant materials are resistant to acid dissolution and have been shown to provide protection along the enamel-resin interface against a caries-like attack (Fig. 31–11). Finally, the enamel-resin interface creates a protective barrier against colonization of the fissure by microorganisms and does not allow passage of nutriments into the fissure (Hicks and Silverstone, 1982a, b).

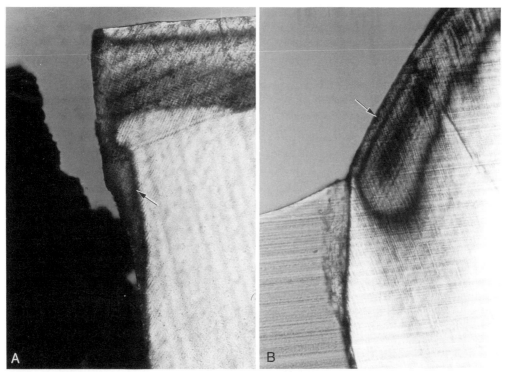

Figure 31 – 11 ■ Caries-like lesion formation adjacent to amalgam and sealant materials (polarized light microscopy; water imbibition). *A,* Secondary caries formation *(arrow)* may be seen along the cavity wall of this amalgam restoration, indicating that microleakage between the restoration and cavity wall has occurred. Fracturing of the restoration occurred during preparation of the section for microscopic examination. *B,* The primary surface lesion *(arrow)* terminates at the point where bonding occurs between the etched enamel and sealant material. No secondary cavity wall lesion exists. Resin tags provide resistance against a cariogenic challenge at the enamel-resin interface.

Caries Susceptibility of Acid-Etched Enamel

Concern has been expressed by dental practitioners regarding whether caries susceptibility is increased when a sealant is lost from the occlusal surface as a result of the fact that the enamel was etched with an acid solution prior to sealant placement. Results from laboratory studies have shown that etched enamel is definitely more susceptible to both acid dissolution and artificial caries formation than sound enamel (Silverstone, 1977, 1984; Hicks and Silverstone, 1982b). This is not surprising, because etched enamel has a greater degree of porosity and an increased surface area for acid to come in contact with than sound enamel does. However, if etched enamel is exposed to saliva for a 24-hour period prior to either demineralization in acid or an artificial cariogenic challenge, acid solubility and the extent of artificial lesion formation in both etched and sound enamel are comparable. This implies that exposure of etched enamel to saliva for a relatively short period of time allows for remineralization of the etched surface, resulting in resistance to demineralization similar to pre-treatment levels. When a previously sealed enamel surface that has had the resin abraded to the point at which the resin can no longer be detected macroscopically is subjected to acid dissolution, adjacent sound enamel is found to have a higher solubility rate than the enamel that had been sealed. These laboratory findings have been supported by clinical studies in which significant reductions in caries were found where partial or even total loss of sealant from the teeth had occurred (Houpt and Shey, 1983). There is no doubt that resin tags remain behind that are not clinically detectable but still provide a caries-preventive function for enamel.

Therefore, should a sealant be lost from an occlusal surface or etched enamel adjacent to a sealant be left exposed following sealant application, the caries susceptibility of the exposed

enamel would be similar to that for adjacent sound enamel. However, this does not mean that if a sealant is lost, reapplication should not occur. In order to ensure that caries formation of clinical significance does not commence, the occlusal surface should be protected by reapplication of sealant material.

Salivary Contamination of Acid-Etched Enamel

Perhaps the greatest reason for failure with sealants is a lack of regard for proper isolation of etched enamel from contamination with saliva. With early sealant studies, the effect of salivary contamination on the success of the acid-etch technique was not known. A high degree of failure with respect to sealant loss and caries development most likely occurred because saliva had contaminated the etched enamel and did not allow resin penetration into the porosities of the etched enamel.

The protection of etched enamel from salivary contamination is now considered to be the key to success with the acid-etch technique. Studies have been completed in order to determine whether enamel surfaces exposed to saliva for short periods of time may simply be rinsed with an air-water spray to remove surface contamination (Silverstone et al, 1985; Silverstone, 1984). It has been demonstrated that a tenacious surface coating that cannot be removed by an air-water spray forms on etched enamel with exposure times to saliva of from 60 seconds to 0.5 seconds (Fig. 31–12). Only when etched enamel is exposed to saliva for less than 1 second can the surface coating be removed from the etched enamel surface. This means that should salivary contamination occur, the tooth surface should be rinsed and dried thoroughly, followed by repetition of the etching step in its entirety prior to placement of the resin.

An additional source of contamination of the etched enamel surface is the air-water syringe. It is possible for oil and/or water to contaminate the air line. If the air line is contaminated, a thin microscopic film of oil and/or water may be deposited on the etched surface, which would interfere with penetration of the resin into the etched enamel. Periodically, the air line should be evaluated for contamination by blowing air onto the surface of a mirror. If oil and/or water droplets form on the mirror surface, contamination of the air line has occurred and filtration to remove the contaminants may be necessary.

Sealing Over Caries

Because caries may be present histologically for a considerable time prior to clinical and radiographic detection, it is quite likely that sealant placement over a clinically caries free surface may result in sealing over caries and sealing microorganisms beneath the sealant. This has caused a great deal of concern with practitioners and dental researchers alike.

The effects of sealant placement on the viability of microorganisms and the clinical ap-

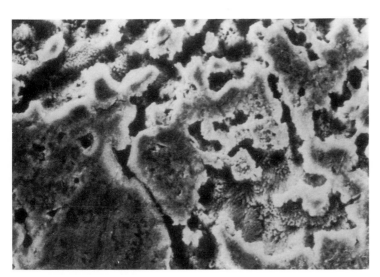

Figure 31–12 ■ Etched enamel that was exposed to saliva for only 10 seconds. A tenacious surface coating, which would interfere with resin bonding, is present, even though the surface was rinsed thoroughly following salivary contamination (scanning electron microscopy).

pearance of caries have been studied (Jensen and Handelman, 1980; Handelman et al, 1976; Mertz-Fairhurst et al, 1979a, b, 1986). Microbiologic studies have been completed, involving sealant placement over carious but intact fissures from molar teeth with radiographic evidence of dentinal involvement. A 23-fold reduction in viable microorganisms from these sealed carious teeth has been reported in as little as 2 weeks following sealant placement. After periods of up to 2 years following sealant placement over dentinal caries, a 99.9% reduction in viable microorganisms was reported. In fact, it has been found that the etching step itself eliminates 75% of viable microorganisms from the fissure.

Of clinical significance was the radiographic appearance of sealed surfaces with caries. The majority of studies have reported that sealed lesions appeared to be arrested and did not progress, whereas control teeth that had not been sealed had lesions that progressed clinically by an average of 640 μm (Mertz-Fairhurst et al, 1979b, 1986). A study that evaluated carious teeth that were sealed for a 5-year period found that sealing over caries resulted in reversal of 89% of the lesions from a caries active to a caries inactive status (Going, 1984). When a sealant was removed to place an amalgam restoration, the affected dentin had a dry, leathery appearance with sclerotic dentin beneath the area of the arrested lesion. The results from sealing over caries involving enamel and dentin emphasize the fact that if sealants are applied properly and are monitored on a continuing basis, one would not expect caries to progress beneath the sealant. If dentinal involvement that is clinically undetectable has occurred, sealing over the incipient lesion may allow for biologic repair of the affected dentin by odontoblasts.

Sealant Utilization

Although the efficacy of sealant placement in reduction of dental caries in pits and fissures has been studied extensively, the dental profession, as a whole, has not adopted sealant usage as would be hoped. In the first American Dental Association (ADA) Survey on attitudes toward sealant usage conducted in 1974, only 38% of the approximately 3500 dentists surveyed used sealants in their dental practice (Gift et al, 1975). At that time, the major reasons for nonutilization of sealants were (1) the effectiveness

of sealants was not substantiated by research, (2) there was the possibility of sealing in decay, and (3) sealants do not last long in the mouth. In 1982, the ADA conducted a similar survey of approximately 3000 dentists in order to determine if changes in attitude and levels of utilization of sealants since the initial survey had occurred (Gift and Frew, 1986). The results were somewhat discouraging. In 1982, at least 58% of dentists surveyed did not use sealants in their practice. Only 10% of dentists felt that sealants were very effective in caries prevention, as opposed to over 77% that believed water fluoridation was very effective in caries prevention. The only group in which the majority of dentists had positive attitudes toward sealant usage was in the group of dentists whose practices consisted of greater than 75% children. In descending order, the most common reasons for not using sealants were (1) sealants do not last long in the mouth, (2) there is the possibility of sealing in decay, (3) placing occlusal restorations is preferred, (4) some patients are unwilling to pay for sealants, (5) sealant use is unsubstantiated by research, and (6) sealants are non-reimbursable by most insurance programs. It appears as though a need for education of the dental profession with respect to the caries preventive potential of sealants exists. In fact, the ADA Health Association has called for education of the general public, as well as the dentist, to the value of sealants in prevention of pit and fissure caries.

Sealants and Amalgam Restorations: A Comparison

Placing an amalgam restoration instead of a sealant on an occlusal surface is preferred by over two thirds of dentists who do not use sealant (Gift and Frew, 1986). This represents at least 39% of dentists. The reason for preferring to place amalgam restorations instead of prevention of caries by sealant placement is based primarily upon the belief that amalgam restorations represent a permanent restoration, whereas sealants are only a temporary measure. However, clinical studies assessing the longevity of amalgam restorations have found only 47% of the restorations to be acceptable after a 5-year period in adults (Hamilton et al, 1981). It has also been shown that 50% of amalgam restorations are replaced usually between 5 and 10 years following insertion (Rob-

inson, 1971; Allan, 1977). With children, the median survival time for amalgam restorations prior to replacement is dependent upon the age of the child at the time the restoration was placed (Walls et al, 1985). The 5-year survival rate for occlusal amalgam restorations prior to replacement has been shown to be 30% for children 5–7 years of age, 43% for children 7–9 years of age, 61% for children 9–11 years of age, and 63% for adolescents 11–15 years of age. It would appear that both sealants and amalgam restorations follow quite similar courses with respect to retention in children and adolescents. The major difference is that with sealant placement a preventive technique has been utilized, whereas amalgam placement represents a restorative technique in which tooth structure is lost. In fact, it has been shown that with replacement of a defective amalgam restoration, the periphery of the cavity preparation increases by 38%, resulting in even greater loss of tooth structure (Elderton, 1976). With sealant loss, reapplication of sealant material may be accomplished with a high percentage of teeth, allowing for continued caries protection and maintenance of an intact tooth.

Two other factors are of concern to dentists who prefer to place occlusal amalgam restorations rather than sealants. The first factor is the belief that sealants require more time to place than amalgam restorations. However, the total amount of time to place a sealant has been shown to be less than 6½ minutes. In one study of occlusal amalgam restorations, the total time for placement was 13 minutes, 51 seconds. With placement and maintenance time over a 4-year period, sealants required a total of only 10 minutes, 2 seconds of time, whereas the time required for amalgam restorations was 14 minutes, 7 seconds (Charbeneau, 1982). The second factor is that dentists who do not use sealants believe that sealants cost more than amalgam restorations to place and maintain. Over a 5-year period, the cost of care for children receiving sealants was $10.23 per child per year, as opposed to $21.15 per child per year for the control group (Simonsen, 1982). More recently, a 10-year retrospective study evaluating the cost-effectiveness of sealant placement and maintenance in a fluoridated community was completed (Simonsen, 1987). It was found that first permanent molars that were not sealed had an 8-fold likelihood that they would become carious, when compared with first permanent molars that had been sealed. The cost of treating the unsealed teeth with the necessary restorations was found to be 1.64 times the cost of

application and maintenance of the sealed teeth. The results from these studies indicate that significant monetary savings may be realized if sealants are placed when indicated, rather than simply monitoring pits and fissures that are considered to be at a relatively high risk for caries development in the near future (Simonsen, 1987).

Perhaps the major factors for the relatively high level of non-utilization of sealants in the pediatric age group are related to the fact that only a small number of insurance programs pay for sealants and that parents are not aware of the benefits of sealants. With insurance programs that pay for sealants, only a small percentage of the sealant fee is paid and the parent must pay the remaining fee. The value of sealants as a preventive agent is not understood either by the insurance profession or by most parents. There is also concern by the insurance profession regarding wholesale utilization of sealants by dental practitioners and placement of sealants on teeth not requiring sealants for the economic gain of the dentist. Until the dental profession accepts a standardized protocol for sealant usage and educates both the insurance profession and the general public regarding the economic benefits of and need for sealants in caries prevention, sealants will continue to be an underutilized preventive service for the pediatric and adolescent population.

REFERENCES

Allan DN: A longitudinal study of dental restorations. Br Dent J 143:87, 1977.

Bell RM, Klein SP, Bohannan HM, Graves RC, Disney JA: Treatment Effects in the National Preventive Dentistry Demonstration Program. Publication No. R-3072-RWS, Santa Monica, CA, The Rand Corporation, 1984.

Bodecker CF: The eradication of enamel fissures. Dent Items Interest 51:859, 1929.

Bohannan HM, Disney JA, Graves RC, Bader JD, Klein SP, Bell RM: Indications for sealant use in a community-based preventive dentistry program. J Dent Educ 48:45, 1984.

Bowen RL: Composite and sealant resins—past, present and future. Pediatr Dent 4:10, 1982.

Buonocore MG: Simple method of increasing the adhesion of acrylic filling materials to enamel surfaces. J Dent Res 34:849, 1955.

Charbeneau GT: Pit and fissure sealants. J Dent 32:215, 1982.

Elderton RJ: The cause of failure of restorations: A literature review. J Dent 4:257, 1976.

Galil KA, Gwinnett AJ: Three-dimensional replicas of pits and fissures in human teeth: Scanning electron microscopic study. Arch Oral Biol 20:493, 1975.

Gift HC, Frew RA: Sealants: Changing patterns. JADA 112:391, 1986.

Gift HC, Frew RA, Hefferren J: Attitudes toward and use of pit and fissure sealants. J Dent Child 42:460, 1975.

Going RE: Sealant effect on incipient caries, enamel maturation, and future caries susceptibility. J Dent Educ 48:35, 1984.

Graves RC, Burt BA: The pattern of the carious attack in children as a consideration in the use of fissure sealants. J Prev Dent 2:28, 1975.

Hamilton JC, Moffa JP, Ellison JA: Ten-year clinical evaluation of two different amalgams. J Dent Res 60:521, 1981.

Handelman SL, Washburn F, Wopperer P: Two-year report on the sealant effect on bacteria in dental caries. J Dent Res 93:967, 1976.

Hennon DK, Stookey GK, Muhler JC: Prevalence and distribution of dental caries in preschool children. JADA 79:1405, 1969.

Hicks MJ: Preventive resin restorations: Etching patterns, resin tag morphology and the enamel-resin interface. J Dent Child 51:116, 1984a.

Hicks MJ: Caries-like lesion formation around occlusal alloy and preventive resin restorations. Pediatr Dent 6:17, 1984b.

Hicks MJ, Flaitz CM: Caries-like lesion formation in occlusal fissures: An *in vitro* study. Quint Int 17:405–410, 1986.

Hicks MJ, Silverstone LM: Fissure sealants and dental enamel: A histological study of microleakage *in vitro*. Caries Res 16:353, 1982a.

Hicks MJ, Silverstone LM: The effect of sealant application and sealant loss on caries-like lesion formation *in vitro*. Pediatr Dent 4:111, 1982b.

Hicks MJ, Flaitz CM, Silverstone LM: The current status of dental caries in the pediatric population. J Pedod 10:57, 1985.

Houpt M, Shey Z: The effectiveness of a fissure sealant after six years. Pediatr Dent 5:104, 1983.

Houpt M, Eidelman E, Shey Z, Fuks A, Chosak A, Shapira J: The composite/sealant restoration. Five-year results. J Prosth Dent 55:164, 1986.

Hyatt TP: Occlusal fissures: Their frequency and danger. How shall they be treated? Dent Items Interest 46:493, 1924.

Jensen OE, Handelman SL: Effect of an autopolymerizing sealant on viability of microflora in occlusal dental caries. Scand J Dent Res 88:382, 1980.

Mertz-Fairhurst EJ, Schuster GS, Fairhurst CW: Arresting caries by sealants: Results of a clinical study. JADA 112:194, 1986.

Mertz-Fairhurst EJ, Schuster GS, Williams JE, Fairhurst CW: Clinical progress of sealed and unsealed caries. Part I: Depth changes and bacterial counts. J Prosth Dent 42:521, 1979a.

Mertz-Fairhurst EJ, Schuster GS, Williams JE, Fairhurst CW: Clinical progress of sealed and unsealed caries. Part II: Standardized radiographs and clinical observations. J Prosth Dent 42:633, 1979b.

National Caries Program, NIDR: The Prevalence of Dental Caries in United States Children, 1979–1980. NIH Publication No. 82-2245, December, 1981.

National Center for Health Statistics: Decayed, Missing and Filled Teeth Among Children: United States. Vital and Health Statistics, Series 11—No. 106, DHEW Publication No. (HSM) 72-1003, Washington, DC, US Government Printing Office, 1971.

National Center for Health Statistics: Decayed, Missing and Filled Teeth Among Youths 12–17 Years: United States. Vital and Health Statistics, Series 11—No. 144, DHEW Publication No. (HRA) 75-1626, Washington, DC, US Government Printing Office, 1974.

Ngano T: Relationship between form of pits and fissures and the primary lesion of caries. Dent Abstr 6:426, 1961.

Robinson AD: The life of a filling. Br Dent J 130:206, 1971.

Silverstone LM: Fissure sealants: Laboratory studies. Caries Res 8:2, 1974.

Silverstone LM: *In vitro* studies with special reference to the enamel surface and the enamel-resin interface. Proc Int Symp on Acid-Etch Technique. Saint Paul, MN, North Central Publishing, 1975, p 39.

Silverstone LM: Fissure sealants: The susceptibility to dissolution of acid-etched and subsequently abraded enamel *in vitro*. Caries Res 11:46, 1977.

Silverstone LM: State of the art on sealant research and priorities for further research. J Dent Educ 48:107, 1984.

Silverstone LM, Hicks MJ, Featherstone MJ: Oral fluid contamination of etched enamel surfaces: An SEM study. JADA 110:329, 1985.

Silverstone LM, Saxton CA, Dogon IL, Fejerskov O: Variation in the etching pattern of acid-etching of human dental enamel examined by scanning electron microscopy. Caries Res 9:373, 1975.

Simonsen RJ: Preventive resin restorations (I). Quint Int 1:69, 1978a.

Simonsen RJ: Preventive resin restorations (II). Quint Int 2:95, 1978b.

Simonsen RJ: Preventive resin restorations: Three-year results. JADA 100:535, 1980.

Simonsen RJ: The clinical effectiveness of a colored pit and fissure sealant at 36 months. JADA 102:323, 1981.

Simonsen RJ: Five-year results of sealant effects on caries prevalence and treatment cost. J Dent Res 61:332, 1982.

Simonsen RJ: Group health white sealant trial: Results after 10 years. J Dent Res 66:830, 1987.

Walls AWG, Wallwork MA, Holland IS, Murray JJ: The longevity of occlusal amalgam restorations in first permanent molars of child patients. Br Dent J 158:133, 1985.

Pulp therapy for young permanent teeth

Gary K. Belanger

Mature teeth are those that have experienced complete apical development, whereas young permanent teeth are identified as those recently erupted teeth in which apical root closure has not been completed. Pulp protection and therapy for young permanent teeth require consideration of many of the same objectives and techniques that are necessary for both deciduous teeth and mature permanent teeth. However, a major additional concern for the young permanent tooth with a diseased or traumatized pulp may be the need either to promote normal apical completion or to stimulate an atypical apical closure. These outcomes are sought in order to ensure that an adequate crown to root ratio is established and so that, if necessary, a definitive root canal procedure can be successfully completed at a later date. Because normal physiologic root closure of permanent teeth may take 2–3 years after the tooth's eruption, young permanent teeth are a developmental stage in children from 6 years of age until the mid-teens.

Numerous factors can affect the pulpal health of teeth, but the two major conditions detrimental to young permanent teeth are deep caries and traumatic injuries. Deep caries is much more likely to affect the posterior teeth, especially the permanent first molars. Trauma is much more likely to affect the anterior teeth, especially the maxillary incisors.

Pulpal Assessment

Assessment of the pulp status of young permanent teeth is divided into the same five categories as for deciduous teeth: (1) patient history, (2) clinical examination, (3) clinical diagnostic procedures, (4) radiographic examination, and (5) direct pulpal evaluation.

PATIENT HISTORY

A child may report complaints of spontaneous dental pain or pain and sensitivity that is

precipitated from external sources such as air, heat, cold, food, and pressure. Spontaneous pain occurs without provocation and is indicative of significant damage to the pulp that is usually irreversible. Precipitated (or stimulated) pain that does not persist after removal of the stimulus is often a more favorable finding, indicating dentinal sensitivity (Seltzer and Bender, 1984).

A complaint of pressure sensitivity may indicate a serious situation, such as total pulpal necrosis, extending to the periodontal ligament and causing extrusion of the tooth from its socket. However, it may also indicate a fairly innocuous situation such as a previously placed restoration or a sealant that is in hyperocclusion. A foreign body (such as a popcorn kernel) that has wedged into the sulcus can also account for sensitivity to pressure. Historical information must be compared with other findings in order to diagnose a child's complaints about pressure pain properly.

Any historical findings regarding dental caries should include an assessment of the length of time that the lesion may have been developing; how long it has been bothersome; whether there is any facial or intraoral redness, swelling, or drainage; and whether there has been any previous treatment. Anything that the child is able to do that reduces or eliminates pain should also be noted. Many children complain of "toothaches" during the eruption of permanent first molars around age 6. In such instances, the dentist should be careful to rule out that the child is really only reacting to a pericoronitis or the biting on an operculum.

In the assessment of a traumatic injury to a young permanent tooth, time is a critical element for the dentist to consider. The longer a pulp has been exposed, the greater the opportunity has been for bacterial infection and degenerative pulpal changes. Thus, conservative techniques (such as direct pulp cap) are possible with a very recently fractured incisor (less than 1 hour), but as the elapsed time increases, progressively more aggressive therapy is required.

CLINICAL EXAMINATION

Young permanent teeth with pulpal involvement that is due to a carious lesion will likely be obvious during clinical inspection. However, some deep lesions progress through poorly coalesced pits, fissures, or hypoplastic enamel and display minimal enamel destruction clinically. Sensitivity to explorer probing, radiographs, and clinical excavation can confirm a suspicion that the lesion is more advanced than it appears (Fig. 32–1).

Traumatized teeth may show evidence of injury in many ways. Fractures may involve enamel, dentin, cementum, or pulp of dental crowns or roots. Displacement injuries affect the periodontal structures and may range from minor loosening to avulsions. In all situations, the pulp is affected to some degree (see Chapter 33 for treatment of traumatized teeth). With some injuries, the effect on the pulp may be neither apparent nor diagnosable and actually may take months or years to become manifested. With severe injuries, however, the pulp will almost always be deleteriously affected and require immediate and/or subsequent treatment.

CLINICAL DIAGNOSTIC PROCEDURES

Heat, cold, and an electrical pulse are classic tests for pulpal sensitivity, vitality, and viability. In young permanent teeth, these measurements can provide some clues as to the histopathologic status of the pulp in a carious or a traumatized tooth in comparison with non-involved teeth. Interpretation of testing data must be cautious, however, since an open apex provides a significantly enlarged vascular supply but an incompletely developed nervous innervation when compared with mature permanent teeth (Bernick, 1964). In traumatized teeth especially, the reactions to pulp tests should not be interpreted literally, since the pulp can be in a state of shock for many days or weeks and may register negatively to tests, then return later to normal status. Nevertheless, testing should be performed, since test results serve as good baseline data for subsequent comparisons and for evaluation of changes over time.

Tests of mobility and percussion sensitivity should also be performed for comparing with antimeres and/or unaffected teeth. Increased mobility in carious teeth is indicative of periodontal ligament involvement. Traumatized teeth often suffer slight to extreme increases in mobility, which indicates damage to the supporting structures and possibly an altered pulp status.

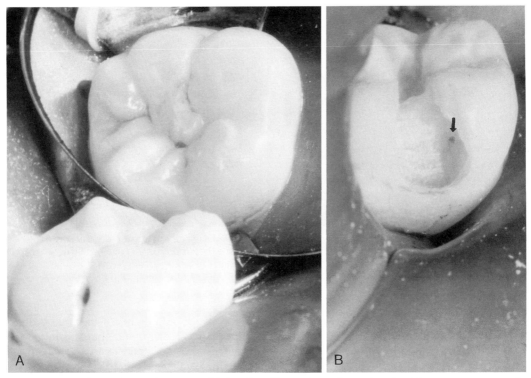

Figure 32 – 1 ■ *A,* Clinical view of permanent first molar with poorly coalesced occlusal fissures and buccal pit but without gross decay. *B,* Same tooth at time of treatment, showing a carious pulp exposure *(arrow).*

RADIOGRAPHIC EXAMINATION

A diagnostically accurate periapical radiograph is essential for correct pulpal evaluation of a deeply carious or traumatized young permanent tooth. The interpretation may be difficult, however, because of a normally large and open apex; the dentist must be careful to never make treatment decisions based on radiographic information alone (Fig. 32 – 2). It is also helpful to have a view of the antimere available for the sake of comparison. Radiographic evaluation should include the same factors as described in the section on primary dentition radiographic examination (see Chapter 20). Several additional factors worthy of consideration are as follows:

1. More than one view of the area of interest, each taken at a different angle, is helpful for locating subtle changes (e.g., root fractures).

2. Pathologic changes should not be confused with normal anatomy (e.g., mandibular canal, mental foramen, incisive fossa, nasopalatine canal, etc.).

3. Internal resorption is possible in perma-nent teeth but is not seen as often as in primary teeth. Pathologic external root resorption is frequently a sequela of severe disruption of the periodontal ligament (e.g., avulsions).

4. Treatment-induced calcification (i.e., bridging or apical closure) may be too thin to visualize radiographically. Clinical probing, although potentially dangerous, may be necessary to confirm development of calcification.

DIRECT PULPAL EVALUATION

As for primary teeth and mature secondary teeth, important information may become apparent at the time of actual clinical treatment. Careful visual inspection, tactile evaluation during instrumentation, and even detection of foul odors given off by a pulp will provide important clues about lesion depth and pulpal status. The texture of carious dentin must be judged, as well as its proximity to the pulp. The quality (color) and quantity of bleeding from a direct exposure of pulp tissue (unintended, planned, or traumatic) must be assessed. The

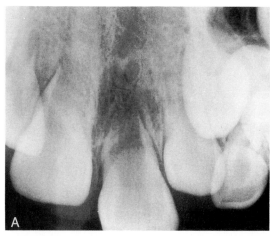 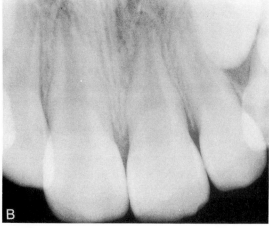

Figure 32–2 ■ *A*, Radiograph of maxillary centrals with apparent radiolucency associated with recently erupted tooth No. 9. However, there was no history of trauma, pain, or excess mobility, and the tooth was within normal limits for all pulp tests; thus, no treatment was begun. *B*, Radiograph of same maxillary centrals 12 months later, showing symmetrical apical development of No. 8 and No. 9 and no evidence of periapical pathosis.

dentist will develop clinical experience and judgment of how these direct findings may confirm or alter planned treatment.

Pulp Treatment Procedures

Young permanent teeth are considered good candidates for many pulp-healing procedures because of their increased apical perfusion, which is thought to enhance the pulp's ability to react to various insults successfully (Massler, 1972). As for primary and mature permanent teeth, protection of exposed dentin during any mechanical preparation or restorative phase of treatment is mandatory. Calcium hydroxide preparations should be placed routinely over dentin in any area that is appreciably deeper than the dentino-enamel junction, either from mechanical preparation, caries excavation, or a coronal fracture involving dentin. This is intended to protect dentinal tubules, odontoblasts, and pulp by sealing the dentin and protecting the pulp through sclerosis of dentinal tubules.

CARIES CONTROL

A child may present with uncontrolled multiple carious teeth, one or more of which can have frank pulp involvement and/or deep dentinal caries encroaching upon the pulp. Rather than trying to complete all pulp and re-

storative procedures in a sequential order, the dentist may recommend that the initial treatment visit be used to try to arrest all deep active carious lesions and halt their advancement towards pulpal involvement. In such a case, under rubber dam isolation, the gross caries is removed followed by calcium hydroxide placement and an interim restoration with a reinforced zinc oxide and eugenol product such as I. R. M.* The goal is to arrest the progression in a caries active mouth and promote a favorable pulpal response. Definitive restorations and further pulp treatment, if necessary, are completed at subsequent visits.

INDIRECT PULP CAP

Given the situation of a deep carious lesion in an asymptomatic young permanent tooth in which a pulpal exposure would most likely occur if total removal of carious dentin were attempted (Fig. 32–3A), in the indirect pulp cap procedure a very thin layer of carious dentin directly over the pulp is left in place. A calcium hydroxide preparation is placed over the soft carious dentin, followed by a reinforced zinc oxide and eugenol interim restoration in order to seal the cavity (Fig. 32–3B). The goal is to promote pulpal healing by removing the majority of infective bacteria and by sealing the lesion, which stimulates sclerosis of dentin and reparative dentin formation (King et al, 1965).

---

* LD Caulk Co, Milford, DE.

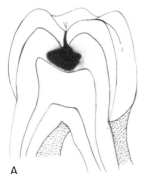 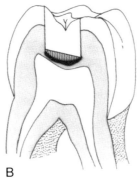 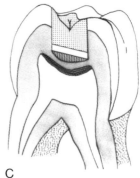

A   B   C

Figure 32–3 ■ Indirect pulp cap. *A*, Carious lesion *(black area)* progressing through enamel and dentin toward pulp; if all carious and decalcified dentin were removed, a pulpal exposure would likely occur. *B*, A small layer of soft dentin is left over pulp, over which a calcium hydroxide preparation *(vertical lines)* is placed directly, followed by reinforced zinc oxide and eugenol interim restoration *(white area)*. *C* shows reparative dentin that has formed *(horizontal lines in pulp chamber roof)*, sclerosis of the dentin that was left, calcium hydroxide, base (or previous interim restoration if it was not totally removed at second instrumentation), and final amalgam restoration *(stippled area)*.

As the procedure was originally practiced, after a minimum of 6 weeks the zinc oxide and eugenol, calcium hydroxide, and remaining carious dentin were removed. It was hoped that this second instrumentation of the tooth would confirm the intended goals and would be followed by placement of a permanent restoration (Fig. 32–3C). For the experienced clinician using good case selection, however, it may be preferable to avoid the second instrumentation (and the potential risk of a pulpal exposure). If the dentist is confident in the case selection and has good technical expertise for the procedure, a final (rather than interim) restoration may be placed and the procedure may be performed in one step. Periodic follow-up of the tooth's history and radiographic appearance are necessary. Indirect pulp capping is an excellent and conservative treatment option for some deep carious lesions in permanent teeth (especially if it avoids complete root canal treatment).

It should be emphasized that the indirect pulp cap procedure is intended to *avoid* a direct carious exposure. Therefore, very cautious caries removal is required prior to calcium hydroxide placement. Unfortunately, some dentists use the term "indirect pulp cap" whenever calcium hydroxide is placed over dentin. The term should truly be reserved for the procedure as described previously.

DIRECT PULP CAP

Actual clinical exposure of the pulp of a young permanent tooth may, in some instances, render it a candidate for a direct pulp capping procedure (Camp, 1983). Several situations in which this would be indicated include the following:

1. If a small mechanical exposure is caused by overpreparation and has occurred with a rubber dam in place.

2. If a small carious exposure occurs in a tooth that has not had any spontaneous pain, redness, swelling, or fever associated with it; shows no radiographic signs of pulp degeneration or changes in the periapical areas; and presents controllable bleeding at the exposure site (see Fig. 32–1).

3. If a traumatic injury has caused a coronal fracture involving the pulp and the exposure is no larger than 2 mm in diameter with the injury having occurred within the past few hours. If time since the injury is longer than that or if the exposure is larger in size than 2 mm, apexogenesis may be indicated or the dentist may choose to remove several millimeters of infected surface pulp and place calcium hydroxide at a slightly more apical level where healthy pulp tissue is encountered (see Chapter 33 for treatment of traumatized teeth).

In any of these situations, the child and parents need to be informed that problems may develop later (with or without symptoms) and that periodic monitoring is necessary. Monitoring should occur every few weeks initially, then less frequently if no signs, symptoms, or radiographic problems develop. After a direct pulp cap of a carious exposure, an interim restoration is indicated (usually a reinforced zinc oxide and

eugenol preparation), followed by a final restoration once success appears to be ensured. A mechanical direct pulp cap is usually restored by whatever final restoration had originally been planned. For trauma cases, a composite "bandage" can be placed over the direct pulp cap and enamel. A final composite restoration is seldom indicated at the same appointment that the direct pulp cap is placed because of two reasons:

1. The additional manipulation necessary to complete a final restoration may be additive to any pulpal and periodontal damages already sustained from the traumatic injury.

2. A final restoration that is esthetically pleasing in a pain free child may discourage the parents from returning for important follow-up monitoring visits.

FORMOCRESOL PULPOTOMY

The formocresol pulpotomy procedure has enjoyed very high clinical success in primary teeth. Dentists have attempted to extrapolate its use in permanent teeth. Results have been equivocal, and the routine use of this procedure cannot be recommended. Given the situation in which (1) deep caries involves an especially critical tooth (e.g., permanent first molar), causing extensive pulpal involvement; (2) the parents have ruled out conventional endodontic treatment; and (3) the dentist wishes to avoid extraction if at all possible, a formocresol pulpotomy may be attempted (Trask, 1972). Although there may be clinical success for several years afterwards, deterioration may occur in time. The procedure should be considered and tried only as a last alternative in attempting to temporarily forestall an eventual need for conventional endodontic treatment.

APEXOGENESIS (CALCIUM HYDROXIDE OR VITAL PULPOTOMY)

If a young permanent tooth has a sufficiently large or long-standing pulp exposure such that its coronal pulp is infected, inflamed, or judged unlikely to retain its viability, the coronal portion of the pulp can be removed and the remaining radicular pulp treated with calcium hydroxide (Fig. 32–4, *left middle*). The goal is to maintain the radicular pulp's viability to allow apexogenesis or apical closure (Dannenberg, 1974). Calcium hydroxide placed directly on

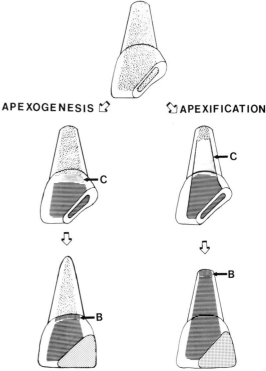

APEXOGENESIS ⬈   ⬉ APEXIFICATION

Figure 32–4 ■ Top diagram indicates that pulp exposure of immature permanent incisor can be treated by apexogenesis *(left arrows)* if radicular pulp is vital, or by apexification *(right arrows)* if radicular pulp is necrotic. For both procedures, "C" indicates the level where calcium hydroxide is placed at initiation of the procedure; "B" indicates the location of a bridge formation with time. Horizontal lines represent the interim restoration and final base; stippled area represents final composite restoration.

the radicular pulp stump stimulates a calcific response immediately adjacent to it, which is seen later on a radiograph as a radiopaque "bridge" over the amputation site (Fig. 32–4, *left bottom*). If degenerative and irreversible coronal pulp changes have not progressed into the radicular pulp, successful root closure can progress to completion (Figs. 32–5 and 32–6). The procedure can be thought of as analogous to a direct pulp cap, only performed at a more apical level.

For apexogenesis candidates, a radiograph should be taken to confirm that no pathologic periapical changes are present. Even though hemorrhage will occur at the amputation site, it should not be profuse or have an abnormal color. Slight pressure for several minutes with a sterile cotton pellet should significantly reduce bleeding. The calcium hydroxide can be either

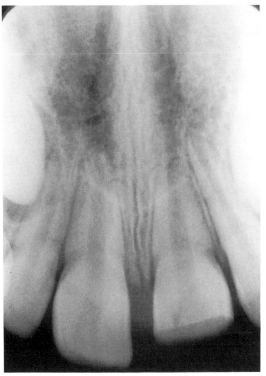

Figure 32-5 ■ Apexogenesis was started on tooth No. 9 several days after a dentino-enamel fracture with pulp exposure; note open apex.

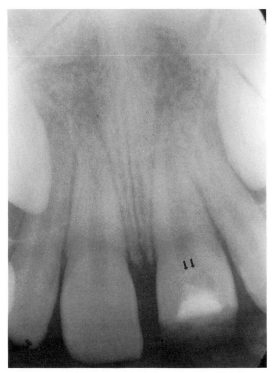

Figure 32-6 ■ Apexogenesis (radiograph taken 6 months after Figure 32-5) showing bridge formation *(arrows)* and apical maturation.

U. S. P. powder or a proprietary calcium hydroxide pulp capping preparation such as Pulpdent.* It is placed directly on the pulp amputation site, then covered with a base and interim restoration. Although a final restoration may be placed, it is preferable to wait until success is evident so that the time and expense of a permanent restoration is warranted.

The child and parent should be informed that there is a risk that the procedure may not be successful and that more aggressive treatment (i.e., apexification) will be necessary later. Also, conventional gutta percha endodontic treatment after the apical closure has occurred is recommended, even in the absence of a problem, because of a concern that complete canal obliteration through continued calcification will progress after apexogenesis and make endodontic procedures impossible later (Fuks et al, 1982).

Apexogenesis is a very useful treatment for saving young permanent teeth with exposed vital but infected coronal pulps. (If the apex is closed, conventional endodontic procedures can be performed.) Periodic clinical and radiographic observation is mandatory.

APEXIFICATION (FRANK PROCEDURE OR ROOT-END CLOSURE)

If a young permanent tooth has a pulp with extensive degeneration or necrosis throughout (usually with clinical and radiographic signs of a periapical reaction), the pulp should be totally débrided and the canal treated with calcium hydroxide (Figs. 32-4, *right*, 32-7, and 32-8). Were a conventional endodontic procedure attempted, it would be compromised as a result of incomplete root formation, a blunderbuss canal (which would be difficult, if not impossible, to seal apically), and a decreased crown to root ratio. Apexification is used to promote root elongation and/or a calcific root closure across the enlarged apex of the tooth (Frank, 1966). Even though the pulp has been necrotic and is removed, Hertwig's epithelial root sheath is thought to persist and be capable of generating the response (Michanowicz and Michanowicz, 1967). A conventional endodontic procedure is done after apexification is complete (Fig. 32-9).

---

* Pulpdent Corporation of America, Brookline, MA.

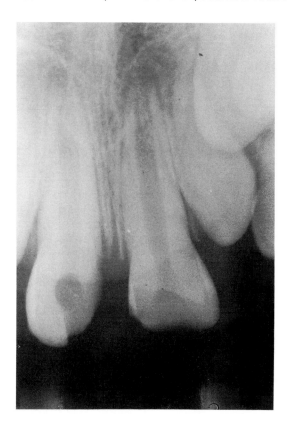

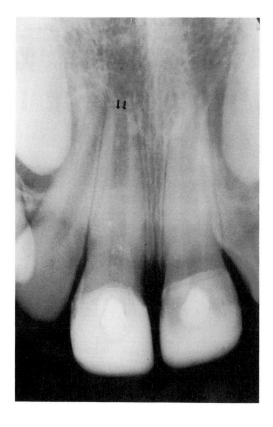

Figure 32–7 ■ Apexification was started on both No. 8 and No. 9 after pulp exposures with necrosis.

Figure 32–8 ■ Apexification (radiograph taken 14 months after Figure 32–7) showing radiographically apical bridging of tooth No. 8 *(arrows)* but not of No. 9. Later, both teeth were obturated with gutta percha when clinical probing confirmed apical closure; note interim composite restorations.

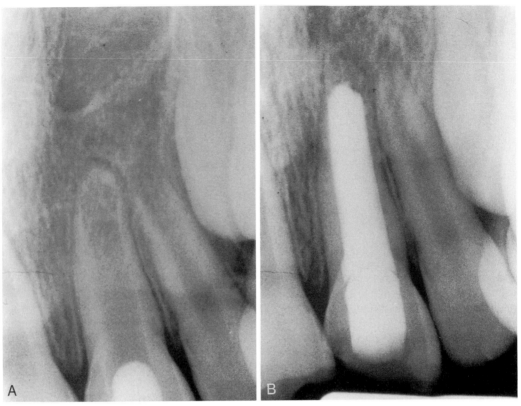

Figure 32–9 ■ *A,* Apical bridge apparent after apexification (but without increase in wall thickness). *B,* Gutta percha obturation of canal.

In apexification, the entire pulp contents are removed to the level of the radiographic apex, using endodontic broaches and files. Care must be taken not to file against the incompletely formed thin and tapered internal walls of the root. Liberal irrigation with a sodium hypochlorite solution or a non-irritating solution (e.g., sterile saline or local anesthetic solution) will help to remove all organic and necrotic tissue. Calcium hydroxide is placed at the apical end of the radicular canal; a proprietry calcium hydroxide preparation (Pulpdent) or a mixture of U. S. P. calcium hydroxide mixed with sterile saline or local anesthetic can be carried to the apical portion of the root, covered with a sterile cotton pellet, and sealed with an interim restoration. The calcium hydroxide gradually washes out; therefore, it must be replaced every several months until apical closure occurs. In 6 months to a year (possibly longer), an apical barrier will develop, against which a conventional gutta percha endodontic procedure can be completed. Although a complete apical closure may be seen radiographically, it may actually be a porous osteo-dentin or cementoid bridge (Goldman, 1974). Careful clinical probing within the root should be performed to confirm closure and the readiness of the tooth for a definitive endodontic filling.

Apexification is analogous to two other conditions in mature permanent teeth for which the entire root canal contents are removed and replaced with calcium hydroxide. This procedure is performed in cases of developing internal or pathologic external root resorption after a traumatic injury in an attempt to halt progressive root destruction (Andreasen, 1981).

REFERENCES

Andreasen JO: Traumatic Injuries of the Teeth, 2nd ed. Philadelphia, WB Saunders Co, 1981.

Bernick S: Differences in nerve distribution between erupted and non-erupted human teeth. J Dent Res 43:406–411, 1964.

Camp JH: Pedodontic-endodontic treatment. *In* Cohen S, Burns RC: Pathways of the Pulp, 3rd ed. St. Louis, CV Mosby, 1983.

Dannenberg JL: Pedodontic endodontics. JADA *18*:367–377, 1974.

Frank AL: Therapy for the divergent pulpless tooth by continued apical formation. JADA *72*:87–93, 1966.

Fuks AB, Bielak S, Chosak A: Clinic and radiographic assessment of direct pulp capping and pulpotomy in young permanent teeth. Pediatr Dent *4*:240–244, 1982.

Goldman M: Root-end closure techniques, including apexification. Dent Clin North Am *18*:297–308, 1974.

King JB, Crawford JJ, Lindahl RL: Indirect pulp capping: A bacteriologic study of deep carious dentine in human teeth. Oral Surg *20*:663–671, 1965.

Massler M: Therapy conducive to healing of the human pulp. Oral Surg *34*:122–130, 1972.

Michanowicz JP, Michanowicz AE: A conservative approach and procedure to fill an incompletely formed root using calcium hydroxide as an adjunct. J Dent Child *34*:42–47, 1967.

Seltzer S, Bender IB: The Dental Pulp: Biologic Considerations in Dental Procedures, 3rd ed. Philadelphia, JB Lippincott, 1984.

Trask PA: Formocresol pulpotomy on (young) permanent teeth. JADA *85*:1316–1323, 1972.

Managing traumatic injuries in the young permanent dentition

Dennis J. McTigue

Injuries to the primary dentition are discussed in Chapter 14. Also covered are the following fundamental areas relevant to managing trauma in children of any age:

1. Classification of traumatic injuries to teeth
2. Medical and dental history
3. Clinical and radiographic examinations
4. Common reactions of teeth to trauma

This chapter deals with injuries to the young permanent dentition, but the reader is strongly advised to review the fundamental areas just noted in Chapter 14. Frequent reference will be made to them.

Etiology and Epidemiology of Trauma in the Young Permanent Dentition

Falls during play account for most dental injuries to young permanent teeth. Children engaging in contact sports are at greatest risk for dental injury, though the use of mouth guards greatly reduces their frequency (see Chapter 39). In the teenage years, automobile accidents cause a significant number of dental injuries when occupants not wearing seat belts hit the

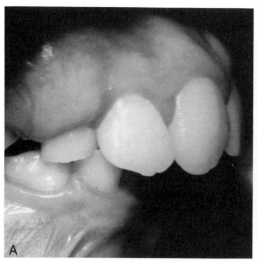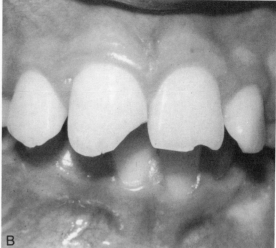

Figure 33 – 1 ■ *A*, Lateral view, showing large horizontal overjet. *B*, Same patient with fractured central incisors. (From McTigue, DJ: Management of orofacial trauma in children. Pediatr Ann *14*(2): 125 – 129, 1985.)

steering wheel or dashboard. As noted in Chapter 14, children with seizure disorders also injure their permanent teeth more frequently.

In contrast to the primary dentition, permanent teeth suffer crown fractures more frequently than luxation injuries. The smaller crown to root ratio and denser alveolar bone in the permanent dentition contribute to this phenomenon. Maxillary central incisors are again most commonly injured, and protruding incisors are at greatest risk (Jarvinen, 1978) (Fig. 33 – 1).

Classification of Injuries to Young Permanent Teeth

Classification of tooth fractures and luxation injuries is discussed in Chapter 14. Refer to Figures 14 – 1 and 14 – 2.

History

The essential elements of the medical and dental history are discussed in Chapter 14. The use of a trauma assessment form to help organize the gathering of historical and clinical data is emphasized (see Fig. 14 – 3). The reader is reminded to determine the status of the child's tetanus prophylaxis and to consult the child's physician if there is any question about its adequacy.

Another issue worthy of review relates to the potential for injury to the central nervous system. Older children are likely to suffer harder blows at play, and thus the dentist should find out if the child lost consciousness or became disoriented or nauseated after the injury. Positive findings indicate immediate medical consultation.

Clinical Examination

Refer to Chapter 14 for a thorough discussion of the clinical examination. An important difference between the primary and permanent dentition exists in respect to vitality testing. Whereas it is not routinely performed in the primary dentition, vitality testing can be a useful diagnostic aid in the permanent dentition. Electrical vitality testing is preferable to heat and cold testing because the former technique utilizes a stimulus that can be gradually increased and precisely recorded. Temperature tests are less exact and elicit "all or none" responses.

The dentist should be aware that electrical pulp testing may not elicit reliable responses from erupting permanent teeth and from those with open apices. Further, recently traumatized teeth may not respond to any vitality test for several months. Positive findings following a traumatic injury are thus more valuable for assessing pulp vitality than are negative responses.

Principles of radiographic diagnosis for permanent teeth do not differ from those for primary teeth. A frequent error made by dentists in diagnosing traumatic injuries is taking an insufficient number of radiographs. In 1981, Andreasen noted that additional views taken from slightly different angles both vertically and horizontally can improve the accuracy of diagnosis significantly (Andreasen, 1981, p 62).

It is important to note the urgency of follow-up radiographs after injury. Reviewing radiographs at 1 month post-injury will detect signs of pulpal necrosis and inflammatory resorption. At 2 months, replacement resorption can be detected.

Pathologic Sequelae of Traumatized Teeth

Refer to Chapter 14 for a discussion of the pathologic sequelae of traumatized teeth.

Treatment of Traumatic Injuries to the Permanent Dentition

The dentist treating a traumatic injury follows essentially the same principles of gathering historical information and completing a clinical examination, regardless of the child's age. Further, the pathologic sequelae of injuries to teeth are similar for both primary and permanent teeth. There are many significant differences, however, in the way that injuries to permanent teeth are treated. As in the primary

dentition, a complete diagnostic work-up (described in Chapter 14) should precede all treatment. Even though a blow may cause little if any obvious injury to a permanent tooth, it may lead to pulp necrosis as a result of disruption of the neurovascular bundle at the apex of the tooth. Post-treatment evaluation is indicated for all traumatic injuries.

ENAMEL FRACTURES

In some cases, minor enamel fractures can be smoothed with fine disks. Larger fractures should be restored using an acid-etch–composite resin technique (see Chapter 38).

ENAMEL AND DENTIN FRACTURES

All exposed dentin should be covered with calcium hydroxide to prevent thermal and chemical insult to the pulp. An acid-resistant calcium hydroxide paste is recommended. The tooth can then be restored with an acid-etch–composite resin technique (Fig. 33–2). If adequate time is not available to restore the tooth completely, an interim covering of resin material can temporize the tooth until a final restoration can be placed. Some dentists routinely place such a partial restoration to ensure an appropriate post-treatment evaluation when the patient returns for the final restoration. In cases in which clinical circumstances such as hemorrhage prevent adequate moisture control, a temporary basket crown can be fabricated by spot welding orthodontic band material over an orthodontic band. This restoration is cemented

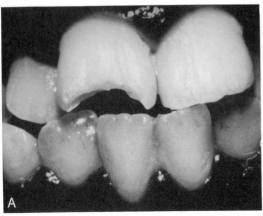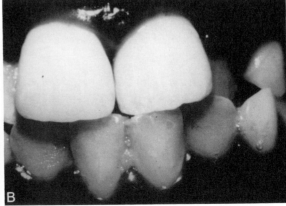

Figure 33–2 ■ A fractured incisor (A) can quickly be restored unsing an acid-etch–composite resin technique (B).

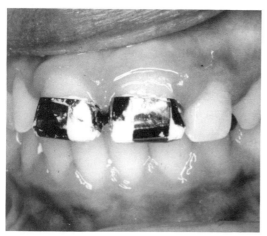

Figure 33–3 ■ Basket crown interim restorations for fractured incisors.

with reinforced zinc oxide and eugenol (Fig. 33–3).

FRACTURES INVOLVING THE PULP

Crown fractures that expose the pulp are particularly challenging to treat (Fig. 33–4). The pertinent clinical findings that dictate treatment include the following:

1. Vitality of the exposed pulp
2. Size of the exposure
3. Time elapsed since the exposure
4. Degree of root maturation of the fractured tooth
5. Restorability of the fractured crown

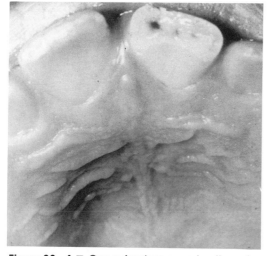

Figure 33–4 ■ Crown fracture exposing the pulp.

The objective of treatment in managing these injuries is to preserve a vital pulp in the entire tooth. This will allow for physiologic closure of the root apex in immature teeth. It is important to note that root end closure does not signal completion of root maturation. Progressive deposition of dentin normally continues in roots through adolescence, making them stronger and more resistant to future traumatic insult. Maintaining a vital pulp in the tooth crown allows the clinician to monitor the tooth's vitality periodically.

It is not always possible to maintain vital tissue throughout the tooth. Three treatment alternatives are available, based on the clinical findings just noted:

1. Direct pulp cap
2. Pulpotomy
3. Pulpectomy

Direct Pulp Cap

The direct pulp cap is indicated in small exposures that can be treated within several hours of the injury. The chances for pulp healing decrease if the tissue is inflamed, has formed a clot, or is contaminated with foreign materials. The objective, then, is to preserve vital pulp tissue that is free of inflammation and physiologically walled off by a calcific barrier.

A rubber dam is applied, and the tooth is gently cleaned with water. Commercially available calcium hydroxide paste is applied directly to the pulp tissue and to all exposed dentin. It is essential that a restoration be placed that is capable of thoroughly sealing the exposure to prevent further contamination by oral bacteria. As in the treatment of dentin fractures, it is acceptable to use an acid-etch–composite resin system for an initial restoration. An acid-resistant calcium hydroxide paste is again recommended. A basket crown sealed with zinc oxide and eugenol is also acceptable as an interim restoration. The calcific bridge stimulated by calcium hydroxide should be evident radiographically in 2–3 months.

In fractures of immature permanent teeth with incomplete root development, a direct cap should be employed only under the most favorable circumstances. Failure in these cases leads to total pulpal necrosis and a fragile root with thin dentinal walls. Thus, the more conservative treatment in fractures of immature permanent teeth is the pulpotomy.

Pulpotomy

The objectives of the pulpotomy technique are to remove only the inflamed pulp tissue and to leave healthy tissue to enhance physiologic maturation of the root. Some authors differentiate between a "complete pulpotomy," wherein all pulp tissue is removed from the crown, versus a "partial pulpotomy," which includes removal of just a portion of the pulp. That distinction will not be made in this chapter. Hence, a "pulpotomy" will indicate removal of any or all tissue from the tooth crown.

As previously noted, this technique is favored for immature permanent teeth with exposed pulps. It is also indicated in large exposures or for pulps exposed for longer than several hours.

Rubber dam isolation to prevent contamination of the pulp with oral bacteria is essential. The inflamed pulp is gently removed with a sterile bur at high speed and with copious irrigation. Calcium hydroxide is then applied to the pulp stump, and the chamber is sealed with zinc oxide and eugenol.

It is difficult to determine clinically how far the inflamed pulp extends. The tooth shown in Figure 33–5 had been fractured for 4 days with a pulp exposure approximately 3 mm in diameter. The dentist elected to remove all tissue in the pulp chamber, with obvious success. Figure 33–5B demonstrates complete maturation of the root, including apical closure and dentinal wall thickening as well as a calcific barrier at the amputation site. Maintaining some pulp tissue in the crown, however, allows the dentist to monitor the vitality of the tooth and is thus preferable when possible.

In 1978, Cvek noted that in most cases of pulps exposed for more than a few hours, the initial biologic response is pulpal hyperplasia. Inflammation in these cases rarely extends beyond 2 mm. In his study involving 60 teeth with pulps exposed from 1 hour to 90 days, Cvek removed only 2 mm of the pulp and the surrounding dentin. He then placed calcium hydroxide as previously noted. His success rate of 96% indicates that this conservative removal of tissue is the treatment of choice.

Pulpectomy

A pulpectomy involves complete pulp tissue removal from the crown and root and is indicated when no vital tissue remains. It is also

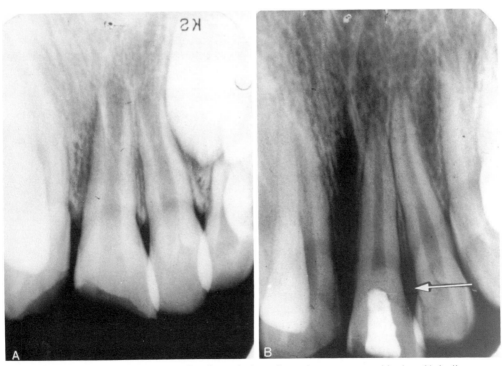

Figure 33–5 ■ (A), Crown fracture exposing the pulp in an immature permanent incisor. Note the open apex and thin dentinal walls in the root. (B), A calcium hydroxide pulpotomy stimulated the formation of a calcific barrier (arrow) and enabled the root to mature.

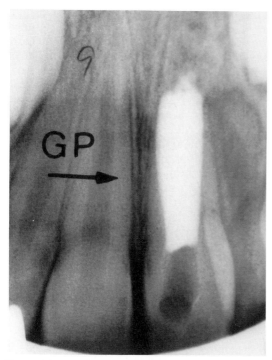

Figure 33–6 ■ An apexification procedure enabled this immature permanent tooth to be obturated successfully with gutta percha (GP). The root, however, will remain fragile and at increased risk to future trauma because no further dentinal wall apposition can occur.

indicated when root maturation is complete and the permanent restoration requires a post build-up. In the absence of inflammatory root resorption, treatment is to obturate the canal with gutta percha. The reader is referred to standard endodontic textbooks for more information on this technique.

One of the greatest challenges facing the clinician is the management of a non-vital immature permanent tooth with an open apex. In this case, an apexification procedure is indicated wherein calcium hydroxide is carried to the root apex to contact vital tissues directly. The calcium hydroxide stimulates the formation of a cementoid barrier against which gutta percha can subsequently be condensed. Even though a good apical seal can be achieved in this manner, no dentinal wall deposition will occur in the root and it will remain thin and fragile (Fig. 33–6). Refer to Chapter 32 for more detailed information regarding the apexification technique.

Criteria for Success

Criteria to judge success of the techniques used to manage pulpal insult in fractured teeth include the following:

1. Completion of root development in immature teeth
2. Absence of clinical signs such as pain, mobility, or fistula
3. Absence of any radiographic signs of pathologic processes, such as periapical radiolucency of bone or root resorption

POSTERIOR CROWN FRACTURES

Posterior crown fractures in the permanent dentition pose a restorative challenge for the clinician. These fractures usually occur secondary to hard blows to the underside of the chin, and vertical crown fractures frequently result (Fig. 33–7). Full coverage with stainless steel or cast metal crowns is frequently the only alternative. The reader is reminded to watch for mandibular symphisis fractures and cervical spine injuries in these cases (Bertolami and Kaban, 1982).

ROOT FRACTURES

The prognosis for teeth with root fractures is best when the fracture occurs in the apical one third of the root. The prognosis worsens pro-

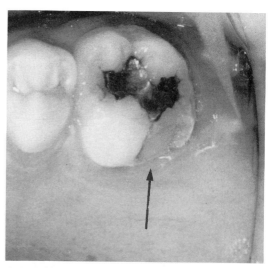

Figure 33–7 ■ A vertical crown fracture of the distolingual cusp *(arrow)* occurred secondary to a blow to the underside of this child's chin.

gressively with fractures that occur more cervically on the root. In 1983, Bender and Freedland reported that over 75% of teeth with intra-alveolar root fractures maintain their vitality.

Appropriate management of root fractures in permanent teeth involves repositioning the coronal portion of the tooth fragment (if it is displaced) and firm immobilization with a splint for 2–6 months. Root canal therapy should not be initiated until clinical and radiographic signs of necrosis or resorption are apparent. Even in those cases, treatment can often be limited to the coronal fragment. In 1980, Jacobsen and Kerekes reported success in treating the coronal fragments of such fractured teeth with calcium hydroxide. The apical fragments were not treated. This treatment technique was successful because in most instances the apical fragments maintain their vitality.

Techniques for splinting teeth are discussed later in this chapter.

MANAGING SEQUELAE TO DENTAL TRAUMA

In Chapter 14, common reactions of the teeth to trauma are described. Three of the most challenging sequelae include calcific metamorphosis, inflammatory resorption (both external and internal), and replacement resorption. These pathologic processes can occur following crown fractures or luxation injuries.

Calcific Metamorphosis

Calcific metamorphosis is a degenerative pathologic process that ultimately leads to obliteration of the pulp canal (see Fig. 14–8B). It was noted previously that most primary teeth resorb normally, and thus treatment for them is usually not indicated. Controversy exists, however, regarding treatment of permanent teeth.

Some clinicians contend that as soon as calcific metamorphosis is diagnosed, a pulpectomy with gutta percha should be performed. This treatment is advocated because of reports of later development of pulpal necrosis and periapical change. Further, the difficulty in completing routine endodontic procedures after pulp canals have calcified is noted. Andreasen counters, however, that necrosis has been reported in only 16% of such cases. Further, he states that endodontic procedures can be successfully completed in a great majority of obliterated canals (Andreasen, 1981, p 368). The dentist is advised, then, to monitor calcific metamorphosis in permanent teeth closely and to initiate endodontic procedures only when periapical changes are noted.

Inflammatory Resorption

Inflammatory resorption can occur externally and/or internally (see Fig. 14–8). It commonly arises following luxation injuries when the periodontal ligament is inflamed and the pulp is necrotic. Odontoclastic activity can occur so rapidly that the teeth are destroyed in a matter of weeks.

Immediate treatment of inflammatory resorption is essential. As soon as this process is detected radiographically, the pulp tissue in the tooth is thoroughly extirpated. Copious irrigation with sodium hypochlorite assists in the dissolution of organic debris in the canal. In permanent teeth, calcium hydroxide is placed in the canal with a technique identical to that used to induce apexification (see Chapter 32). Here the objective is not to induce apical closure but to create an environment unfavorable for the resorptive process. It is theorized that calcium hydroxide has antiseptic properties because of its extremely alkaline pH. This medicament apparently percolates through the dentinal tubules to the areas of resorption at the periodontal ligament and halts its progress.

Depending upon the severity of the inflammatory resorption, calcium hydroxide may need to be retained in the tooth for 6–24 months. Repeated applications may be necessary if the resorption progresses. When radiographs confirm that the process is not continuing, gutta percha is placed as the final filling material.

Replacement Resorption (Ankylosis)

Replacement resorption occurs most commonly following severe luxation injuries like avulsions or intrusions in which periodontal ligament cells are destroyed. Alveolar bone directly contacts cementum on the involved tooth and becomes fused with it. Then as the bone undergoes its normal, physiologic, osteoclastic, and osteoblastic activity, the root is resorbed or "replaced" with bone (Fig. 33–8).

This type of resorption cannot be treated once the tooth is firmly immobilized by the process. In young children with rapid bone turnover, teeth are completely resorbed in 3–4 years. In adults, the process may take up to 10 years. Replacement resorption can be pre-

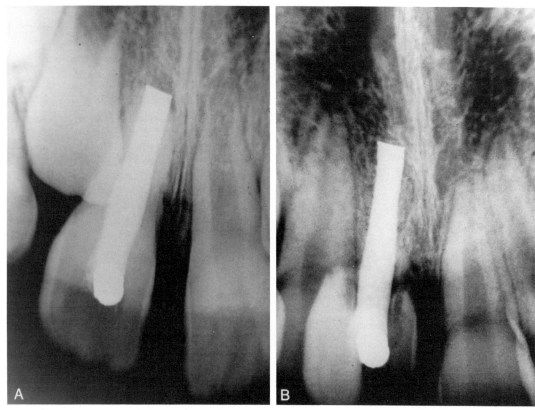

Figure 33–8 ■ (A), A permanent incisor that had been avulsed for 3 hours was filled with gutta percha prior to reimplantation. (B), Three years later, replacement resorption has completely destroyed the root.

vented only by prompt and appropriate treatment of luxation injuries.

TREATING LUXATION INJURIES IN THE PERMANENT DENTITION

The reader is referred to Chapter 14 for the definition of the various types of luxation injuries. Luxation injuries damage the supporting structures of the teeth, that is, the periodontal ligament and alveolar bone. Additionally, in mature teeth with closed apices, the pulp frequently becomes necrotic. Pulp necrosis occurs less frequently when immature teeth with open apices are luxated.

Vitality of the periodontal ligament is far more important than pulp vitality in determining the prognosis of luxated teeth. The objective of treatment in these injuries is to *maintain periodontal ligament vitality*.

Concussion

Concussion injuries in permanent teeth must be followed closely. Although the prognosis is normally good, pulp necrosis and root resorption have been reported. Involved teeth can be carefully taken out of occlusion if the child complains of pain.

Subluxation

Pulp necrosis occurs far more commonly in subluxated permanent teeth than in primary teeth. These teeth should be monitored closely with radiographs for at least 1 year, and root canal therapy should be instituted at the first sign of pathologic change. Immature teeth with open apices are less likely to undergo pulpal necrosis. Splinting subluxated teeth should be avoided.

Intrusive Luxation

The prognosis for intruded permanent teeth is not good. These teeth frequently undergo pulpal necrosis, root resorption, and alveolar bone loss.

The treatment of choice is to reposition the intruded teeth orthodontically, using light

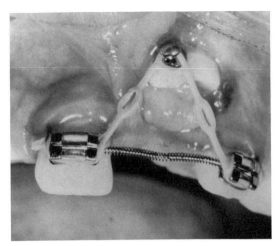

Figure 33–9 ■ Orthodontic repositioning of intruded permanent incisor prevents replacement resorption and alveolar bone loss.

forces (Fig. 33–9). The pulp should be extirpated within 1 week following the injury, and calcium hydroxide should be placed in the root canal using the same technique as described for apexification in Chapter 32. Radiographic monitoring of the tooth should occur for at least 1 year, and the calcium hydroxide in the canal should be replaced if signs of root resorption persist.

As opposed to the primary dentition, the author does not wait for the intruded permanent tooth to re-erupt. Permanent teeth with closed apices do not re-erupt and will undergo replacement resorption (Turley et al, 1984). Those with open apices may re-erupt but the process would take several months, in which time the root could be badly resorbed.

Immediate surgical repositioning of intruded permanent teeth is also contraindicated. This enhances both root resorption and alveolar bone loss.

Extrusion

Extruded permanent teeth should be repositioned and splinted for 2–3 weeks (see Fig. 14–2A). It normally takes the periodontal ligament fibers this period of time to reanastomose. Extruded permanent teeth with closed apices will undergo pulpal necrosis; therefore, root canal therapy should be initiated after the teeth are splinted. Extruded teeth with open apices have a chance at maintaining their vitality, and so the decision to initiate therapy can be delayed until clinical or radiographic signs indicate necrosis.

Lateral Luxation

Alveolar bone fractures frequently occur in lateral luxation injuries and can complicate their treatment (see Fig. 14–2B). In the most severe cases, periodontal ligament and marginal bone loss occurs. Treatment is to reposition the teeth and alveolar fragments. A splint should then be applied for 3–8 weeks, depending upon the degree of bone involvement. With good oral hygiene, alveolar bone regeneration can occur in children in approximately 8 weeks. If the apices are closed, the pulp will become necrotic; therefore, endodontic therapy should be instituted after the teeth are splinted. Again, teeth with open apices should be monitored until signs of necrosis are evident.

Avulsion

The prognosis for long-term retention of an avulsed permanent tooth worsens the longer that the tooth is out of its socket. The primary therapeutic concern is to maintain the vitality of the periodontal ligament. Such teeth that are reimplanted within 30 minutes stand a 90% chance of survival (Andreasen and Hjorting-Hansen, 1966). Few teeth reimplanted after 2 hours survive. It is thus imperative that the tooth be immediately reimplanted by the first capable person, whether that person be a parent, teacher, or sibling.

The procedure for reimplantation is as follows:

1. The tooth should be held by the crown to prevent damage to the periodontal ligament.

2. It should be gently rinsed off with tap water. No attempt should be made to scrub or sterilize the tooth.

3. The tooth should be manually reimplanted in the tooth socket.

Owing to a variety of circumstances, it is sometimes not possible to reimplant a tooth immediately. Research has shown that the best transport medium for avulsed teeth is milk (Blomlof, 1981; Courts et al, 1983). It is readily available, relatively aseptic, and its osmolality is more favorable to maintaining the vitality of the periodontal ligament cells than is saline, saliva, or tap water. Thus in these cases, with the tooth stored in milk, the patient should be taken to the dentist as soon as possible.

Because root resorption is so closely correlated with the extraoral period, the dentist should immediately reimplant the tooth in its socket. In mature teeth with closed apices, a

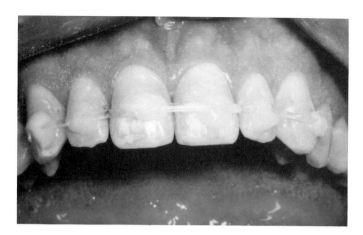

Figure 33-10 ■ An esthetic, flexible splint is easily fabricated using 80 pound monofilament fishing line retained with composite resin.

splint should be applied for 7-10 days. Calcium hydroxide should be placed in the tooth after 1 week. This will prevent the initiation of inflammatory root resorption. Root canal therapy should not be performed in the hand prior to reimplantation. This extends the extraoral period and places the periodontal ligament at greater risk to injury as a result of the additional manipulation of the tooth. In immature teeth with open apices, the tooth should be splinted for approximately 2 weeks. This will give the neurovascular tissues an opportunity to reanastomose. Success in these cases has been reported, and thus dentists should await clinical or radiographic signs of necrosis prior to initiating root canal therapy.

When the splint is removed, the dentist will note that the tooth is quite mobile. This mobility is preferable to long-term rigid splinting, as the latter has been correlated with an increased incidence of replacement resorption. The mobility of the tooth physiologically interrupts areas of incipient resorption on the periodontal ligament, allowing it to heal normally.

Splinting Technique

Various methods of splinting teeth have been advocated, but it is apparent that the ideal splint should possess the following characteristics. It should

1. Be passive and atraumatic
2. Be flexible
3. Allow for vitality testing and endodontic access
4. Be easy to apply and remove

The composite resin–retained arch wire splint has been advocated as the best system to meet these criteria. To allow for flexibility, a light orthodontic arch wire or an 80 pound test monofilament fishing line can be used (Fig. 33-10).

Summary

Advances in dental research have greatly improved the ability of dentists to ensure long-term retention of traumatized teeth in children. It is the dentist's responsibility to stay abreast of this new information and to be available to his or her patients when they are in need of urgent treatment.

REFERENCES

Andreasen JO: Traumatic Injuries of the Teeth, 2nd ed. Philadelphia, WB Saunders Co, 1981.

Andreasen JO, Hjorting-Hansen E: Replantation of teeth. I. Radiographic and clinical studies of 110 human teeth replanted after accidental loss. Acta Odont Scand 24:263, 1966.

Bender IB, Freedland JB: Clinical considerations in the diagnosis and treatment of intra-alveolar root fractures. JADA 107:595, 1983.

Bertolami CN, Kaban LB: Chin trauma: A clue to associated mandibular and cervical spine injury. Oral Surg 53:122, 1982.

Blomlof L: Storage of human periodontal ligament cells in a combination of different media. J Dent Res 60:1904, 1981.

Courts FJ, Mueller WA, Tabeling HJ: Milk as an interim storage medium for avulsed teeth. Pediatr Dent 5:183, 1983.

Cvek M: A clinical report on partial pulpotomy and capping with calcium hydroxide in permanent incisors with complicated crown fracture. J Endo 4:232, 1978.

Jacobsen I, Kerekes K: Diagnosis and treatment of pulp necrosis in permanent anterior teeth with root fracture. Scand J Dent Res 88:370, 1980.

Jarvinen S: Incisal overjet and traumatic injuries to upper permanent incisors: A retrospective study. Acta Odontol Scand 36:359, 1978.

Turley PK, Joiner MW, Hellstrom S : The effect of orthodontic extrusion on traumatically intruded teeth. Am J Orthod 85:47, 1984.

chapter *34*

Treatment planning and treatment of orthodontic problems

John Christensen □ Henry Fields

By the time that orthodontic treatment is considered, the patient's data base has been gathered. A list of orthodontic problems is generated from this data base, and the problems are ranked in order from most to least severe. Severity is a balance of patient, functional, and esthetic concerns. The clinician is specifically trained to identify functional and esthetic problems but does not always consider the concerns of the parent and child. These concerns should be listened to carefully. Many times, the motivation for treatment can be elicited from these concerns. If the child patient desires to have treatment, cooperation will usually be good during treatment and little parental support will be necessary. This is called internal motivation. External motivation, motivation supplied by the parent for treatment, will require continuous parental support to complete treatment. It is also possible for the chief complaint or reason for seeking treatment to rank low on the treat-

ment priority list. An explanation should be provided to the child and parent to justify this situation.

After the problem list has been generated and each problem has been ranked in order of severity, a list of possible solutions to each problem should be made. The solution list should be comprehensive, that is, all reasonable solutions should be considered for each specific problem without regard for the other problems. After the solution list has been constructed, the clinician should look for similar solutions that are listed for more than one problem. In some cases, the best solution for one problem is the best solution for all problems, and the treatment plan is easily derived. Unfortunately, in most cases, a solution for one problem is not the solution for the others and, worse, may actually magnify the second problem. Treatment planning is not entirely scientific and depends on clinical wisdom to decide on a plan in these cases.

Skeletal Problems

Orthodontic problems in the preadolescent patient are generally thought of in terms of being dental or skeletal in origin. The complexity of the problem varies tremendously. Many dental problems are well within the treatment domain of the general practitioner. Skeletal problems, as diagnosed from the facial profile analysis, are best treated by a specialist. However, the general practitioner should have an understanding of how skeletal discrepancies are treated. Three basic alternatives to treat skeletal discrepancies exist: growth modification, camouflage, and orthognathic surgery. Growth modification attempts to change skeletal relationships by using the patient's remaining growth to alter the size and/or position of the jaws. Camouflage and orthognathic surgery usually are considered only in the non-growing or adult patient. The camouflage type of orthodontic treatment is aimed at hiding a mild skeletal discrepancy by moving teeth within the jaws so they will fit together. The skeletal discrepancy still exists but is disguised by a normal occlusion and acceptable facial esthetics. Orthognathic surgery places the jaws and teeth in normal or near normal position through the use of surgical procedures and pre- and post-surgical orthodontics.

Three assumptions are made when growth modification is undertaken. First and most obvious, the patient must be growing. The normal child in this age group is actively growing; however, there is a wide variation in the amount of growth occurring at one time. Treatment is ideally planned to coincide with the patient's maximal growth spurt so that the greatest amount of modification can occur in the shortest amount of time. Numerous investigators have tried to determine if the peak growth spurt can be predicted or anticipated by dental development, skeletal development, or chronological age. There is a weak relationship between the peak growth spurt and each of the three indicators, but this relationship is one that is not very useful clinically. The clinician should use all three indices and a thorough past medical history that includes a history of growth to make an educated decision as to whether the child is growing at a fairly rapid rate. Females tend to enter the adolescent growth spurt between the ages of 9 and 11, and males are best treated between ages 11 and 13. The discrepancy between dental development and maximum growth velocity may create situations in which the patient may be ready for growth modifica-

tion but not ready for orthodontic dental treatment, and vice versa.

The second assumption made when growth modification is undertaken is that the practitioner can accurately diagnose the source of the skeletal discrepancy and then design treatment that will apply the appropriate amount and direction of force to correct the discrepancy. Diagnosis is not an exact science, and the discrepancy may be due to a number of small skeletal problems rather than to one easily identified discrepancy. Force delivery to dental and skeletal structures is also inexact, and the clinical impression often dictates the amount and direction of force applied to modify growth.

The third assumption made is that growth modification is usually only the first phase of a two phase treatment plan. The appliances used to modify growth are basically designed to alter skeletal structures rather than teeth. Although the appliances are capable of tooth movement, they are not as precise as fixed orthodontic appliances. Therefore, the majority of growth modification treatment is followed immediately or at some later time with traditional fixed orthodontic appliances to move the teeth into ideal position.

Three theories are offered to explain how growth modification works to achieve the desired results. The first theory suggests that growth modification appliances change the absolute size of one or both jaws. For example, a Class II skeletal profile may be treated by making a deficient mandible larger to fit a normal-sized maxilla or by limiting the size of an over-sized maxilla. Some investigations on animals have shown that absolute size change is possible, but clinical application in humans has not been as successful. Certain individuals do show dramatic size changes, but there appears to be large variability in patient response to growth-modifying appliances, with moderate changes being the rule rather than the exception.

Growth modification may work by accelerating the desired growth but not changing the ultimate size or shape of the jaw. A deficient mandible may not end up larger than it ultimately would have been but may achieve its final size sooner. This allows the clinician to make some final dentoalveolar changes to establish an ideal occlusion and shorten total treatment time. This type of growth modification response also exhibits large individual variability.

A third possibility is that growth modification may work by changing the spatial relationship of the two jaws. The ultimate size of the

jaw and its rate of growth are not changed, but by modifying the orientation of one jaw a more balanced profile may result. For example, an individual with a convex profile and an increased lower facial height could be made more proportional if the vertical growth of the maxilla could be inhibited and the mandible allowed to rotate upward and forward. The profile would become less convex and the vertical relations more ideal. Jaw reorientation would be successful in a concave Class III short face patient if the mandible could be rotated downward and backward (more vertical) to create a more acceptable profile. Reorientation does not work well in Class II short face or Class III long face patients because making one problem better makes the other problem worse.

GROWTH MODIFICATION APPLIED TO ANTEROPOSTERIOR PROBLEMS

Anteroposterior skeletal problems are Class II and Class III in nature. These descriptions are not very informative, however, because the source of the discrepancy may be either the maxilla, the mandible, or a combination of the two. Therefore, the first step in patient evaluation is to identify the source of the problem and then design a treatment plan to resolve the problem.

Class II Maxillary Protrusion

The Class II maxillary protrusive patient is best treated by headgear therapy to restrict or redirect maxillary growth. Headgear places a distal force on the maxillary dentition and the maxilla (Fig. 34-1). Theoretically, the relative movement of dental and skeletal structures is dependent on the amount and time of force application. In actual practice, it is probably not possible to move selectively only teeth or bones. However, more tooth movement occurs if the headgear is worn greater than 16 hours per day at force levels of 12 ounces or less. Conversely, more orthopedic or skeletal effect is expected if the headgear is worn between 8 and 12 hours per day at force levels of 16 ounces or more. The vertical direction of force exerted by a headgear varies according to the type of headgear chosen. One should avoid using a headgear that tends to extrude posterior teeth in a long face individual. However, the same type of headgear would be useful in a deep bite, short face patient.

A Class II maxillary protrusive patient may also be treated with a functional appliance. Al-

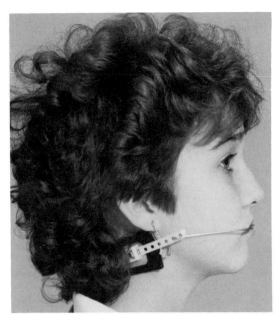

Figure 34-1 ■ The Class II maxillary protrusive patient is best treated by headgear therapy to restrict or redirect maxillary growth. This patient is being treated with a cervical headgear that places a distal and extrusive force on both maxillary skeletal and dental structures. The force is provided by a neck strap attached to the outer bows of the headgear.

though a functional appliance is primarily designed to stimulate mandibular growth, studies have indicated that it has a secondary effect of restricting maxillary skeletal and dental movement. This happens because the mandible, which is postured forward, returns to a more distal position as a result of distal muscle and soft tissue forces transmitted through the appliance to the maxilla and the maxillary teeth. The maxillary teeth tend to tip lingually rather than to move bodily, and the mandibular teeth tip facially.

Class II Mandibular Deficiency

The mandibular deficient patient is usually treated with a functional appliance that positions the mandible forward in an attempt to stimulate or accelerate mandibular growth (Fig. 34-2). Controlled clinical studies have shown that these appliances can produce a small average increase in mandibular projection (2-4 mm per year) (Remmer et al, 1985; McNamara et al, 1985). There is a great amount of variability in patient response. In most cases, this increased growth will not totally correct the Class II skeletal problem for several reasons. First, the amount of growth is not enough to overcome

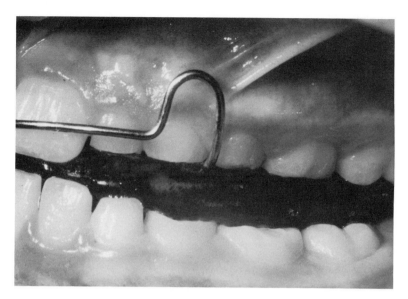

Figure 34–2 ■ The Class II mandibular deficient patient is usually treated with a functional appliance that positions the mandible forward in an attempt to stimulate or accelerate mandibular growth. Because functional appliances also have tooth-moving effects, dental aspects of the malocclusion must also be considered during treatment planning.

the discrepancy. Second, all the available growth would need to be used to produce anteroposterior change. This is usually not the case, because some eruption and vertical growth occurs. This interaction of anteroposterior and vertical dimensional changes decreases mandibular projection and Class II correction because the mandible grows downward and forward and not straight forward. The rest of the anteroposterior discrepancy is made up by restricting maxillary growth, tipping maxillary teeth back, and tipping mandibular teeth forward. Different appliances can be prescribed that will exaggerate the secondary responses of maxillary restriction and dental movement if desired. There are some studies that indicate headgear treatment may cause a small increase in mandibular growth, but it is unlikely that the amount of mandibular stimulation by this method would be of clinical significance (Baumrind and Korn, 1981).

Class III Maxillary Deficiency

True midface deficiency can be treated by using a reverse pull headgear or face mask to exert anteriorly directed force on the maxilla (Fig. 34–3). The ideal time to attempt this treatment is between ages 6 and 8 if skeletal change is desired. Because the face mask applies force to the maxilla through an appliance (either removable splint or fixed appliance) attached to the teeth, tooth movement also occurs. In fact, after age 8 this type of appliance will have a tendency to exert a predominately tooth-moving force. Functional appliances designed to

stimulate maxillary growth do not seem to be effective. The improvement in facial profile obtained by using these appliances in patients with very minor Class III problems is the result of a downward and backward rotation of the

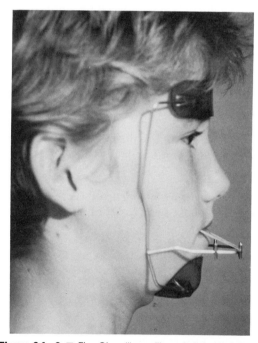

Figure 34–3 ■ The Class III maxillary deficient patient is treated by using a reverse pull headgear or face mask to exert anteriorly directed force on the maxilla. The force is provided by rubber bands attached from the face mask to intraoral hooks or wires. The ideal time to attempt this treatment is between 6 and 8 years of age if skeletal change is desired.

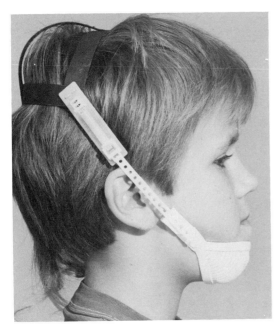

Figure 34–4 ■ The Class III mandibular protrusive patient has been historically treated with chin cup therapy. The chin cup was designed to apply a distal and superior force through the chin to inhibit growth at the condyle. In clinical practice, this has not proved to be routinely successful, although chin cup therapy does cause a distal rotation of the mandible. Therefore, the chin cup may be useful to treat mild mandibular protrusion with short to normal vertical proportions.

mandible. The occlusion improves as a result of facial tipping of the maxillary incisors and lingual tipping of the lower incisors.

Class III Mandibular Excess

The Class III mandibular protrusive patient has been historically treated by chin cup therapy (Fig. 34–4). The strategy of chin cup therapy is to apply a distal and superior force through the chin that will inhibit or redirect growth at the condyle. Again, studies in animals have shown some change in absolute mandibular size, but clinical application in humans routinely has not been as successful. The typical response to chin cup therapy is a distal rotation of the mandible and lingual tipping of the lower incisors. Therefore, chin cup therapy is well tolerated in patients with mild mandibular protrusion and short to normal vertical proportions. It is contraindicated, however, in an individual with a long lower face because the anteroposterior correction would come at the expense of an increased vertical dimension. Functional appliances designed to treat Class III mandibular excess show the same

changes as those in instances of Class III maxillary deficiency.

GROWTH MODIFICATION APPLIED TO TRANSVERSE PROBLEMS

The most common transverse problem in the preadolescent is maxillary constriction and posterior crossbite. Treatment of maxillary constriction should begin as soon as the problem is discovered and when the child is mature enough to accept treatment. Three basic appliances are used to correct the constriction, but the appliances are not interchangeable.

In Chapter 26, the quad helix and W-arch were introduced for treatment of maxillary constriction. The appliances provide both skeletal and dental movement in the 3- to 6-year-old. As the patient grows older, more dental change and less skeletal change occur. This is because the midpalatal suture, which was open at an early age, has developed bone interdigitation that makes it difficult to separate. More force is required to separate the suture and obtain true skeletal correction than a quad helix or W-arch can deliver.

In the older preadolescent patient, in whom there is a chance that the midpalatal suture is closed, an appliance that can deliver large amounts of force is necessary to correct the skeletal constriction. Rapid palatal expansion is a term given to the procedure in which an appliance cemented to the teeth is opened 0.5 mm per day to deliver 2000–3000 gm of force (Fig. 34–5). In the active phase of treatment, there is little dental movement because the periodontal ligament has been hyalinized, which limits dental movement, and the force is transmitted almost entirely to the skeletal structures. During retention, however, the skeletal structures begin to relapse toward the midline. Because the teeth are held rigidly by the appliance, there is some compensatory dental movement to maintain the same width. Depending on the amount of expansion needed, active treatment normally takes 10–14 days. A similar approach to skeletal expansion is slow rather than rapid palatal expansion. Essentially the same appliance is used, although force levels are calibrated to provide only 900–1300 gm of force. Coupled with a slower activation rate, slow palatal expansion widens the palate by dental and skeletal movement. Although the final position of the teeth and supporting structures is approximately the same in rapid and slow expansion,

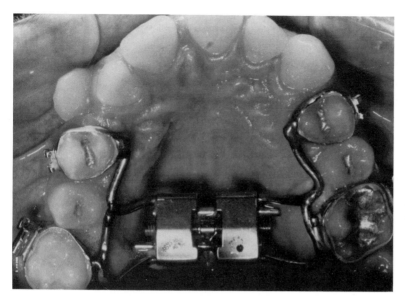

Figure 34–5 ■ Rapid palatal expansion is used to treat maxillary constriction and posterior crossbite when there is a chance that the mid palatal suture is partially closed. The jackscrew in the appliance provides approximately 2000–3000 gm of force when opened 0.5 mm per day. Depending on the amount of expansion needed, the appliance is normally activated two times each day for 10 days to 2 weeks.

proponents of slow expansion maintain that slower expansion is more physiologic and stable.

Transverse growth modification can also be accomplished by means of acrylic or wire buccal shields attached to functional appliances. The buccal shields relieve the teeth and alveolar structures from the resting pressure of the cheek muscles and soft tissues. Transverse expansion of 3–5 mm can be achieved, although the changes are quite variable. Whether the movement is dental or skeletal and whether it will remain stable are still under question because there are no controlled experimental studies to provide answers.

GROWTH MODIFICATION APPLIED TO VERTICAL PROBLEMS

Vertical skeletal problems become manifest as long and short facial heights and are located below the palatal plane (Fields et al, 1984). The short face individual has a reduced mandibular plane angle and undererupted teeth. In the long face patient, the mandibular plane angle, lower facial height, and amount of dental eruption are increased compared with the normal face patient. Vertical skeletal problems certainly may be successfully treated with growth modification techniques; however, maintaining the cor-

rection is extremely difficult. The face grows vertically for a long time, and there is a tendency for the original growth pattern and growth problem to return.

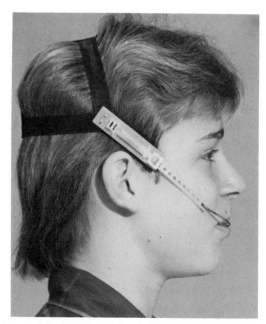

Figure 34–6 ■ The patient with vertical skeletal excess is best treated with a high pull headgear. The force, generated by the strap resting on the head, is applied in a superior and distal direction and is intended to inhibit vertical development of the maxilla and eruption of the maxillary posterior teeth.

Vertical Excess

Vertical skeletal excess may be treated by extraoral force, intraoral force, or a combination of the two. Extraoral force is delivered by means of a high pull headgear through the maxillary first molars. The force is applied in a superior and distal direction and is designed to inhibit vertical development of the maxilla and eruption of the posterior maxillary teeth (Fig. 34–6). Because no force is applied to the mandibular teeth, they are free to erupt and compensate for the lack of vertical development in the maxilla. This compensatory eruption can eliminate all the positive effects of the high pull headgear and lead to downward and backward rotation of the mandible instead of forward projection.

A second alternative to control vertical development is to block the eruption of the maxillary and mandibular teeth. A functional appliance can be designed that will posture the mandible open in an increased vertical position. The force of the mandible attempting to return to its original position will be transmitted to the maxilla and the teeth in both arches. This will result in all mandibular growth being directed forward, because no dental eruption has occurred to increase the vertical dimension (Fig. 34–7). To supplement the effect on the maxilla, a headgear may be attached to the functional appliance that will allow the headgear and functional appliance to be worn at the same time (Fig. 34–8). Recent developments in rare earth magnetics may also prove to be of value in restricting vertical facial development. Magnets placed in repulsion in each arch may provide enough force to restrict vertical eruption and skeletal growth. By whatever means vertical excess is treated, excellent patient cooperation

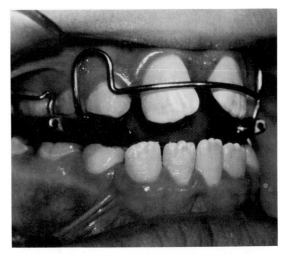

Figure 34–7 ■ Vertical skeletal excess can also be treated with a functional appliance designed to inhibit the eruption of the maxillary and mandibular teeth. The appliance is constructed so that the mandible is postured open in an increased vertical position. The force of the mandible attempting to return to its normal, more closed vertical position will be transmitted to the maxilla and to the teeth in both arches.

is necessary because treatment must be continued as long as the patient is growing.

Vertical Deficiency

Vertical skeletal deficiencies can be treated with either headgear or functional appliances. The force vector from the headgear should direct the maxilla distally and extrude the maxillary posterior teeth. Functional appliances are typically designed to inhibit eruption of upper and lower anterior teeth and promote eruption of the posterior teeth. As in vertical skeletal ex-

Figure 34–8 ■ In some cases, a headgear tube is added to the functional appliance described in Figure 34–7. This allows the patient to wear the functional appliance and the high pull headgear at the same time to restrict vertical skeletal and dental growth further.

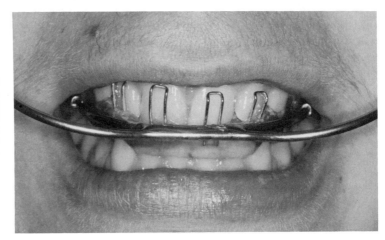

cess, the original growth pattern tends to recur, and retention should be designed to prevent this recurrence.

Dental Problems

SPACE MAINTENANCE

Space maintenance philosophy and the appliances used to maintain space in the primary dentition are discussed in Chapter 24. The same philosophy and appliances apply to space maintenance in the 6–12 age group. However, treatment of early loss of primary teeth in the mixed dentition requires some additional thought and consideration. Loss of posterior teeth in the primary dentition is a nearly universal indication for space maintenance therapy. In the mixed dentition, the timing of permanent tooth eruption, timing of tooth loss, presence of succedaneous teeth, and the extent of crowding must also be taken into account.

Premature loss of a primary molar at a very early age will delay the eruption of the permanent tooth. On the other hand, premature loss of a primary molar at a later age may actually accelerate the eruption of the permanent tooth and make space maintenance unnecessary. In general, the permanent tooth will be delayed in eruption if the primary molar is lost before age 8, whereas it will tend to erupt earlier than normal if the primary molar is lost after age 8. A more accurate method of determining delayed or accelerated eruption of permanent teeth is to examine the amount of root development and alveolar bone overlying the unerupted permanent tooth from panoramic or periapical films. The succedaneous tooth will begin to erupt when root development is approximately one-half completed. In terms of alveolar bone coverage, roughly 6 months' time should be anticipated for every millimeter of bone that covers the permanent tooth. If it is apparent that the tooth will be delayed in erupting, space maintenance is absolutely indicated. Because space loss usually occurs within the first 6 months after the premature loss of a primary molar, space maintenance should be undertaken, unless the tooth will erupt within 6 months or unless there is enough space in the arch that a 1 or 2 mm space reduction will not compromise the eruption of the permanent tooth.

A second factor to consider is the amount of time that has elapsed since the primary tooth was lost. At one extreme is the case of a primary molar scheduled for extraction. At the other extreme is the case of a primary molar already missing for 6 months or longer. In the first case, space maintenance is certainly indicated to prevent space loss when the tooth is extracted. In the second case, the majority of space loss has already occurred and space maintenance may not be indicated. The clinician should complete space and profile analyses and make a decision based on those findings. If there is adequate space in the arch or if so much space has been lost that extraction of permanent teeth is inevitable, space maintenance is contraindicated. A space maintainer is indicated to prevent any more space loss if there is only marginally adequate space remaining to allow the permanent tooth to erupt.

The absence of a permanent successor also complicates space maintenance in the mixed dentition. The second premolar is the most commonly missing posterior tooth in the permanent dentition, excluding the third molars. If the primary second molar is lost prematurely, the clinician is faced with a decision regarding the space that the missing second premolar would have occupied. Two choices can be made. One alternative is to maintain space in the arch and eventually construct a fixed prosthetic replacement. This is feasible only if the skeletal and dental relationships are Class I, there is no crowding, and there is good interarch occlusion. The advent of resin-bonded bridges has made this option more popular. The other alternative is to allow or encourage the space to close. Factors that would favor this solution would include crowding within the arch, protrusive incisors and lips, and possibly other missing teeth.

The amount of crowding in the arch is a very important factor in the space maintenance decision, and it is predicted from the space analysis and put in perspective by the facial form analysis. If the incisor position is normal and there is adequate space or minor crowding (less than 5 mm) in the arch, space maintenance should be initiated. However, early loss of a primary molar in an arch with more than 5 mm of crowding must be considered carefully. Space maintainers alone will not solve a problem of this magnitude. Either permanent teeth will need to be extracted, or the arches will need to be expanded. Expansion is possible only if the incisor position is normal or retrusive. If expansion is contemplated, space maintainers should be placed. In some cases, however, crowding of this magnitude is treated by extracting two first premolars and closing the remaining space orthodontically. If no space maintenance is im-

plemented and tooth movement as a result of drifting occurs prior to the first premolar extractions, less space remains to be closed later. Consultation with a specialist is usually desirable before this type of decision is made.

If the crowding approaches 10 mm per arch, space maintainers should be placed, even though permanent tooth extraction is inevitably required. The average width of a premolar is approximately 7 mm; therefore, the extraction of two premolars would effectively gain 14 mm of arch length. If further space is lost in an arch that is already severely crowded, a two premolar extraction may not resolve all of the crowding. Space maintainers would ensure that no further decrease in arch length occurs. In some instances, timed extraction, called serial extraction, can alleviate the crowding and relieve the demands of subsequent orthodontic treatment.

Probably the most significant difference between space maintenance strategy in the mixed dentition versus that in the primary dentition is bilateral loss of teeth in the mandibular arch. In the primary dentition, two band and loop appliances are indicated; in the mixed dentition, the lingual arch is preferred if all lower incisors have erupted. Primary second molars or permanent first molars may be used as abutment teeth. If oral hygiene is a problem, it is recommended that primary second molars be banded. This is done so that if decalcification under bands occurs as a result of poor oral hygiene, it will be on teeth that will eventually exfoliate.

Space maintenance in the mixed dentition requires close supervision as permanent teeth erupt and primary teeth exfoliate. When primary abutment teeth exfoliate, an appliance may need to be remade, using permanent teeth as abutments. Space-maintaining appliances obviously should be removed when the permanent tooth erupts into proper position.

POTENTIAL ALIGNMENT AND SPACE PROBLEMS

Ectopic Eruption

Problems associated with ectopic eruption of the permanent first molar are discussed in the previous section. A 3- to 6-month observation period is the best initial therapy, because there is a possibility that the molar may spontaneously self-correct or "jump" distally and erupt into normal position. Intervention is necessary if the molar is still blocked from erupting at the end of the observation period. The goal of treatment is to move the ectopically erupting tooth away from the tooth it is resorbing. If a small amount of movement is needed and little or none of the permanent molar is clinically visible, a piece of .020 inch brass wire can be passed around the contact between the permanent molar and the primary second molar. The brass wire is tightened every 2 weeks. When the wire is tightened, the periodontal ligament space is compressed and the molar is forced distally until it can slip past the primary molar and erupt (Fig. 34–9). In some cases, a steel spring clip separator may be used to dislodge the molar but only in cases in which there is minimal resorption of the primary molar. It may be difficult to seat the spring if the contact point between the molars is below the cemento-enamel junction of the primary molar. Elastomeric separators have been advocated by some dentists but are not recommended by most dentists because they may dislodge in an apical direction and cause a periodontal abscess. Some elastomeric separators are not radiopaque and can be quite difficult to locate.

A second method of moving the permanent molar back is to band the primary second molar and apply a distal force to the permanent molar through an .028 inch helical spring attached to the band. This type of tooth movement requires that the occlusal surface of the permanent molar be visible so that force can be applied to move the tooth distally. A small ledge of resin or a metal button can be bonded to the occlusal surface to serve as the point of force application (Fig. 34–10). However, salivary contamination of the occlusal surface makes bonding a frustrating and difficult procedure in some cases.

Occasionally, the primary second molar will need to be removed if the permanent molar has caused extensive resorption of the primary root structure. In these cases, loss of arch length is certain, and some plan of treatment for the impending space deficiency should be considered in advance unless there is a congenitally missing second premolar and arch length is to be reduced purposefully, or unless premolar extractions and mesial movement of the molars is anticipated. To manage the space, a distal shoe can be placed to guide eruption of the permanent molar. A distal shoe will maintain space but will not regain space lost prior to the primary molar extraction. An alternative plan is to allow the permanent molar to erupt and then regain the space with a space-regaining appliance (described shortly). After the space is regained, a space maintainer should be instituted.

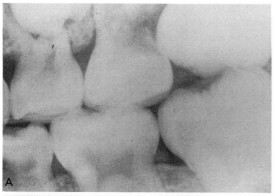

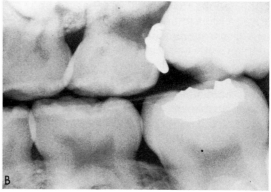

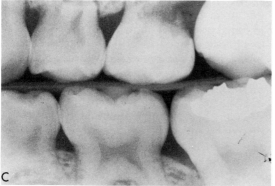

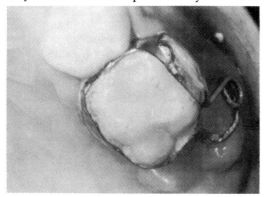

Figure 34–9 ■ *A,* This radiograph shows an ectopically erupting permanent maxillary left first molar. *B,* Because only a small amount of movement is required to correct the ectopic eruption, a piece of .020 inch brass wire is slipped around the contact point between the permanent molar and primary second molar and is tightened. *C,* After the wire has been tightened three times at 2-week intervals, the molar is dislodged and begins to erupt into normal position. (From Fields HW, Proffit WR: Orthodontics in general practice. *In* Morris AL, Bohannan HM, Casullo DP: The Dental Specialties in General Practice. Philadelphia, WB Saunders Co, 1983.)

Ectopic eruption of lateral incisors is usually an early indication of crowding but may only be the result of aberrant tooth positioning. If a primary canine exfoliates prematurely as a result

Figure 34–10 ■ A band and helical spring appliance is used to treat an ectopically erupting permanent molar that requires a large amount of movement. The primary second molar is banded, and a helical spring is soldered to the band. A small ledge of composite resin, a metal button bonded to the occlusal surface of the permanent molar, or a small preparation can serve as a point of force application. The spring is reactivated at monthly intervals until the permanent molar is dislodged. (From Fields HW, Proffit WR: Orthodontics in general practice. *In* Morris AL, Bohannan HM, Casullo DP: The Dental Specialties in General Practice, Philadelphia, W.B. Saunders Co, 1983.)

of ectopic eruption, the lower incisors typically drift to that side of the arch, creating a midline discrepancy. If the laterals cause resorption and exfoliation of both primary canines, the incisors usually tip lingually and decrease arch length. It appears that the space problem is corrected, but this is only temporary and the space shortage will become apparent again when the permanent canines begin to erupt. Whether the loss of primary canines is unilateral or bilateral, the clinician should determine if there is an arch length inadequacy and assess anteroposterior lip and incisor position. This information will help determine if space maintenance, space regaining, or more extensive treatment is needed.

The goal of treatment should be to prevent a midline shift. This can be accomplished by placing a lingual arch with a soldered spur distal to the lateral incisor to hold the midline if adequate space is present and the incisors are in good position. If the midline has already shifted, the contralateral primary canine can be removed to promote spontaneous midline correction. If space loss cannot be tolerated, a lingual arch should be placed following extraction. If there is sufficient crowding, so that space maintenance is contraindicated, or if the incisors are considered too protrusive and

should not be maintained in this position, no lingual arch should be placed following the extraction of the contralateral primary canine. In situations in which both canines exfoliate prematurely as a result of ectopic eruption, similar treatment decisions should be made, although the clinician does not normally need to worry about a midline shift.

Missing Permanent Teeth

The absence of permanent teeth creates many treatment problems for the clinician, and most treatment decisions are best made by a specialist. The maxillary lateral incisor and the mandibular second premolar are the most common missing teeth in the permanent dentition. Treatment decisions are based not only on the missing tooth but also on arch length, incisor position, and lip and profile esthetics.

Treatment of missing maxillary lateral incisors varies, depending on whether one or both incisors are absent and on the position of the permanent canine when it erupts into the arch. The canine will either erupt into the normal canine position or resorb the primary lateral incisor and spontaneously substitute for the missing lateral incisor. If the canine erupts into its proper position, the primary lateral incisor will eventually need to be removed because it does not make an esthetic substitute for the permanent lateral and because the root will eventually resorb. The missing lateral incisor can be replaced with a resin-bonded or conventional bridge. A bridge is the treatment of choice when the occlusion, incisor position, and profile are nearly ideal and when closing space orthodontically is not appropriate.

If the permanent canine erupts into the lateral incisor position, the primary canine must be extracted and the space closed or the permanent canine must be moved back into the correct position and a bridge constructed for the lateral incisor. Crowding or protrusive incisors usually call for space closure and substitution of canines for lateral incisors. These canines require recontouring by enamel removal and resin addition to improve the esthetics of the teeth. Canine substitution cases are considered quite difficult to treat well. Normal pretreatment occlusion favors bridge placement.

Arch length, incisor position, and facial esthetics must be thoroughly evaluated before a treatment plan is generated when a premolar is congenitally missing. Unlike primary canines and laterals, a primary molar may be a reasonable substitute for a missing premolar. The size, shape, and restorative status of the primary molar give some indication of the possibility of maintaining the tooth for a period of time. Ankylosis and advanced root resorption are signs to remove the primary molar. Most clinicians favor removing the primary molar and closing space orthodontically, but in certain situations a resin-bonded or conventional bridge may be more ideal treatment. These situations are rare and usually occur in skeletal and dental Class I individuals with ideal or near ideal occlusions.

If the arch is crowded enough for teeth to be extracted, the incisors too protrusive, or the profile too full, the retained primary molar should be removed and the case treated in a manner similar to that for a four premolar extraction case. Typically, first premolars are removed in an extraction case, but the majority of congenitally missing premolars are second premolars. If it can be determined that the second premolar is missing and that extractions are necessary to resolve the arch length inadequacy, the primary molar can be removed early, allowing the space to close by mesial drifting of the permanent first molar and distal drifting of the anterior teeth. Unfortunately, congenital absence of the second premolar may not be definitively determined at an early age, and this delays the extractions. The longer the extractions are delayed, the less drifting and spontaneous space closure will occur.

Supernumerary Teeth

A supernumerary tooth may create space and eruption problems. It can cause permanent teeth to erupt into malalignment or even prevent eruption. Treatment is usually directed at removing the supernumerary before it causes any eruption problems. Management of the supernumerary varies, depending on the size, shape, and number of supernumeraries and the dental development of the patient. Typically, the supernumerary is detected on a panoramic radiograph or an anterior occlusal film unless there is clinical evidence of an extra tooth at an earlier age. If the supernumerary is conical and is not inverted, there is a chance that it will erupt, at which time it should be removed. If the supernumerary is inverted, tubercular in shape, or significantly impeding eruption of the adjacent teeth, it should be surgically removed. Ideally, the surgery is timed so that removal of the supernumerary tooth does not interfere with permanent tooth development. However, the earlier that the supernumerary can be removed,

the more likely it is that the permanent teeth will erupt normally. Surgery to remove a supernumerary is often complicated, especially if there are multiple supernumerary teeth or if access to the supernumerary is limited, and these cases are appropriately referred to a specialist.

Tooth Size Discrepancies

Isolated tooth size discrepancies can cause alignment problems. The maxillary lateral incisor commonly creates this type of problem because it is undersized or pegged in shape. Occasionally, the lateral incisor can be restored to its normal size with composite resin and no other treatment. As discussed in the section on tooth size analysis, sometimes the peg lateral requires a combination of tooth movement and restorative dentistry to achieve ideal occlusion. Depending on the size of the discrepancy, the peg lateral can be treated in one of three ways (Fig. 34–11). If the lateral incisor is only slightly smaller than normal, all the space can be closed.

An alternative for a marginally small incisor is to move the lateral incisor orthodontically until it contacts the central incisor and leave space distal to the lateral. The canine is not brought forward to close the space, because this would put the canine in an end-to-end relationship and disrupt the occlusion. This solution is generally not esthetic unless only a small space is left distal to the lateral. A third solution, usually reserved for incisors with considerable size problems, is a combination of orthodontic tooth movement and resin bonding to reshape the crown. The lateral incisor needs to be positioned so that the resin addition will be esthetic and restore near-normal crown anatomy. This type of treatment is best performed under the auspices of a specialist. Fusion and gemination in the permanent dentition are even more difficult to treat and should be referred to a specialist.

Dens evaginatus and incisor talon cusps provide interesting challenges in securing ideal occlusion (Fig. 34–12). In most cases of dens evaginatus, a fine, thread-like pulp extends from

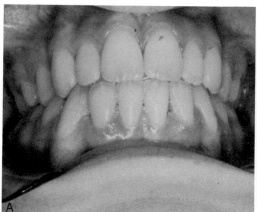
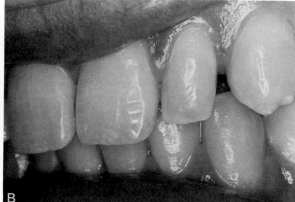
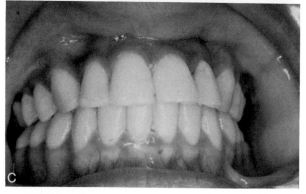

Figure 34–11 ■ Isolated tooth size discrepancies such as a maxillary peg lateral can cause alignment problems that can be treated in one of three ways. A, If the lateral incisor is only slightly smaller than normal, all the space is closed orthodontically. This leaves the patient with minimal overjet and overbite. B, An alternative is to move the lateral incisor until it contacts the central incisor and to leave space distal to the lateral incisor. The canine is not moved forward to close the space because it would place the canine in an end-to-end relationship and disrupt the occlusion. This alternative is generally not esthetic unless only a small amount of space is left distal to the lateral incisor. C, A third solution is a combination of orthodontic tooth movement and resin bonding to reshape the crown of the tooth. The lateral incisor is positioned so that the resin addition will be esthetic and restore near normal crown anatomy. This patient had two peg laterals treated with orthodontic tooth movement and resin addition.

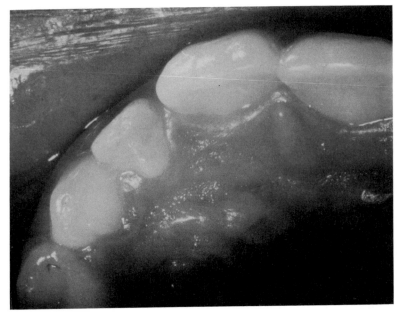

Figure 34–12 ■ Dens evaginatus and incisor talon cusps create problems in the development of good occlusion. The talon cusp on this maxillary right lateral incisor has interfered with the normal positioning of the mandibular right lateral incisor.

the main pulp chamber into the evagination, and the location of this pulp tissue extension should be determined radiographically. Most cases in the posterior region do not require treatment because the force of mastication slowly wears the evagination down and reparative dentin is formed. In the anterior region, however, this slow attrition must be accomplished mechanically with a handpiece and bur. A small amount of tooth structure is removed at each appointment, and after each session calcium hydroxide paste is applied to the exposed dentin to stimulate the reparative process. Usually the tooth can be treated at monthly appointments without permanent injury to the pulp. When treatment is complete, the exposed dentin is covered with a calcium hydroxide base and a resin restoration is placed.

ALIGNMENT PROBLEMS

Anterior and posterior tooth irregularity should be thought of differently than anterior and posterior space shortage. Tooth irregularity alone is due to rotated and tipped teeth in which there is no shortage of arch length. Arch length discrepancies also result in tooth irregularity, but the two conditions are not always related.

Tooth irregularity can be treated with either a fixed or a removable appliance. If a simple tipping force will align the tooth, a removable appliance with a finger spring is an appropriate appliance choice. An infinite variety of remov-

able appliances exist; however, several essential components need to be included in the design. The appliance needs to be retentive so that the force applied to the tooth will not dislodge the appliance. Adams clasps are often prescribed and are very retentive, although they can be difficult to adjust and may interfere with the occlusion. A minimum of two clasps, one on each side of the arch, should be employed. An additional amount of retention and stability is gained from the palatal acrylic in maxillary appliances. An .022 inch finger spring incorporated into the palatal acrylic delivers a light, continuous force. The spring should be activated 1–2 mm to move the tooth approximately 1 mm per month (Fig. 34–13).

Fixed appliances can be used to correct irregularity as well and are indicated when bodily movement of teeth or rotational control is necessary. Orthodontic appliances have evolved to a point at which specific brackets have been designed for specific teeth. The brackets have been constructed to provide proper crown and root positioning when precisely placed on the teeth. Before the appliances can be placed, the facial surfaces of the teeth selected for treatment are thoroughly cleaned (Fig. 34–14A). Then the teeth are isolated with either cotton rolls or specially designed retractors to provide a field free of salivary contamination with optimum access. Using the acid-etch technique, etching solution is painted on the facial surfaces of the teeth. The solution is restricted to the area that will eventually be covered by the bracket

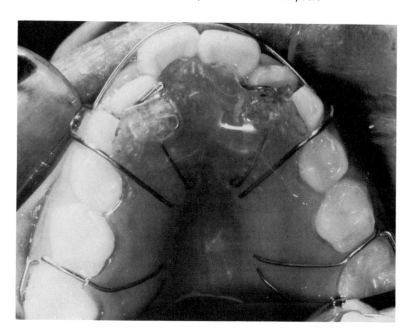

Figure   34–13 ■ Localized tooth irregularity is treated with either a removable or a fixed appliance. In this case, both maxillary lateral incisors erupted slightly rotated. A removable appliance with .022 inch finger springs is used to align the rotated lateral incisors. The springs are activated 1–2 mm per month to correct the irregularity.

(Fig. 34–14B). After the enamel is etched for 1 minute, the facial surfaces are thoroughly washed with water and dried. If the enamel surfaces appear to be well etched, a bonding agent is applied to the teeth and the excess is blown away with an air syringe. A two paste, autopolymerizing composite resin is mixed, and a small amount is placed on a single bracket pad (Fig. 34–14C). The bracket is placed on the tooth and moved into proper position. Proper position is dictated by the manufacturer's specifications and is based on the long axis of the crown, the long axis of the root, or the incisal edge (Fig. 34–14D). After the bracket is in position, it is firmly seated in place with a scaler or explorer. The excess composite resin expressed from underneath the bracket pad is carefully removed before it is fully polymerized (Fig. 34–14E). Removal of this excess flash will ensure that the bracket slots can be fully engaged and will also eliminate a source of plaque retention. This process is repeated until all the brackets have been properly placed. Finally, an arch wire is selected, placed in the brackets, and ligated with steel ligatures or elastomeric modules (Fig. 34–14F). The clinician should understand the physical properties of wires, because a wire must be selected that is strong enough to withstand the force of occlusion in the posterior segments yet flexible enough in the anterior region to be deflected into the brackets and deliver light, continuous force. Usually loops must be bent into the arch wire to allow anterior flexibility and posterior strength, but some of the

newer alloys can provide ample strength and flexibility.

Retention is essential following the correction of irregularity because of the strong propensity for teeth to relapse. Gingival fibers reorganize very slowly following these types of movements, and in some cases irregularity returns even if retention was well conceived. If the periodontium is healthy, it is suggested that a circumferential supracrestal fibrotomy be performed to reduce relapse. When treatment is complete or near completion, the supracrestal gingival fibers are cut with a scalpel and a No. 12B blade, using local anesthesia. Theoretically, the stretched gingival fibers will not need to reorganize but will reattach in a new position after being cut. Care should be taken if this procedure is used in patients with a thin gingival covering.

Many children exhibit a midline diastema in the mixed dentition, and it is considered a normal stage of development. Occasionally, a large midline diastema is present that is due to a mesiodens, protruding incisors, or a tooth size problem. A diastema caused by a midline supernumerary tooth is treated by removing the supernumerary. The supernumerary should be removed as early as possible without causing injury to the adjacent permanent teeth. Early removal of the mesiodens will allow the permanent teeth to erupt normally and close the space spontaneously.

In some cases, a large diastema may be due to facio-lingual, rather than mesio-distal, posi-

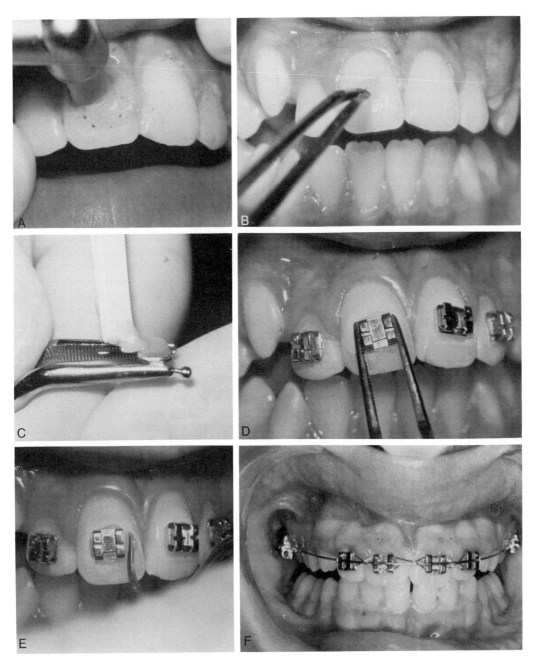

Figure 34–14 ■ *A*, Orthodontic appliances are designed to provide proper crown and root positioning when precisely placed on the teeth. Therefore, it is imperative to follow the appropriate sequence when placing the appliances. Before the appliances are placed, the teeth selected for treatment must be thoroughly cleaned. *B*, After the teeth have been cleaned and isolated to provide a field free of salivary contamination, etching solution is painted on the facial surfaces of the teeth. After the enamel has been etched for 1 minute, washed, and dried, a bonding agent is applied to the teeth. *C*, A two paste, autopolymerizing composite resin is mixed, and a small amount is placed on a single bracket pad. *D*, The bracket is placed on the tooth and is moved into proper position. Proper position is based on the long axis of the crown, the long axis of the root, or the incisal edge. *E*, After the bracket is positioned properly, it is firmly seated in place. The excess resin expressed from beneath the pad is carefully removed before it is fully polymerized. *F*, This process is repeated until all the brackets have been properly placed. At this point, the arch wire is selected, placed in the brackets, and ligated with steel ligatures or elastomeric ties.

tioning of the incisors. Flared incisors are un-esthetic and are at a greater risk of traumatic injury (Andreasen and Ravn, 1972). If the teeth can be tipped back into ideal position to close the diastema and if the overbite will not hinder tooth movement, a removable appliance is recommended. The appliance is designed to include at least two clasps for retention, palatal acrylic, and an .028 inch labial bow with adjustment loops (Fig. 34–15). The labial bow is activated to tip the incisors lingually by closing the adjustment loops. At the same time, acrylic must be removed from the lingual side of the appliance to allow for tooth movement and excess gingival tissue. The labial bow is activated approximately 1.5 mm per month until the diastema is closed and the teeth are in ideal position.

Fixed orthodontic appliances are suggested for treating patients if the incisors are so protrusive that bodily movement is required to close the diastema. The molars are banded, and the incisors are bonded with orthodontic brackets. The teeth initially are aligned, if necessary, with small, round arch wires and then are retracted, using a larger rectangular wire with closing loops or elastomeric chain. Rectangular arch wires are necessary to provide bodily control of tooth position during retraction. Headgear is prescribed at the same time to supplement anchorage because of the strong tendency of the molars to come forward while the incisors are retracted. The choice of headgear is based on the vertical dimensions of the patient.

If the diastema is due to a tooth size discrepancy between upper and lower teeth, treatment usually requires adding resin to the interproximal surfaces of the maxillary incisors. Closing space via orthodontic procedures will eventually result in relapse, because the occlusion will force the space open again.

Treatment to close a midline diastema that is not associated with an anteroposterior position or tooth size problem is usually initiated if the diastema is greater than 3 mm or if the diastema is still present after the permanent canines have fully erupted. A diastema larger than 3 mm will usually inhibit or disturb eruption of the lateral incisors and should be closed before these teeth emerge. Both of these types of diastemata are due to faulty mesio-distal positioning of the incisors, but the choice of an appliance is still based on the type of tooth movement required to close the space. If the central incisors can be tipped together to close the diastema, a removable appliance should be used. Finger springs are either incorporated into the palatal acrylic or soldered to the labial bow and engage the distal of the incisor crown (Fig. 34–16). The springs are activated 2 mm per month, and closure should not take more than 2 months.

Brackets are bonded on the facial surface of the central incisors if the teeth require bodily mesio-distal movement to close the diastema. After initial alignment, a large segmental or full rectangular arch wire is placed in the brackets and the teeth are moved together, using elastomeric chain. The chain is attached only to the

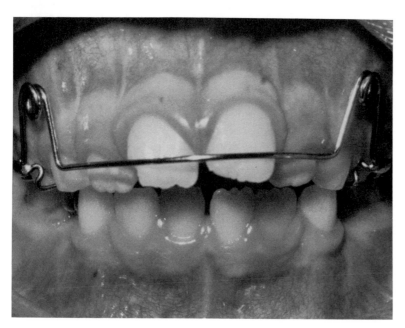

Figure 34–15 ■ A large diastema that is due to excessively protruding incisors is sometimes treated with a removable appliance if the overbite will not interfere with incisor retraction. The appliance incorporates a labial bow with adjustment loops that are activated to tip the incisors lingually. By tipping the incisors lingually, both the diastema and the incisor protrusion are corrected.

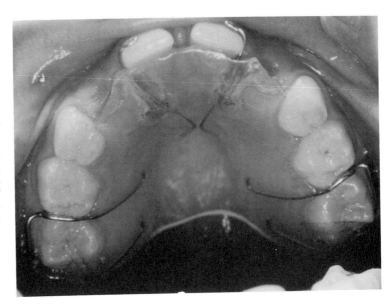

Figure 34–16 ■ In this case, a midline diastema is due to the mesio-distal positioning of the maxillary central incisors. A removable appliance with finger springs is incorporated into the palatal acrylic, and the finger springs are activated 2 mm per month to close the diastema by tipping the teeth together. (Reproduced by permission from Fields HW: Treatment of nonskeletal problems in preadolescent children. *In* Proffit WR, et al: Contemporary Orthodontics, St. Louis, 1986, The C. V. Mosby Co.)

mesial wings of each bracket to prevent the teeth from rotating when the space is closed (Fig. 34–17).

No matter which type of treatment is used to close a midline diastema, retention can be a problem and should be planned. In most cases, a removable appliance will maintain the space closure. The appliance will need to be adjusted periodically if the diastema is closed before the lateral incisors and canines are erupted fully. If the diastema reopens during or following retention, the incisors should be realigned. At that time, a surgical procedure, a frenectomy, can be completed if the frenum is suspected to be the cause of reopening the diastema. The frenectomy is performed after the space is closed be-

cause the scar tissue created by the procedure may actually impede closure if the surgery is accomplished first. If the diastema again reopens following retention and the surgical procedure, an .0175 inch multistranded wire can be bonded to the lingual surface of the incisors to keep the teeth together. The only contraindication to a bonded wire retainer is an excessively deep bite and poor oral hygiene.

CROWDING PROBLEMS

The first sign of crowding in the mixed dentition usually coincides with the eruption of the permanent incisors. Arch length insufficiency

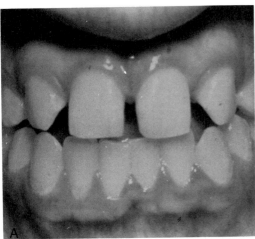
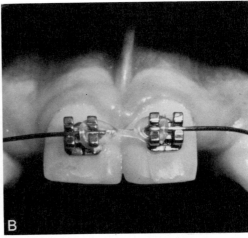

Figure 34–17 ■ *A,* If bodily mesio-distal movement is needed to close a diastema, fixed appliances are placed on the teeth. *B,* After initial alignment, either a segmental or a full arch wire is placed in the brackets and the teeth are moved together with an elastomeric chain.

may be manifest as slight incisor rotation and irregularity all the way to gross incisor malalignment. The first step should be to perform a space analysis and determine the extent of the arch length inadequacy.

Mild Crowding

An arch length discrepancy of 0–2 mm may not be apparent or may be manifest as mild crowding. This mild crowding is considered normal. Longitudinal study of individuals with ideal occlusions shows that there is a period when up to 2 mm of transitional crowding occurs early in the mixed dentition (Moorrees et al, 1969). Observation is usually the best treatment. Some patients with very small overall space shortages demonstrate noticeable crowding during incisor eruption. Treatment may be indicated for these children if lateral incisors erupt lingual to their proper position or in very irregular positions. If treatment is deemed necessary, interproximal enamel can be removed from the mesial surface of the primary canines to provide space. Disking may be accomplished with a hand-held strip, a sandpaper disk in a slow speed handpiece, or a tapered bur in a high speed handpiece. The procedure is performed without anesthesia so that the child can indicate any discomfort. Discomfort usually indicates that sufficient enamel has been removed to cause the pulpal tissues to react. Typically, careful disking may yield 2–4 mm of space. A professional strength topical fluoride preparation should be applied to the mesial surface of the canines after disking to reduce postoperative sensitivity.

If it is apparent that disking will not alleviate the anterior crowding, it may be appropriate to extract the primary canines and place a lingual arch. For the most part, this therapy is undertaken in the mandibular arch, although there are a few situations in which it is indicated in the maxilla. A lingual arch is necessary because the lower incisors tend to upright and tip lingually without the support of the primary canines. This results in further loss of arch length. In this situation, the lingual arch is placed in a passive state, that is, the arch does not exert any force to move the incisors and increase the space. The clinician should communicate to the parent that this treatment requires close supervision and that the primary first molars may need to be disked or extracted when the permanent canines erupt. The lingual arch remains in place until the second premolars have erupted

or until it is evident that there will be sufficient space for all the permanent teeth to erupt.

Moderate Crowding

Treatment of a moderate arch length discrepancy of less than 5 mm is based on the facial profile and incisor position as well as on the amount of crowding. If the profile is straight, with good anteroposterior or slightly retrusive position of the lips and incisors, a small amount of expansion can be tolerated to accommodate all the teeth. Expansion is not a good treatment option if the incisors are already protrusive. The clinician must always keep in mind the interaction between crowding, incisor position, and profile because they are essentially part of the same problem, expressed in a different way.

Moderate crowding can be either localized or generalized. Localized crowding may be the result of space loss following extraction or premature exfoliation of a primary tooth. If space loss is 3 mm or less, the adjacent tooth can be tipped into proper position with either a removable appliance or an active lingual arch. After the space has been regained, arch length should be near ideal and can be maintained. For example, a removable appliance with a finger spring can tip a permanent maxillary first molar distally following removal of a primary second molar compromised by ectopic eruption (Fig. 34–18). After the space has been regained, a band and loop appliance or a lingual arch can be placed to maintain the space.

If localized crowding is confined to the canine-premolar region of the arch, permanent tooth impaction is likely. Orthodontic tooth movement is necessary to increase the space and allow room for eruption. Fixed orthodontic appliances are placed on the entire arch, and the arch is aligned with light, flexible arch wires. After alignment, a heavy arch wire is placed to maintain good arch form during space-regaining movements. A compressed coil spring provides the force necessary to open the space (Fig. 34–19A). After the space has been opened, it may be necessary to expose the crown of the tooth surgically if it does not erupt within a 6-month period. Surgical exposure of the crown requires the elevation and repositioning of soft tissue to provide adequate keratinized tissue around the impacted tooth (Fig. 34–19B). Adequate attached gingiva is essential for good periodontal support and esthetics. If the clinician is not well versed in surgical exposure, the patient is best referred to a spe-

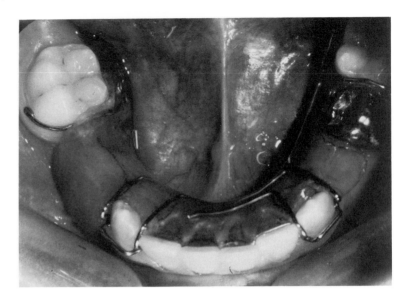

Figure 34-18 ■ Localized crowding is often the result of prematurely exfoliating primary teeth. In this case, the primary right second molar was lost prematurely, allowing the permanent first molar to drift mesially. A removable appliance has been designed to tip the permanent first molar back with a finger spring. The spring is activated until the molar is correctly positioned. Then a band and loop or lingual arch can be placed.

cialist. When the crown is exposed, an orthodontic attachment is bonded to the crown and the tooth is moved with traction into the arch (Fig. 34-19C).

Patients characterized by anterior or generalized crowding of less than 5 mm present difficult treatment decisions. As stated earlier, incisor and lip position provide important guides as to whether arch length can be created by expansion. Upright or lingually inclined incisors may be moved facially into correct alignment if the lips are retrusive. However, the risk associated with generalized arch expansion is instability of the new position. Movement of teeth facially may upset the existing equilibrium balance and result in relapse after appliances are

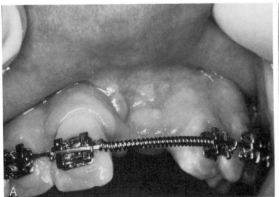

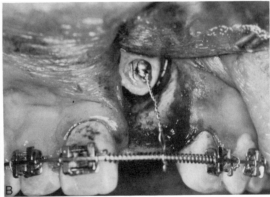

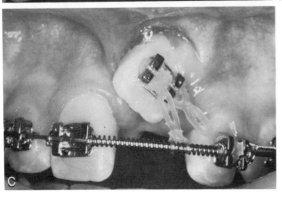

Figure 34-19 ■ A, If localized crowding is confined to the anterior or premolar region, tooth impaction is likely. Orthodontic tooth movement is necessary to create space for eruption of the impacted tooth. In this case, the permanent maxillary left central incisor was impacted and a coil spring was placed to open up space for the tooth to erupt. B, The tooth did not erupt within 6 months; therefore, the crown of the tooth was surgically exposed, bonded, and ligated to the base arch wire. C, After the soft tissues have healed sufficiently, orthodontic forces are applied to the tooth to bring it into the arch.

removed. Not all cases relapse; some maintain increased arch dimensions and remain stable after treatment is complete. However, there does not seem to be a good method to predict stability. Unfortunately, clinical judgment must be relied upon in many cases.

If the clinician elects to alleviate arch length inadequacy by expansion, several approaches may be taken. An active lower lingual arch can be constructed with adjustment loops to tip incisors facially if the overbite is not prohibitively deep to prevent facial incisor movement (Fig. 34–20) and perhaps to move molars distally a small amount. The adjustment loops, located mesial to the molars, should not be activated beyond 1 mm, because the activation of such a large wire (.036 inch) places extremely large forces on the teeth. When the appliance is properly activated, the wire contacts the tooth high on the cingulum of the incisors. The direction of force is apical, but it will tip the incisors facially because of the inclination of the lingual surface of the teeth. In 4–6 weeks, the appliance can be activated another millimeter. This is repeated until there is adequate arch length available for the permanent dentition. Primary canines may need to be disked or removed as discussed previously if the crowding is located in the anterior region.

A lip bumper, a wire appliance inserted in tubes on the lower molars, may be used to decrease lower lip pressure and achieve generalized arch expansion (Fig. 34–21). The lip bumper removes resting pressure of the lips and cheeks from the teeth in the incisor and canine regions. The incisors and canines move forward as a result of lack of lip pressure and the force of resting tongue pressure. The pressure from the lower lip may tip the molar distally.

Arch expansion may also be accomplished using a functional appliance with buccal shields in the vestibule. The buccal shields disrupt the equilibrium between the tongue and cheek and allow the teeth to move facially (Fig. 34–22). Some investigators claim that properly constructed buccal shields actually stretch the underlying periosteum of the bone and cause skeletal remodeling in the transverse dimension. Although this claim has not been substantiated in careful investigation, there is no doubt that enough expansion can be created in this manner to relieve minor to moderate crowding.

Fixed orthodontic appliances may be used to increase arch length in situations in which bodily movement of incisors is necessary to alleviate crowding and align the teeth. A variety of arch wire designs can be used to expand the arch, and they are pictured in Figure 34–23. After the expansion has been completed, a lower lingual arch is placed to retain the expansion. In most cases, further treatment will be necessary to align the remaining permanent teeth when they erupt. In addition, distal movement of the maxillary molars may be required, because the leeway space was used to align the mandibular teeth and cannot be used for the mesial molar shift. Therefore, multibonded appliances should be used sparingly and generally only in cases in which the molars are already Class I and there is some increased overjet. Re-

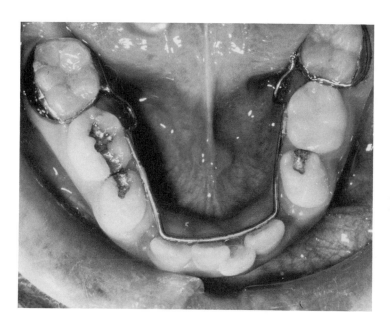

Figure 34–20 ■ Generalized crowding of less than 5 mm is occasionally treated with an adjustable lingual arch if the overbite is not too deep to prevent facial movement of the mandibular incisors. The appliance is activated by opening the adjustment loops.

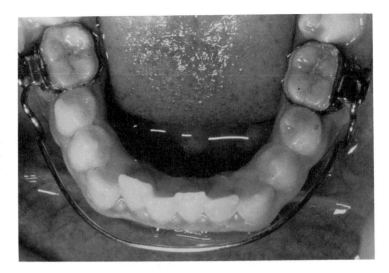

Figure 34–21 ■ A lip bumper is also used to treat generalized crowding of less than 5 mm. The lip bumper is designed to decrease lower lip pressure on the teeth and to allow generalized expansion by facial movement of the teeth.

gardless of which appliance is selected, expansion comes at the expense of incisor position and profile.

Severe Crowding

Crowding greater than 5 mm is considered to be severe. This amount of crowding is treated either by generalized arch expansion or by removal of selected permanent teeth. Generalized arch expansion can be accomplished with different appliances, but it usually requires bodily tooth movement with fixed appliances. Retaining the expansion often is very difficult. Incisor position, profile, and periodontal status

will all influence whether the patient should be treated without extraction. This type of patient is most appropriately referred to a specialist.

The decision to extract teeth is based on factors listed previously and is further influenced by the location of the crowding, the position of the dental midline, and the dental and skeletal relationships of the patient. After careful case analysis, appropriate teeth may be removed to make subsequent tooth movement easier to accomplish and to minimize the effects of extraction on the profile. The permanent first premolar is most often selected for extraction, because it is located at a midpoint in the arch and because the space it occupies can be used to cor-

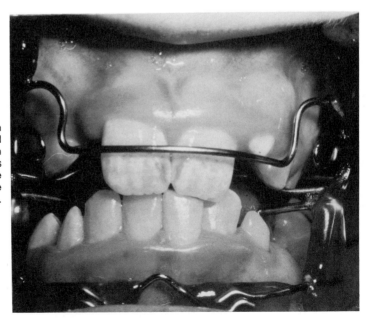

Figure 34–22 ■ Generalized arch expansion can also be accomplished using a removable appliance with buccal shields. The buccal shields disrupt the equilibrium between the facial musculature and the tongue and allow the teeth to move facially.

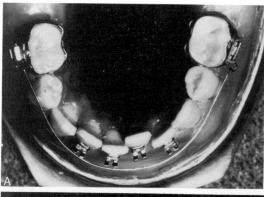
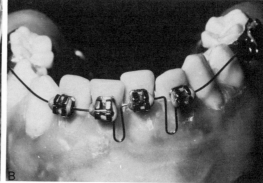
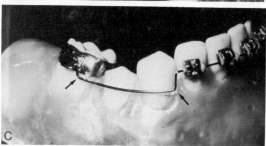

Figure 34–23 ■ *A,* Fixed orthodontic appliances are used to increase arch length when bodily movement or rotation of teeth is required. One way to expand the arch is to place an arch wire with loops that abut the molar buccal tubes. The loops are purposely placed so that the arch wire is 1 mm in front of the brackets and must be compressed to be engaged. Full bracket engagement provides the necessary force to expand the arch. *B,* If only a single tooth needs bodily movement, such as this mandibular left central incisor, loops are placed on either side of the tooth in an otherwise ideal arch wire. The portion of the arch wire between the loops is placed into the central incisor bracket slot. This activation provides the force necessary to bring the tooth into ideal position. *C,* Fixed orthodontic appliances can also be used to create more space for posterior teeth to erupt. In this example, the premolar requires more space to erupt into the arch properly. After initial alignment, a square arch wire is activated by making the bends *(arrows)* in the arch wire less acute. This will tip the molar distally and the incisors facially and will create space for the premolar to erupt.

rect midline problems, incisor protrusion, molar relationship problems, and crowding. Other teeth can be removed, depending on the specifics of the case and the mechanotherapy to be used. Extraction cases are best treated by a specialist.

In some children, crowding is so severe in the mixed dentition that expansion is not feasible and extractions are necessary to obtain a suitable occlusion that is in harmony with the supporting structures and facial profile. In these cases, planned sequence of extractions of primary and permanent teeth can benefit the patient by reducing incisor crowding and irregularity in the early mixed dentition, which will make subsequent orthodontic treatment easier and quicker. The extractions also make room for teeth to erupt over the alveolus and through keratinized tissue rather than being forced buccal or lingual into positions that may affect the periodontal health of the teeth. *Guidance of eruption* and *serial extraction* are terms used to describe this sequence of extractions (Hotz, 1970; Kjellgren, 1947). Guidance of eruption was originally developed to treat severe crowding without orthodontic appliances but now is

viewed as the first step of treatment culminating in fixed orthodontic appliance therapy. For this reason, the clinician should consult with a specialist before embarking on a planned extraction sequence.

Guidance of eruption should be considered an option in a situation in which crowding is greater than 10 mm per arch, which should be confirmed by a space analysis after the permanent lateral incisors have erupted. In addition, the patient should exhibit a Class I dental and skeletal pattern with good lip and incisor position, because guidance of eruption does not treat the skeletal problem. Guidance of eruption begins in the early mixed dentition with the eruption of the lateral incisors. If a significant arch length discrepancy is predicted, the primary canines should be removed. This will allow the incisors ample room to erupt and align. Typically, the incisors will also tip lingually and upright, causing the bite to deepen. Facio-lingual incisor displacement usually improves, but rotations are more resistant to spontaneous correction.

The child is then observed for 2 years or until it appears that the canines and premolars are

ready to erupt. At that time, another space analysis should be completed to ensure that the arch length deficiency is still great enough to warrant permanent tooth extraction, and a radiograph should be obtained to determine the position of the unerupted teeth. The goal of treatment is to encourage the eruption of the permanent first premolar so that it can be extracted before the eruption of the permanent canine. Unfortunately, the mandibular canine erupts first nearly one half the time in the mandibular arch. If it appears that the canine is ahead of the premolar and will erupt facially, the primary first molar should be removed when one half to two thirds of the first premolar root is formed. At this stage of root development, premolar eruption will be accelerated and it will erupt before the canine enters the arch. This makes removal of the first premolar much easier. In the maxillary arch, the first premolar normally erupts before the canine and this is not a problem.

In some cases, the primary first molar is removed but the permanent canine still erupts before the first premolar. This can lead to impaction of the first premolar, requiring surgical removal. Similarly, it may be apparent that the permanent canine will erupt before the first premolar regardless of the extraction sequence. In this situation, the primary first molar and first premolar are both removed at the same time. This procedure is termed *enucleation* because the premolar is removed from within the alveolar bone. Surgical removal of teeth from within the alveolar bone should be avoided if feasible because of the potential for creating bone and soft tissue defects. These occur if the alveolar bone is fractured or removed. New alveolar bone will not be stimulated to form, because no tooth will erupt through this area. Surgical soft tissue defects resolve infrequently.

An alternative extraction sequence has been advocated to prevent lingual tipping of the lower incisors and the subsequent increase in overbite, but this sequence is recommended only when incisor crowding is limited. The primary canine is not removed when the lateral incisor erupts. Instead, the primary canine is retained and the primary first molar is extracted to accelerate the eruption of the permanent first premolar. This allows some anterior crowding to resolve. The premolar is extracted when it erupts into the arch. The primary canine is often extracted at the same time as the premolar, or it is left to exfoliate when the permanent canine erupts. The drawback of this alternative is that substantial incisor crowding is not readily resolved, which somewhat defeats the goal of selective tooth removal to encourage good dental alignment.

ANTEROPOSTERIOR DENTAL PROBLEMS

Anterior Crossbite

Anterior crossbite in the mixed dentition is not an uncommon finding. The clinician should determine if the crossbite is skeletal or dental in origin from the profile analysis and intraoral findings. Skeletal problems should be referred to a specialist, whereas dental problems can be addressed immediately.

The most common cause of non-skeletal crossbite is a lack of space for the permanent maxillary incisors to erupt. A space analysis will verify the space shortage. Anterior crossbite develops because the permanent tooth buds form lingual to the primary teeth. When space is inadequate, the incisors are forced to erupt on the lingual side of the arch. If it is apparent that the permanent incisors are beginning to erupt lingually, the adjacent primary teeth should be disked or removed to provide space for the permanent incisors. If space is provided as the incisors are just beginning to erupt, they will migrate facially out of crossbite and appliance therapy may not be necessary.

If the incisor fails to erupt facially or the anterior crossbite is not diagnosed early in the mixed dentition, appliance therapy is needed to correct the crossbite. Space for the incisors is gained by either disking or extracting the adjacent primary teeth. At this point, a decision must be made as to whether the teeth should be tipped into position or bodily moved into place. If tipping will accomplish treatment goals, either a removable appliance or a fixed appliance can be used to correct the crossbite. As described earlier in the chapter, a removable appliance can be used to tip one or more teeth into proper alignment. The appliance is constructed of palatal acrylic with at least two Adams clasps for retention and a .022 inch finger spring to move the teeth (Fig. 34–24). The spring is of a double helical design that provides a physiologic amount of force over an extended range of action. The spring is activated 2 mm to provide 1 mm of tooth movement per month. As with all removable appliances, the child must cooperate by wearing the device full-time for the appliance to accomplish the desired tooth movement.

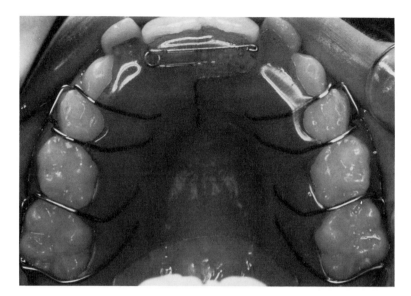

Figure 34–24 ■ If an anterior crossbite can be corrected by tipping the teeth facially, a removable appliance is designed to accomplish this goal. In this case, a single finger spring is tipping both maxillary central incisors out of crossbite.

Anterior crossbite with an accompanying deep overbite does not automatically require a biteplane or bite-opening device. Most individuals habitually posture with the mandible open and occlude only during swallowing and parafunctional movements. If the crossbite has not improved after 3 months of active treatment, it may be necessary to open the bite by adding acrylic that covers the occlusal surfaces of the posterior teeth to the appliance. This limits closure and keeps the anterior teeth apart, which allows uninhibited incisor movement. In most cases, the crossbite will correct quickly and the biteplane can be removed. Extended use of a biteplane is discouraged, because the teeth not

in contact with the appliance will continue to erupt and will create a vertical occlusal discrepancy.

Fixed appliances can also tip teeth out of crossbite and do not require as much cooperation from the child. If bonded to each individual tooth, a fixed appliance can also provide precise control of tooth movement in all three planes of space by using rectangular wires (Fig. 34–25). The disadvantage of either a labial or lingual fixed appliance is the patient's inability to clean around the teeth and appliance thoroughly, which can result in marginal gingivitis and caries.

A maxillary lingual arch is a suitable appli-

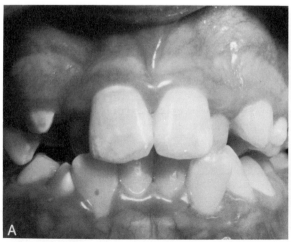
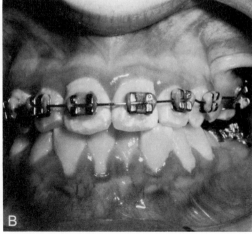

Figure 34–25 ■ *A,* Fixed appliances may also be used to tip teeth out of anterior crossbite. This patient had both maxillary lateral incisors in anterior crossbite. *B,* After the brackets were placed, progressively larger round wires were used to tip the teeth out of crossbite. A rectangular arch wire will be used to achieve proper crown and root position.

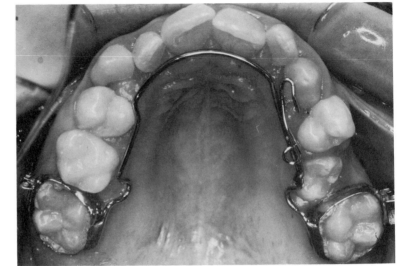

Figure 34-26 ■ Fixed lingual appliances can also be used to tip teeth out of anterior crossbite. This patient required facial movement of the maxillary left canine to correct the crossbite. A small finger spring was soldered to the base lingual arch and was activated to provide the force necessary to move the tooth.

ance to correct an anterior crossbite if teeth require tipping movement. The maxillary arch is constructed of .036 inch wire, with adjustment loops similar to those in a lower lingual arch. Finger springs made of .022 inch wire provide the tooth-moving force. The springs are usually soldered on the opposite side of the arch from the tooth being moved in order to increase the length and range of the spring (Fig. 34-26). The springs are activated approximately 3 mm before the appliance is cemented into place. During cementation, the springs are tied with steel ligature to the lingual arch so that they will not interfere with the seating of the appliance. After the excess cement has been cleaned away, the ligature is cut away to activate the springs. In some cases, the spring will slip over the incisal edge of an incisor that is not fully erupted. In these cases, a stainless steel guide wire is soldered to the lingual arch at the midline to prevent the spring from slipping incisally. Three millimeters of activation provides one millimeter of tooth movement per month. The appliance should be removed, reactivated, and recemented at 4- to 6-week intervals until the crossbite is corrected.

In older patients, space may need to be created for crossbite correction by arch expansion because there are no primary teeth to disk or extract. In this situation, the permanent molars should be banded and the incisors should be bonded with orthodontic brackets.

An anterior crossbite that requires bodily movement of teeth to correct the problem is best treated with bonded brackets and a planned sequence of arch wires. Initially, teeth can be

tipped out of crossbite. Usually an arch wire is selected that is strong enough to withstand the force of occlusion in the posterior segments yet flexible enough in the anterior region to engage the brackets of the malaligned teeth. This generally requires a stainless steel arch wire with loops bent mesial and distal to the tooth in crossbite (Fig. 34-27). Loops in the anterior region are designed to provide horizontal and/or vertical tooth movement and exert optimum force. After alignment is completed, an arch wire is placed into the brackets that is capable of delivering a root-positioning force to the tooth previously in crossbite. The purpose of such a force is to move the root into proper position so that the entire tooth has essentially moved forward out of crossbite.

Retention must be planned in all cases, regardless of the appliance selected. Active tooth movement is usually continued until the crossbite is slightly overcorrected. The correction should be retained with a passive removable appliance for 2 months if there is a positive overbite. If there is not adequate overbite, retention should be continued until adequate overbite develops. A circumferential supracrestal fibrotomy should also be considered if rotational movement was made during treatment.

In a small number of cases, the anterior crossbite is caused by excessive spacing and flaring of the mandibular incisors. A removable appliance can be constructed with an adjustable .028 inch labial bow to retract the lower incisors and close space. The appliance should be activated 1 mm per month and treatment continued until the space is closed and there is positive

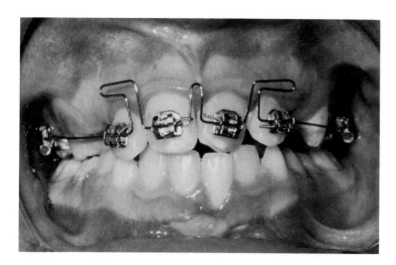

Figure 34–27 ■ In some cases, anterior teeth need bodily movement to correct a crossbite. This requires that fixed appliances be placed to position the teeth properly. Initially, an arch wire is selected that is strong enough to withstand the force of occlusion in the posterior segments and flexible enough to engage the brackets of the malaligned teeth. Often it is necessary to place loops in the arch wire to provide enough flexibility to engage the brackets properly. After the teeth have been tipped out of crossbite, a rectangular wire is used to position the roots.

overbite and overjet. The tooth movement can be retained with the same removable appliance, which is made passive.

Incisor Protrusion

Incisor protrusion in the mixed dentition is a serious esthetic problem for the preadolescent patient. Protrusive incisors not only are unesthetic but are more prone to dental injury than incisors of normal angulation. For those reasons, treatment is usually undertaken to move the incisors lingually into a more suitable position if the overbite is not prohibitively deep. This is treatment for a dental problem, not a skeletal problem. Skeletal problems should be referred to a specialist for growth modification.

Treatment of incisor protrusion has already been discussed in the section on treating diastemata in the mixed dentition. To summarize, teeth that can be tipped back into ideal alignment should be treated with a removable appliance that incorporates an active labial bow. The bow is activated by means of an adjustment loop to provide a lingual tipping force to the flared incisors. One to two millimeters of palatal acrylic is removed from the appliance to allow the crown to move lingually and to accommodate the palatal tissue that tends to bunch up behind the tooth being moved. The retention schedule should be full-time wear for 3 months.

In some cases, bodily movement of teeth is necessary to correct incisor protrusion. The maxillary first molars should be banded and brackets bonded to the anterior permanent teeth. A small, round, flexible arch wire is placed in the brackets to align the teeth initially. Anterior tooth retraction is accomplished on a rectangular arch wire with a closing loop or elastomeric chain. A headgear and/or a transpalatal arch is usually used during retraction to supplement anchorage. The choice between cervical, combination, or high pull headgear is based on the patient's vertical dimensions. A cervical headgear is generally used when the patient has normal vertical facial proportions, whereas a high pull headgear is indicated when the patient has increased lower facial height. The clinician should follow the progress of a patient undergoing incisor retraction carefully, to prevent problems associated with retraction. A complication encountered during incisor retraction is moving the root of the permanent lateral incisor into the path of the unerupted permanent canine. The lateral incisor root either will impede eruption of the canine or may be resorbed. The wire should be bent or the bracket placed so that the lateral incisor root is upright or even tipped slightly to the mesial.

TRANSVERSE DENTAL PROBLEMS

Posterior crossbite correction in the mixed dentition can be difficult and confusing. The clinician must rely on a well-documented data base to determine whether skeletal or dental correction is necessary. The presence of a mandibular shift is also important. A posterior crossbite with an associated mandibular shift should be treated as soon as possible to prevent possible asymmetrical facial growth and dental compensation. Crossbites can be corrected with a W-arch or a quad helix in the primary and early mixed dentitions. Skeletal and dental movements both occur with these appliances, and it is difficult to preferentially effect one or

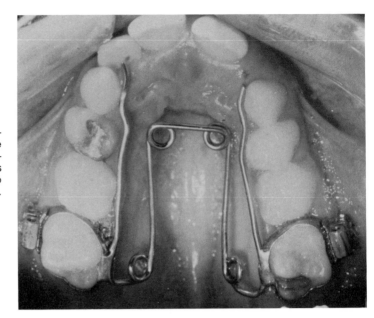

Figure 34–28 ■ Generalized posterior crossbites of dental origin in the mixed dentition are treated with either a W-arch or a quad helix. In this situation, a quad helix is being used to correct a bilateral posterior crossbite.

the other. In the late mixed dentition, the midpalatal suture may be more interdigitated and the clinician can make primarily dental or skeletal changes, depending on the appliance selected to treat the case. Skeletal problems should be referred to a specialist, but the clinician should treat dental problems without referral. Posterior dental crossbites are either generalized or localized.

Generalized crossbites of dental origin are usually bilateral and are corrected with a W-arch or a quad helix (Fig. 34–28). If the crossbite is due to a unilateral dental constriction, an unequal W-arch (made of .036 inch wire) or a quad helix (made of .038 inch wire) can be used to expand the arch. Alternatively, a lower lingual arch can be used to stabilize the lower teeth and cross-elastics can be worn to the maxillary arch to correct the crossbite unilaterally. These appliances have been discussed in previous sections, and the reader should review those sections.

Localized crossbites are usually due to displacement of single teeth in one or both arches. For example, a maxillary lingual crossbite involving the permanent first molars is usually the result of the lingual displacement of the maxillary molar and/or the facial displacement of the mandibular molar. If only one tooth is causing the problem, a removable appliance with a finger spring can be used (Fig. 34–29). If teeth in opposing arches are at fault, it is easy to correct the problem using a simple crossbite elastic. The offending teeth are fit with ortho-

dontic bands without attachments. After the bands are fitted, they are removed and a button is welded to the opposite surface of the band from the direction the tooth is to be moved. In the example just noted, a button is welded to the lingual surface of the maxillary band and to the buccal surface of the mandibular band. After the bands have been welded and cemented, a medium weight (3/16 inch, 6 ounces) is attached from button to button through the oc-

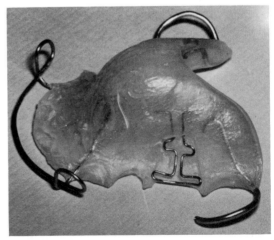

Figure 34–29 ■ Localized posterior crossbites are usually caused by the malalignment of a single tooth in one or both arches. This removable appliance was designed to correct a lingually displaced primary second molar with a T-spring. The spring tips the displaced tooth facially.

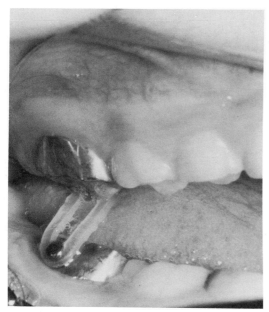

Figure 34–30 ■ If teeth are at fault in both arches, a simple crossbite elastic is used to correct the crossbite. Bands can be placed on both permanent right first molars and buttons welded to the lingual of the maxillary band and to the facial of the mandibular band. A medium weight elastic (4–6 ounce) is attached from one button to the other and provides the force required to correct the crossbite.

clusion (Fig. 34–30). The elastic should be worn full-time, except when the patient is eating, and should be changed at least one time per day. The elastic should be worn until the crossbite is slightly overcorrected. It may be prudent to leave the bands in place and discontinue use of the elastic for 1 month to ensure that the teeth will not relapse into crossbite. When the occlusion is stable, after 4–6 weeks without elastic force, the bands can be removed. Buttons are now available that can be bonded directly to the tooth, making bands unnecessary, but there is a risk of bond failure and appliance aspiration.

VERTICAL DENTAL PROBLEMS

Vertical problems in the mixed dentition are primarily open bite or deepbite malocclusions. Dental open bite is most often the result of an active digit habit that has impeded eruption of the anterior teeth. In some cases, the digit habit has been discontinued but the open bite has been maintained because the tongue rests between the teeth and prevents eruption. Treat-

ment is essentially the same as that described for digit habits in the late primary and early mixed dentitions. If non-appliance therapy is unsuccessful, a palatal crib is effective if the patient desires to stop the habit. It reminds the child to refrain from the habit and blocks the tongue from being postured forward. Therapy will be successful in the majority of cases unless the child is unwilling to abandon the habit. Skeletal open bite treatment has been described, and these patients should be referred to a specialist.

Dental deep bite is caused by the over-eruption of the anterior teeth or under-eruption of the posterior teeth. It should be distinguished from skeletal deep bite that is characterized by a flat mandibular plane angle and a short vertical dimension as well as by over- and under-erupted teeth. In a normal incisor to lip relationship, 2 mm of the maxillary central incisor is exposed when the lip is at rest. If more than 2 mm of incisor is exposed, maxillary anterior over-eruption must be considered. In the mandibular arch, over-eruption is difficult to diagnose; however, the curve of Spee may provide some

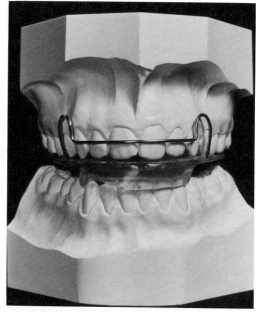

Figure 34–31 ■ In this age group, a deep overbite can be treated with a removable appliance designed to inhibit anterior eruption and allow posterior eruption. This appliance is blocking maxillary and mandibular anterior eruption and maxillary posterior eruption. The mandibular posterior teeth are free to erupt and decrease the overbite. This type of treatment alone for deep overbite is infrequently prescribed.

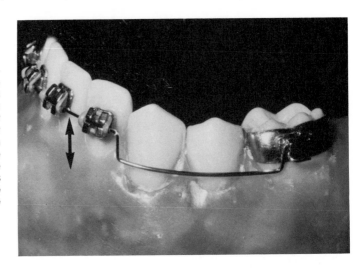

Figure 34–32 ■ Fixed orthodontic appliances are also used to treat deep overbites in the mixed dentition. In this case, the patient exhibits a deep curve of Spee and would best be treated by intruding the mandibular incisors. A utility arch wire is bent so that it rests passively in the mandibular or buccal vestibule. The arch wire is activated by lifting the wire up and placing it into the incisor brackets (arrow). This creates a light intrusive force on the anterior teeth and a light extrusive force on the molars.

clue. An excessive curve of Spee (2 mm or more) is suggestive of mandibular incisor over-eruption.

Treatment in a growing patient can usually be incorporated into comprehensive orthodontic treatment. Occasionally, mixed dentition treatment is aimed at preventing further anterior eruption and encouraging or allowing posterior eruption. In these cases, incisor teeth are blocked from erupting with a removable appliance. The appliance is constructed so that acrylic touches the upper and lower incisors but allows the posterior teeth to erupt (Fig. 34–31). The appliance must be worn full-time for correction to take place and then must be worn as a retainer to maintain the correction until the patient stops growing vertically.

If the deepbite is deemed to be the result of maxillary incisor over-eruption or a combination of maxillary and mandibular over-eruption, fixed orthodontic appliances are placed on the teeth. A utility arch, a wire that connects the permanent first molars with the incisors, is constructed to exert a very light intrusive force on the incisors (Fig. 34–32). Because there is an equal and opposite reaction to every force placed on the teeth, the molars experience an extrusive force. Specifically, the molar will erupt and tip distally and facially. Facial movement of the molars can be counteracted by a transpalatal arch or a lower lingual arch, but neither will prevent the distal tipping. The util-

ity arch is a deceptively simple appliance but it may create more orthodontic problems than it remedies unless it is used with thought and care. Often this is the first phase of comprehensive orthodontic treatment, and consultation with a specialist is appropriate.

REFERENCES

Andreason JO, Ravn JJ: Epidemiology of traumatic dental injuries to primary and permanent teeth in a Danish population sample. Int J Oral Surg 1:235–239, 1972.

Baumrind S, Korn EL: Patterns of change in mandibular and facial shape associated with the use of forces to retract the maxilla. Am J Orthod 80:31–47, 1981.

Fields HW, Proffit WR, Nixon WL, Phillips C, and Stanek E: Facial pattern differences in long-faced children and adults. Am J Orthod 85:217–223, 1984.

Hotz RP: Guidance of eruption versus serial extraction. Am J Orthod 58:1–20, 1970.

Kjellgren B: Serial extraction as a corrective procedure in dental orthopedic therapy. Trans Euro Ortho Soc, pp 34–47, 1947–1948.

McNamara JA, Bookstein FL, Shaughnessy TG: Skeletal and dental changes following functional regulator therapy on Class II patients. Am J Orthod 88:91–110, 1985.

Moorrees CFA, Gron AM, Lebret LML, Yen PKJ, Frohlich FJ: Growth studies of the dentition: A review. Am J Orthod 55:600–616, 1969.

Remmer KR, Manandras AH, Hunter WS, Way DC: Cephalometric changes associated with treatment using the activator, the Frankel appliance, and the fixed appliance. Am J Orthod 88:363–372, 1985.

SUMMARY FOR SECTION III

The dentist who follows a child from age 6 to age 12 will have had the opportunity to see many changes in the child. The physical changes will be dramatic, and those that have to do with facial form, occlusion, the advent of the permanent teeth, and the esthetics of these permanent teeth are the professional responsibility of the dentist. He or she must supervise the exfoliation of the 20 primary teeth in the 6-year-old and supervise through the 6 years the eruption of the 28 permanent teeth that are found in most 12-year-olds. The dentist must provide answers to parents concerned about the appearance of their child, intercept those developing malocclusions that are within his or her treatment talents, and refer when appropriate those malocclusions that need specialist care.

As in previous age groups, the prevention of both hard and soft tissue diseases is very important. The repair of trauma and pulpal therapy, and the effective restoration of carious teeth, both primary and permanent, are also important to children 6–12 years of age. One thing significantly different during the transitional years is the increase of information regarding the ultimate occlusion of the child. The dentist is responsible for making sure that in the later stages of the transitional dentition and in the early permanent dentition, the dental and facial esthetics of the child have been anticipated, any apparent problems have been diagnosed correctly, and in problem cases treatment has been planned and performed according to the most desirable timing and techniques. Another demand of this age group is pulpal and restorative care of the young permanent teeth.

As is true for children between ages 3 and 6, so it is true for children between 6 and 12 — they are generally as a group very fun to treat. Obviously, the management modalities and type of conversation that one would have with a 6-year-old will necessarily have to be refined and sophisticated over the years, since the mental functioning of a 12-year-old is for all practical purposes the same as that of an adult. The only thing his mind lacks is the continuing education and experience that school and life will give to him.

The dentist that can deliver the child from age 12 to adolescence with no amount or just a modest amount of hard tissue disease, no remarkable soft tissue diseases, allegiance to prevention and developed home care habits, and harmonious dento-facial relationships has indeed mastered the ultimate obligations in treating this age group.

section IV

Adolescence

Adolescence represents an extremely important time in the dental care of the child patient. Certainly, prevention of dental diseases is one of the pivotal concerns of the dentist who cares for adolescents. Adolescence marks a time in which the role of the parent in the child's dental home care needs to be minimized and the responsibility of the adolescent for managing his or her own oral health program must be emphasized. Some adolescents will be able to do this easily and will seem to be inherently motivated to practice proper oral hygiene on a day-by-day basis. However, there are certainly exceptions to this finding, and some of these exceptions can be extremely stubborn. The dentist must play a role in educating and motivating such patients, for not only is caries a problem but also periodontal disease and its unfortunate implications become increasingly important as the child proceeds to the later years of adolescence.

Another preventive concern is the fact that adolescents, particularly those older adolescents who have their own transportation, sources of money, and freedom to choose their own diet, may stray away from the diet that was maintained in their home and go to a regimen containing many more snacks and a possibility of much more sugar ingestion. This can predict increased dental disease.

Adolescence is also a time very likely to impose upon a child stressful life situations and anxieties regarding social circumstances. This, paired with fatigue, a poor diet, and increasing responsibilities at school and in life in general, may bring about enough stress to predict the onset of certain stress-related oral diseases, such as necrotizing ulcerative gingivitis.

Another concern of the dentist who treats adolescents is their dentofacial esthetics. More so than at any other age, the adolescent will want a dentition that is esthetic. Previous irregularities in the dentition or in the color of the teeth that are visible during conversation or smiling may become of deep concern to the child, and demands may be put upon the dentist to make sure that these problems are corrected. However, crown and bridge procedures in the adolescent as well as other restorative techniques may be more difficult than at later ages because of the height of the gingiva on the clinical crown and the relatively large size of the pulpal tissues. Although acid-etch techniques have given dentists a revolution in the way that dentistry can handle anterior esthetic problems, the crown and bridge are still needed to resolve certain problems. In certain cases, the dentist may need to employ an interim treatment plan until there has been sufficient reduction of the pulpal chamber.

IV

A certain percentage of adolescents will be athletically involved, and this, paired with their larger bodies and the possibility of more velocity when they play their sport, predicts that dental trauma for certain sports is very high. A dentist who has athletes among his or her child patient population must be aware of the prevention concerns and needs that this group presents.

Third molar extractions may become needed in late adolescence. The dentist will need to follow the development of these molars and assess their position in the jaws to determine if and when extraction is needed.

Lastly, adolescence represents a relatively long period of life in our society. The dentist must be well versed in understanding the different characteristics of adolescence as they relate to age. Obviously, the conversation that a dentist would have with a 13-year-old would be substantially different than that with an 18-year-old. The dentist needs to be acutely aware of these differences and be able to be versatile in his or her communication style with this age group.

chapter 35

The dynamics of change

CHAPTER OUTLINE

■ **PHYSICAL CHANGES**
   Body
   Head and Neck
   Dental Changes

■ **COGNITIVE CHANGES**

■ **EMOTIONAL CHANGES**

■ **SOCIAL CHANGES**

PHYSICAL CHANGES

BODY

J. R. Pinkham

Adolescence in some societies is a very short transitional period that marks the arrival of a child to full citizenship within his or her respective tribe and culture. In a technological society such as Europe or North America today, adolescence is a time of enormous transition and is certainly not of a short duration. Hence, the term *teenager* has become synonymous with the term *adolescent* in our society. Literature describing the adolescent may portray the adolescent as an old child or a young adult. Certainly, it is an in-between age in our society and needs to be understood as something independent of either childhood or adulthood.

Critical to the definition of adolescence regardless of culture and to the understanding of the adolescent physically is the concept of puberty. Puberty is the landmark in physical development when sexually an individual is capa-

ble of reproduction. In common law, this has been established in our society historically to be age 14 for boys and age 12 for girls. The advent of puberty is paralleled with the development of genital tissue and secondary sexual characteristics, such as the development of hair in the area of the genitals.

It is also a time when there is increase of the mass of muscles, a redistribution of body fat, and an increase in the rate of skeletal growth. There is a growth spurt associated with this time of life. This growth spurt follows two different forms, depending upon sex. In females, when compared with males, it appears early. The average onset in males is 2 years later than in females. It appears that the fact that males experience their growth spurt later than females and therefore have a longer pre–growth spurt maturation period is one of the reasons why the total height of males generally exceeds the height of females. The earlier growth spurt of females also accounts for a period of time when mean height of a group of young female adolescents may exceed the mean height of the males. It is important to realize also that in females

451

menarche serves as a signal that growth is ending, but for males there is no such marker.

The magnitude of the velocity of change during the growth spurt also differs between the sexes. In 1975, Tanner and colleagues concluded that females peak at 9 cm change per year at age 12, and that males peak at just over 10 cm at age 14.

REFERENCE

Tanner, JM, Whitehouse RH, Marshall WA, et al: Assessment of Skeletal Maturity and Prediction of Adult Height: TW 2 Method. New York, Academic Press, 1975.

HEAD AND NECK

Jerry Walker

During adolescence, subtle changes in skeletal growth of the face and skull take place to give the individual the final adult appearance. The postpubertal or adolescent period shows no increase in the brain case. However, there is a slow increase in the height of the face, accompanied by an increase in prognathism (Behrents, 1985). In the adolescent, the nose and chin become more prominent. In 1947, Bjork concluded from his cross-sectional study that in adolescence the face increases in height and in prognathism. The mandible exhibits a greater prognathic change than the maxilla. The circumpubertal growth spurt is generally recognized to take place between the ages of 10 and 12 in the female and 12 and 14 in the male (Behrents, 1985) (Table 35 – 1).

The chin becomes more prominent by bone deposition. The convex profiles in the lip region of children tend to be reduced by these growth changes. The brow area becomes larger as a result of pneumatization of the frontal sinuses and apposition on the glabella (Ranly, 1980). The maxillary sinuses, which have since birth expanded laterally and vertically, occupy the space left by the permanent teeth as they erupt, and the sinuses grow downward. By puberty, the sinuses are usually fully developed, although they may continue to enlarge. There are considerable variations in size of the maxillary sinuses from one age to another and from person to person. They are also not necessarily symmetrical.

There is an average increase in the palatal vault of approximately 10 mm from birth through adolescence, but simultaneously the palate moves downward as a result of appositional growth. In 1966, Bjork concluded that in some cases sutural growth as well as appositional growth provide a large contribution to the increase in height of the maxillary body. The nose becomes more protrusive, and the tip of the nasal bone comes to lie well ahead of the basal bone of the premaxilla.

The growth of the jaws continues during this period. This growth may be sufficient to develop room for third molars. In many cases, the growth is inadequate and these molars become impacted. The marked mesial inclination of the posterior permanent teeth diminishes somewhat as the mandible completes its growth from under the maxilla, and the lower incisors tend to become more upright. Often some crowding in the lower incisors is the result (Ranly, 1980).

Table 35 – 1 ■ Growth of the aging skeleton: sexual dimorphism in craniofacial growth

	Females	**Males**
Circumpubertal growth spurt	10–12 years	12–14 years
Mature size	Growth plateaus at 14 with increases to 16 years	Active growth to 18 years
Supraorbital ridges	Absent	Well developed
Frontal sinuses	Small	Large
Nose	Small	Large
Zygomatic prominences	Small	Large
Mandibular symphysis	Rounded	Prominent
Mandibular angle	Rounded	Prominent lipping
Occipital condyles	Small	Large
Mastoid processes	Small	Large
Occipital protuberance	Insignificant	Prominent

(From Behrents RG: Growth in the Aging Craniofacial Skeleton. Ann Arbor MI, Center for Human Growth and Development, University of Michigan, 1985; modified from Broadbent BH Jr: Bolton Standards of Dentofacial Developmental Growth. Cleveland, Bolton–Brush Growth Study Center, Case Western Reserve University.)

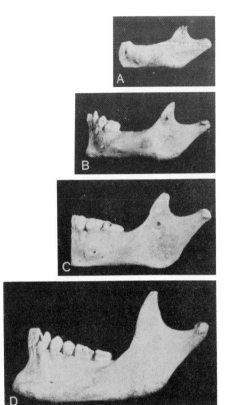

Figure 35 – 1 ■ Four stages in the development of the mandible. *A*, At birth. *B*, At 18 months. *C*, At 4 years. *D*, At 16 years. (From Sicher's ORAL ANATOMY, 8th Edition, by E. Lloyd DuBrul, Ishiyaku EuroAmerica, Inc., St. Louis, Missouri, 1980.)

The stages in the development of the mandible from birth through 16 years of age are shown in Figure 35 – 1 (DuBrul, 1980). Mandibular growth has taken place at the condyles in the same mode as interstitial cartilage growth. Such growth imparts an increase in the vertical height of the ramus of the mandible, and it also becomes more upright. The elongation of the ramus accommodates the massive vertical expansion of the nasal region and the eruption or completion of the permanent dentition. The lower jaw catches up with the maxilla and matches most or all of the early growth in this area. The alveolar bone in the adolescent becomes more protrusive and proportionally more massive than in the infant and young child. The whole face is a great deal longer vertically and more sloping as a result of the many changes (Enlow, 1968, Ranly, 1980) (Fig. 35 – 2).

Figure 35 – 3 illustrates that the adult facial skeleton is literally twice as large as that of the newborn but that the brain case differs in size by only 50%.

Figure 35 – 4, a magnification of the child's skull, demonstrates the change in the form and proportions of the skull from childhood through adolescence. It is evident that the brain case of the newborn is much larger in relation to the facial skeleton than that of the adult (Lundstrom, 1960).

Figure 35 – 2 ■ Serial tracings of an individual superimposed in the S-N plane with the sella as the reference point. (From Ranly DM: A Synopsis of Craniofacial Growth. E Norwalk, CT, Appleton-Century-Crofts, 1980.)

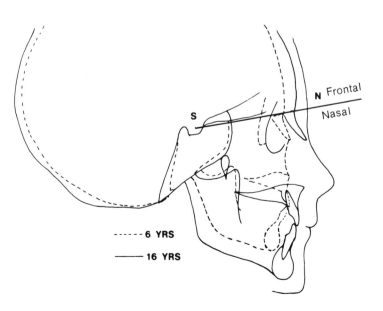

N Frontal

Nasal

S

S

------ 6 YRS

——— 16 YRS

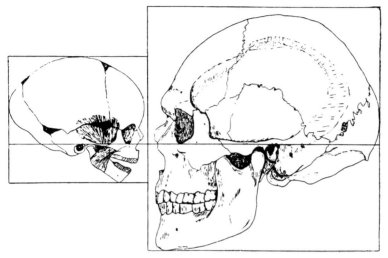

Figure 35–3 ■ Skulls of a new-born child and an adult contrasted in lateral view. They are oriented on the Frankfort plane (upper margin of external auditory meatus and lower margin of orbit) and are in their natural proportion to each other. (From Brash JC: Five Lectures on the Growth of the Jaws Normal and Abnormal in Health and Disease. Dental Board of the United Kingdom, 1924.)

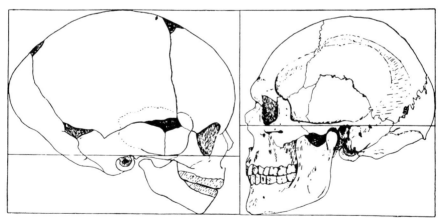

Figure 35–4 ■ The same skulls as in Figure 35–3. Relative to the adult, the child's skull is magnified twice in all directions. (From Lundstrom A: Introduction to Orthodontics. New York, McGraw-Hill Book Co, Inc, 1960.)

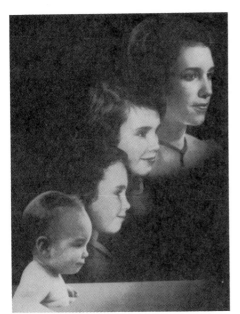

Figure 35–5 ■ Changes in the skull from infancy to the completion of adolescence. (Courtesy of William L. Briedon. From Enlow DH: The Human Face. New York, Harper and Row, 1968.)

By completion of adolescence, the 27 bones (5 single and 8 pairs, excluding the hyoid and ear bones) that originally made up the skull have become 22 bones (6 single and 8 pairs, excluding the hyoid and ear bones) and are so closely adapted that the skull can be considered as a single bone. Although growth will continue throughout one's lifetime, the variations that give each of us our individuality have become dominant (Enlow, 1968) (Fig. 35–5).

REFERENCES

Behrents RG: Growth in the Aging Craniofacial Skeleton. Monograph 17, Craniofacial Growth Series, Ann Arbor, MI, Center for Human Growth and Development, 1985.

Bjork A: The face in profile. Sven Tanalak Tidskr *40*:Suppl 5B, 1947.

Bjork A: Sutural growth of the upper face studied by the implant method. Acta Odontol Scand 24:109–127, 1966.

DuBrul EL: Sicher's Oral Anatomy, 8th ed. St. Louis, Ishiyaku EuroAmerica, Inc, 1980.

Enlow DH: Handbook of Facial Growth. Philadelphia, WB Saunders Co, 1982.

Lundstrom A: Introduction to Orthodontics. New York, McGraw-Hill Book Co, 1960.

Ranly DM: A Synopsis of Craniofacial Growth. New York, Appleton-Century-Crofts, 1980.

DENTAL CHANGES

C. A. Full

All of the permanent teeth generally will have erupted by age 12, except possibly the four second molars, which may erupt as late as age 13, and the third molars, which usually erupt between the ages of 17 and 21.

Except for the third molars, the dentist should be concerned about any unerupted permanent tooth after age 13 and should examine the area in question radiographically.

The roots of all the teeth are considered to have been completed by age 16, except for those of the third molars, which could achieve completion as late as age 25.

COGNITIVE CHANGES

J. R. Pinkham

The adolescent continues his or her cognitive development and by middle to late adolescence is capable of extremely sophisticated intellectual tasks. High ability at abstract thinking allows the adolescent to deal with complex and difficult vocational and educational challenges. Formal operational thinking and the ability to store information in the memory after perceiving it are hallmarks of the maturation of cognitive ability for adolescents.

The new information available to the adolescent, along with more sophisticated ways of analyzing this information, often makes him or her appear to be a rebel, a complainer, and an

accuser. This age often ascertains the possible and becomes discontent, even angry, with the real. Kiell pointed out in 1967 that Aristotle, more than 2000 years ago, concluded that adolescents "are passionate, irascible, and apt to be carried away by their impulses."

It has been noted that the thoughts of adolescents are both *introspective* and *analytical*. They are also *egocentric*. This dwelling upon one's self may make an individual overly self-conscious. Clothes, cars, hairstyle, music tastes, and identity with certain people or groups probably reflect the adolescent's involvement in self-consciousness.

In summary, by mid- to late adolescence, most young people are capable of formal operational thinking and can, both in and out of school, master subject material that is extensive, difficult, and abstract. Many will have matured into skillful, enthusiastic communicators and conversationalists. Many will also be opinionated and perhaps argumentative. These last two characteristics may make for some trying times for parents, teachers, and dentists also.

REFERENCE

Kiell N: The Universal Experience of Adolescence. Boston, Beacon, 1967.

EMOTIONAL CHANGES
J. R. Pinkham

The very rapid and dramatic changes that happen to adolescents can be paralleled with many emotional circumstances. The self-confidence and personal identity of the adolescent may be compromised if his or her feelings about body image are wrong. In 1984, Mussen and colleagues noted the following issues as having the possibility of misinterpretation and anxiety for this age group:

● Being attractive or unattractive
● Being loved or unloved
● Being strong or weak
● Being masculine or feminine

For females, the onset of menstruation may also present circumstances that can be anxiety provoking. This does not have to be so, but chances of anxiety rise if there is a prevailing negative reaction to the menstrual process by family and peers, if the child is showered with sympathy, or if there is considerable pain before and during menses. Anyone who works with postmenarcheal females should be aware that some percentage of them will display, at times, irritability and/or depression.

The advent of puberty and the hormones associated with puberty lead to sexual feelings and urges. The timing of this process, the nature and magnitude of the sexual arousal process, and what the adolescent wishes to do or chooses to do about these feelings and urges are handled differently from one adolescent to another. Family guidance, the adolescent's own values, the values of peers, and the value system of the person that the adolescent first loves are just a few of the factors that ultimately predict how he or she will deal with these new feelings.

One last emotion is critical to understanding adolescents. This is the emotion of love. Adolescents are capable of great commitment to one another, and some of these relationships are of natural and paralleling concern and can be a long-term commitment. Unfortunately, many of the relationships do not last, as one partner becomes disinterested. This can lead to genuine depression for the abandoned partner. The term "puppy love" is a terrible misnomer and belies exactly how painful these broken relationships can be.

REFERENCE

Mussen PH, Conger JJ, Kagan J, Huston AC: Child Development and Personality, 6th ed. New York, Harper and Row, 1984.

SOCIAL CHANGES

J. R. Pinkham

Adolescence represents the final transition socially from childhood to adulthood. When it is over, if everything proceeded as it should, the emerging young adult will be able to establish and maintain loving and sexual relationships with a partner, be independent of the parents, be capable of working with peers, and be self-directed. These are formidable social challenges, and some adolescents cannot master them. Delinquency, attempted or successful suicide, alcohol and drug use and abuse, running away from home, teenage prostitution, and dropping out of school are some of the frequently cited instances of adolescent failure to socialize properly.

Peers are very important social agents in large, technological societies, in which children of the same age group are often kept together. It can be argued that as relationships and dependencies upon parents start to decline, the importance of peers escalates. Increasingly, the adolescent may find that it is difficult to share secrets, thoughts, and fantasies with his or her parents. In these situations, the close friend becomes the adolescent's confidant. In such cases, the peer is a valuable and useful audience.

Despite the obvious value of peers, there are peer relationships that are not so fortunate for the involved adolescent. For example, to avoid rejection or ridicule from peers an adolescent may try drugs, participate in criminal acts, or defy authority.

Another important social change in the adolescent is an increase in the size and range of acquaintances. Children younger than adolescence tend to limit their friends to those of their neighborhood, school, and perhaps church. Adolescents, on the other hand, can have individual friends, belong to a clique of friends, and can identify with larger groups such as an Explorer troop or a football team. An adolescent's ability to sustain relationships with all three groups is indicative of good social skills and that the socialization process is going well.

Popularity is a very important desire for adolescents. There are few adolescents who are not preoccupied with acceptance by peers. The following qualities in an adolescent seem to correlate with desirable social acceptance:

- Friendly — likes other people
- Energetic and enthusiastic
- Flexible and forgiving
- Laughs — good sense of humor
- Outgoing
- Self-confident but not conceited
- Appears natural
- Tolerant of the shortcomings of others
- Shows leadership qualities
- Others feel good when this person is around

The adolescent who gets along with his or her peer group seems to relate successfully with adults. Those who do not get peer acceptance seem to have more difficulty with adults and grow up to have a variety of social and emotional difficulties (Hartup, 1983).

REFERENCE

Hartup WW: The peer system. In Mussen PH (ed): Handbook of Child Psychology, Vol 4, edited by EM Hetherington. Personality and Social Development, 4th ed. New York, John Wiley and Sons, 1983.

chapter *36*

Examination, diagnosis, and treatment planning for general and orthodontic problems

Paul Casamassimo □ John Christensen □ Henry Fields

CHAPTER OUTLINE

- **THE PATIENT HISTORY**
- **THE EXAMINATION**
  Behavioral Assessment
  General Appraisal
  Head and Neck Examination
  Facial Examination
  Intraoral Examination
  Radiographic Evaluation

- **TREATMENT PLANNING FOR NON-ORTHODONTIC PROBLEMS**

- **TREATMENT PLANNING AND TREATMENT FOR ORTHODONTIC PROBLEMS**
  Skeletal Problems
  Dental Problems

The classic portrayal of adolescence as a time of rising hormones, rebelliousness, and fads contrasts vividly with how dentistry has viewed adolescent oral health. Dentistry for children abruptly ends with eruption of the permanent premolars and canines. Adult dentistry begins at its earliest with consideration of what to do with third molars. For many dental professionals, the one intervention that comes to mind for the adolescent is orthodontic care, which is often begun during the preadolescent transitional period.

Quite to the contrary of prevailing beliefs about the quiescence of the teenage years is the reality of a rapidly changing patient challenging his or her environment head-on and learning to cope in the process. The implications of these changes for dentistry (Cassamassimo et al, 1979) are highlighted as follows:

1. *Rapid, unpredictable, and irregular skeletal and dental growth.* The adolescent growth spurt is associated with accompanying facial growth of up to 35% of total height of the face. More than a dozen teeth, primary and permanent, erupt and exfoliate from age 10 to age 13 years. Immunologic changes, hormonal shifts, and other subtle and not so subtle physical developments alter the oral cavity.

2. *The environmental challenges, with obstacles and pitfalls.* Few adults would choose to return to adolescence. Drugs, smoking, sexually transmitted diseases, peer pressure, acne, more competitive education, career decisions, alcohol, and family pressure make up some of the challenges facing today's adolescent. Perhaps the most poignant statement on this aspect of the teenage years is that accidental death is the leading cause of mortality. Dental professionals see trauma, oral manifestations of sexual activity, hormonal gingivitis, smokeless tobacco–induced hyperkeratosis, non-compliance to dental recommendations, and drug-related behaviors, to mention a few points of observation.

459

3. *Learning to cope, make decisions, and become independent.* It isn't surprising that primitive cultures associated emerging manhood with a challenge of survival or the first hunt. Adolescence has always been a time to make decisions, seek independence from families, deal with sexuality, and choose a career. The dentist often sees this turmoil in poor oral hygiene compliance or refusal of treatment. The missed appointment is just one of many ways to say, "I am too involved in my search for self, my changing values, and handling my environment to worry about my teeth."

The Patient History

The health history of the adolescent is constantly changing and must be kept current. An adult history format will capture both of these elements. More important, perhaps, from the standpoint of accuracy is the process of obtaining information from the teenager. The following are some considerations when the history is taken from the adolescent patient:

1. *The health history should address smoking, recreational drugs and alcohol, pregnancy, and sexually transmitted diseases.* The controversy over inclusion of these issues is easily quieted by the simple realities of adolescent life in the United States. Consider the facts:

● Every day, approximately 3000 teenagers start smoking.
● Out-of-wedlock births have increased by 50% in the last decade. Radiation and medications used in dentistry can be dangerous to a fetus.
● The majority of adolescents now try drugs or alcohol before leaving high school. Untoward interactions between licit and illicit medications can be fatal.
● Sexually transmitted diseases are epidemic in the adolescent age group. Dentists have contracted a variety of infectious diseases from these patients.

Inadequate surveying of these elements of the health history puts both dentist and patient at risk. These issues can be addressed forthrightly by including them as choices dispersed with others on a health history form. Another less threatening approach is to word these questions in the past tense or to associate a risk with them to alert the patient to their importance.

2. *The process should allow privacy and encourage disclosure.* An accurate history taking may mean allowing the adolescent to assume greater participation in the process. The desired yield on the adolescent history from this perspective is information that might not be available from or known to a parent, such as those items described previously. The dentist may be caught in a double bind by providing an environment that fosters disclosure if pregnancy or illicit drug use is uncovered and the parents are unaware. This is a risk that requires counseling and resolution prior to dental treatment, and the dentist's responsibility is to help direct the family to address the issue. Unfortunately, the adolescent may see this as betrayal or breach of confidence, and the relationship between dentist and patient may be jeopardized. No easy way exists to deal with this type of problem, but the dentist treating adolescents should be aware of the responsibilities to the situation. It also may mean delaying treatment until resolution of the problem.

The dentist can do some things both to facilitate an accurate history and to deal consistently with identified problems of a serious nature:

● Encourage parents to complete histories *with* adolescents, not *for* them.
● Allow the adolescent the opportunity to contribute alone, which can be done in the context of a final check prior to treatment at chairside.
● Never treat an adolescent minor without a consenting parent available.
● Explain suspicions or concerns to both parent and adolescent.
● Have a policy on deferral of treatment and dealing with identified problems of a serious nature that is consistent and medico-legally sound.
● Have resources available in the event that consultation with a specialist is needed. It is far better to have an established relationship than to seek help from a stranger.

The Examination

The techniques of clinical examination remain the same for the adolescent, but with closer attention to identification of problems specific to this group, such as occlusal disharmonies, periodontal conditions, and temporomandibular joint disorders. Table 36–1 addresses some clinical findings peculiar to adolescent patients.

Table 36–1 ■ Possible clinical findings in examination of the adolescent

Structure	Finding	Comment
Extraoral Evaluation		
Skin	Acne	May be painful locally
		Adolescent may take antibiotics
		Can show up as radiopacity on some radiographs if calcification occurs
	Cosmetic use	Can complicate evaluation of skin;
		Can cause local allergic response
Neck	Hematoma	From suction; indicates sexual activity
Ears	Healing or scarred punctures	Multiple ear piercing common in both sexes
Hair	Coloring and preparation	Can complicate examination of scalp
Intraoral Examination		
Mucosa	Generalized erythema	Effect of smoking
		Sexually transmitted disease
Buccal Mucosa	Erythema, hyperkeratosis	Use of smokeless tobacco
Tongue	Coating, odor	Smoking; poor hygiene; fungal overgrowth from medication
Breath	Acetone; alcohol	Excessive dieting; alcohol abuse; metabolic disorders (e.g., diabetes)
Gingiva	Inflammation	Hormonal change
	Pregnancy tumor	Use of oral contraceptives
		Pregnancy
Teeth	Erosion	Bulimia
	Wear facets	Temporomandibular joint disorders/bruxism
	Excessive stain	Tobacco use
	Discoloration	Existing pulpal pathosis from trauma

BEHAVIORAL ASSESSMENT

The access to dental care for most healthy Americans has made it unlikely that a teenager will present for a first visit at that period in life, although first visits during adolescence *are* possible. Most people have at least one visit or more to a dentist before adolescence. Personality changes and other behavioral aberrations can suggest problems for the adolescent. Extremes in behavior, such as depression or overt flirting, may indicate sexual abuse in the adolescent female, especially if the child demonstrates a reluctance to oral examination. Depression, manifested in severe introversion, can also be a sign of suicidal tendency, family dysfunction, or even drug use. It isn't the dentist's purview to diagnose or manage these kinds of problems, but the dentist should be aware of the impact of the problem on the child and comment to parents about noticeable changes in behavior. Few behavioral problems should be encountered that will preclude care delivery, yet exceptions

do occur. The following are case situations that may require behavior management:

1. *Sexual abuse.* The young adolescent female or male who has been sexually abused with oral penetration may exhibit reluctance in accepting dental care from a dentist of the same sex as the perpetrator. Aids in uncovering this situation are a good history of previous compliance, behavioral cues such as depression, and overt refusal of care when oral contact is made. Nonetheless, confirmation is difficult, since the abuse may be unknown to parent or parents. It may be the limit of the dentist's role to recommend counseling for a child to uncover reasons for refusal of care with the idea that intervention may uncover the cause.

2. *Rampant caries.* Clinicians have noted that in rampant caries—a condition of rapid onset and progression of decay in an adolescent (more often female)—personality problems are often associated (Fig. 36–1). The typical pattern is a shy, reluctant, introverted individual who is passive to treatment. The behavioral manifes-

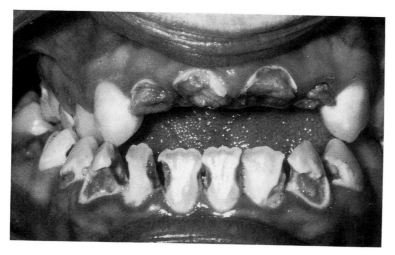

Figure 36–1 ■ This treatment photograph illustrates a 14-year-old female with rampant caries, which is a distinct clinical entity with rapidly progressing decay, multiple pulpally involved teeth, and short onset. Patients may attest to a low caries history prior to development of overt signs of decay.

tations can be varied, with a girl crying silently or not saying a word during the appointment. In some cases, treatment appointments can degenerate as the child whimpers and finally loses composure. Time and engagement in conversation are often the most successful behavioral management keys in dealing with these adolescents. Dramatic changes in behavior occur with the dentist's verbal reinforcement of improved hygiene and provision of even temporary esthetic anterior restorations that allow the patient to smile and experience a more positive self-image.

3. *Extreme anxiety.* Pinkham and Schroeder (1975) describe the behavioral management of the child who exhibits extreme anxiety at the thought of dental treatment. Desensitization by psychological intervention may hold the key to development of acceptable clinical behavior from that child. Tools available for the dentist are use of non-invasive therapies at first, reinforcement of positive accomplishments, positive peer interaction, and involvement with a psychologist. The poorly managed or unmanaged adolescent phobic may become the adult dental phobic.

4. *Anorexia nervosa.* The treatment of the child with an eating disorder can be difficult. Experience indicates that these patients, mostly females, will develop dependency on a male authority figure. They will also require a dentist's full attention during office visits and, unless counseled, will demand time outside scheduled appointments.

5. *Illicit drug use.* Clinicians have noted bizarre behavior on the part of adolescents and young adults who present for treatment after taking unprescribed medications. A number of untoward reactions to dentist-administered medications have been associated with prior ingestion of drugs or alcohol by a young patient. Manifestations of drug ingestion can be varied from a slight mental dissociation or drifting to outright verbal aberrations or extreme changes in personality.

The management of behavioral problems in the adolescent can be complex and often involves parents and other professionals. On the other hand, a number of adolescents will exhibit age appropriate behavior that may be disruptive to delivery of care. Most practitioners treating adolescents will try to treat them alone rather than in a setting of other peers. This one-on-one situation provides necessary attention to the patient and prevents disruptive interaction. Any dentist who has worked with a group of seventh or eighth grade students will appreciate this recommendation. The teenager who is acting up but simply expressing healthy emotions will respond to reason and provide compliance.

An important part of behavior management in this age group relates to simple transfer of information. A good communicator will be aware of the characteristics of adolescence, which will enhance the ability to relate to teens. They are the following:

1. *Peers are important.* The adolescent's relationship to those outside the nuclear and extended family becomes important. Friends, classmates, teammates, and popular persons of similar age are all involved in the life of the teenager. A dentist can enhance his or her ability to communicate with the adolescent by asking about peer interaction and by knowing who is involved in the teen's life.

2. *Fads and experimentation are part of adolescence.* Successful adolescent practitioners are those who are aware of trends, popular fads, and the celebrities of interest to teens. A clear demonstration of this to teens is the operatory with posters or contemporary music. The dentist who knows the trends and interests of the adolescent has an edge in establishing communication, in reaching the teen at a level that is non-authoritarian. It is an entrée into the teen's world that can be fostered and that can lead to discussion of more significant issues with a sense of relationship. Contrast that access to the barrier that arises when both teen and dentist see themselves as worlds apart.

3. *Teens are trying to establish independence, searching for identity, needing to make educational or career choices, and finding sexuality.* All of these involve a certain degree of stress. Within that stressful period are times of anxiety, satisfaction, anger, excitement, and a host of other emotions. The dentist is a small part of the adolescent's world but is a mirror of it. How the practitioner fosters the healthy development of personality in a child and counsels toward independence and career may be important — both in terms of the teen's life and in terms of his or her dental health. In talking with teens, it is helpful to remember their "problem list" and to empathize with the stress of their lives, which is real to them.

The office visit should be a mirror of life. It should provide a respite from pressures, and be a cameo of the role that the adolescent will have as an adult patient. The relationship that the dentist would like to have with the adolescent as an adult should be fostered.

4. *The basis of success in adolescent-adult interactions is a good relationship.* The most significant factor in successful compliance and communication is the quality of the relationship between dentist and adolescent. In earlier periods of life, the child could be successfully motivated with reason, praise, or other approaches. The changing values and their short-term intensity in adolescence belie the use of these approaches in long-term motivation. A feeling of trust, good communication, and a perception of sincere interest by the teenager will provide a strong motivator for compliance.

GENERAL APPRAISAL

The general appraisal of the adolescent is obfuscated by the timing of physical growth changes, especially in the early teenage years. Within a group of young teenagers, girls can tower over boys and look far more like adults than their male peers. Similarly, within a group of boys, variations in voice tone, skin condition, amount and distribution of fat, and skeletal proportion are often remarkable. Differentiation of growth disorders is difficult at best.

Determining Developmental Status

Ideally, orthodontic treatment would be much easier and less unpredictable if a biologic marker could be identified that provided information about the developmental status of the patient. Growth modification could be started if the marker indicated that there were an impending growth spurt or sufficient remaining growth to alter skeletal relationships. To be clinically useful, this biologic marker would need to be reliable, easily identified, recognized in both sexes, and closely correlated to the growth of the facial bones. Unfortunately, a single biologic marker of this description is not available. A number of clinical markers have been identified. However, studies have indicated that the relationship between the markers and facial growth, although statistically significant, is not so precise that growth can be predicted accurately. Because of the limited predictive value of the markers, one marker or another may be used to determine if there is remaining growth, but it is extremely difficult to determine the extent of any remaining growth.

Height and weight measurements are often used to determine the patient's growth status. Measurements are plotted on standardized growth charts and indicate the relative size of the patient. An average-sized child is located near the 50th percentile, and a large child is somewhere near the 90th percentile. A single measurement does not provide the clinician with all pertinent growth information, but it does give some idea about where the patient is developmentally compared with other children at this time point. A series of measurements, which may be available from the patient's physician or school nurse, provide much more information. The measurements can be plotted in one of two ways. The first way is to plot the measurements on a cumulative growth chart (Fig. 36–2). This provides information about the total amount of growth the patient has had up to the last measurement. The normal growth curve is sigmoidal in shape, and the pubertal growth spurt corresponds to the steepest portion of the slope. Because growth charts are

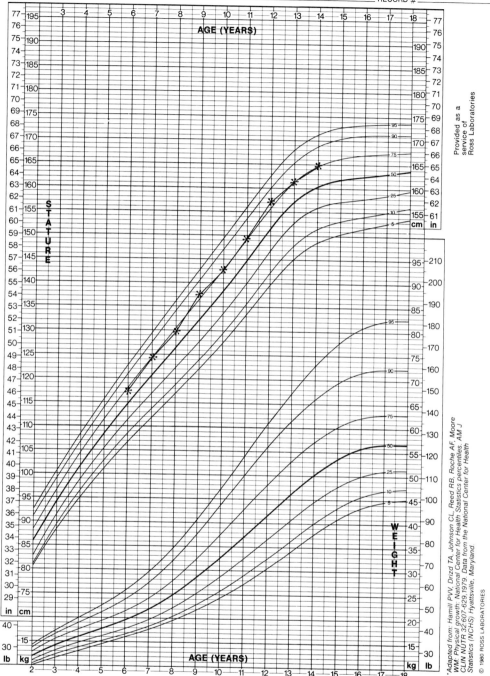

Figure 36–2 ■ A standardized growth chart is used to indicate the relative size of the patient. A single measurement does not provide the clinician with all pertinent growth information, but it does give some idea about where the patient is developmentally compared with other children at a particular time. A series of measurements plotted on a standardized growth chart provides much more information than a single measurement. The measurements may be plotted in one of two ways. One method is to plot the measurements on a cumulative growth chart. This provides information about the total amount of growth the patient has had up to the last measurement. This female patient has been measured yearly, starting at age 6, and is roughly following the 75th percentile line. (Adapted from Hamill PVV, Drizd TA, Johnson CL, Reed RB, Roche AF, Moore WM: Physical growth: National Center for Health Statistics percentiles. AM J CLIN NUTR 32:607–629, 1979. Data from the National Center for Health Statistics (NCHS), Hyattsville, Maryland. Courtesy of Ross Laboratories.)

based on mean growth rates, the individual patient may show an accelerated or delayed growth spurt if the individual's growth rate is not coincident with the mean growth rate. More importantly, some concern should be expressed if the patient is not following the percentiles, for example, dropping from the 50th to 40th to 30th percentile over time. This suggests there may be a physical or psychological problem requiring medical attention.

Height and weight measurements can also be plotted as yearly growth increments rather than as total growth achieved to that point (Fig. 36–3). By plotting measurements this way, changes in the growth rate can be easily identified. A sharp rise in height usually signals the start of the pubertal growth spurt, and growth modification treatment should be initiated immediately if it is required.

Height and weight measurements also can be compared with the height and weight of the patient's natural parents and siblings. Although the interaction between environment and heredity is not clearly understood, there is some familial influence on ultimate size and it may be possible to glean useful information from the comparison.

Hand-wrist radiographs are used by some investigators to judge the skeletal age and development of the patient (Fig. 36–4). The size and maturational stage of certain hand and wrist bones are compared with published standards of normal bone development and skeletal age

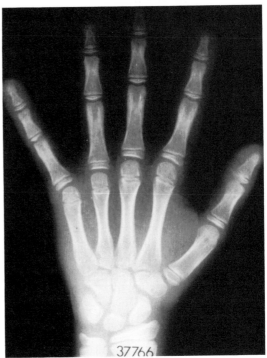

Figure 36–4 ■ A hand-wrist film is used occasionally to judge the skeletal age and development of the patient. The size and stage of certain bones are compared with published standards of normal bone development and skeletal age.

(Gruelich and Pyle, 1959). Unfortunately, the correlation between the appearance of reliable bone markers (skeletal growth status) and mean maximum mandibular growth velocity is not perfect and should not serve as the only index of facial growth.

Secondary sexual characteristics provide some information about the amount of growth the patient is yet to experience. In females, breast stage development and menarche are markers that can be used to assess developmental status. Breast development determination is obviously not practical in the dental office and is of little clinical use. Menarche, however, can be determined from the health history questionnaire or from an interview at the initial patient examination. Unfortunately, the pubertal growth spurt precedes menarche by over 1 year (Tanner, 1978). Therefore, menarche is basically used to decide whether growth modification is still feasible.

In the male, there is no single indicator, such as menarche, by which to judge developmental status. The amount and texture of facial hair and the patient's general physical appearance are two highly variable indicators of male de-

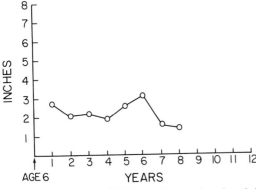

Figure 36–3 ■ Growth information can be also plotted as yearly growth increments rather than as total growth achieved to a certain point. The growth data on the female patient described in Figure 36–2 are plotted here incrementally, beginning at age 6. By plotting measurements this way, changes in the growth rate can be easily identified. A sharp rise usually signals the start of the pubertal growth spurt, and growth modification should be initiated immediately if it is required.

velopmental status and maturity. Facial hair usually appears near or following peak statural growth.

For an individual with an obvious skeletal problem, more than one cephalometric head film of the patient may be available. These head films can be superimposed to provide information about the amount and direction of growth that has occurred over time (Fig. 36–5). Although past growth tendencies do not guarantee that the patient will continue to grow or will grow in the same pattern, comparing head films provides a great deal of information about the patient. It is unlikely, however, that the average patient would have a series of head films available for pre-treatment review.

The patient's developmental status can also be judged from the developmental stage of the dentition. Panoramic or periapical radiographs can be used to determine the stage of development of individual permanent teeth. The results can then be compared with standards relat-

ing dental development to chronological age (Moorrees et al, 1963). However, studies indicate that the relationship between dental age and skeletal maturation is very weak and clinically useless (Chertkow, 1980).

In summary, the clinician has a number of biologic markers available to assess the developmental status of the patient. Unfortunately, no one marker by itself will provide definitive information about the patient's growth potential. The most logical approach is to gather all available information and make an educated estimate of the patient's growth potential and suitability for growth modification.

HEAD AND NECK EXAMINATION

The principles of the head and neck examination of the teen are similar to those for the adult or child. The variations from normal can be caused by a variety of factors, the most notable

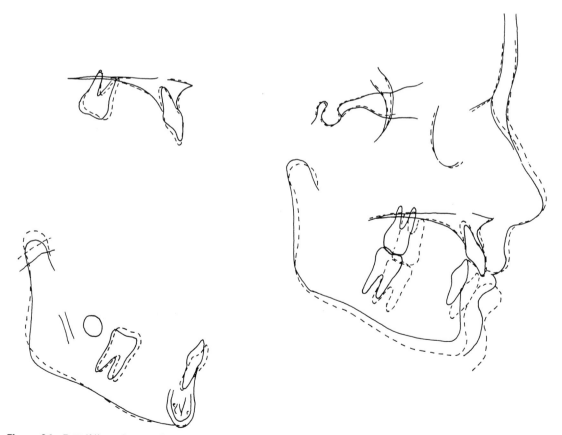

Figure 36–5 ■ If there is more than one cephalometric head film of the patient available, the head films can be superimposed to provide information about the amount and direction of growth that have occurred over time. Although past growth tendencies do not guarantee that the patient will continue to grow or grow in the same pattern, superimpositions provide a great deal of information about the patient.

of which are growth and developmental changes and effects of the adolescent's environment.

The physical changes and habits in the teen require modification of the procedures used in children. On the positive side, the loss or redistribution of body fat and elongation of the neck provide the ability to perform a better lymph node evaluation. These changes facilitate a thorough head and neck and cancer examination.

FACIAL EXAMINATION

The facial examination analyzes the soft tissue profile and the face from a frontal view. During adolescence, the face is beginning to assume adult-like features, and treatment decisions can be based more on the current rather than projected facial appearance. This does not mean that growth is complete, only that it has slowed considerably from its previous pace during the early adolescent growth spurt. The adult profile tends to be more straight than that of the adolescent because of continued mandibular skeletal growth. In addition, the soft tissue chin increases slightly in thickness. The nose also continues to grow, both horizontally and vertically. Most of this growth is horizontal, but the nasal tip tends to drop down a small amount. The lips are less protrusive in the adult owing to continued growth of the nose and soft tissue chin as well as to a slight thinning of the soft tissue thickness of the lips.

For patients with Class I skeletal and dental characteristics, the facial profile examination should provide an adequate basis for analysis when minor orthodontic treatment is considered. For the patient with a skeletal problem, again, a cephalometric radiograph and analysis is required to diagnose the problem definitively and prescribe treatment. When physical growth is occurring, usually facial growth is also occurring. Treatment of skeletal orthodontic problems during pre- or early adolescence, when the adolescent growth spurt is still active, can result in growth modification. The preadolescent patient is assumed to be growing and is expected to experience a pubertal growth spurt. The early adolescent still has enough growth remaining to make significant skeletal changes with treatment. The adolescent, by definition, has experienced the pubertal growth spurt and is on the down side of the growth rate curve. Adults, on the other hand, have such limited facial growth that it has little therapeutic potential. These differences in growth potential have a large impact on how skeletal malocclusion is treated in the adolescent. The point is that as the individual becomes more skeletally mature, less skeletal growth modification can be accomplished. Therefore, during the orthodontic evaluation of the adolescent patient, it is essential to establish the growth or developmental status of the patient in order to plan sensible treatment.

INTRAORAL EXAMINATION

The larger oral cavity of the adolescent permits good visualization. Also, normal intellectual status and reasonable behavior provide cooperation in functional assessment of occlusion and temporomandibular joint disorders. On the negative side, there are more teeth to evaluate, gingival and periodontal issues are present that were not critical in early childhood, and unpredictable growth changes can occur. The clinician should approach the adolescent as an adult, especially in the later teen years. For the first visit, the dentist may choose to "walk" the adolescent through the examination, using a hand mirror to explain procedures and normal findings.

Periodontal Evaluation

In the adolescent, more emphasis is placed on the periodontal examination. The prevalence of periodontal disease begins to increase in this age group (Poulsen, 1981). The reason for this increase in periodontal disease is unknown at this time. Therefore, a thorough evaluation of the supporting structures is an absolute necessity. A periodontal probe is used to measure pocket depths, the width of keratinized gingiva, and the amount of attached gingiva, and for probing to establish a bleeding index (Fig. 36–6). Periodontal probing should be confined to fully erupted teeth. Mobility tests may reveal slightly increased mobility in erupted teeth without complete root formation. The use of disclosing agents to reveal plaque, although helpful, may be discontinued at the patient's request. If a panoramic radiograph is used for diagnosis, selected periapical films may be needed if the clinical examination detects any unusual periodontal findings. Referral to a specialist is suggested if significant periodontal disease is evident. During orthodontic treatment, gingival, plaque, and bleeding indices should be established at regular intervals to detect newly active periodontal disease.

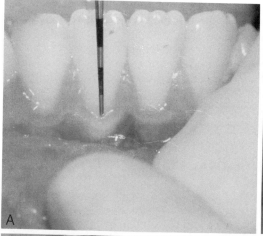

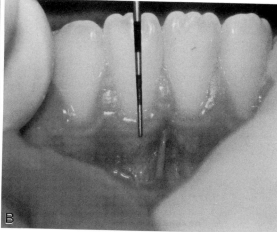

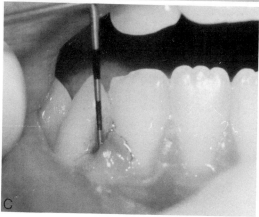

Figure 36–6 ■ The prevalence of periodontal disease begins to increase in the adolescent patient; therefore, a thorough evaluation of the periodontium is absolutely necessary. A periodontal probe is used to measure pocket depths (A), to measure the width of keratinized gingiva (B), and for probing to establish a bleeding index (C). The amount of attached gingiva is determined by subtracting the pocket depth from the width of keratinized gingiva.

Related Hard and Soft Tissue Problems

A number of pathologic conditions occur in adolescence that may be first noticed in this period. One is smokeless tobacco use, described further in Chapter 40. Another is temporomandibular joint dysfunction, also described in more detail in that chapter.

Anorexia nervosa will often show up in enamel erosion of all teeth if vomiting is a regular component of this psychiatric disorder (Brady, 1980). Bulimia describes those afflicted who vomit regularly to purge themselves of food in a misdirected attempt to control their weight. Bulimia affects far more girls than boys, but boys can exhibit similar behavior. The regurgitated stomach contents, which are highly acidic, erode the enamel of teeth in a process called perimyolysis (Fig. 36–7). Dentin is exposed, making teeth sensitive and encouraging decay. Enamel will flake off, leaving sharp edges. Restorations will appear to have grown out of their preparations as enamel and dentin

dissolve around them. During clinical examination, these problems will speak for themselves; however, in the early bulimic, they may be absent. It may help to air-dry teeth to look for etching of surfaces.

Treatment of bulimia is a psychiatric problem. Treatment of the teeth is equally difficult and expensive. Pulpal pathosis, elongated clinical crowns, gingival recession, and loss of vertical dimension are a few of the treatment issues noted in bulimia. Unless the vomiting is stopped, extensive treatment may be futile. The dentist should work with a psychotherapist to deal with this problem.

Another pathologic problem is dental trauma. The clinical and radiographic examination should address tooth crazing, chips, or discoloration with adjunctive radiographs to clarify the status of teeth. Not all teeth that appear sound clinically are healthy (Fig. 36–8), and not all trauma is to hard tissues. Identification of the effects of smoking and oral sexual activity (Fig. 36–9) may occur during examination.

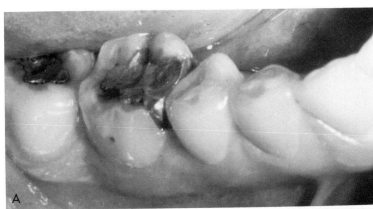

Figure 36–7 ■ A series of photographs of the dentition of a bulimic female. *A,* Loss of occlusal enamel with exposure of dentin. *B,* Ragged incisal edges as a result of fracturing of enamel. *C,* Lingual exposure of dentin highlighted by outlines of remaining enamel and exposed surfaces of restorations. (From Casamassimo P, Castaldi C: Considerations in the dental management of the adolescent. Ped Clin North Am 29:648, 1982.)

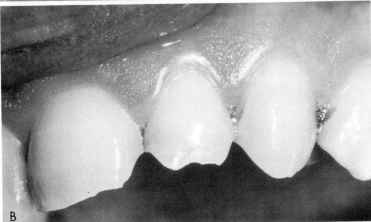

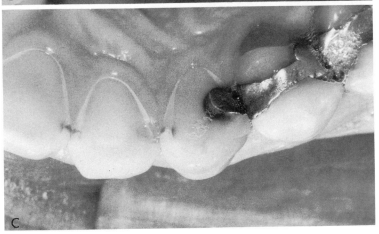

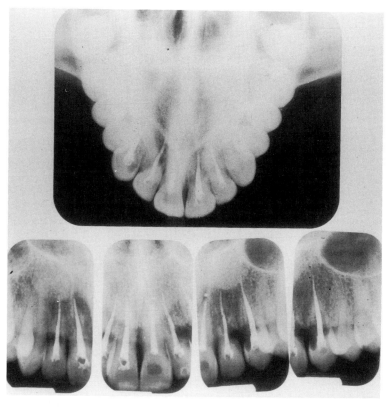

Figure 36–8 ■ Severe resorption of roots secondary to trauma is evident on radiographic examination. These teeth were remarkably stable clinically despite the amount of root resorption.

Evaluation of third molars is usually completed during the mid- to late-adolescent period. Commonly asked questions by parents are what to do with third molars or why extract them. The reasons for extraction of third molars include impaction or failure to erupt; possible or existing pathosis, such as cysts or ameloblastoma; decay; post-eruption malposition; nonfunction as a result of an absent opposing tooth; difficulty with hygiene; and recurrent pericoronitis. If any of these are considerations, third molars should be removed during adolescence.

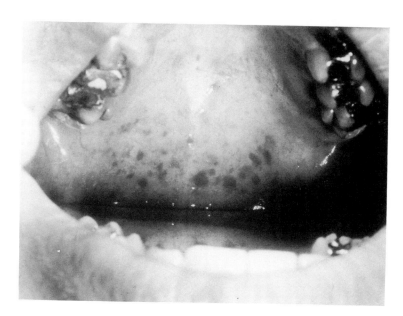

Figure 36–9 ■ This patient exhibits palatal hematomas secondary to oral sex. Negative intraoral pressures cause blood to be pulled to the surface of the palatal tissue.

The concept of anterior crowding as the result of forward pressure from third molars is currently unproved and is not a reason to extract. Surgical access and root development are important issues in determining when to extract. Some root development is desired to stabilize teeth, but complete root development can make extraction more difficult and may increase the likelihood of root fractures. Females using oral contraceptives can also run a high risk of post-surgical dry socket.

Occlusal Evaluation

Evaluation of the occlusion in three spatial planes is similar to the intraoral examination described in previous chapters. The major difference is that arch length deficiencies are no longer predicted from space analyses but are measured directly from the casts, because all the permanent teeth usually have erupted by this age. The first step is to measure the arch circumference by dividing the arch into segments extending from the mesial of the permanent first molar to the mesial of the contralateral first molar (Fig. 36–10A). Each segment is measured over the contact points and incisal edges of the teeth. The segments are added together to yield the total arch circumference. Next, the mesio-distal width of each individual permanent tooth is measured and the widths are added together (Fig. 36–10B). The difference between the arch circumference and the sum of the mesio-distal widths indicates the amount of crowding or spacing within the arch. If one or two primary teeth have not exfoliated, the width of the contralateral erupted permanent tooth can be substituted for the unerupted permanent tooth.

Careful attention should be paid to teeth adjacent to edentulous areas, because these teeth may need to be repositioned orthodontically prior to restorative treatment. The pulpal and restorative status of these teeth will help determine the direction of treatment.

Once again, the interaction between facial profile and dental crowding should be considered. Committing the patient to treatment based solely on dental characteristics can have a disastrous effect on the facial profile.

The anteroposterior, transverse, and vertical occlusal components should be evaluated as described in Chapter 29.

RADIOGRAPHIC EVALUATION

The adolescent radiographic examination ranges from a transitional to an adult multi-film survey, depending upon the child's dentition. The issues surrounding radiographic examina-

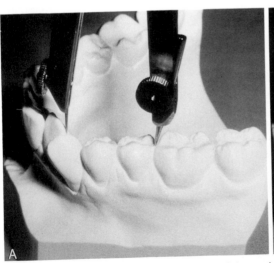
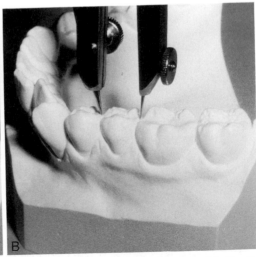

Figure 36–10 ■ *A,* Arch length analysis in the adolescent patient is measured directly from the casts rather than by using mixed dentition space analysis prediction tables because all the permanent teeth have usually erupted by this age. The first step is to measure the arch circumference by dividing the arch into segments extending from the mesial of the permanent first molar to the mesial of the contralateral first molar. *B,* Next, the mesio-distal width of each individual permanent tooth is measured and the widths are added together. The difference between the arch circumference and the sum of the mesio-distal widths indicates the amount of crowding or spacing within the arch.

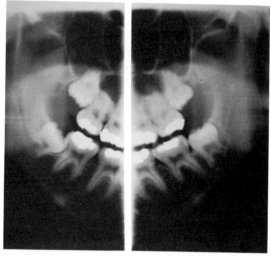

Figure 36–11 ■ In late adolescence, the presence and developmental status of unerupted third molars are evaluated by using periapical radiographs or a "third molar" panoramic radiograph as shown here.

tion in the adolescent are related to the type and frequency of exposure.

The types of films used in adolescent radiography should be determined by the number of teeth present and the reason for radiographic examination. For the new adolescent patient with major dental care needs, a survey should include, at the minimum, three to five anterior maxillary periapical films, three mandibular anterior films, a periapical film of each posterior quadrant, and right and left bitewing films. The

anterior films should be adult size No. 1, whereas posterior films should be No. 2 size films. It is also recommended that all tooth-bearing areas be surveyed within 2 years of the eruption of the permanent second molars. This can be achieved with a full mouth survey or a panoramic radiograph combined with bitewing radiographs.

The radiographic examination in this age period often addresses largely growth and development issues: the eruption status of unerupted premolars and canines. Later in adolescence, a final issue is third molar development. The development of these teeth can be evaluated by using periapical radiographs or a third molar panoramic radiograph (Fig. 36–11).

Even as early as age 12, the adolescent should be able to tolerate size No. 2 intraoral films. For the child with a small oral cavity, techniques to aid in positioning are described in the radiographic section of Chapter 29.

Multiple or serial periapical radiographs will be required for diagnosis of pathosis or for management of conditions that require significant follow-up such as endodontic therapy on traumatized incisors.

Bitewing radiography during early adolescence is affected by the developing occlusion and lack of contacts. It may be that most, if not all, posterior surfaces can be adequately visualized until full eruption of premolars. The benefit of exposing bitewing films to examine two or four interproximal surfaces should be weighed against the risk. In these cases, a longstanding

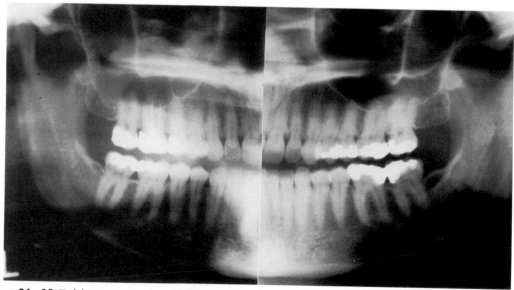

Figure 36–12 ■ A large mucosal cyst in the sinus is evident in this panoramic film of a 21-year-old. The cyst is possibly a reaction to pulpal pathosis in the permanent maxillary first and second molars.

history of decay incidence and a thorough clinical examination will help determine if films are necessary.

The panoramic film has a role in adolescent dentistry as a full mouth radiograph survey for a new patient who does not have major treatment needs. For this adolescent, who is essentially clinically disease free, the panoramic film and bitewing survey may be adequate to determine dental health. The panoramic film will reveal bone pathosis as well as orient the examiner to the presence and position of third molars. The panoramic film also grossly displays sinuses and the temporomandibular joint (Fig. 36–12), which may be more poorly displayed on a multi-film intraoral survey.

Table 36–2 summarizes issues in radiography of the adolescent patient.

Table 36–2 ■ Radiographic issues in the adolescent

Aspect	Recommendation
Frequency	
Full mouth survey	No suggested frequency or interval
Bitewing radiographs	No suggested frequency or interval: Should be taken if clinical caries noted Should be taken if multiple interproximal restorations present and are being followed Should be taken if incipiencies noted on previous films and are being followed Interval for these situations should be individualized and re-evaluated at each periodic examination
Periapical radiographs	No suggested frequency or interval: Pathosis or treatment needs should dictate frequency To determine developmental status of third molars
Panoramic radiographs	Possible component of a full mouth survey for a disease free new patient "Third molar" panoramic radiograph to determine developmental status of third molars
Type	
Full mouth survey	Number of films included to be based on tissue coverage needed *Early adolescence (12–14 yr):* Maxillary and mandibular periapicals (No. 1 size) Canine periapicals (No. 1 or 2) Bitewings (2 films, No. 2 size) Four posterior quadrant periapicals (No. 2 size) to include premolars and erupted molars *Late adolescence (16–21 yr):* Complete set (21 film) survey
Bitewing radiographs	Size determined by oral access, but No. 2 size used if possible One film sufficient until eruption of second molars Position will vary with the location and number of posterior contacts
Periapical radiographs	Should be adult No. 1 size films rather than No. 2 size, used as occlusal film as in primary tooth survey. An exception to this would be use of No. 2 film as initial trauma screen.
Panoramic radiographs	Can be used with bitewings for a full mouth survey and is desirable in caries free and pathosis free patients after a clinical examination "Third molar" panoramic radiograph can be used to determine developmental status of third molars

Treatment Planning for Non-orthodontic Problems

In the adolescent patient, attention must be made to the long-term consequences of immediate treatment. Although the transitional dentition is addressed in terms of its *effect* on the adult, the adolescent dentition must be addressed as *being* that of the adult. In other words, there are no teeth to follow, only substitutes.

All phases of treatment planning should be addressed. The adolescent depicted in Figure 36–13 illustrates the complexity of problems, requiring preventive, periodontal, restorative, and endodontic management.

All adolescents should receive a preventive plan that addresses the particular needs of the adult dentition, such as flossing. In addition, a preventive plan should address environmental concerns, such as smoking, diet, trauma prevention, and the effect of medications on the periodontium and teeth.

Periodontal and gingival concerns are now solidly tied to restorative care. In the child, the minor inflammation around a stainless steel crown on a primary tooth that is due to grossly adjusted margins is tolerated. In the adolescent, with a cast crown, the tissues must be completely healthy.

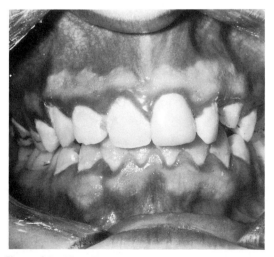

Figure 36–13 ■ The dentition of a 19-year-old male. The final treatment problems included caries, bone loss, defective crowns, and pulpal involvement of two anterior maxillary teeth.

Restorative treatment planning for the teen is characterized by a number of issues (Castaldi and Brass, 1980):

1. Pulp size is large, affecting choice of coronal coverage.
2. Anterior teeth continue to erupt, requiring consideration of various types of esthetic restorations for traumatized or defective teeth to prevent exposure of margins.
3. Esthetic awareness by the patient may force treatment of congenital or acquired discoloration or require repeated treatment of teeth, if transitional procedures are used.
4. Partially erupted posterior teeth may not serve as good abutments for protheses.
5. Decreased chewing efficiency as a result of loss of a posterior tooth may force interim replacement with a removable appliance, although this may not be the treatment of choice.
6. Planned or active orthodontic treatment may delay restoration of missing teeth.
7. Active athletic involvement may require interim replacement of teeth.

The use of acid-etch composite resins has greatly improved the treatment of adolescent restorative needs by providing esthetically acceptable, reasonably priced interim restorations. Their use as a treatment option in restorative treatment planning is a must.

The two remaining elements of importance in adolescent treatment planning are interrelated. They are consent and compliance. The adolescent under the age of majority requires consent of parents for treatment. The payment for services also demands clarification of consent. Explanation of proposed treatment is best done with both parent and adolescent present, whereas actual delivery of care can be done with the adolescent alone in the operatory. A good one-on-one dialogue during active treatment will help ensure compliance. Some general guidelines for communication to maximize success are the following:

1. Show the adolescent the same respect and interest as you would the adult.
2. Be sincere.
3. Treat the adolescent in privacy as an adult, separate from younger children.
4. Outline procedures and explain reasons for them.
5. Minimize or eliminate authoritarian posturing, using your knowledge rather than age as a reason for your role as a dentist.

6. Be flexible enough to adapt to a changing relationship.

Treatment Planning and Treatment for Orthodontic Problems

Adolescent orthodontic problems create difficult treatment decisions for the general practitioner and the specialist. The nature of the malocclusion heavily influences how the case will be treated.

SKELETAL PROBLEMS

If the malocclusion is skeletal, treatment is aimed at altering the relationship or orientation of the jaws and teeth. This can be accomplished by growth modification, camouflage, or orthognathic surgery. Because the physical maturity of the adolescent patient varies from individual to individual of the same age, any one of three treatments may be appropriate. If the developmental assessment of the patient suggests that the patient is actively growing, growth modification is a viable treatment alternative. Growth modification, previously discussed, attempts to change the actual size, shape, or orientation of the jaws to obtain an acceptable occlusion. Functional appliances and extraoral traction are used to secure these changes.

In the non-growing, physically mature individual, skeletal malocclusion is appropriately treated by camouflage or orthognathic surgery. Camouflage is the orthodontic movement of teeth without changing the underlying skeletal malocclusion. Camouflage should only be considered when the soft tissue profile is acceptable and when tooth movement will not change or compromise the profile. Teeth are tipped or bodily moved on the denture base to positions considered less than ideal but acceptable for normal occlusion. For example, a mild Class II mandibular deficiency with a relatively prominent bony pogonion can be treated by camouflage (Fig. 36–14). To camouflage this type of problem, the upper teeth are tipped backward and the lower teeth tipped forward to bring the teeth together and disguise the skeletal problem. In conjunction with the tipping of teeth for camouflage, teeth can be extracted in the maxillary arch to provide more space to tip the upper

teeth backward. Although a small amount of soft tissue change may occur and the final position of the mandibular incisors may be less than ideal, a functional occlusion is achieved without surgery. Camouflage of Class II skeletal problems is more acceptable in women and camouflage of Class III problems is more acceptable in men, because the respective convex and straight profiles are more acceptable for these groups.

Skeletal malocclusion in the non-growing patient can also be treated with orthognathic surgery. The specialist works with an oral and maxillofacial surgeon to reposition one or both jaws into proper alignment surgically. Typically, the orthodontic treatment plan calls for a pre-surgical period of orthodontic tooth movement to align teeth in both arches so that they will fit together following the surgery. Orthognathic surgery is performed under general anesthesia, and the maxilla, mandible, or both jaws are repositioned. It is possible to move the entire jaw or individual segments of the jaw in nearly any direction within the constraints of the soft tissue covering. Following the surgical procedure, the jaws are immobilized with wires or with bone plates and screws and are allowed to heal in the new position for several weeks. After healing is demonstrated, a short period of post-surgical orthodontic procedures is necessary to settle the teeth into an ideal occlusion.

DENTAL PROBLEMS

If the orthodontic problem in the adolescent is strictly dental in nature, conventional orthodontic treatment can be used to treat the malocclusion. Identification and treatment of dental orthodontic problems has already been discussed and basically does not change with the age of the patient. However, there is one aspect of dental orthodontic treatment that has not been discussed and should be mentioned in this section. Despite the preventive efforts of the dental profession, some individuals continue to lose permanent teeth to either decay or trauma. When this occurs, a combination of orthodontic tooth movement and restorative dentistry is recommended to obtain an optimal esthetic and functional result.

In the anterior region, orthodontic treatment is often designed to move teeth to simplify prosthetic treatment. To provide precise control of tooth movement, orthodontic brackets should be bonded to all the anterior teeth and bands

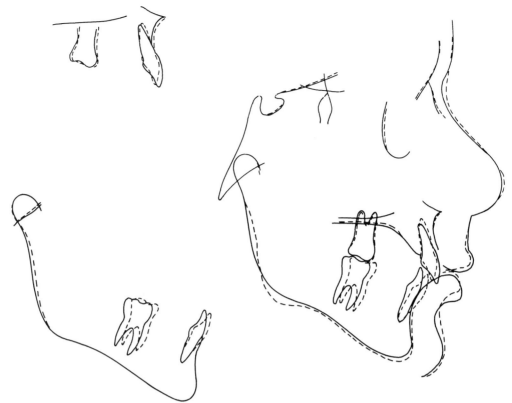

Figure 36-14 ■ In the nongrowing, physically mature patient, skeletal malocclusion is appropriately treated by camouflage or orthognathic surgery. Camouflage is the orthodontic movement of teeth without changing the underlying skeletal malocclusion. The patient represented in these diagrams exhibited a mild Class II mandibular deficiency with a relatively prominent bony chin. The skeletal problem was camouflaged by tipping the maxillary incisors backward and by tipping the mandibular incisors forward. Although a small amount of soft tissue change may occur and the final position of the mandibular incisors may be less than ideal, a functional occlusion is achieved without surgery.

should be placed on the permanent first molars. Treatment must be carefully planned so that only the teeth that require movement are affected and the other teeth remain stationary. This means that molar, canine, and midline relationships should be carefully studied and controlled during treatment. For example, if the patient is missing one lateral incisor or if the

lateral incisor is peg-shaped, the space between the central incisor and canine on that side should equal the distance between these two teeth on the other side. This will ensure that the restored width of the lateral incisor matches that of the contralateral lateral incisor. Elastomeric chain, arch wire loops, and open coil springs can be used to open and close space (Fig.

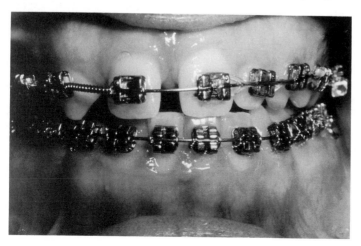

Figure 36-15 ■ Orthodontic treatment is often necessary to move teeth to simplify prosthetic treatment. In this patient, an open coil spring is used to open space for a missing permanent maxillary right lateral incisor and to position the maxillary right central incisor in its correct midline position. Elastomeric chain is used on the left side of the maxillary arch to close space and promote midline correction.

36–15). Once the space has been opened and is nearly ideal, a closed coil spring or loops bent into the arch wire are used to hold or maintain the space until the restorative or prosthetic treatment is completed. Although this type of treatment sounds simple, close attention to detail is necessary. Uncontrolled tooth movement can result in unanticipated changes in the midline, overjet, and overbite.

In the posterior region, orthodontic treatment may be necessary to upright teeth that have tipped into extraction sites after loss of permanent teeth. Typically, the permanent first molar is lost as a result of carious or periodontal involvement, and the second molar tips mesially into the extraction site while the second premolar tips distally. Both teeth next to the edentulous area may need to be uprighted to improve the periodontal and restorative potential. Orthodontically uprighting of teeth will (1) facilitate more conservative, ideal restorations; (2) eliminate plaque-forming areas; (3) improve the alveolar ridge contour; (4) improve the crown to root ratio; and (5) re-establish long axis force loading of the teeth. This is best accomplished with limited, single arch, fixed appliance treatment. Bonded brackets or bands are placed on the canine and first and second premolars. The second molar is banded. In addition, an .032 inch wire is bonded to the lingual surface of both canines to provide additional anchorage and stability during molar uprighting. There is a possibility that the arch form could change or

that other teeth could move inadvertently without the lingual wire in place.

After the appliance has been placed, either segmental or continuous arch wire mechanics can be used to upright the teeth. Selection of mechanics depends on the severity of the tipping. If the tooth is not severely tipped, a light, round, continuous arch wire can be placed from the molar to the canine. Next, the occlusion on the molar should be adjusted by reducing the length of the crown with a bur to allow the molar to erupt and upright. Finally, any periodontal defects around the tipped teeth should be thoroughly curetted to reduce inflammation and loss of attachment during treatment. Occlusal adjustments and curettage should be performed at each appointment. At subsequent appointments, the size of the arch wire is progressively increased until it is of sufficient size and strength to upright and position the teeth ideally. Sometimes a coil spring placed between the premolar and molar is required to tip the molar distally and increase the edentulous space.

If the molar is too tipped for a continuous arch wire to be placed, segmental mechanics are employed. The canine-premolar segment is aligned independent of the molar with a progression of arch wires similar to that just described. When initial alignment of this segment is completed, an uprighting spring is bent out of .0195 × .025 inch stainless steel wire (Fig. 36–16A). A helix is bent in the spring to provide

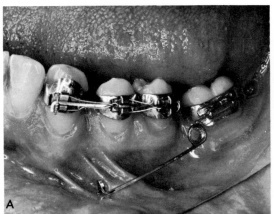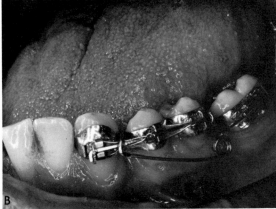

Figure 36–16 ■ Occasionally, adolescents and young adults are missing a permanent first molar and require molar uprighting before prosthetic treatment can begin. The canine and premolar teeth are stabilized independently with a large segmental rectangular wire. The canines are usually further stabilized, using a bonded or banded lingual wire. After stabilizing the anterior teeth, the molar can be uprighted using a .0195 × .025 inch helical spring placed in a bonded or banded tube on the tipped molar. *A*, The spring is passive prior to engagement of the arch wire. *B*, The spring engaged on the arch wire delivers the uprighting and extrusive forces to the tipped molar. Reduction of occlusal interference is necessary to allow the molar to move freely. (From Fields HW, Proffit WF: Orthodontics in general practice. *In* Morris AL, Bohannan HM, Casullo DP: The Dental Specialties in General Practice. Philadelphia, WB Saunders Co, 1983, p 327.)

more flexibility and a greater range of activation. In addition, a hook is bent into the end of the uprighting spring so that the spring can be attached to the segmental wire just distal to the canine bracket to allow the uprighting spring room to move distally along the segmental wire as the molar uprights (Fig. 36–16B). The force of activation should provide approximately 75–100 gm of force to upright the molar.

After the molar has been ideally positioned, tooth movement must be retained until a prosthetic replacement can be fabricated. The clinician can use either a fixed or a removable retainer. A fixed retainer is simply a .021 × .025 inch rectangular wire that rests on the occlusal surfaces of the abutment teeth. The wire should be bent down in the edentulous area to remain out of occlusion. Small rests can be placed in the occlusal surfaces of the abutment teeth with a high speed handpiece, especially if the abutment teeth are scheduled for full-coverage restorations. The wire can be retained with either composite resin or amalgam. The major problem with wire retainers is bond and wire breakage under the stress of occlusion. If the patient does not return to have the wire repaired, relapse will occur quite rapidly. A removable appliance also can be used as a retainer. The edentulous area is filled with acrylic, and clasps are placed on either molars or premolars, depending on retention needs. Again, the removable appliance must be worn faithfully until the restorative treatment is completed.

Adolescent orthodontic treatment is a challenging exercise in problem solving. A good data base and growth assessment are necessary to make the proper decisions about treatment alternatives. Unless the orthodontic problem is obviously the result of dental malalignment, the patient should be referred to a specialist because of the difficulty in managing skeletal discrepancies in patients of this age.

REFERENCES

Brady WF: The anorexia nervosa syndrome. Oral Surg 50:509–513, 1980.

Casamassimo PS, Pinkham JR, Steinke D: Dental needs of the adolescent. Pediatr Dent 1:129–137, 1979.

Castaldi CR, Brass GA: Dentistry for the Adolescent. Philadelphia, WB Saunders Co, 1980.

Chertkow S: Tooth mineralization as an indicator of the pubertal growth spurt. Am J Orthod 77:79–91, 1980.

Greulich WW, Pyle SI: Radiographic Atlas of Skeletal Development of the Hand and Wrist. Palo Alto, CA, Stanford University Press, 1959.

Moorrees CA, Fanning EA, Hunt EE, Jr: Age variation of formation stages for ten permanent teeth. J Dent Res 42:1490–1502, 1963.

Pinkham JR, Schroeder CS: Dentist and psychologist: Practical considerations for a team approach to the intensely anxious dental patient. JADA 90:1022–1026, 1975.

Poulsen S: Epidemiology and indices of gingival and periodontal disease. Pediatr Dent 3:82–88, 1981.

Tanner JM: Foetus Into Man. London, Open Books Publishing Ltd, 1978.

Prevention of dental disease

Arthur Nowak □ James Crall

The time of adolescence has been described as the period between childhood and adulthood. It has also been described as a period of change, rebellion, friction, and problems. It is a period when the patient emerges from junior high into senior high school and then off to college, the military, or the work force. It is a period of preference for peer group relationships and avoidance of all other associations, either societal or familial.

The period witnesses the completion of growth and development in both the female and male. All permanent teeth will have erupted, except for the congenitally missing or impacted third permanent molars. The occlusion will have stabilized, either on its own or with orthodontic intervention. Most studies show a gradual but general increase in the incidence of dental caries through this period. Periodontal disease becomes clinically evident because of fewer routine and supervised home care sessions as well as fewer professional interventions.

It is also known that dietary habits undergo dramatic changes during this period. As a female patient completes her maximum growth and development and begins the long process of "figure development," she may begin many dietary experiments and modifications. It is known that some of these modifications can lead to the serious pathologic conditions of anorexia nervosa and bulimia. In the male patient, similar modifications in dietary habits are also observed. During this period, the male's skeletal growth and body weight usually undergo dramatic changes, which peak around age 16–18. Caloric requirements increase dramatically, and large amounts of protein and carbohydrates are consumed. For both sexes, irregular eatings, fast food eating, frequent snacking, and unusual patterns of eating are all common.

With these adolescent characteristics so frequently described and routinely observed, how is the dentist and his or her providing professional dental care affected? Fortunately, if this population has had the advantages of both systemic and topical fluorides, the problem of caries will usually be confined to occlusal surfaces of posterior teeth. Nevertheless, with the eruption of the posterior teeth in an environment of increased plaque secondary to reduced cleaning and the frequent consumption of foods, which are usually high in carbohydrates and retentive to the teeth, the immature enamel of the smooth surfaces will be at high risk for caries.

Therefore, periodic professional visits, with emphasis on continuing home care, optimal use of topical fluorides, and assistance in dietary management, will be the goals and challenges of the dentist with the adolescent patient.

Dietary Management

As with younger age groups, the overall recommendations on dietary management for adolescents should concentrate on balanced intake, reduction of frequency of snacking, and selection of foods that will not be retentive to the teeth and soft tissues.

Unfortunately, these recommendations are often in conflict with the lifestyles of adolescents. Because of their gaining independence; rebellious posture to established social systems; acceptance of recommendations from television, radio, and movie idols; and peer group pressure, it is a difficult task for the dentist and his or her staff to convey these recommendations and expect compliance.

Fortunately, with increasing social development in the middle years of adolescence, there is a strong desire to look attractive, and the mouth, being the center of the face, takes on significant importance to the teenager's vanity. The challenge dentists have is to somehow make the daily care of teeth, including dietary regulations, motivational to this group.

For the patient who has been at high risk to dental disease during the early years and has had caries in the primary dentition, dietary management is again recommended. Depending on the patient's present oral status, emotional and psychological maturity, and parental influences, the counseling can be performed with the patient only or, if indicated, with the parent and patient. At this age, the adolescent may enjoy independence from the involvement of the parent. The dentist will have to make this decision whether or not to include the parents and how to inform the parents of the results of the counseling if they were not directly included.

Initially, a 24-hour dietary history will probably be sufficient. Based on the information provided from the history as well as the information from the patient as to usual daily schedules and academic, athletic, and social obligations, the dentist or staff members responsible for counseling can assist in creating a dietary plan with the patient.

Having the patient recognize the problem and agreeing either orally or in writing to a solution will improve compliance. During the periodic examination, progress or lack of progress can be evaluated. Plans may have to be modified frequently, depending on the patient's changing needs. With food preference, social pressure, and growth changes taking place daily, this plan has to allow for flexibility.

For the patient with active lesions in the developing permanent dentition, dietary management and modifications are definitely indicated, along with a comprehensive program of oral cleaning and application of topical daily fluorides. It is best to elicit a complete understanding from the patient of the importance of this information and a willingness to cooperate. If these criteria are not met, the history taking will only be a paper exercise and a waste of time for both parties involved. If the patient is found to be interested and willing to cooperate, a dietary history is indicated.

Although a 24-hour diet history will be helpful, more information will be provided from a 5- or 7-day history, including the weekend days. For the history to be accurate, the patient should complete the first day with the dentist, paying particular attention to include all liquid and solid foods for both mealtimes and between meals. Information on how much of the food was consumed and where the food was eaten will be helpful.

Once the dietary history is received, the dentist or a staff person assigned to counseling responsibilities should carefully review the history with the patient. Foods high in refined carbohydrates or retentive to the oral tissues should be circled. Intake of fresh fruits and vegetables should be noted. Overall balance of the diet should be evaluated. Unusual foods or dietary patterns should be listed.

The patient should then be asked to list the problem areas and prioritize them as to the problems that will be easy to change, followed by those that will be more difficult. With the problems identified and written in a sequence most acceptable for modification, the patient has to agree to a plan. It is important that it be the patient's plan and not the dentist's. It is the dentist's role to guide the patient to develop a realistic plan and a plan that will be built on successes. Periodic review will determine the status of the dietary modifications. Reinforcements and rewards from the dentist will be helpful, but the patient's own perception of success will be the most rewarding.

For the patient with a developmental disability, the challenge will be great. Depending on the severity of the disability, dietary habits may or may not be affected. For the severely disabled patient with a neuromuscular involvement, diet and eating methods will have been modified. Parents or caretakers must be made aware that potential problems—holding the food in the mouth, slow passage from the mouth into the digestive tract, and rumination—are all potentially devastating to the mouth and teeth. If regulation of the diet is not possible, efforts should be made on more frequent and thorough cleaning, as well as daily use of topical fluorides.

Home Care

Personal hygiene, like any established societal activity, will be met with varying responses during adolescence. Nagging by the parent or dentist will probably lead to a negative response. When the patient understands the importance of oral hygiene and is ready to make a daily commitment, the dentist can assist him or her in developing a routine of oral hygiene that will be acceptable to the patient as well as maintain a healthy oral environment.

During this period, dental flossing should become a part of the daily oral hygiene routine. Adolescents should have well-developed eye-hand coordination and fine motor activity. For those still having difficulty in the traditional method of flossing, a floss holder may be helpful.

The goal of the patient should be one thorough cleaning each day. Prior to bedtime is the preferred and ideal time. The patient must be informed of the importance of thoroughness and why a period before bed should be set aside for the routine of brushing and flossing. A vigorous rinsing of the mouth with water after meals should be encouraged. If orthodontic appliances are present, additional time will be necessary, as well as modifications of the routine to remove not only the plaque but also the debris around the brackets and wires. Additional massaging of the marginal gingiva is also important.

For the adolescent patient with a developmental disability, daily home care is equally important. Again, depending on the severity of the disability, either the patient, parent, or aide will be responsible for the care. In patients unable to keep the mouth open, a mouth prop will be helpful.

Fluoride Administration

APPROACH TO THE ADOLESCENT PATIENT

Although most adolescents possess the ability to carry out effective oral hygiene procedures, many neglect to perform these activities on a regular basis. The key to promoting effective caries prevention during what can be a very hectic and trying stage of life often depends upon recognizing the predominant motivational factors operating in this age group and adopting an approach that is based upon less than ideal compliance. The focus on personal appearance and hygiene in this age group can be used as a powerful motivator for developing preventive activities. Another strategy involves appealing to the adolescents' desires to be viewed as autonomous and capable of taking care of themselves.

Irrespective of the psychological basis for the motivation, time should be taken to ensure that adolescents understand the nature of the disease processes that the preventive programs are addressing and the general mechanisms by which the prescribed measures are thought to counteract these processes. This emphasis on education is more likely to be accepted and produce better long-term outcomes than a more authoritarian or condescending approach.

CARIES ACTIVITY DURING ADOLESCENCE

In spite of a well-documented decline in caries levels in children in the United States and other Western countries, adolescence still represents a period of significant caries activity for many individuals. Cross-sectional data from the 1979–1980 survey conducted by the National Institute of Dental Research (The Prevalence of Dental Caries in United States Children, 1981) showed that the mean number of decayed, missing, and filled permanent tooth surfaces increased from 5.41 for 13-year-olds to 11.04 for 17-year-olds. The results of that study indicated that the 17-year-olds who were examined had experienced an average of 1.2 additional lesions on buccal and lingual surfaces, 1.7 additional lesions on interproximal sur-

faces, and 2.7 additional occlusal lesions, compared with the 13-year-olds. Thus, fluoride administration should continue to be an important concern during this stage of high caries susceptibility.

Topical fluorides (along with occlusal sealants) become the primary preventive agents during adolescence, since the entire permanent dentition except for the third molars normally will have erupted by age 13 (Bell et al, 1982). Most studies have shown that fluorides reduce the incidence of smooth surface caries to a greater extent than that of occlusal caries (Backer-Dirks et al, 1961). Therefore, the combination of fluoride therapy and occlusal sealants can be used to provide optimal protection for all surfaces of the teeth.

HIGH FREQUENCY–LOW CONCENTRATION FLUORIDE APPLICATIONS

As with younger children, the daily use of a fluoride dentifrice should form the basis of a sound personal preventive dentistry program, regardless of whether the individual lives in a fluoridated or non-fluoridated community. Additional protection can be provided on a daily basis by the use of a 0.05% sodium fluoride rinse. Frequent rinsing would seem particularly advisable for very busy teenagers who do not take the time to practice thorough plaque removal. Frequent exposures to fluoride may help to suppress the cariogenic potential of the oral flora and can help to establish an environment that may inhibit demineralization or promote remineralization (DePaola, 1980). Fluoride mouthrinses also are indicated for individuals who have difficulty removing plaque because of the presence of orthodontic appliances or for those with a predisposing medical condition.

APPLICATIONS OF MORE CONCENTRATED FLUORIDE AGENTS

Daily applications of more concentrated fluoride gels may be indicated for some teenagers who exhibit poor oral hygiene or who continue to exhibit high levels of caries between recall examinations. These gels can be applied by brushing or via customized plastic trays. Custom trays are easily fabricated using vacuum-forming devices to adapt the plastic tray material over stone models of the patient's maxillary and mandibular arches. The best time to apply the gels is just before bedtime, in order to allow the fluoride to remain in contact with the teeth for a longer period of time. Professional topical fluorides should continue to be applied at least every 6 months during adolescence, especially for those patients with a history of caries activity or those who are perceived to be at greater risk to develop caries.

Adolescence is a time of heightened caries activity for many individuals as a result of increased intake of cariogenic substances and inattention to oral hygiene procedures. Because fluorides have been shown to exert a greater anti-caries effect in individuals with higher baseline levels of caries activity and because the concurrent use of various forms of fluoride often produces greater caries reductions than when the agents are used separately (Wei, 1974), multiple exposures to a variety of fluoride sources should be encouraged during this period in an attempt to control the caries process.

REFERENCES

Backer-Dirks O, Houwink B, Kwant GW: The results of 6½ years of artificial drinking water in the Netherlands: The Tiel-Culemborg experiment. Arch Oral Biol 5:284–300, 1961.

Bell RM, Klein SP, Bohannan HM, Graves RC, Disney JA: Characteristics of the data analysis population. *In* Results of Baseline Dental Exams in the National Preventive Dentistry Demonstration Program. Santa Monica, CA, Rand Corporation, 1982, p 26.

DePaola PF: The anticaries effect of single and combined topical fluoride systems in schoolchildren. Arch Oral Biol 25:649–653, 1980.

National Caries Program, National Institute of Dental Research: Summary of findings. *In* The Prevalence of Dental Caries in United States Children—1979–80, NIH Publ. No. 82–2245, December 1981, pp 5–8.

Wei SHY: The potential benefits to be derived from topical fluorides in fluoridated communities. *In* Forrester DJ, Schultz EM, Jr (eds): International Workshop on Fluorides and Dental Caries Reductions. Baltimore, University of Maryland, 1974, pp 178–240.

Esthetic restorative dentistry for the adolescent

John W. Reinhardt

A pleasing, attractive appearance is a dream of most adolescents in our society. Great effort and expense is invested in gaining or maintaining that appearance through means such as dieting, use of cosmetics, and selection of apparel. An important component of the idealized physical appearance is a radiant smile displaying teeth that are attractive in shape and color and do not distract during speaking and smiling.

The use of dental techniques and materials to help young people obtain the most attractive appearance possible is a clinical challenge requiring knowledge, disciplined attention to detail, and skill. In return for their efforts, dentists may receive the satisfaction of seeing a young person develop a healthy self-image, which can have a positive effect upon his or her maturation into adulthood.

Newly developed and improved composite resins, along with the acid-etch technique, have made the conservative restoration of esthetic defects possible. The use of visible light–cured composite resins has made the job easier. A multitude of composite resins are available and offer a choice of physical properties such as viscosity, opacity, and surface smoothness.

Fundamentals of Material Selection

Choice of materials is an important consideration for dental esthetics. For optimum attachment of composite resin to tooth structure, a bonding agent developed for dentin and enamel should be used.

Because it is easier to confine the etchant to the precise area of enamel desired, gel etching agents are preferred over liquids. The colorant added to gel etchants makes it easy to see where the etchant is placed.

Because there are a variety of products available with slightly differing physical properties, choice of composite resins for esthetic restorations can be confusing. Basically, the three types of composite resins that could be used are

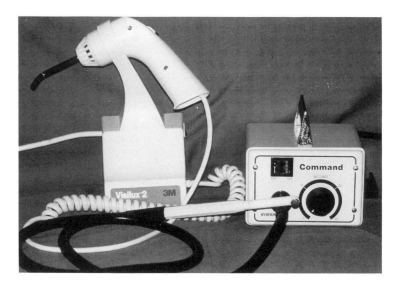

Figure 38-1 ■ Gun-type *(left)* and cable-type visible light polymerization units.

(1) traditional (those with filler particles ranging in size from 0.1 μm and upward, usually with an average particle size of 1.0-5.0 μm), (2) microfilled (those will filler particles of less than 0.1 μm in size, often pre-polymerized into larger masses), and (3) hybrid (a blend of microfilled and traditional particles). The primary advantage of traditional composites is strength, because they contain a higher percentage of filler particles and are therefore more resistant to fracture. With their extreme smoothness, microfilled composite resins can be polished to an enamel-like luster. The hybrid composites were developed as a compromise between the traditional and microfilled types, as materials that have greater strength than microfilled compos-

ite resins and a smoother surface than traditional composite resins.

Regardless of whether a traditional, microfilled, or hybrid composite resin is chosen, the use of visible light-curing products is recommended. Besides the convenience of extended working time and rapid polymerization, these materials also have lower porosity and are less likely to become discolored than the chemically cured (spatulated two paste) systems.

Polymerization of light-cured composite resins is accomplished by using an intense blue light with a peak wavelength of approximately 470 nm. This light may be transmitted by a unit with the light source (bulb) contained in a box located somewhat remotely from the patient

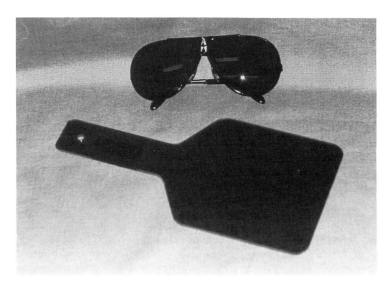

Figure 38-2 ■ Filtering devices designed to provide eye protection when using visible light-curing techniques.

and conducted to the restoration via fiberoptic bundles. Such a unit offers the convenience of a compact handpiece that is light and easy to maneuver. However, the danger of fiber breakdown in the cable, which leads to decreased intensity and polymerization, is a distinct disadvantage. Another type of light-curing unit uses a gun-type handpiece that is larger and contains the bulb and cooling fan (Fig. 38–1). This instrument is slightly more cumbersome to use but offers a short light transmission tube, which is less likely to become damaged during repeated use.

Be sure to protect your eyes when using the curing lights, as direct viewing of the light may be detrimental to vision. Amber filters, which block the intense blue component of the light, are commercially available and can be handheld or worn as eyeglasses (Fig. 38–2). In the absence of specific protective devices, make an effort to avoid looking directly at the light.

Fundamentals of Clinical Technique

Shade selection is the first step in a successful esthetic restorative procedure. The teeth to be matched should be cleaned with a rubber prophylaxis cup and flour of pumice. Moisten the shade guide and hold it near the tooth to be matched, using only room light or indirect sunlight. Do not use the high intensity operatory light to select shades. The proper value (whiteness) may be better selected by squinting. If shade selection takes more than a few seconds, one may need to resensitize the eyes by staring momentarily at a dark blue object. Many clinicians allow the patient to make the final decision between two similar shades. Be aware that the composite resin shade guide may vary from the actual shade of the composite paste. One way to verify the actual shade is to put a small portion of composite resin on the tooth surface and polymerize it, observe the "correctness" of that shade, and then remove it with a hand instrument. Do *not* etch the tooth prior to doing this. It is generally best not to combine shades of composite resin by mixing, as porosity may be introduced into the paste.

It is extremely important to maintain a dry field during the insertion of composite resins. The most reliable way to control moisture is through the use of a well-adapted rubber dam. If not using a rubber dam, one should place cotton rolls and 2×2 inch gauze sponges to prevent moisture contamination. Another technique for maintaining a dry field involves using a commercially available lip and cheek retractor (Fig. 38–3). This plastic device, when used in conjunction with gauze sponges, provides excellent access and good field control. Retractors such as this are especially helpful when anterior esthetic dentistry is performed with a dental assistant.

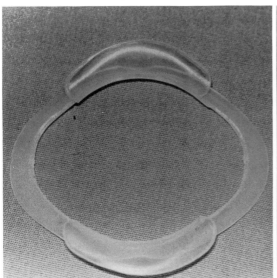 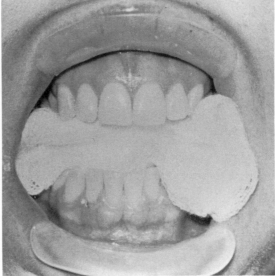

Figure 38–3 ■ ■ Isolation of anterior teeth may be enhanced through the use of a lip-retracting device.

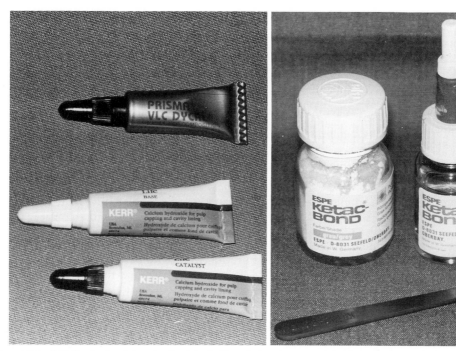

Figure 38–4 ■ Typical calcium hydroxide (*left* and glass ionomer (*right*) basing and lining products commonly used with composite resins.

Use of a base or liner to protect dentin from the effects of acid-etching and composite resin chemical irritation is important. A calcium hydroxide paste should be used in deep areas of a cavity preparation that are believed to be within 1.0 mm of pulpal tissue. The remaining dentin, which is directly between the composite resin and pulpal tissue, should be covered with a glass ionomer liner (Fig. 38–4). The liner provides pulpal protection from the etchant and composite resin, chemical adherence to tooth structure, slow release of fluoride, and the possibility of mechanical retention to the glass ionomer after acid-etching. The etchant should contact the glass ionomer only briefly (15 seconds), to prevent destruction of the liner.

Following enamel etching (60 second etch and 30 second rinse), build-up the light-cured composite resin in layers no greater than 2.0 mm in thickness, using 40 seconds of polymerization time per layer. Thin layers and adequate length of time for light exposure help ensure the maximum degree of polymerization. Maximum polymerization provides optimum strength and color stability of the restoration. It is important to cover the light-curing composite resin on the mixing pad so that room light does not start the polymerization process. In addition, it may be necessary to lessen the intensity of the operating light.

Use plastic or metal instruments for material placement and contouring. Fine sable brushes allow easy contouring and blending of composite resin into the proper form. To prevent composite from adhering to the brushes and instruments, lightly lubricate them with gauze sponges moistened with bathing alcohol.

Following the polymerization process, contour and finish the composite resin restoration, using carbide finishing burs, ultrafine diamond burs, or finishing disks. Use fine-pointed burs to contour areas that are difficult to reach, such as embrasures. Rounded burs may be used on concave surfaces, and disks may be used on flat or convex surfaces. After contouring and finishing, polish the restoration with a series of polishing disks or rubber abrasive instruments. Finish and polish interproximal areas with abrasive strips.

Fundamentals of Tooth Color and Form

The most ideal esthetic restoration is one that looks so natural it is difficult to discern from the surrounding tooth surface or adjacent teeth. Color and translucency must be considered together to achieve an optimum result. Areas of

discoloration on a tooth may be altered by applying color modifiers or opaquing agents to improve the appearance, then covering those areas with composite resin.

Composite resins with greater opacity, such as traditional, hybrid, and microfilled opaque pastes, should be used in most situations. The reason for this selection is that excessive translucency can often allow intraoral darkness to show through a restoration and cause the unpleasant esthetic result of a dark restoration.

Highly translucent materials such as nonopaque microfilled pastes should be used only for Class III restorations and small Class IV restorations on highly translucent teeth, or for Class V restorations when the underlying base is dentin colored.

Form and anatomy of anterior esthetic restorations are also dictated by making the restoration look natural. In general, embrasure spaces should be symmetrical whenever possible and contours should match those of the adjacent teeth. Adolescent anterior teeth usually show very little evidence of wear and display prominent incisal embrasure spaces, rounded incisal point angles, and developmental characteristics such as mamelons on incisal edges. These characteristics are especially noticeable with young women and should be used whenever possible to enhance a feminine smile.

Restorations for Fractured Anterior Teeth

Trauma to the anterior dentition can often result in tooth fractures involving incisal edges.

Injuries such as these can present pulpal as well as esthetic problems, and should be carefully evaluated through clinical and radiographic means. Clinical findings may range from little or no dentin exposure with minimal thermal and pressure sensitivity, to the acute pulpitis of a pulp exposure. Radiographs help diagnose the presence or absence of root fractures. Treatment must begin with pulpal therapy as a first consideration, and if pulpectomy or pulpotomy is necessary, it should begin simultaneously with the restorative procedure.

Some clinicians consider the Class IV composite resin restoration an interim restoration for adolescents, until the time when a more permanent ceramic crown can be fabricated. However, with modern materials and techniques, the strength and color stability of composite resin Class IV restorations are such that they can be considered ''final'' restorations that will provide many years of service. For early adolescents with severely fractured anterior teeth, these restorations can provide years of service, allowing maturation of the teeth so that pulpal involvement during crown preparation is less likely.

CLINICAL TECHNIQUE

Acid-etching techniques have lessened the need for extensive mechanical retentive design in Class IV restorations. The primary retentive feature is a bevelled enamel cavosurface margin, which should be a minimum of 1.0 mm in length (Figs. 38–5 to 38–7). Bevelling will allow maximum bond strength and minimum

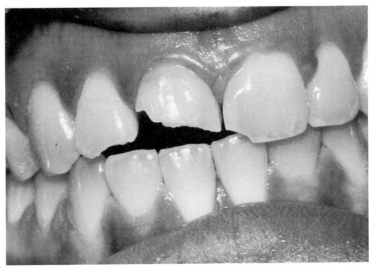

Figure 38–5 ■ Teeth 7–9 were fractured as the result of a sports injury.

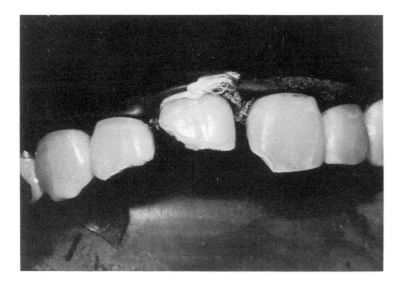

Figure 38–6 ■ Isolation and preparation (smoothing and bevelling) of teeth 7–9 (see Fig. 39–5).

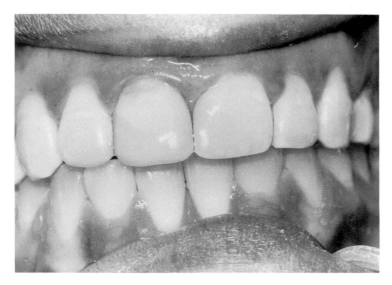

Figure 38–7 ■ Adhesively retained (bonded) composite resin restorations of the fractured teeth seen in Figures 38–5 and 38–6.

leakage, by virtue of exposing the ends of the enamel rods to etching. Because anterior restorations are sometimes subject to strong shearing forces that can be greater than the bond strength of the restoration to the tooth, features such as grooves, retentive points, or pins may be used to gain additional retentive strength in some cases.

After administering anesthesia, placing the rubber dam, and preparing the bevel (using a medium grit diamond bur), apply base or liner to exposed dentin. The etchant, bonding agent, and composite resin application is performed as described previously. A wedged celluloid matrix strip can prevent etching and bonding of an adjacent tooth. After placing, finishing, and polishing the composite resin, remove the rubber dam and carefully check the restoration with articulating paper or ribbon for interferences in all excursive movements. Occlusal stresses should be minimized on the restoration.

Restoration of Diastemata

Many adolescents, as well as adults, consider spaces between anterior teeth (diastemata) to be unattractive. Historically, the only restorative treatment to fill these spaces has been the construction of crowns larger than the original teeth. Even though many patients disliked their appearance with diastemata, most were unwilling to undergo the trauma and expense of crowning sound teeth simply for esthetic improvement. Improved composite resin materials and acid-etching technology now allow restoration of diastema spaces with a method that is non-destructive, reversible, and considerably less expensive than the alternative crowns. However, patients should be forewarned that fracture and staining are possible drawbacks of composite resin diastema closures, and that replacement may be necessary after 5–10 years.

When an adolescent patient wants a diastema closure, whether the spaces are the result of natural development or post-orthodontic discrepancies, careful evaluation and planning is necessary prior to treatment. If the patient is nearing completion of orthodontic therapy but is still undergoing treatment, the restorative dentist may advise the orthodontist about the optimum arrangement of anterior teeth for diastema closure. The orthodontist may then complete active treatment and place the patient into a retention phase prior to diastema closure. It is best to allow a minimum of a few months between the end of active orthodontic treatment and diastema closure therapy so that anterior teeth will be more stable and will settle into their final position. The use of impressions and diagnostic study casts is highly recommended for evaluation and treatment planning. A trial wax-up of the proposed restorative treatment can aid both the patient and clinician in envisioning the probable esthetic result.

Important considerations before treatment is begun include the size and location of the space or spaces and the size (length and width) and shape of the teeth to be restored. Normally, composite resin is added to the teeth on both sides of the space. For patients who are still in orthodontic treatment, decide if the remaining space would best be left in one place, such as the midline between teeth Nos. 8 and 9, or distributed over interproximal areas throughout the anterior segment. Also, consider the length and width of the teeth to be restored. If the width becomes greater than the length, those teeth appear increasingly "square" causing an esthetic result that is unnatural and may be as displeasing as the original diastema. Because of occlusal patterns and chewing stresses, teeth cannot be lengthened using composite resin without a high probability of resin fracture. However, light reflections can be used to create the illusion of a tooth being longer and narrower when the composite resin is extended to cover most or all of the facial surface of a tooth. To create the illusion of a more narrow tooth, form mesial and distal line angles in composite resin that are nearer the center of the tooth and add definite vertical anatomic highlights (developmental depressions). For some patients, the best treatment is partial diastema closure, in which an existing space is made smaller by enlarging the teeth with composite resin, but not making the teeth so large that they become displeasing. In summary, esthetic possibilities must be carefully evaluated and explained to the patient before treatment is begun.

CLINICAL TECHNIQUE

Following cleaning, shade selection, and isolation (as described previously), treatment should begin on one tooth at a time. The space to be eliminated should be carefully measured using a periodontal probe or Boley gauge, because when one tooth is restored in an effort to

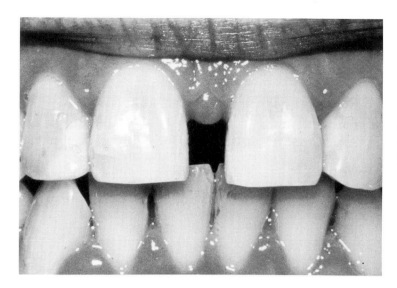

Figure 38-8 ■ A preoperative view of a large maxillary midline diastema, which the patient found unattractive.

eliminate one half the space, it is usually difficult to determine how much of the space has actually been restored. The entire labial surface of the tooth should be etched and bonding agent applied, since most of the labial surface will be covered with a thin layer of composite to allow a subtle color transition from composite to tooth. In addition, covering most of the labial surface allows the use of visual illusions, causing the tooth to look narrower or longer, as described previously. Composite resin (preferably one that is quite viscous and opaque) should be applied, beginning at the gingival margin of the interproximal area. Using instruments and brushes, shape the material to allow a smooth-flowing gingival embrasure without creating an overhanging ledge. The entire proximal sur-

face, along with the labial, can be built up and polymerized at once or incrementally. Following that build-up, finish the interproximal area to the proper contour and polish. Next, restore the second tooth in a similar fashion. A celluloid matrix and wedge are usually inserted after the gingival increment is polymerized, to retain the composite resin and to prevent bonding the restorations together. Upon completion, the matrix is removed and contouring and polishing are finished (Figs. 38-8 to 38-11).

Anterior teeth that are unusually small, such as peg lateral incisors, may be restored in the same manner as teeth requiring both mesial and distal diastema closure restorations. Again, careful treatment planning is advised. Use sound judgment in determining whether the

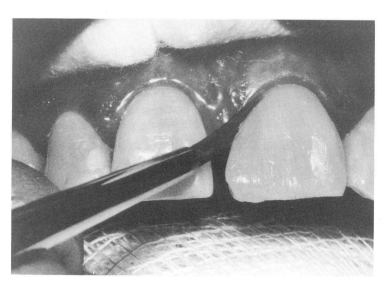

Figure 38-9 ■ The initial increment of composite resin being contoured with a sable brush prior to polymerization (see Fig. 38-8).

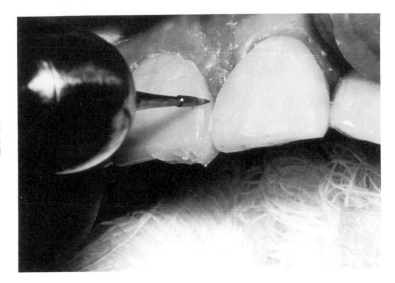

Figure 38–10 ■ Contouring and removing excess composite resin following build-up of the second tooth (see Figs. 38–8 and 38–9).

restorations should be done only on the smaller tooth or on both the small and adjacent teeth for maximum cosmetic benefit. Preoperative diagnosis is again necessary to determine if lengthening is feasible. Warn the patient that the possibility of restoration fracture increases as length increases.

Restoration of Discolored Teeth

Although there are many causes of tooth discoloration in adolescents, the most common discolorations are the result of trauma, enamel hypoplasia (such as occurs from fluorosis), and the administration of tetracycline antibiotics during childhood. These lesions vary from small white or yellowish flecking of the surface enamel to the deep intrinsic bluish-gray color often seen in tetracycline staining.

TREATMENT OF HYPOPLASTIC SPOTS

Discrete hypoplastic white or yellow-brown spots can be improved by making shallow, saucer-shaped preparations in enamel to remove the intensely colored tooth structure and then restoring the enamel with composite resin. Using a large, round bur in a high speed handpiece, the preparation can normally be made

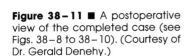

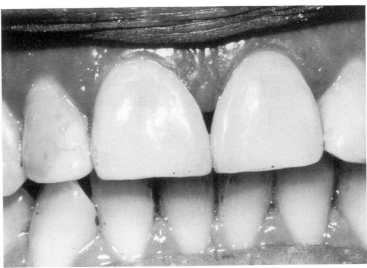

Figure 38–11 ■ A postoperative view of the completed case (see Figs. 38–8 to 38–10). (Courtesy of Dr. Gerald Denehy.)

without anesthesia. The composite resin can be contoured with brushes to proper form, so that little finishing is required.

VENEERS

Composite resin or porcelain veneers provide a treatment option for patients who have moderate to severe staining of one or more teeth. Veneers are usually more successful on maxillary teeth than on mandibular teeth. Most patients are more concerned about the appearance of their maxillary teeth, especially the anteriors, since they are more visible in speaking and smiling. In addition, mandibular teeth are less likely to be successfully veneered because of limited space (insufficient overjet) and unfavorable forces at the junction of tooth and veneer during normal chewing. Thus, mandibular veneers are usually discouraged. For veneer treatment to be successful, the patient must have excellent periodontal health, because the placement of veneers will result in contours and margins that require good oral hygiene to maintain gingival health. In addition, patients should be warned that biting on hard objects, such as raw carrots or pencils, can dislodge or break veneers.

Although the predicted longevity of an esthetic veneer restoration is somewhat less than that of a porcelain fused-to-metal crown, the cost is also considerably less. In addition, veneers can be placed with little or in some cases no tooth preparation, thus preserving the natural dentition. Veneers may be made by direct build-up of composite resin in the mouth or by indirect procedures (constructed on laboratory models) using composite resin or porcelain.

Laboratory-Constructed Veneers

The indirect veneer technique has the advantage of requiring less total chair time, since the veneers are constructed in the laboratory. Excellent esthetic contours can be achieved, using porcelain or composite resin laboratory techniques. Disadvantages include the necessity of two appointments, laboratory expense, and the possibility of excess bulk of restorative material.

The clinical indirect technique usually requires the removal of some enamel (0.5–1.0 mm) from the facial surface to provide space for the veneer. This is best accomplished with a medium grit diamond bur, with the goal of producing a chamfer finish line throughout the surfaces to be covered. This preparation extends to the proximal surfaces but does not include the contact points. Gingivally, the preparation must extend far enough to cover the stained enamel sufficiently to improve the color. For better periodontal health, the finish line should be kept supragingival whenever possible.

Following the preparation(s), make an accurate impression of the teeth using standard techniques and an elastomeric impression material such as polysulfide or silicone, and pour a stone model.

At the second appointment, isolate the teeth and clean them with pumice. Acid-etch the teeth individually and bond the veneers to

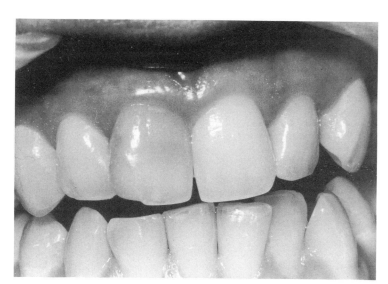

Figure 38–12 ■ Preoperative view of a discolored and rotated tooth No. 8.

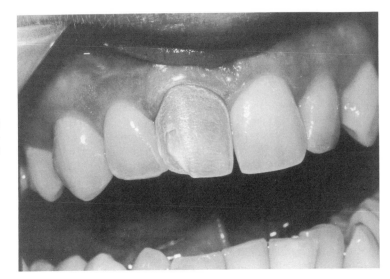

Figure 38–13 ■ Preparation of tooth No. 8 for an indirect (laboratory-fabricated composite resin) veneer.

place, following the manufacturer's instructions. Use celluloid matrices to protect adjacent teeth. Light-cured resins of moderate viscosity are preferred for bonding, and excess resin may be removed prior to polymerization. Use adequate polymerization time (40–60 seconds) in each area, since the veneers will shield some of the light transmission. Finishing and polishing are usually necessary only at the margins, and may be done with abrasive strips and burs (Figs. 38–12 to 38–14).

Direct Veneers

Veneers made of light-cured composite resins can be constructed directly in the mouth. Compared with the indirect type, direct veneers offer the advantages of better margins, placement in one appointment, and no laboratory fee. The disadvantages include the fact that direct veneers require more time, greater skill, and more patience on the part of the clinician. Also, results are more difficult to predict.

The clinical direct technique may be performed with or without any enamel removal. Darkly stained teeth usually require some enamel removal, because more composite resin is needed to mask the underlying enamel. The teeth are then pumiced and individually etched, and bonding agent is applied. Again, celluloid matrices are used between adjacent teeth. Opaquing agents may then be painted on, to cover more intensely stained areas or entire surfaces, although the use of opaquers can

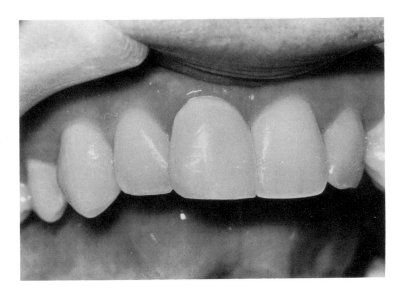

Figure 38–14 ■ Finished veneer bonded to tooth No. 8.

cause an unesthetic flat appearance in the color of the final restoration. For that reason, opaquers should be used minimally and with care. Next, the composite resin (microfilled, opaque) should be applied in a layer 1.0–1.5 mm in thickness, and contoured using brushes. The gingival one third of the restoration should be a yellow shade, such as YO, and the remaining enamel should be covered with GO or UO, with the shades overlapped and blended to create a natural-looking, gentle color transition.* In many cases, a non-opaque shade can be used on the incisal one fourth to allow a natural translucency (Fig. 38–15). After all composite resin has been added to a single tooth and contouring with brushes is complete, polymerize the material by exposing each area to 40–60 seconds of curing light. Be careful to overlap the light for each period of exposure, since narrow-tipped lights may require four or five separate periods to cover the entire labial surface. Finish and polish with burs and disks, as described before.

Bonded Bridges and Splints

Cast metal appliances can be bonded to enamel, using composite resins. This procedure, in which the inner surfaces of metal are etched in the laboratory to create micro-mechanical retentive areas, is very useful for attaching bridges and splints to etched enamel. Bridges constructed by this technique offer two advantages over conventional bridgework: greater conservation of tooth structure and less expense. Splints can be made, using the same

---

* YO = yellow opaque; GO = gray opaque; UO = universal opaque.

technique for patients requiring fixed post-orthodontic stabilization.

Diagnosis and treatment planning should include careful observation of occlusion of teeth receiving the retainer portion of a bridge or splint. Ideally, the retainers would cover 80–90% of the lingual enamel surfaces of those teeth in order to provide maximum retention. Anterior teeth with markedly translucent incisal edges may not allow coverage to extend near those edges, since metallic or resin coverage can cause an unnaturally opaque appearance. Diagnostic study models are helpful. The teeth must have adequate enamel for bonding, because the presence of exposed dentin or restorations can significantly decrease retentive strength. Enamel may be reduced (0.5 mm) to provide space for the metal retainer, and occasionally opposing teeth may also be reduced slightly. For anterior bridges and splints, a slight reduction of lingual enamel can be prepared with diamond burs, ending in a supragingival chamfer. Shade selection for pontics should be made prior to preparation.

Make an impression of the prepared arch with an accurate elastomeric impression material such as polysulfide or silicone rubber, and pour the model with a type IV die stone. Using a sharp red pencil, outline extensions of the preparations on the working model. It is helpful to ask the laboratory technician to provide incisal rests that serve as guides for accurate seating of the appliance. These guides can be removed with carbide burs following cementation of the appliance.

Try-in the appliance and make any necessary adjustments of shade, contour, or occlusion. Then isolate the teeth with a rubber dam while the appliance is cleaned in an ultrasonic water bath. Clean and etch the abutment teeth. Mix the composite resin luting cement (autopoly-

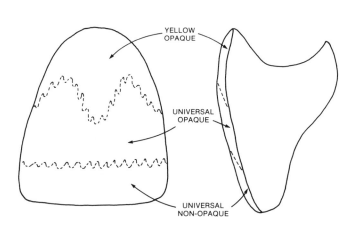

Figure 38–15 ■ The use of overlapping shades of composite resin to create a natural-looking directly placed veneer.

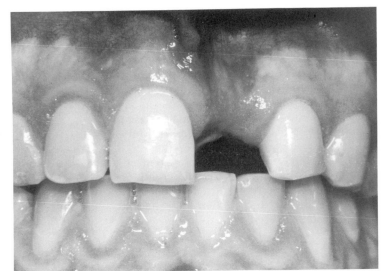

Figure 38–16 ■ Preoperative view of a patient missing tooth No. 9.

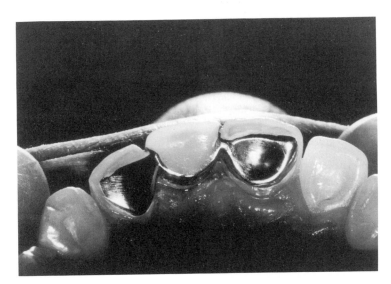

Figure 38–17 ■ Incisal view of a bonded bridge replacing tooth No. 9 (see Fig. 38–16).

Figure 38–18 ■ Labial view of the finished case (see Figs. 38–16 and 38–17). (Courtesy of Dr. Gerald Denehy.)

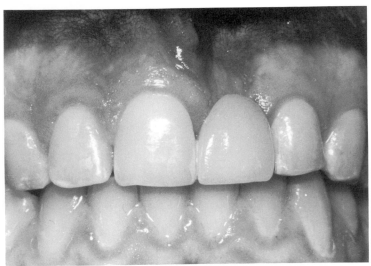

merizing), and apply it to the appliance. The appliance must be seated and held with firm pressure for several minutes while the resin cement hardens; otherwise, the rubber dam may push the appliance incisally and result in incomplete seating. Following cementation, carefully cut the rubber dam with a scissors and remove it. Excess cement may be removed with diamond or carbide burs (Figs. 38–16 to 38–18).

In the unlikely and unfortunate event of a retainer loosening from an abutment tooth, remove the appliance and return it to the laboratory for re-etching. It may then be reattached, using the same procedure.

BIBLIOGRAPHY

Bagheri J, Denehy GE: Effect of enamel bevel and restoration lengths on Class IV acid-etch retained composite resin restoration. JADA 107:951–953, 1983.

Black JB, Retief DH, Lemons JE: Effect of cavity design on retention of Class IV composite resin restorations. JADA 103:42–46, 1981.

Christensen GJ: Veneering of teeth. Dent Clin North Am 29:373–391, 1985.

Fan PL, Leung RL, Leinfelder KF: Visible light–cured composites and activating units. JADA 110:100–103, 1985.

Ham WT: Ocular hazards of light sources: Review of current knowledge. J Occup Med 25:101–103, 1983.

Hormati AA, Fuller JL, Denehy GE: Effects of contamination and mechanical disturbance on the quality of acid-etched enamel. JADA 100:34–38, 1980.

Jordan RE, Suzuki M, Gwinnett AJ, Hunter JK: Restoration of fractured and hypoplastic incisors by the acid etch technique: A three-year report. JADA 95:795–803, 1977.

Leinfelder KF: Composite resins. Dent Clin North Am 29:359–371, 1985.

Lutz F, Phillips RW: A classification and evaluation of composite resin systems. J Prosthet Dent 50:480–488, 1983.

McLean JW: Status report on the glass ionomer cements. JADA 99:221–226, 1979.

McLean JW, Powis DR, Prosser HJ, Wilson AD: The use of glass-ionomer cements in bonding composite resins to dentine. Br Dent J 158:410–414, 1985.

Mount GJ: Restoration with glass-ionomer cement: Requirements for clinical success. Oper Dent 6:59–65, 1981.

Onose H, Sano H, Kanto H, Ando S, Hasuike T: Selected curing characteristics of light-activated composite resins. Dent Mater 1:48–54, 1985.

Prevost AP, Fuller JL, Peterson LC: The use of an intermediate resin in the acid-etch procedure: Retentive strength, microleakage, and failure mode analysis. J Dent Res 61:412–418, 1982.

Reinhardt JW, Denehy GE, Jordan RD, Rittman, BRJ: Porosity in composite resin restorations. Oper Dent 7:82–85, 1982.

Schaefer ME, Reisback MH: A three-year study of a small particle light cured composite resin. Can Dent Assoc 11:53–57, 1983.

Sockwell CL, Heymann HO: Tooth-colored restorations. In Sturdervant CM, Barton RE, Sockwell CL, Strickland WD (eds): The Art and Science of Operative Dentistry, 2nd ed. St. Louis, CV Mosby, 1985, pp 267–311.

Sockwell CL, Heymann HO, Brunson WD: Additional conservative and esthetic treatments. In Sturdervant CM, Barton RE, Sockwell CL, Strickland WD (eds): The Art and Science of Operative Dentistry, 2nd ed. St. Louis, CV Mosby, 1985, pp 312–372.

Sports injuries/mouth protectors

William Olin

Each year, more and more athletes are wearing some form of mouth protection while participating in contact sports. Some athletes who are not in contact sports are also wearing mouth protectors for sports such as gymnastics and weight lifting. Dentists who are professionally involved with sports recommend that mouth protectors be used for any activity in which mouth structures could be injured.

The mouth protector is made for the maxillary dental arch. It provides a cushion effect that softens the shock from a blow by distributing the shock over a large number of teeth in a way that minimizes all types of injury to the structures involved.

There is very little written regarding the history of intraoral mouth protectors prior to 1950. However, mouth protectors were used as far back as 1913 in English boxers to protect the oral tissues from violent blows to the mouth and teeth.

Actual research concerning injuries obtained from athletics was first performed in 1929 on football players. During the following years, the emphasis was placed on making better pads and helmets, while protection for the mouth and face was neglected. In the early 1950's, a

new interest surfaced in protecting the teeth in different kinds of sports, including boxing, ice hockey, basketball, and football. Watts and colleagues (1954) reported the number of football injuries and discussed a program in Chicago in which 26 members of a Chicago high school football team were fitted with mouth protectors made of velum rubber. Dental injuries were reduced 100%, whereas opposing teams without mouth protectors suffered an average of two injuries in and about the mouth in the same game.

Another study conducted with the Notre Dame football team by Stenger and coworkers (1964) showed a distinct reduction in the number of concussions and neck injuries after all members of the team were provided with custom-fitted mouth protectors.

Mouth injuries composed 50% or more of all football injuries in the 1950's. In the late 1950's, a joint committee was formed by the American Dental Association and the American Association of Health, Physical Education and Recreation to investigate dental and oral injuries. In 1962, the National Alliance Football Rules Committee formulated the following regulation for high school football players:

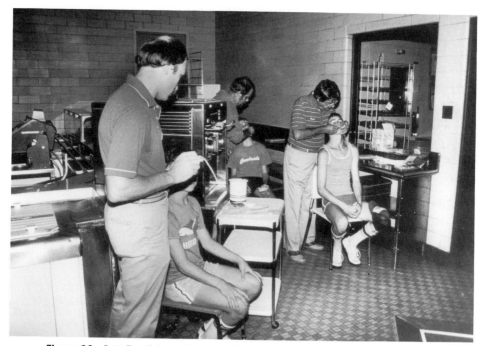

Figure 39–1 ■ Dentists making mouth-formed guards for high school athletes.

Each player shall wear an intraoral mouth and tooth protector which includes an occlusal (protecting and separating the biting surfaces) and a labial (protecting the lips) portion.

In response to this regulation, many dental societies throughout the United States organized programs to provide area high school football players with mouth protectors. The author's local dental society (Johnson County of Iowa), working with volunteer dentists, set up a program to fit athletes with mouth protectors in August, before the football season begins. As the program is run now, the fittings are performed at a high school cafeteria, involve 15–20 dentists, and entail 2–3 hours per night (Fig. 39–1). In that amount of time, 350–400 mouth protectors can be made. The dental society is at present utilizing a mouth-formed plastic protector with a strap. The cost for each protector is approximately 35 cents. Recently, a new program has been instituted by the dental society for other athletes at risk for oral and dental injuries.

Even though mouth injuries have all but been eliminated in football, other sports are still reporting injuries. This was emphasized by means of a study completed in Texas by Drs. Robert M. Morrow and William A. Kuebker from the University of Texas Sports Dentistry Program (personal communication). This study

was undertaken among Texas high schools in 1984. It was conducted for high school male and female athletes. Six hundred and twenty-six schools responded for male athletes. The injury rate for individual sports revealed that the greatest number of injuries occurred in soccer, closely followed by basketball. Of the football athletes, 92.4% wore mouth protectors; however, only 6.7% of soccer players wore mouth protectors, and only 1.58% of basketball players used the devices. Six hundred and five schools reported on injuries to female athletes. Soccer was reported as having the greatest number of injuries, followed by basketball. Less than 1% of female athletes were fitted with mouth protectors.

It is obvious that all participants in sports that may cause an injury to the mouth or face should be fitted with a mouth protector, and this should be accomplished when the athlete first participates in sports, even if this is as early as 6 or 7 years of age (Fig. 39–2).

Types of Mouth Protectors

Three types of mouth protectors are used by athletes (Fig. 39–3). These are stock mouth

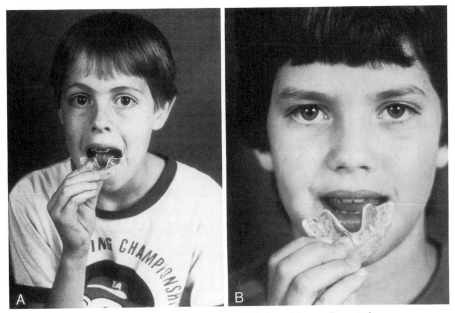

Figure 39-2 ■ *A* and *B,* Young athletes with mouth guards.

protectors, mouth-formed protectors, and custom-fitted mouth protectors.

STOCK MOUTH PROTECTORS

The stock mouth protector can be purchased from sporting goods stores. It is purchased in various shapes and sizes, depending on the age of the patient. This type of protector will offer only a minimal amount of protection. It is very difficult to retain because it can only be held in place when the mouth is closed, and it makes breathing and talking very difficult. These type of protectors are not recommended by sports dentists.

MOUTH-FORMED PROTECTORS

The mouth-formed protector is made from a thermoplastic material and can be purchased by

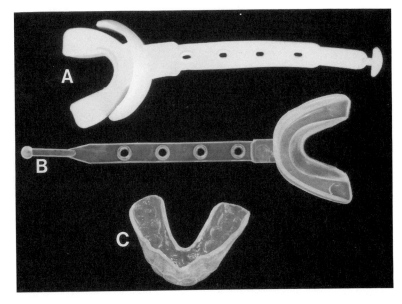

Figure 39-3 ■ Three types of mouth guards. *A,* Stock mouth guard. *B,* Mouth-formed protector. *C,* Custom fit mouth guard.

the athlete in most sporting goods stores. This mouth protector is fabricated by being immersed in boiling water for 15–45 seconds, depending on the type. Care is taken so that it cools sufficiently before being placed in the mouth. The protector is then placed in the mouth and is adapted to the teeth. The athlete is urged to close the lips and suck to aid in adapting the protector to the teeth and gingival tissues.

These protectors should be made by a dentist and are the type used by the author's dental society for high school football players. This protector is widely used today because it has a minimal amount of bulk, has a satisfactory fit, and is reasonable in price. Straps can be attached to retain the protector with the face mask of the football helmet.

CUSTOM-MADE MOUTH PROTECTORS

Custom-made mouth protectors are fabricated on a dental cast of an athlete's maxillary dental arch that is taken by a dentist. This is by far the most satisfactory mouth protector. In the past, various materials were used. However, the most common type used today, which is a polyvinyl acetate–polyethylene product, is widely regarded as the best. This material is supplied in square sheets approximately 5 × 5 inches in size, with a thickness of approximately 3.8 mm, or .150 inches. The same thickness should be used for all sports. Anything thinner results in a mouth protector that does not offer maximum protection (Fig. 39–4).

In the past few years, color-tinted mouth guards have become increasingly popular. Not only are they easier to find if dislodged; they also provide coaches and referees easier visual information that an athlete's mouth is protected.

Construction of the Custom-Made Mouth Protector

Making the impression ■ An alginate impression is made of the maxillary arch only. The impression should include all of the teeth and hard palate and should extend to the height of the vestibule. The impression must be muscle trimmed, paying special attention to the frenal attachments. Overextension can cause problems for the athlete. All removable appliances should be removed. Usually, removable appliances are not worn during competition. Compensation must be made for fixed orthodontic appliances.

Making the model ■ A stone model should be poured immediately and the model properly identified. These strong casts can be used more than once if this is necessary. If the athlete is

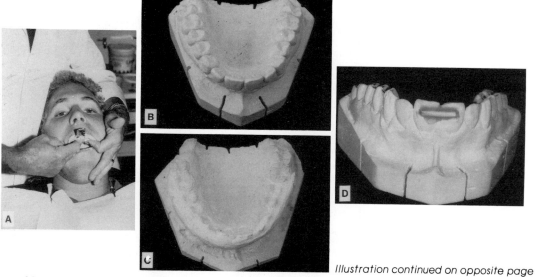

Illustration continued on opposite page

Figure 39–4 ■ Making a custom fit mouth guard. *A* to *D*, Securing a good working model. *E* to *H*, Vacuum forming and gross trimming of the protector. *I* to *M*, Final finishing.

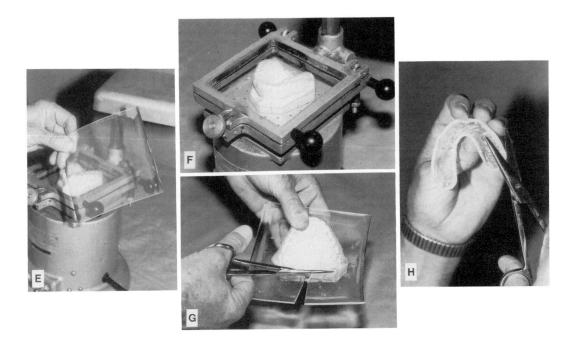

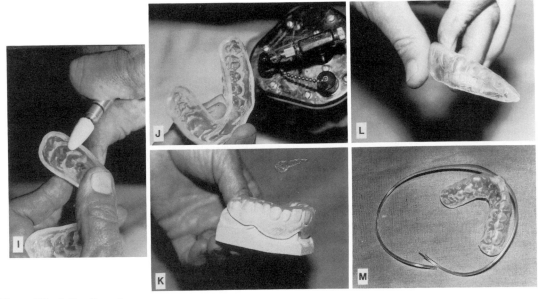

Figure 39–4 *Continued*

wearing a fixed orthodontic appliance, it should be blocked out on the stone model with plaster.

Vacuum-forming the protector ■ The sheet of polyvinyl acetate–polyethylene is placed on a heating–vacuum unit, such as the Omnivac.* The material is softened and vacuum formed over a wet, cold model (instructions come with the Omnivac). As soon as the vacuum starts, the protector is additionally hand adapted, using a wet paper towel. This improves the fit of the protector. The mouth protector is then allowed to cool, to prevent distortion.

Trimming and finishing ■ Care should be taken when the protector is removed from the model, so as not to fracture any teeth. A cut up the middle of the palate will help. All of the excess material is trimmed with sharp scissors. Proper extension is very important, and all frenum attachments must be sufficiently relieved. The protector should be extended just short of the muco-buccal fold. The protector should include the second molars in most cases. The edges should then be smoothed with a stone, and the edges should be flamed with an alcohol torch and smoothed with wet fingers on the stone model.

Athlete's name ■ The name of the athlete should be placed on each mouth protector. On the buccal surface in the area of the first molar tooth, a small amount of material is removed with a small stone. The name is typed on a piece of paper. This small piece of paper (3 × 6 mm) is placed in the shallow indentation after the area has been heated. A thin piece of vinyl is then placed over the area and is heated with an alcohol torch; the edges are then sealed with a hot spatula.

Strap ■ Many football players desire having a strap attached to their mouth protector. This is done by waxing a piece of cotton appli-

cator wood approximately ½ inch long on the labial surface of the central incisors (see Fig. 39–4D). When the mouth protector is vacuum formed, an area on the labial surface with a slight labial bulge results. At each end, a small hole is made with a No. 8 round bur. A piece of polyethylene tubing approximately 2 mm in diameter (0.30 inch inside diameter) and 14–16 inches in length is attached to the mouth protector through the small holes on the labial. The tubing is then joined with a small piece of 0.36 inch round stainless steel orthodontic wire. One end of the wire is rounded. This will allow the strap to come apart if pulled on and thereby will prevent injury to the athlete.

Instructions for care ■ After the mouth protector has been issued to the athlete, instructions should be given regarding proper care. The mouth protector should be thoroughly cleaned after each use and stored in an identifiable container. Commercially available mouthwashes can be used as lubricants and fresheners.

> As mentioned previously, mouth injuries have been reduced to less than 1% of all injuries in football. It is now time that mouth protectors be made mandatory for all contact sports or for any activity that could cause injury to the mouth or teeth. They should be made as early as the athlete participates in these various activities.

REFERENCES

Watts G, Woolard A, Singer CE: Functional mouth protectors for contact sports. JADA 49:7–11, 1954.

Stenger JM, Lawson EA, Wright JM: Mouthguards: Protection against shock to head, neck and teeth. JADA 69:273–281, 1964.

---

* Omnidental, Chicago, IL.

Periodontal disease and temporomandibular joint disorders

Paul S. Casamassimo □ **Sidney L. Bronstein**
John Christensen □ **Henry Fields**

CHAPTER OUTLINE

- **NORMAL PERIODONTAL STRUCTURES**
- **PERIODONTAL DISEASE IN ADOLESCENTS**
- **SPECIFIC DISEASE ENTITIES**
  Puberty Gingivitis
  Eruption Gingivitis
  Pericoronitis
  Acute Necrotizing Ulcerative Gingivitis
  Localized Juvenile Periodontitis

Gingival and Periodontal
  Manifestations of Venereal Disease
Mouthbreathing
Effects of Smokeless Tobacco

- **TEMPOROMANDIBULAR JOINT DISORDERS**
  Diagnosis and Treatment of
  Temporomandibular Joint Problems

The hallmark of gingival inflammation in childhood is reversibility, but in adolescence, the human organism begins to lose its ability to prevent permanent breakdown of tissues. The reasons for this change are not fully understood but can be seen at the clinical and microscopic level. Research has identified distinct cellular differences in the body's response to local irritants in the adult dentition. The immune system has matured. The permanent dentition is in function with an established periodontal apparatus. The skeletal system, including the alveolar bone, is approaching adult proportions, and the hormonal influence on the oral cavity and the body in general is far different from a few short years earlier.

The cumulative effect of these changes is unclear, except in general terms. During adolescence, for example, the number of people who develop irreversible bone loss increases. Adolescent gingivitis appears with both a hormonal and local cause. According to the data from the National Health Survey, the periodontal index and oral hygiene problems also tend to worsen during this period (1974). Adolescence becomes a period of critical importance in periodontal management. It is truly a turning point. Decisions made and habits fostered in adolescence may mean prevention of periodontal destruction in later life.

Normal Periodontal Structures

The dentition of the adolescent is similar to that of the adult in many ways. The periodontal tissues are adult tissues for all practical purposes. With completion of eruption (minus

503

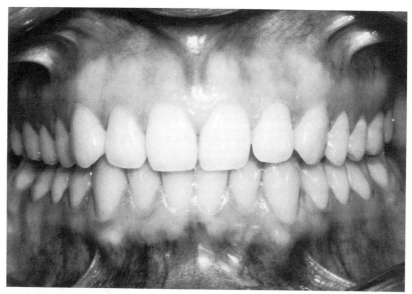

Figure 40 – 1 ■ Normal healthy gingival and periodontal tissues of a patient in late adolescence.

third molars) of teeth, the alveolar bone has reached maximal height. The interdental areas are finer projections of bone than those found in the primary dentition. The alveolar bone, although still resilient, is beginning to increase in calcification, a process that will result over decades in decreased vascularization, increased brittleness, and slower healing. Dry socket following extraction of third molars is one manifestation of these changes.

The gingival tissues are different both in form and contour. The increased fiber content and decreased vascularity per unit volume make the tissues a paler pink. Rete attachments to the underlying tissue create stippling. Sulcus depth has stabilized at 2 – 3 mm, and the gingival cuff is firmer and more adherent to the crown. Interdentally, a depression has formed, the gingival col, and the interdental papilla is more pointed and fine. The periodontal ligament has stabilized, unless the patient is under orthodontic care. Figure 40 – 1 shows a healthy late adolescent periodontium.

Periodontal Disease in Adolescents

The clinical and histologic manifestations of gingival and periodontal disease in adolescents are similar to those in the adult. Bone loss from periodontitis does occur in a small percentage of teenagers, but the predominant condition noted in this age group is gingivitis. The clinical manifestations of gingivitis include marginal inflammation, loss of stippling, edema, and bleeding on stimulus or spontaneously. The histologic picture of a mature gingival lesion is different from that of the child and is more like that of the adult, with a major preponderance of plasma cells in the affected area (Ranney et al, 1981).

The bone loss from periodontitis (as differentiated from localized juvenile periodontitis) that occurs in a small percentage of teenagers by age 18 may be a signal of a change in host resistance. The histologic variation between childhood and adolescent gingival response, the more significant response to local factors by the adolescent gingivae, and the identification of bone loss that results from the gingivitis to periodontitis progression for the first time in adolescence suggest strongly that this is a period of transition in terms of body response.

The long-term clinical consequence of chronic gingivitis in adolescence is not clear. The gingivitis experienced in the primary dentition seems to have no impact on the adult dentition. On the other hand, chronic inflammation around mandibular or maxillary incisors through adolescence may for some patients be inconsequential, yet for others it may result in fibrotic tissues, recession, and crestal bone loss.

Adolescence becomes a transitional period in management of the periodontium. Good oral hygiene may be the leverage to prevent irreversible periodontal changes from occurring during this period. Emergence from the teenage

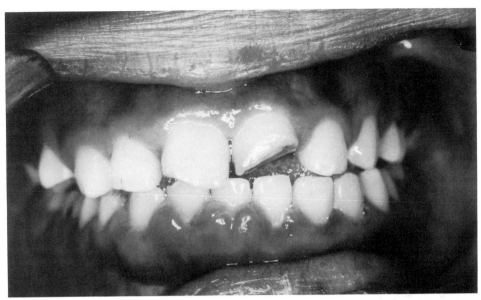

Figure 40–2 ■ Puberty gingivitis in a 14-year-old black female. Note inflamed and enlarged interdental papillae. Professional cleaning of calculus and good oral hygiene led to amelioration of this condition.

years with a healthy periodontium and good hygiene skills should help prevent periodontal disease in the adult.

Specific Disease Entities

In addition to routine gingivitis and periodontitis clearly associated with local factors, the adolescent can develop a number of gingival and periodontal problems, of both an acute and chronic nature.

PUBERTY GINGIVITIS

Exacerbation of gingival inflammation by hormonal fluctuation is a recognized phenomenon in female adolescents. Gingival inflammation with enlargement of interdental areas, spontaneous or easily stimulated bleeding, and a response beyond that expected from local factors characterize this condition (Fig. 40–2).

The response of the gingival tissues to hormonal changes in adolescence is similar to that seen during pregnancy or during a regimen of oral contraception. The hormones and local factors tend to combine to cause aggravated gingivitis. Therapy for this condition is by necessity local in nature. Removal of calculus is a first step. Good personal hygiene will also help

relieve some swelling. For the majority of adolescents, this therapy will cause major improvement. A typical regimen is daily brushing and flossing for 1 week, after professional removal of gross calculus. A 1-week follow-up will (1) help identify problem areas, (2) provide the opportunity for reinforcement of oral care, and (3) allow fine scaling without problems of pain and hemorrhage. Some patients may have areas that remain refractory to intervention, in which case time will usually bring an equilibrium to hormonal levels and the gingivitis should recede. By age 18, the hormonal effect will usually have subsided. In rare cases, untreated puberty gingivitis regresses to leave fibrotic interdental areas that may require surgical recontouring.

An aggravating factor in gingival problems in this age group is the orthodontic appliance. Today's bonding techniques have reduced the problem significantly, but whenever orthodontic appliances serve as harbors for plaque, the gingivae are at greater risk. Good oral hygiene, hygienic appliance design, and regular professional monitoring are critical to prevent gingival problems (Fig. 40–3).

When hormonally stimulated gingivitis is the result of medication or pregnancy, termination or regulation of either should bring relief. Oral contraceptives can be changed if gingival tissues do not respond, but this is seldom necessary.

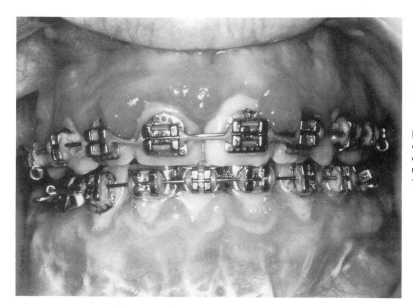

Figure 40-3 ■ Gingivitis associated with orthodontic appliances in a 12-year-old patient undergoing surgical orthodontic procedures.

ERUPTION GINGIVITIS

The young adolescent may demonstrate inflammation around erupting teeth (Fig. 40–4). The process of eruption causes at first a rupture of tissue with an inflammatory response. The accompanying sensitivity and tooth position make hygiene poor, and inflammation continues or worsens as plaque accumulates. Eruption gingivitis subsides with attainment of normal occlusal position. Good oral hygiene is the treatment of choice for eruption gingivitis, since some inflammation normally accompanies eruption of teeth. Unless a particular situation demands it, such as a rare local abscess, no more aggressive treatment should be instituted.

PERICORONITIS

Pericoronitis occurs when an operculum develops over a third molar (Fig. 40–5). Food impaction, stress, and trauma have all been implicated in its acute etiology. Pericoronitis can and does occur with acute necrotizing ulcerative gingivitis. Symptoms include pain and limited jaw closure as a result of sensitivity over the flap. Bad breath may be present as well, owing to inadequate oral hygiene. The opercular area will be swollen, edematous, and sensitive. Food impaction may be present under the tissue cover. Swelling can extend deeper into tissues, and a surface ulceration may be noted from the offending opposing tooth.

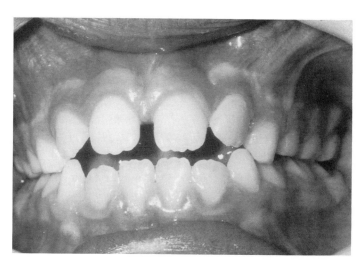

Figure 40–4 ■ Inflammation around erupting permanent teeth. This problem is a combination of local inflammatory response to tooth movement, generation of new gingival structures, and plaque accumulations.

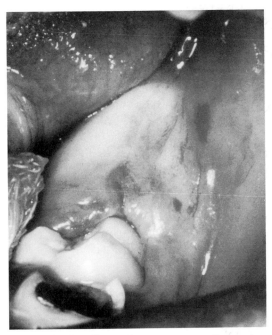

Figure 40–5 ■ Operculum over an erupting molar.

The treatment for pericoronitis depends on its severity. In some cases that are minor, the involved tooth can be extracted to relieve impingement. In other cases, when swelling and pain are significant, definitive treatment may be deferred until inflammation subsides and until good anesthesia can be obtained for extraction of the third molars. Palliative treatment includes gentle irrigation to remove food debris, reduction of the opposing tooth, and saline mouthrinses. Antibiotics may be needed if inflammation is extensive. Extraction of functionless third molars should follow when symptoms subside, to preclude recurrence.

ACUTE NECROTIZING ULCERATIVE GINGIVITIS

Acute necrotizing ulcerative gingivitis (ANUG) is an acute infection, usually attributed to stress, a decreased host resistance, or some other condition, that alters the host-bacteria relationship between humans and *Borrelia vincentii*. ANUG is also called trench mouth or Vincent's infection. Three clinical manifestations are considered classic, with pain, foul odor, and punched-out gingival lesions characteristic of ANUG (Fig. 40–6). The pain associated with ANUG is continuous and strong. Gingival tissues are sensitive to touch and manipulation. The patient's breath is noticeably bad, owing to bacterial accumulation and necrotic tissue. The lesions usually affect the interdental papillae. These usually pointed, pink projections are blunted and covered with a white pseudomembrane that can extend along the gingival margin. The condition is also often accompanied by generalized complaints — lymphadenopathy, malaise, and low grade fever.

The treatment of ANUG involves both local and systemic therapy. Removable of gingival necrosis with gentle mechanotherapy should be a first step. The patient begins gentle daily oral hygiene, using a toothbrush and oxygenating agent such as peroxide, which can help restore balance to the oral flora. Gentle oral irrigation with oxygenating compounds may also help. Systemic treatment utilizes antibiotics such as penicillin or erythromycin taken four times a day in doses of 250 mg for 5 days. Metronidazole has become more popular as a method to eliminate the acute symptoms rapidly (Mitchell, 1984). This drug is a strong agent

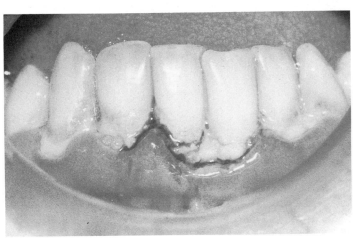

Figure 40–6 ■ Gingival manifestations of acute necrotizing ulcerative gingivitis. Note punched out or blunted interdental papillae.

that should not be used with alcohol because of its Antabuse-like effect, or used during pregnancy because of its possible effect on the fetus.

LOCALIZED JUVENILE PERIODONTITIS

Localized juvenile periodontitis (LJP) is a distinct clinical entity that has also been called periodontosis in the past. LJP is characterized by a rapid, clinically undetectable breakdown of the periodontal apparatus with localized bone loss and destruction of the periodontal ligament. The condition is believed to be caused by the organism *Actinobacillus actinomycetemcomitans* (AA, alternatively called *Haemophilus actinomycetemcomitans*, or HA).

LJP tends to occur in families, but no clear genetic pattern has emerged. Very recent evidence suggests that the commonality among family members may be in a shared neutrophil function disorder. Pubescent and adolescent children are at greatest risk in the 10- to 15-year age range. Clinical examination of a child with LJP shows a localized bone loss with pockets usually around incisors and first permanent molars. Gingival health may appear good on visual examination, with the infection confined to the gingival sulcus. Probing may stimulate bleeding from involved pockets. Without treatment, the disease can progress to severe bone loss, tooth movement, and mobility and loss of involved teeth (Fig. 40–7).

Treatment of incipient LJP involves both chemo- and mechanotherapy. The scaling, root planing, and curettage of infected tissues are directed at eliminating reservoirs of organisms in diseased hard and soft tissues in affected areas. Periodontal surgery may be necessary to eliminate hard and soft tissue deformities. Chemotherapy using tetracycline (1 gm per day) is recommended, for a prolonged period of time, well past the point at which the organism is rendered undetectable in the sulcular area. The shortest regimen recommended is 2 weeks, but some authors suggest that therapy continue over several months with continued laboratory testing for the presence of HA (Zambon et al, 1986).

Long-term management of LJP may involve reconstructive periodontal surgery; tooth extraction; root amputation; or orthodontic repositioning, if irreversible damage has occurred. Frequent follow-up at bi-monthly intervals can prevent recurrence, which is a distinct possibility for many children.

GINGIVAL AND PERIODONTAL MANIFESTATIONS OF VENEREAL DISEASE

The early and active sex life of some adolescents can lead to venereal disease. Oral-oral and oral-genital contact provide the vehicles for transmission and manifestation of some of these conditions in the oral cavity. The oral manifestations of venereal disease are highly variable, ranging from a single isolated lesion of the mucosa to stomatitis. The significance of these lesions is two-fold: They represent a sign of infection for the patient as well as a risk for the practitioner. Table 40–1 lists some of the oral manifestations of and treatments for venereal diseases. Some examples of oral lesions are depicted in Figure 40–8.

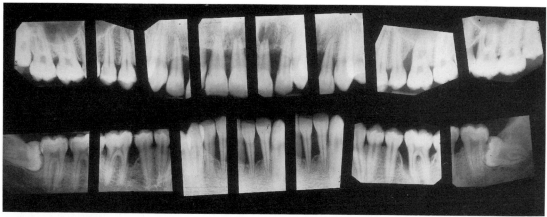

Figure 40–7 ■ Radiographic appearance of localized juvenile periodontitis showing cratering in molar and incisor regions.

Table 40–1 ■ Mucosal and periodontal manifestations of sexually transmitted diseases

Condition/Causative Agent	Oral Manifestations	Sites	Differential Diagnosis	Management
Acquired immune deficiency syndrome (AIDS) *Human T-cell lymphotropic virus III*	ANUG*-like periodontitis Fungal infection	Gingiva Mucosa, palate	ANUG* Immune deficiency Blood dyscrasia Immunosuppression	Palliative
Condyloma acuminatum (venereal wart) *Verruca vulgaris*	Cauliflower-like pedunculated pink lesion on keratinized surface	Lips, gingiva, palate, tongue	Papilloma	Excision
Gonorrhea *Neisseria Gonorrhoeae*	Tonsillitis Pharyngitis Diffuse erythema Mucosal ulceration Vesiculopustular lesions of skin	All oral and perioral structures	Upper respiratory infection Pharyngitis Scarlet fever "Strep" throat Tonsillitis Impetigo (skin)	Antibiotics
Herpes labialis *Herpes simplex virus I*	Vesicles becoming ulceration	Keratinized tissues, including lips, gingiva, palate, tongue	Aphthous ulcer Herpangina Exanthems	Palliative
Syphilis *Treponema pallidum*	Chancre Beefy red gingival lesion, possibly ulcerated	Point of inoculation	Aphthous ulcer Traumatic ulcer	Antibiotics
	Mucous patch Maculopapular rash of skin of face and palms, soles Pharyngitis Lymphadenopathy	Mucosa	Upper respiratory infection Pharyngitis	
Trichomonas vaginitis *Trichomonas vaginalis*	Pharyngitis	Throat	Upper respiratory infection	Appropriate antimicrobial

*Acute necrotizing ulcerative gingivitis.

MOUTHBREATHING

A consequence of mouthbreathing is anterior gingivitis secondary to desiccation of tissues (Fig. 40–9). The management of the problem is complicated by the cause of the condition, which may be a complex of airway and craniofacial problems requiring comprehensive management by an orthodontist and otolaryngologist. The treatment of the immediate problem of gingivitis is often accomplished by lubrication of tissues with petrolatum or use of an oral screen that covers the tissues during sleep. Mucus and plaque become more tenacious in these cases; therefore, good oral hygiene is critical. Bad breath is often a presenting complaint, for which the most effective treatment is good oral care by the patient. Elimination of the problem of mouthbreathing may be more difficult than control of the symptoms.

EFFECTS OF SMOKELESS TOBACCO

It is estimated that up to 60% of adolescent males aged 12–17 years try smokeless tobacco at least once per year and that about 10% use it regularly. The effects of the habit on gingival and periodontal tissues include gingival recession, gingivitis, abrasion, hyperkeratosis of the mucosa adjacent to quid placement, and possible increased risk for oral carcinoma (Greer et al, 1986). Oral examination will often reveal a patchy hyperkeratosis in the muco-buccal fold area, with a constellation of signs just listed (Fig. 40–10). Shreds of tobacco will often be found in sulcular or interdental areas. The management of the oral conditions are both local and generalized, with cessation or control of the habit being the first step. Individualized defects of gingiva are managed as needed. Hyperkera-

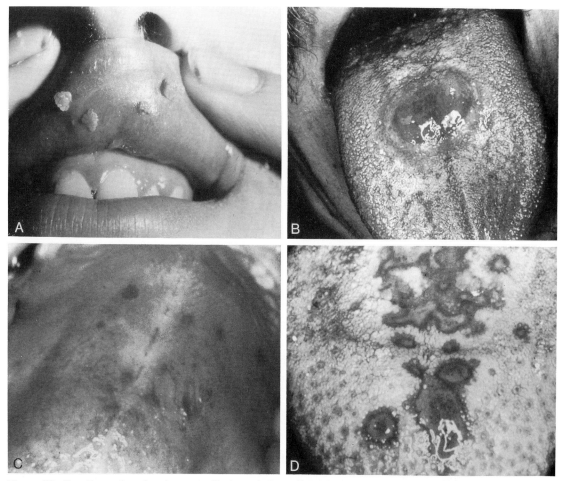

Figure 40–8 ■ Examples of oral venereal lesions. *A*, Condyloma acuminatum (venereal wart). *B*, Mucous patch of syphilis. *C*, Maculopapular palatal lesions of syphilis. *D*, Gonococcal glossitis.

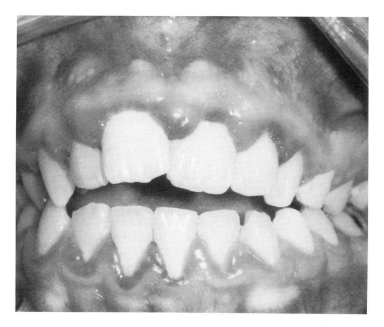

Figure 40–9 ■ Gingivitis associated with chronic mouthbreathing.

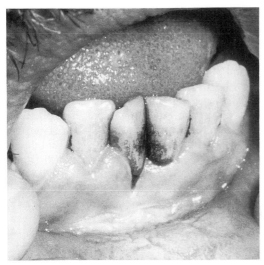

Figure 40–10 ■ Constellation of effects of smokeless tobacco use, including staining of teeth, gingival clefting, and hyperkeratosis of mucosa.

tosis is often reversible, and biopsy is not routinely recommended in this age group.

Temporomandibular Joint Disorders

The stresses of adolescence evoke numerous physiologic responses, one of which can be masticatory and temporomandibular joint–related dysfunction. The actual prevalence of temporomandibular joint (TMJ) dysfunction in the adolescent population is not clear. A number of authors (Grosfeld et al, 1985; Nilner, 1983) have conducted large scale cross-sectional epidemiologic studies to describe the occurrence of TMJ dysfunction and to characterize signs, symptoms, and predilection characteristics. Because many studies simply screen for signs and symptoms within the study population, it is unclear how extensively TMJ dysfunction occurs in adolescence and childhood. In addition, much of the epidemiologic data available have been obtained by interview in schools, rather than in clinics or treatment facilities from people seeking care. Much of what is known about TMJ disorders in this age group can be summarized as follows:

1. Functional signs (occlusal wear, deviation on opening, TMJ clicks, opening limitation) are common and may occur in as many as 50% of adolescents.

2. Pain associated with functional signs is far less common, with an occurrence in about 3–5% of adolescents, although even a smaller percentage actually seek care for the problem.

3. Adolescence appears to be a transitional period in TMJ dysfunction. Prior to adolescence, true TMJ dysfunction is rare, except from trauma or inflammatory-infectious involvement. During adolescence and early adulthood, the number of signs and symptoms of TMJ dysfunction steadily increases.

4. There is a weak association between TMJ dysfunction and certain malocclusions. Class II, division 2; Class III; and open bite malocclusions may predispose the patient to later TMJ problems.

5. The correlation between parafunctional habits and TMJ problems is not strong.

DIAGNOSIS AND TREATMENT OF TMJ PROBLEMS

The evaluation of a teenager for a TMJ disorder begins with an historical review of factors leading up to onset and the current status of the problem. Parents may help provide the corroborating information for the adolescent, who is minimally helpful as a result of pain or reluctance. Unlike the adult patient who is usually the instigator of care, the adolescent may be present because of parental pressure. A precipitating event such as chewing a jawbreaker, chronic gum or ice chewing, or bruxing during a stressful period of examinations may be identified. The adolescent may take enjoyment at demonstrating a loud click as a contribution to the diagnostic process. Trauma; removal of impacted third molars; or psychological problems resulting in stress (Belfer and Kaban, 1982), headaches, and bruxing may also be significant historical findings.

Clinical examination of the patient involves a thorough evaluation of hard and soft tissues, looking at both functional and anatomic relationships. The musculature associated with mastication should be evaluated for pain, soreness, and tender areas of myospasm. The joint itself should be palpated and evaluated for clicking, popping, or crepitus; symmetry of form and function; and tenderness. The maximum voluntary opening, the amount that a patient can comfortably open the mouth, should be recorded. The maximum forced opening is determined by forcing the patient's mouth open beyond maximum voluntary opening with digital pressure. Restricted opening can be caused

by coronoid hyperplasia as the coronoid strikes the zygomatic arch during opening; therefore, the restriction of opening coincident with a dull noise should be noted.

The examination of the TMJ should involve an evaluation of movements of the mandible. Limitation of opening and ranges of motion are assessed by asking the patient to open and close the mouth and engage in excursive movements. Deviation of the mandible during opening, locking of the joint, limitation of opening, and reduced range of motion may be indications of disk problems and internal derangement.

Internal derangement of the TMJ and muscle dysfunction are the most common causes of TMJ problems. An internal derangement is defined as an abnormal relationship of the articular disk to the mandibular condyle, fossa, and articular eminence (Fig. 40–11). In most cases, the disk is displaced anteriorly. Pain and restriction of movement are variable findings. Disk displacement is further classified into displacement with and without reduction. In reducible anterior displacement, the disk is displaced anteriorly in the closed mouth position but reduces to a normal relationship to the condyle during opening or translation. The disk will click or produce a sharp cracking sound when it reduces. Usually the disk will slip back off the condyle as the patient closes the mouth, producing a second or reciprocal click. In disk dis-

placement without reduction, the disk is displaced in the closed mouth position and does not reduce during opening but remains anterior to the condyle. This normally causes restricted opening and associated pain. Many times, it is difficult to distinguish non-reducible displacement from degenerative arthritis or ankylosis without appropriate radiographs and other information. In some cases of disk displacement, the posterior portion of the disk is actually torn or perforated and the condylar head articulates with the glenoid fossa. Myofascial pain dysfunction (MPD) is a term used to describe muscular pain resulting from spasm or hyperactivity of the muscles of mastication, face, and neck. The cause of MPD is elusive: stress, occlusal interferences, bruxism, and certain malocclusions all have been suggested to precipitate MPD. Whether actual joint pain is part of the dysfunction is under debate.

Ankylosis of the joint is classified as either true or false ankylosis. True ankylosis is characterized by a lack of joint translation or lateral excursions. The patient's maximum voluntary opening is equal to the maximum forced opening. The ankylosis is either fibrous or bony in nature, and pain is a variable finding. In false ankylosis, translation and lateral excursion are possible, although the maximum voluntary opening is restricted. Pain accompanies muscle fibrosis, and the maximum forced opening is

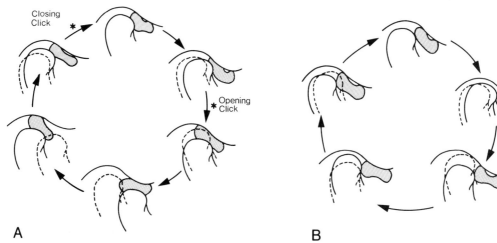

A, Disk displacement with reduction is illustrated in this figure. In reducible anterior displacement, the disk is displaced in the closed mouth position but reduces to a normal relationship to the condyle during opening or translation. The disk will click when it reduces. Usually, the disk will slip back off the condyle as the patient closes the mouth, producing a reciprocal click. **B**, In disk displacement without reduction, the disk is displaced in the closed mouth position and does not reduce during opening but remains anterior to the condyle. No click is present. (Redrawn from Tucker M: Treatment of temporomandibular joint disorders: Concepts for the general practitioner. The North Carolina Dental Review, published by the School of Dentistry and the University of North Carolina Dental Alumni Association, Volume 2, Number 1, Spring 1984, page 7.)

Figure 40–11 ■

greater than the voluntary opening. Ankylosis can be the result of a developmental problem or trauma.

Arthritic disorders such as degenerative and rheumatoid arthritis create muscle and joint pain. There is restricted voluntary opening and usually pain and deviation of the jaw to the affected side. In most cases, the patient's mouth can be forced open beyond the maximum voluntary opening. These arthritic disorders are reasonably uncommon in children and adolescents, but when present, they cause very tender joints.

The intraoral examination should address occlusal and tooth-related aspects of TMJ dysfunction. The occlusion should be evaluated for prematurities and the presence of a centric occlusion–centric relation (CO-CR) slide. Tooth sensitivity may be indicative of bruxing. The occlusal surfaces of teeth should also be evaluated for wear facets indicative of heavy use and biting pressures. Attempts at placing the patient's mandible in a retruded position may reveal joint tenderness secondary to posterior capsulitis and the presence of gross occlusal discrepancies. Some cases of TMJ dysfunction manifest as severe open bites when the condyles are in improper relationship to the disk and fossa and the patient attempts mandibular closure. Impressions and a centric relation recording should be made so that the casts can be mounted on an adjustable articulator to review clinical findings. In some cases, muscular pain and joint dysfunction may be so severe that an accurate centric relationship cannot be determined. Therapy may need to be initiated to decrease or relieve symptoms to a point at which an accurate and reproducible occlusal registration can be made.

Radiographic confirmation of the type and extent of a TMJ disorder is a complex procedure best done by those actively involved in TMJ

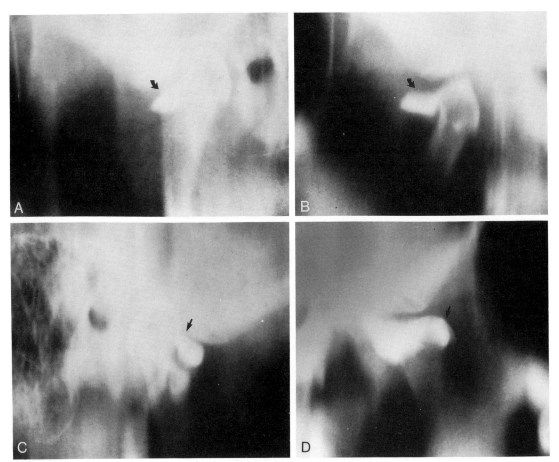

Figure 40–12 ■ Arthrotomogram of left joint in closed (A) and open (B) positions, indicating non-reducing anteriorly displaced disk (arrows); right joint in closed (C) and open (D) positions, indicating incompletely reducing anteriorly displaced disk (arrows). Radiopaque contrast medium outlines inferior disk surface.

evaluation. The array of radiographs involved in a complete diagnosis includes a full mouth survey or panoramic film to rule out dental or other contributory pathosis, multidirectional tomograms to provide a multi-layer picture of the joint and arthrograms, and using a radiopaque contrast medium to demonstrate disk relationships more clearly (Figs. 40–12 and 40–13). CT scanning and nuclear magnetic resonance (NMR) studies also utilized in a noninvasive manner aid in diagnosis (Katzberg et al, 1985). At the writing of this text, ultrasound techniques for diagnosis of TMJ disorders are only beginning to be evaluated. Their role is as yet undetermined, yet they also present the po-

tential for non-invasive evaluation of the resting and functioning TMJ.

The treatment of TMJ disorders in adolescents follows the same principles as treatment in the adult, with a minimally invasive, reversible initial treatment as the first choice. The acute symptoms are addressed first. A splint is often the first treatment performed, and may serve as both a therapeutic and diagnostic modality. A variety of designs can be used, each of which involves impressions and custom construction with adjustment to the patient's occlusion at the insertion visit. Initial management may also involve physical therapy, psychological counseling, medications such as

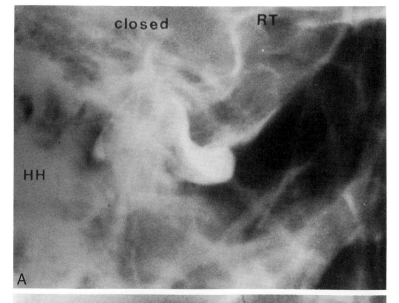

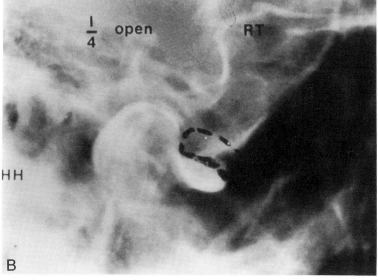

Figure 40–13 ■ Arthrogram of right joint, indicating non-reducing disk in closed (A) and early opening (B) positions. Disk is outlined in B.

muscle relaxants, diet regulation, or a combination of all these methods.

If the pathophysiology of the problem is suspected to be internal disk derangement, arthroscopy may be indicated to confirm diagnosis and alleviate the derangement. Surgery to correct a disk or joint problem is indicated in refractory or late stage cases.

Some special treatment considerations in the adolescent should involve the dentist's counseling of patients and parents. These include the following:

1. Identification and discussion of covert issues such as school-related problems, drug use, family dysfunction, and other adolescent concerns. The dentist may not be the best person to initiate therapy for these problems, and help from a psychologist or other therapist may be necessary.

2. Continued aggravation of a physically caused problem by active sports activities or habits. The adolescent may be involved in situations contributing to TMJ problems that he or she views as priorities in this period of life.

3. Lack of compliance to treatment measures. The adolescent may be a reluctant recipient of care. Compliance with splint use, medication, diet, exercises, and other treatment approaches may be limited by the patient, despite claims to the contrary. Adolescents may also have difficulty in establishing a constructive relationship with the dentist.

4. Coping with issues of growth or concurrent therapy. The dentist may have to wait to address the problem definitively because of ongoing orthodontic therapy. In cases of multiple concurrent treatments, it may be advisable for the dentist to work in conjunction with other therapists.

5. Early recognition of cause, establishment of a diagnosis, development of a treatment plan, and initiation of treatment as soon as possible will minimize development of bone disease and facial growth problems.

REFERENCES

Belfer M, Kaban L: Temporomandibular joint dysfunction with facial pain in children. Pediatrics 69:5, 564, 1982.

Greer RO, Poulson TC, Boone ME, Lindenmuth JE, Crosby L: Smokeless tobacco–associated oral changes in juvenile, adult and geriatric patients: Clinical and histomorphologic features. Gerodontics 2:87, 1986.

Grosfeld O, Jackowska M, Czarnecka B: Results of epidemiological examinations of the temporomandibular joint in adolescents and young adults. J Oral Rehab 12:95, 1985.

Katzberg R, Tallents R, Hayakawa K, Miller T, Goske M, Wood B: Internal derangements of the temporomandibular joint: Findings in the pediatric age group. Radiology 154:125, 1985.

Mitchell DA: Metronidazole: Its use in clinical dentistry. J Clin Periodontol 11:145, 1984.

Nilner M: Relationships between oral parafunctions and functional disturbances and diseases of the stomatognathic system among children aged 7–14 years. Acta Odontol 41:167, 1983.

Ranney RR, Debski BF, Tew JG: Pathogenesis of gingivitis and periodontal disease in children and young adults. Pediatr Dent 3:89, 1981.

Sanchez M: Periodontal disease among youths 12–17 years. Vital and Health Statistics, Data from the National Health Survey, Series 11, No. 141, 1974.

Zambon JJ, Christersson LA, Genco RJ: Diagnosis and treatment of localized juvenile periodontitis. JADA 113:295, 1986.

SUMMARY FOR SECTION IV

At all four age levels of a patient, the dentist has responsibilities specific to the age level. From conception to age 3, the ultimate goal is to bring a child to his third birthday caries free with paralleling good gingival health. The ultimate goal from 3–6 years of age is to supervise the primary dentition; keep it caries free; treat the teeth and their pulps when necessary; keep the periodontal tissues healthy; maintain the integrity of the primary dental arches; and develop an accepting, unafraid dental patient. From age 6–12, the need for emphasizing hard tissue and gingival health is maintained, treatment of both the primary and permanent dentition and pulps remains, increasing attention is given to a transition of home care responsibility from the parent to the child, and, lastly, more diagnostic and treatment emphasis is placed on harmonious dental arches and dental facial esthetics.

For the adolescent, the ultimate challenge to the dentist is just as formidable as before, if not more so. In late adolescence, the child will begin a process of leaving his last ties of health supervision by his parents. As the adolescent blends into adulthood, he will make decisions about when he will seek professional care. He will have exclusive control over his diet. It will be his decision based upon his own internal motivation as to how he wishes to practice home oral care procedures.

It would appear that the dentist who has over the years instilled a sense of the importance of good dental and gingival health and has delivered a young adult with a dentition that is sincerely an asset to him or her in function and in terms of the social self-confidence brought about by the esthetics of the teeth and face has done the job well. Furthermore, if this young adult will continue in regular supervision of his or her dental health, all the responsibilities of dentistry for children have, in fact, been executed successfully, expertly, and applaudably by that dentist.

Index

Note: Numbers in *italics* refer to figures; numbers followed by (t) represent tables. Also, please note that age-related subentries are arranged in alphabetical order rather than numerical order (e.g., *6- to 12-year-old* is listed before *3- to 6-year-old*).